Comprehensive Healthcare Simulation

Series Editors

Adam I. Levine
Department of Anesthesiology
Mount Sinai Medical Center
New York, USA

Samuel DeMaria Jr.
Department of Anesthesiology
Mount Sinai Medical Center
New York, USA

This new series focuses on the use of simulation in healthcare education, one of the most exciting and significant innovations in healthcare teaching since Halsted put forth the paradigm of "see one, do one, teach one." Each volume focuses either on the use of simulation in teaching in a specific specialty or on a cross-cutting topic of broad interest, such as the development of a simulation center. The volumes stand alone and are also designed to complement Levine, DeMaria, Schwartz, and Sim, eds., THE COMPREHENSIVE TEXTBOOK OF HEALTHCARE SIMULATION by providing detailed and practical guidance beyond the scope of the larger book and presenting the most up-to-date information available. Series Editors Drs. Adam I. Levine and Samuel DeMaria Jr. are affiliated with the Icahn School of Medicine at Mount Sinai, New York, New York, USA, home to one of the foremost simulation centers in healthcare education. Dr. Levine is widely regarded as a pioneer in the use of simulation in healthcare education. Editors of individual series volumes and their contributors are all recognized leaders in simulation-based healthcare education.

More information about this series at http://www.springer.com/series/13029

Lindsay C. Johnston • Lillian Su
Editors

Comprehensive Healthcare Simulation: ECMO Simulation

A Theoretical and Practical Guide

Springer

Editors
Lindsay C. Johnston
School of Medicine
Yale University
New Haven, CT
USA

Lillian Su
School of Medicine
Stanford University
Stanford, CA
USA

ISSN 2366-4479 ISSN 2366-4487 (electronic)
Comprehensive Healthcare Simulation
ISBN 978-3-030-53843-9 ISBN 978-3-030-53844-6 (eBook)
https://doi.org/10.1007/978-3-030-53844-6

This Springer imprint is published by the registered company Springer Nature Switzerland AG
The registered company address is: Gewerbestrasse 11, 6330 Cham, Switzerland

I would like to thank my husband Stephen, my beautiful children, and my parents Mary Ann and Charles Callahan for a lifetime of love, encouragement, and support. This book would not have been possible without the tremendous impact you have each had upon my life, and I am eternally grateful.

– Lindsay C. Johnston

This book is dedicated to Dr. Lang-pao Su and Naoko Su who instilled in their children a lifelong love of learning.

– Lillian Su

Foreword

Medicine is one profession where teamwork is key. Learning how to best work together as a team has been recognized as an important component of providing optimal patient care, increased job satisfaction, and identifying areas of communication strength and weakness. Situations of critical illness, high stress, and relatively low frequency are areas that have been cited to be prone to adverse events related to poor communication and lack of teamwork. As technology has grown to become an integral part of critical care medicine, so too has the need for interaction between multiple disciplines. Extracorporeal life support, more commonly referred to as ECMO, is a great example of high stress, relatively infrequent critical care that requires team interaction at the highest level. As many new ECMO programs are arising, technology is advancing, and patient populations expanding, augmenting team performance is even more important. The use of simulation to help train both novice ECMO personnel, refresh experienced providers with new technology or expanded patient groups, or keep low-volume centers refreshed and up to date has been shown to help in training, team communication, and performance. The ability to provide almost-real-life scenarios from which teams can practice and perform, as well as debriefing sessions to evaluate what aspects of team performance went well and what needs improvement, and allow feedback and conversation from participants, has been shown to improve communication and teamwork and can help reduce stress during actual events. While it may seem easy, simulation requires understanding of how folks learn, how best to convey information, and what steps to take to initiate the best simulation effort to achieve the optimal results. The information provided in this comprehensive text will help you and your center become more knowledgeable about simulation and how it can advance training at your site and improve team performance of the life-saving intervention that ECMO can provide. I have been part of the ECMO community for many years and have seen the evolution and adoption of simulation in ECMO programs. It is a very exciting time and I hope this book helps programs deliver the high quality ECMO care we all strive to provide to our sickest patients.

Heidi J. Dalton, MD, MCCM, FELSO,
Director, Program Development and Research, ECLS
INOVA Fairfax Medical Center INOVA Heart and Vascular Institute, Pediatrics
Falls Church, VA, USA

Preface

Simulation is now utilized commonly in medical training and continuing education to ensure that providers are able to recognize and respond appropriately to clinical situations with varying degrees of time pressure and levels of stress, communicate effectively with all members of the interprofessional team, and assess for barriers or latent safety threats in the actual clinical environment. Simulation for Extracorporeal Membrane Oxygenation (ECMO) was developed more recently, but this educational modality has rapidly gained popularity for training of individuals and teams caring for the most critically ill patients using this specialized and highly technical equipment. Great promise also exists around the ability of ECMO simulation to contribute to improve patient safety and quality improvement through assessment of latent safety threats, standardization of provider training, improvement of workflow, and assurance of individual provider performance standards. Given the novelty of ECMO simulation, this book was conceptualized out of a desire to clarify its optimal applications as part of an institution's interprofessional ECMO educational curriculum, to discuss nuances in curricular design and debriefing, to address specific alterations in the typical simulation equipment to accommodate interactions with the circuit, and to discuss specific applications of this educational technique for providers working with different patient populations (ranging from neonatal to adult) and in varying settings.

Authors with expertise in a number of areas, including ECMO patient care, medical simulation, and ECMO simulation, as well as experts in team science were invited to contribute chapters to this work. Extensive review of the literature was performed to ensure that information presented is timely and accurate. Topics covered a wide range of items related to ECMO simulation, spanning from theoretical aspects of utilizing simulation from adult learning and psychological perspectives to practical items necessary to plan, set-up, orchestrate, and debrief ECMO simulations for different types of learners in different settings. We hope that this work will be a valuable resource for novice ECMO simulationists as they are figuring out the logistics involved in setting up a new program, as well as seasoned educators who are seeking to optimize existing programs. Through this effort, we are excited to play a part in improving the care delivered to patients requiring ECMO across the globe. We are immensely grateful to all of our authors for dedicating the time to produce such high-quality, evidence-based work as well as the editorial team at Springer.

New Haven, CT, USA — Lindsay C. Johnston
Stanford, CA, USA — Lillian Su

Contents

Contributors

Anne M. Ades, MD, MSEd Division of Neonatology, Children's Hospital of Philadelphia, Perelman School of Medicine at the University of Pennsylvania, Philadelphia, PA, USA

Peta M. A. Alexander, MBBS, BSc(Hons), FRACP, FCICM Department of Cardiology, Boston Children's Hospital and Department of Pediatrics, Harvard Medical School, Boston, MA, USA

Catherine K. Allan, MD Department of Cardiology, Boston Children's Hospital and Department of Pediatrics, Harvard Medical School, Boston, MA, USA

SIMPeds, Boston Children's Hospital Simulator Program, Boston Children's Hospital and Harvard Medical School, Boston, MA, USA

Cory M. Alwardt, CCP Department of Critical Care Medicine, Mayo Clinic College of Medicine, Mayo Clinic, Phoenix, AZ, USA

Department of Surgery, Clinical Perfusion, Mayo Clinic, Phoenix, AZ, USA

Tim Antonius, MD Division of Neonatology, Department of Pediatrics, Radboudumc Amalia Children's Hospital, Nijmegen, The Netherlands

Dorothy M. Beke, MS, RN, CPNP-PC/AC Cardiac Intensive Care Unit, Boston Children's Hospital, Boston, MA, USA

Steven Brediger, RRT-NPS ECMO Program/Respiratory Care Department, Boston Children's Hospital, Boston, MA, USA

Brian C. Bridges, MD Division of Pediatric Critical Care, Department of Pediatrics, Vanderbilt University School of Medicine, Nashville, TN, USA

Christie J. Bruno, DO Department of Pediatrics, Yale University School of Medicine, New Haven, CT, USA

Hannelisa E. Callisen, PA-C Department of Critical Care Medicine, Mayo Clinic College of Medicine, Mayo Clinic, Phoenix, AZ, USA

Rachel L. Chapman, MD Fetal and Neonatal Institute, Division of Neonatology, Children's Hospital Los Angeles, Los Angeles, CA, USA

Department of Pediatrics, Keck School of Medicine, University of Southern California, Los Angeles, CA, USA

Rys Chapple, PT, BSc(Hons) Vancouver General Hospital, Intensive Care Unit, Vancouver, BC, Canada

Heidi J. Dalton, MD, MCCM, FELSO Program Development and Research, ECLS, INOVA Fairfax Medical Center, INOVA Heart and Vascular Institute, and Department of Pediatrics, Falls Church, VA, USA

Mehul Desai, MD Department of Critical Care Medicine, INOVA Fairfax Medical Center, Falls Church, VA, USA

Summer Elshenawy, MD Department of Pediatrics, Emory University School of Medicine, Atlanta, GA, USA

Katie Fitzpatrick, BSc Boston Children's Hospital, Simpeds (Simulation Program), Boston, MA, USA

Christine D. Franciscovich, MSN, CRNP, NNP-BC The Children's Hospital of Philadelphia, Philadelphia, PA, USA

Heather M. French, MD, MSEd Division of Neonatology, Department of Pediatrics, The Children's Hospital of Philadelphia, Perelman School of Medicine at the University of Pennsylvania, Philadelphia, PA, USA

Evan F. Gajkowski, RN, BSN, CCRN Department of Cardiology, Geisinger Medical Center, Danville, PA, USA

Kristen M. Glass, MD Department of Pediatrics, Penn State Health Milton S. Hershey Medical Center/Penn State College of Medicine, Hershey, PA, USA

Megan M. Gray, MD Department of Pediatrics, University of Washington, Seattle, WA, USA

Louis Patrick Halamek, MD Division of Neonatal and Developmental Medicine, Department of Pediatrics, Stanford University, Palo Alto, CA, USA

Roberta L. Hales, MHA, RRT-NPS, RN, CHSE Center for Simulation, Advanced Education and Innovation, The Children's Hospital of Philadelphia, Philadelphia, PA, USA

Peggy Han, MD Division of Pediatric Critical Care Medicine, Department of Pediatrics, Stanford University School of Medicine, Palo Alto, CA, USA

Annette Imprescia, RN, BSN, CCRN Cardiac Intensive Care Unit, Boston Children's Hospital, Boston, MA, USA

Ozzie Jahadi, CCP Lucile Packard Children's Hospital, Palo Alto, CA, USA

Lindsay C. Johnston, MD, MEd Department of Pediatrics, Yale University School of Medicine, New Haven, CT, USA

Kelly D. Kadlec, MD, MEd Department of Pediatric Critical Care, University of Nebraska College of Medicine, Children's Hospital and Medical Center, University of Nebraska Medical Center, Omaha, NE, USA

Simmie Kalan, RN, BSN, CNCC(C) Vancouver General Hospital, Intensive Care Unit, Vancouver, BC, Canada

Hussein D. Kanji, MD, MSc, MPH, FRCP(C) Department of Critical Care Medicine, Vancouver General Hospital, Vancouver, BC, Canada

Seth Kaplan, PhD Department of Psychology, George Mason University, Fairfax, VA, USA

Amanda Key, BSN, RN Department of Nursing, Intensive Care Unit, Mayo Clinic, Phoenix, AZ, USA

Jennifer C. King, PharmD, MD Department of Pediatrics, Monroe Carell Jr. Children's Hospital at Vanderbilt University, Nashville, TN, USA

Kimberly W. Kyle, MSN, RN, CCRN ECMO Department, Children's Hospital Los Angeles, Los Angeles, CA, USA

Department of Pediatrics, Keck School of Medicine, University of Southern California, Los Angeles, CA, USA

Dianne Lee, DO, MBA Department of Pediatrics, Yale University School of Medicine, New Haven, CT, USA

Amelia A. Lowell, RT Department of Critical Care Medicine, Mayo Clinic College of Medicine, Mayo Clinic, Phoenix, AZ, USA

Mary E. McBride, MD, MEd Divisions of Cardiology and Critical Care Medicine, Department of Pediatrics and Medical Education, Ann & Robert H Lurie Children's Hospital of Chicago, Chicago, IL, USA

Michael-Alice Moga, MD, MSc Division of Cardiac Critical Care, Department of Critical Care Medicine, The Hospital for Sick Children, The Labatt Family Heart Center, Toronto, ON, Canada

Department of Critical Care Medicine, University of Toronto, The Hospital for Sick Children, Toronto, ON, Canada

Katie M. Moynihan, MBBS Department of Cardiology, Boston Children's Hospital and Department of Pediatrics, Harvard Medical School, Boston, MA, USA

Lara P. Nelson, MD ECMO Department, Children's Hospital Los Angeles, Los Angeles, CA, USA

Department of Pediatrics, Keck School of Medicine, University of Southern California, Los Angeles, CA, USA

Division of Critical Care Medicine, Department of Anesthesiology Critical Care Medicine, Children's Hospital Los Angeles, Los Angeles, CA, USA

Bhavesh M. Patel, MD, RDMS Department of Critical Care Medicine, Mayo Clinic College of Medicine, Mayo Clinic, Phoenix, AZ, USA

Jack Pottle, BSc, BMBCH, MRCP Oxford Medical Simulation, London, UK

Susanna Price, MBBS, BSc, FRCP, EDICM, PhD Department of Cardiology and Intensive Care, Royal Brompton Hospital and Departments of Cardiology and Intensive Care, Imperial College London, London, UK

Danielle J. W. Reed, MD Division of Neonatology, Department of Pediatrics, Children's Mercy-Kansas City, University of Missouri-Kansas City School of Medicine, Kansas City, MO, USA

David L. Rodgers, EdD Clinical Simulation Center, Penn State Health Milton S. Hershey Medical Center, Hershey, PA, USA

Kathleen R. Ryan, MD Division of Pediatric Cardiology, Department of Pediatrics, Lucile Packard Children's Hospital at Stanford, Stanford University Medical Center, Palo Alto, CA, USA

Loren D. Sacks, MD Department of Pediatrics – Cardiology (CVICU), Stanford University, Palo Alto, CA, USA

Miheer Sane, MD Department of Pediatrics, Hospital-Based Medicine, Ann & Robert H Lurie Children's Hospital of Chicago, Chicago, IL, USA

Taylor Sawyer, DO, MEd Department of Pediatrics, Seattle Children's Hospital, Seattle, WA, USA

Ayan Sen, MD Department of Critical Care Medicine, Mayo Clinic College of Medicine, Mayo Clinic, Phoenix, AZ, USA

Paul Shuttleworth, CCP, BSN, MBA Lucile Packard Children's Hospital, Palo Alto, CA, USA

Justin Sleasman, MS, CCP Lucile Packard Children's Hospital, Betty Irene Moore Children's Heart Center, Palo Alto, CA, USA

Lillian Su, MD School of Medicine, Stanford University, Stanford, CA, USA

Justyna Swol, MD, PhD Department of Respiratory Medicine, Allergology and Sleep Medicine, Intensive Care, General Hospital Nuremberg, University Hospital of Paracelsus Medical University, Nuremberg, Germany

Mary J. Waller, PhD Neely School of Business, Texas Christian University, Fort Worth, TX, USA

Elizabeth A. Wetzel, MD, MS Division of Neonatal-Perinatal Medicine, Riley Hospital for Children at Indiana University Health, Indiana University School of Medicine, Indianapolis, IN, USA

Susan B. Williams, MSN, RNC-NIC, CIT The Children's Hospital of Philadelphia, Philadelphia, PA, USA

Vamsi V. Yarlagadda, MD Division of Pediatric Cardiology, Department of Pediatrics, Lucile Packard Children's Hospital at Stanford, Stanford University Medical Center, Palo Alto, CA, USA

Bishoy Zakhary, MD Division of Pulmonary and Critical Care Medicine, Oregon Health & Science University, Portland, OR, USA

Jill Zalieckas, MD Department of Surgery, Boston Children's Hospital, Boston, MA, USA

Department of Surgery, Harvard Medical School, Boston, MA, USA

Jenny Zhou, MA Edu & Tech, BS Biol Engr Oxford Medical Simulation, London, UK

Part I

History of ECMO & ECMO Simulation

ECMO from Conception to Execution

1

Heidi J. Dalton and Mehul Desai

Learning Objectives

1. The reader will have an improved understanding of history of extracorporeal life support (ECLS) and the role researchers played even prior to World War II.
2. The reader will have improved understanding of how membrane lungs were developed and how evolutional changes have improved performance.
3. The reader will have an improved understanding of how heparin was discovered and its role in ECLS.
4. The reader will be able to identify current patient populations for ECLS and general outcomes related to their category of support.

Introduction

Extracorporeal life support (ECLS) has come a long way since the days of fantasy to become an everyday reality. This chapter will review the history of ECLS to the current day. Future thoughts will also be provided.

Birth of an Idea

> But if the place of the heart could be supplied by injection- and if, for the regular continuance of this injection, there could be furnished a quantity of arterial blood, whether natural or artificially formed, supposing such a formation possible- then life might be indefinitely maintained in any portion; and consequently, after decapitation, even in the head itself, without destroying and any functions peculiar to the brain. Not only life might thus be kept up both in the head and in any other portion separated from the body of an animal, but might also be reproduced after its entire extinction. It might be restored likewise to the whole body, and thereby a complete resurrection be performed in the full extent of the word. – Cesar Julien Jean Le Gallois, 1812

Contrary to belief, most great discoveries are not one of a "eureka" moment but rather the culmination of many ideas that come together. In 1812, Le Gallois suggested that organs could be preserved by artificial circulation [1, 2]. In 1828, James Phillip Kay evaluated the efficacy of blood delivery to the abdominal aorta to produce muscular contractions in the lower extremities [3]. Of importance, he noted that arterial blood was more favorable in producing muscular contractions than venous blood but that even infusion of venous blood induced muscular contraction for a significantly longer period compared to the absence of any arterial flow. Thus, some difference between venous and arterial blood seemed to be important.

Early investigators recognized that the substance that seemed to be important in the blood was oxygen to support life. Breathing of air was already recognized as important for life. As far back as the Bible, this concept is described: "And the Lord God formed man of the dust of the ground, and breathed into his nostrils the breath of life; and man became a living soul" (Genesis 2:7).

As the role of oxygen was recognized, investigation into how to deliver it by artificial means advanced during World War II by use of hand bellows and other devices to push air into a person's lungs. Perhaps, one of the most famous descriptions of artificial respiration arose from the Copenhagen polio epidemic in 1952, whereby 200 medical students hand-ventilated polio victims with respiratory paralysis for many hours (shift-work was present even back then!) until their muscle strength recovered [4]. The drop in mortality from 95% to about 25% spurred others to develop other means of supporting such patients. External devices, such as vests which could expand and deflate the thorax and

H. J. Dalton (✉)
Program Development and Research, ECLS, INOVA Fairfax Medical Center, INOVA Heart and Vascular Institute, and Department of Pediatrics, Falls Church, VA, USA

M. Desai
Department of Critical Care Medicine, INOVA Fairfax Medical Center, Falls Church, VA, USA

L. C. Johnston, L. Su (eds.), *Comprehensive Healthcare Simulation: ECMO Simulation*, Comprehensive Healthcare Simulation,
https://doi.org/10.1007/978-3-030-53844-6_1

the iron lung, appeared, and the era of mechanical ventilation development began in earnest [5].

As the interaction between oxygen and circulating blood became more apparent, more research into how to best introduce oxygen artificially into the blood became a focus of investigation. In the 1600s, Hooke described his efforts as follows:

> I shall shortly further try, whether the suffering the Blood to circulate through a vessel, so as it may be openly exposed to fresh air, will not suffice for the life of an Animal; and make some other Experiments, which, I hope, will thoroughly discover the Genuine use of Respiration; and afterwards consider what benefit this may be to Mankind. – Robert Hooke, 1667

Marrying the two concepts of blood flow and oxygen delivery to support life was noted by Brown Sequard in 1858 who evaluated the ability to revive the arms of decapitated criminals by injecting blood with a syringe [2]. He attempted artificial oxygenation of blood by agitating "black" blood in atmospheric air and thereby transforming it to red blood. By injecting the red blood in the arteries of separated dog heads, he could elicit nerve reflexes. Focused experiments in cardiac resuscitation were conducted by Benjamin Ward Richardson, MD, in the 1860s [6]. Attempts were made to force a current of pure oxygen, in order to provide a column of oxygenated blood to the left ventricle and the coronaries, and thereby have it distributed to the systemic circulation. The initial results were promising, with the right ventricle and right auricle demonstrating brisk rhythmic contraction, however contraction was never sufficient to produce blood flow through the pulmonary system. These findings led Richardson to infer that resuscitation could be possible with further experimentation.

Development of Perfusion Technology

In 1862, Ernst Bidder constructed a primitive perfusion apparatus to provide blood flow to the kidneys, in which arterial blood pressure was controlled through the use of a glass cylinder filled with mercury which ended in a glass basin containing blood [7]. Defibrination and oxygenation was obtained by stirring the blood with a rod and then filtering it through fine linen.

In 1882, Waldemar von Schroder constructed an apparatus which allowed for oxygenation of the blood through use of an air current [8]. This experimental work was the first form of bubble oxygenation; however, the direct gas/blood interface resulted in foaming that was an inherent problem. The first closed circulation perfusion system was created by Max von Frey and Max Gruber from the Physiological Institute at Leipzig [9, 10]. The system utilized a 10 ml injecting syringe to imitate the heart and two valves. The key advancement was the development of a film oxygenator, which utilized a rotating cylinder to create a thin blood film that was introduced to atmospheric oxygen. The damage to blood by contact with air limited the time such a device could be utilized and was a significant hurdle to be overcome. Johann Carl Jacobj created a closed perfusion system in 1890, which he later modified by incorporating a physiologic membrane from natural lung tissue which was artificially aspirated [11–13]. As clotting of the blood in artificial systems was a large problem, his inhibition of coagulation by the use of leech extract was another advancement in the field. Leeches have been used for a multitude of purposes since the days of the Roman Empire and even earlier, but their specific function of inhibiting platelet function and coagulation became a focus during development of cardiopulmonary support devices. The discovery of heparin in 1916 by McLean and Howell represented another major breakthrough. Noted as an anticoagulant by a second-year medical student from Johns Hopkins (McLean), the protein was named "heparin" as it was found in canine liver tissue ("hepar" is Greek for liver) [14]. Further research identified the protein sequence of heparin and allowed it to become manufactured for use by the 1930s.

Although the discovery of heparin helped with the problems of coagulation of blood, difficulties with complications associated with the mixing of defibrinated blood with air continued. Multiple theories for development of a system to provide perfusion-based resuscitation were put forward. Zeller noted during multiple experiments that inadequate numbers of blood cells would reduce in poor oxygen delivery and death of the central nervous system organs. Thus, having a pump which could generate enough power to propel blood forward was needed. While the majority of historical reference credits John Gibbon with development of the first cardiopulmonary bypass machine, work in Russia had also resulted in similar devices being patented. In 1927 in Moscow, Sergei Brukhonenko reported his experiments with artificial circulation, using a system of two pumps [15–18]. This device, called the autojector, consisted of one mechanically driven diaphragm pump which brought venous blood to a set of donor lungs (usually from dogs or pigs) and a second pump which delivered oxygenated blood from the lungs to the systemic circulation. Multiple experiments were performed with this device, including demonstrations that it could provide systemic oxygenated blood to isolated heads and neurologic function could be elicited, even to the point of opening eyes and swallowing a piece of cheese. The ability to provide circulatory support to a failed heart was recognized on November 1, 1926, when Brukhonenko maintained artificial circulation to an animal with a stopped heart for 2 hours. Nikolai Terebinski used this device to allow open-heart operations on over 200 dogs between 1929 and 1937 but recognized that it would not be applicable to clinical use as the donor lungs were from animals [19]. Brukhonenko also developed a bubble oxygenator, which when combined with his pump machine allowed cardiopulmonary resuscitation in animals who had circulatory arrest. A patent for the heart-lung machine developed by Brukhonenko and Terbinski was given in Russia in 1941–1942, but the intervening of World War II restricted further advancement of Brukhoenko's work, and it was never used in clinical practice.

At the same time, John Gibbons, while a surgical resident in Boston, faced despair and helplessness as he watched one of his patients expire from a massive pulmonary embolism [20]. He recognized that if he could have bypassed the patient's lungs and provided oxygenated blood systemically while the embolus was being removed, his patient might have survived. This experience resulted in his life-long work, along with his wife Mary, to develop a machine that would allow full cardiopulmonary support. The development of an oxygenator which would not result in destruction of red blood cells was a major effort. In addition, oxygenation was inherently inefficient due to limitations of mass transfer. The Gibbons found that agitating blood around the oxygen source improved oxygenator efficiency and this phenomenon (called the "boundary layer phenomenon") improved performance. By increasing turbulence, blood at the core of laminar flow was brought in contact with the membrane increasing O_2 coupling. A roller-pump device was used to propel blood to the oxygenator, which consisted of vertical stainless-steel sheets over which the blood was passed. Turbulence provided good gas exchange, and the sheets were contained within a plastic shell into which oxygen was provided. Gibbons was also one of the first to comment on the need for adequate carbon dioxide removal by the membrane lung. Gibbon's initial trials provided complete cardiopulmonary support to cats whose pulmonary arteries were occluded. Subsequent refinement of the Gibbons' device was enhanced by financial support provided by IBM, and work on larger animal models such as dogs resulted. In 1953, the Gibbons' heart-lung machine, described as the size of a spinet piano, was deemed ready for clinical use, and the first successful bypass operation was performed on an 18-year-old girl with an atrial septal defect [20]. Following this successful operation, however, subsequent cases did not survive, and Gibbons started to concentrate on teaching rather than focusing on further heart-lung bypass development himself.

DeWall and Lillehei introduced the bubble oxygenator to the field of cardiopulmonary bypass (1955), and it was deemed the safest and most efficient device for many years worldwide [21–24]. Support times were limited, however, due to the direct blood-gas interface and resultant hemolysis. Priming volumes for the device were also high, taking multiple units of blood (up to 4 liters). In 1944, a nephrologist working on renal dialysis, William Kolff, noted that the use of cellophane tubes allowed not only for efficient clearance of solutes but that "oxygen is reabsorbed very rapidly: already after a few windings one sees the blue blood get red" [25]. Further development of membrane lung technology occurred in 1955–1957 by Clowes and others, using sheets of polyethylene as the membrane [26]. Although not as permeable to oxygen as to carbon dioxide and requiring a large surface area, this device was used in 1956 clinically. In 1957, Kammermeyer noted that dimethylpolysiloxane transferred oxygen and carbon dioxide at a rate 10 times that of earlier materials [27]. Kolobow, Lande, Pierce, and others began using this plastic (which came to be called silicone) for membrane lung development [28]. The Kolobow membrane lung, manufactured by Sci-Med (Medtronic Inc), was a silicone sheet wrapped around a polycarbonate spool with wire mesh that allowed gas transfer to occur. Its cylindrical shape was contained within a plastic outer sheet. Different surface area sizes could be selected based on presumed gas exchange needs for the patient. The devices were small enough to be used easily both within the OR and to be expanded to areas outside the operating theater. When placed within the bypass circuit, deoxygenated venous blood and membrane gas flowed in countercurrent directions: venous blood entered at the bottom of the device, while oxygenation and carbon dioxide removal was provided via flowing gas from the top of the device. Partial pressure differences between the gas and the venous blood flowing in countercurrent directions augmented removal of carbon dioxide and addition of oxygen [29]. The oxygenated (and decarboxylated) blood then was delivered to the patient's circulation. This device was (and remains) one of the only devices approved for ECMO by the US Food and Drug Administration. The Kolobow membrane lung was very efficient and was/is used for many years in both adult and pediatric bypass surgery and ECMO. Drawbacks to the Kolobow lung included a fairly high resistance to blood flow through the cylindrical design, which made use of roller-pump devices necessary to generate adequate blood flow, need for priming of at least 20 minutes and the development of clotting within the device that eventually resulted in gas exchange failure [30]. The desire for more low-resistance oxygenators with low priming volumes, excellent gas exchange, and longevity resulted in continued research and the introduction of various other membrane lungs. The development of microporous membranes that had low resistance and smaller surface area which could be primed in only several minutes, maintained excellent gas exchange and allowed for coatings to reduce platelet aggregation and clot formation has resulted in hollow-fiber technology, which rapidly replaced the silicone-membrane lung [31]. Almost overnight, the workhorse of membrane lungs, the silicone oxygenator, disappeared in favor of hollow-fiber devices. Today, the Quadrox polymethlypentene membrane lung, manufactured by Getinge, has almost captured the market, although other devices with similar properties are arriving on the scene. While these devices still fail over time, their longevity is greatly enhanced over previous generations, and expanding research will likely provide even better membrane lungs to be developed in the future [32–36]. Such research is spurred on by the quest for an artificial lung which can be clinically applied to both adults and children, since transplantation is plagued by inadequate organ supply, need for anti-rejection medication lifelong, and a relatively short lifespan of transplanted organs. Additionally, long-term support with ECMO is invasive, costly, and associated with continued complications of bleeding, thrombosis, and infection [37–39].

As the membrane lung field advanced, so too did technology in pump development. While servo-regulated roller head devices owned the field for many years, they had disadvantages that left clinicians searching for something better. Roller head pumps work by generating semi-occlusive pressure by the rotating head pushing against the circuit tubing, which is contained in a stainless steel "box". The rotating heads advance blood forward to the membrane lung where gas exchange occurs and the oxygenated blood is then returned to the body. Roller head devices use gravity to generate inflow to the pump head [40]. This requires longer circuit lengths and also means that the patient must be elevated above the pump head. As the roller heads rotate, negative pressure is created on the side bringing fluid (blood) to the pump head box (usually referred to as the raceway area), and positive pressure is created on the tubing leaving the box. Both excessive amounts of negative pressure, which can result in hemolysis, and positive pressure, which can result in tubing disruption if forward flow is restricted for some reason, are major concerns with roller head devices. Tubing disruption can occur instantaneously both from roller head friction causing weakening of the tubing in the raceway or from acute occlusion of the circuit distal to the roller heads. These potential complications create a necessity for careful observation, usually in the form of a person at the bedside to watch the device, need for replacement of tubing in the raceway area periodically, and long circuit lengths which result in a system which is cumbersome to move around [29].

The development of centrifugal pumps, which avoid the issue of generation of high positive pressure and eliminate tubing disruption as a major concern, seems like a great advance in technology. Early versions, however, were unpopular as the spinning head was supported by a ball bearing which developed heat as it turned and resulted in hemolysis. When used at low flow rates, the blood spends more time in the pump head, and severe hemolysis can occur, which limited centrifugal pump use in small children and infants. Today, the majority of centrifugal pumps use a magnet, which allows the head to be levitated and not rest on a ball bearing. Heat buildup is minimized. Pump heads have also been miniaturized so that priming volumes are very small, and even at low flow rates, hemolysis is greatly reduced. Another potential advantage of centrifugal pumps is that they will not generate high line pressure if tubing distal to the pump head becomes occluded. While the pump head will spin (and hemolyze blood in the head), tubing rupture from pressure buildup will not occur. Centrifugal pumps generate "suction" on the inlet side of the circuit and thus do not rely on gravity. This feature allows for short circuits to be created, which reduces priming volumes, and makes the system easy to setup and move around. The suction effect can generate high negative pressure in the inlet side of the pump, which can create hemolysis and air entrainment from any open stopcock or similar can also easily occur [41]. Risk of air embolus to the patient (which can be lethal) often mandates use of air bubble detectors, which will stop pump flow if air is detected. Combined with the ease of low-resistance, hollow-fiber membrane lungs, centrifugal systems have rapidly become favorites for ECMO, ventricular assist devices (which do not need a membrane lung), and bypass as well. While complications from thrombosis still exist and failure of both pump head and membrane lungs can occur, the ease of use of these devices has allowed many programs to shift from having a specialist at the bedside 24/7 to watch the circuit to either a nurse-driven single caregiver model, in which both patient care and monitoring of the centrifugal system are provided by 1 person, or intermittent monitoring of the system by a circulating perfusionist or specialist. This has the potential to greatly reduce expense related to use of these devices for ECMO and similar modalities. It is of interest that even though centrifugal systems have many theoretical advantages, there is little evidence that centrifugal ECMO systems are "better" than roller-head setups, and some studies have even suggested they are worse in children regarding development of renal failure, hemolysis, and risk of mortality. Nonetheless, the majority of centers have switched to centrifugal pumps. The only patient group which still often receives ECMO with roller-head support are neonates because of lingering concern for hemolysis and the long and successful history of roller-head support in infant ECMO. Centrifugal pumps require an understanding of physiology, as they are both preload and afterload dependent. Adequate preload is needed for forward flow to the pump head, and afterload must be overcome to generate flow from the pump head. Failure to provide enough forward flow can actually result in blood from the patient flowing backwards into the circuit—increasing the revolutions per minute of the spinning head will generate more forward flow pressure and overcome the patient's afterload.

While technology has greatly advanced in the last decade, anticoagulation is still required to prevent clotting in the devices. Although much effort has been put forth to develop the optimal range of anticoagulation, the best monitoring scheme for adjusting anticoagulation and methods to coat the systems to prevent thrombosis from occurring and eliminate anticoagulant need, this area remains the most frustrating and poorly agreed upon portion of ECMO care. While heparin has been the mainstay of anticoagulation since its appearance in the 1930s, new direct thrombin inhibitors are also being used. To date, there is no universally agreed upon, optimal method for providing anticoagulation during ECMO, making bleeding and thrombosis the major risks of the procedure [42, 43]. Once these issues can be solved, the field of extracorporeal support will likely be open to even more patients and embraced with more enthusiasm.

As experience with extracorporeal support systems in the operating theater grew, clinicians began to apply them outside the OR. The first neonate receiving ECMO was treated by Dr. Bob Bartlett, a pioneer in the field, in California. The infant, named Esperanza (which means hope) by the nursing staff after her mother abandoned her following birth, had what we would now know as persistent pulmonary hypertension of the newborn and was dying from hypoxemia. Dr. Bartlett and colleagues took their extracorporeal system from the lab where they were doing experimental work, received a compassionate use agreement by the institutional review board (of which they were members), and applied this device to the infant. Her survival formed the basis from which a multitude of ECMO support in neonates began. Today, Esperanza has grown to have children of her own and is a frequent return visitor to the annual extracorporeal life support organization (ELSO) meetings [44]. The adult world had also had some success with ECMO, with Hill describing one of the first cases where a motorcycle accident victim was supported [45]. Using a roller head device and a large plate oxygenator which took over 4 liters of blood to prime, this patient survived. Randomized trials of ECMO versus conventional mechanical ventilation in infants with respiratory failure found benefit to ECMO, and it became a fairly accepted modality for use in tertiary centers. The National Institutes of Health sponsored a randomized trial of Adult ECMO for respiratory failure, but the bleeding complications in both ECMO and control groups were massive. No adjustment in conventional ventilation was performed once ECMO was initiated either, and mortality was extremely high in both control and ECMO groups [46]. Adult ECMO was largely abandoned for many years. As success with neonatal, pediatric, and cardiac patients with ECMO expanded, the adult world began to again look at ECMO as a supportive tool. The combination of the arrival of new generations of centrifugal pumps, hollow fiber membrane lungs, and another randomized trial of adult ECMO versus conventional ventilation in the United Kingdom which was favorable to ECMO created new interest in its use [47]. At about the same time, the H1N1 flu epidemic occurred, and many young, previously healthy adults received ECMO with good results, and the adult world opened up once again to ECMO support [48]. Since that time, nearly a decade ago now, ECMO has grown exponentially in the adult realm, and adults currently form the largest patient group receiving this therapy worldwide. The use of ECMO in respiratory failure, following cardiac surgery to support heart recovery and in other forms of cardiac failure, and even as a resuscitation tool in refractory cardiac arrest is now commonplace [49, 50]. The extracorporeal life support organization, founded in 1989, is the largest database repository of ECMO patients. Patient populations and outcomes are shown in Table 1.1.

Clinicians yearn for a method to select the most appropriate patients for ECMO support, and several predictive scoring systems have been developed. None, however, are completely accurate and require more refinement before they can be established as the optimal measures. Today, almost every patient placed on ECMO is decided on a case-by-case discussion with the referring team, the ECMO experts at the center and in conjunction with the family. With the exception of severe neurologic injury, expected lifespans of 6 months or less, or advanced directives which do not include "extraordinary" supportive measures, there are few absolute contraindications to ECMO. Even patients with head injury and intracranial bleeds, who would not have received ECMO in the past for fear of expanding hemorrhage, are now reported [51]. The ability of ECMO to be provided without anticoagulation, especially at higher flow rates used in adults, for hours to days has also allowed patients with bleeding diatheses to receive ECMO support. Cancer patients, trauma patients, pregnant women, cardiac arrest victims, and those with septic shock are but a few of the expanded horizons for ECMO support [52–54]. While bone marrow transplant patients with respiratory or circulatory failure still have excessive mortality even with ECMO support (and form a group to which ECMO is not offered in many centers), improved understanding of pathophysiology and less toxic medication regimens may change the approach to these patients in the future [55, 56].

Table 1.1 Outcomes of ECMO patients

	Total runs	Survived ECLS	Survived to DC
Neonatal			
Pulmonary	31,591	27.779 (87%)	23,119 (73%)
Cardiac	8,252	5,684 (68%)	3,529 (42%)
ECPR	1,864	1,315 (70%)	775 (41%)
Pediatric			
Pulmonary	9,487	6,797 (71%)	5,573 (58%)
Cardiac	11,377	8,155 (71%)	5,980 (52%)
ECPR	4,361	2,628 (60%)	1,858 (42%)
Adult			
Pulmonary	19,482	13,453 (69%)	11,565 (59%)
Cardiac	19,627	11,628 (59%)	8,381 (42%)
ECPR	6,190	2,580 (41%)	1,827 (29%)
TOTAL	**112,231**	**80,019 (71%)**	**62,607 (55%)**

Adapted from International ELSO Registry, Jan 2019, With permission

The development of small, easy-to-use, and perhaps safer systems has also coincided with the concerns of delirium and excessive sedation in the ICU environment. ECMO care now encourages patients to be awake and mobile and even to perform rehab on ECMO to maintain muscle strength and perhaps hasten recovery. ECMO is now also being used a bridge to support patients to heart and/or lung transplant (and as a support modality if needed after transplant) [57]. Patients with circulatory failure who do not require gas-exchange assistance also now have a variety of centrifugal-based systems for ventricular support as well [52].

Expanding areas of ECMO-related research are focusing on premature infants by developing an artificial placenta in which premature lambs are enclosed in an amniotic fluid environment and umbilical vessels are used for blood supply. This research is advancing well and may advance to clinical trials in the near future [58]. The use of ECMO perfusion has also allowed ischemic times for organs being harvested for transplantation to be shortened, and excellent results for transplanted kidneys, livers, and pancreas with this support have been described. While ethical considerations remain important (when does resuscitation from cardiac arrest become support for organ transplantation, for instance), the application of ECMO to patient groups never imagined 20 years ago is now a reality [59].

The final frontier for ECMO relates to long-term outcome, quality of life, and expense. If the dream of an artificial lung which can support patients outside the hospital environment is realized, then many of the cost concerns can be reduced. Few centers have long-term follow-up clinics, mainly related to lack of funding for such efforts, and long-term outcome is an essential part of helping to refine optimal patient selection, care, and management. Currently, the rapid expansion of ECMO and its non-regulated use may be developing an unsustainable market in terms of cost. The lack of specific credentialing for ECMO centers and clinicians is also a risk factor for substandard care to be provided, as there is no mandate for reporting of outcomes. While the ELSO registry contains over 100,000 patients, there are MANY hundreds of ECMO centers which do not report patient data to any registry for quality improvement. This lack of transparency and reporting is a major concern as the overall use and outcomes of ECMO cannot be ascertained worldwide. As miniaturization of ECMO and related systems continues to occur, and the problems of anticoagulation are solved, a world where such modalities are quickly and easily available for patients with severe respiratory or cardiac failure is easily imagined. The use of simulation to augment training for patient care, device operation, and quality improvement has a major role to continue to move the field forward.

Conclusions

ECLS has undergone many years of research and development. Today, it is a standard support system in many centers. As the field continues to expand, new technologies may open ECLS to even more patient groups. If the continued need for anticoagulation could ever be eliminated, the use of ECLS could someday replace invasive mechanical ventilation, provide support for premature infants, and become a first-line modality rather than a rescue therapy. The use of simulation will continue to play a vital role in advancing ECLS safely and efficiently. Simulation is playing an increasingly important role in educating new ECLS centers and maintaining competencies in those already established.

References

1. Le Gallois JJC. Experiments on the principle of life, and particularly on the principle of the motions of the heart, and on the seat of this principle: including the report made to the first class of the Institute, upon the experiments relative to the motions of the heart. Philadelphia: Published by M.Thomas, William Fry, printer; 1813.
2. Brown-Sequard E. Recherches experimentales sur les proprietes physiologiques et les usages du sang rouge et du sang noir et leurs principaux elements gazeux, loxygene et lacide carbonique. Journal de la Physiologie De l'Homme et des Animaux. 1858;1:95–122, 353–67, 729–35.
3. Kay J. Physiological experiments and observations on the cessation of the contractility of the heart and muscles in the asphyxia of warm blooded animals. Edinb Med Surg J. 1828;29:37–66.
4. Lofstrom JB. The polio epidemic in Copenhagen in 1952--and how the anaesthetist came out of the operating room. Acta Anaesthesiol Scand. 1994;38:419.
5. Wackers GL. Modern anaesthesiological principles for bulbar polio: manual IPPR in the 1952 polio-epidemic in Copenhagen. Acta Anaesthesiol Scand. 1994;38:420–31.
6. Richardson BW. An inquiry in to the possibility of restoring the life of warm-blooded animals in ceratin cases where respiration, the circulation and the ordinary manifestations of organic motion are exhausted or have ceased. Proc R Soc Lond. 1865;14:358–71.
7. Bidder E. Beitrage zur Lehre von der Function der Niere. Inaugural Dissertation Dorpat; 1862.
8. von Schroder W. Ueber die Bildungsstatte des Harnstoffs. Archiv fur Experimentelle Pathologie und Pharmakologie. 1882;15:364–400.
9. von Frey M, Gruber M. Untersuchungen über den Stoffwechsel isolirter Organe. Ein Respirationsapparat für isolirte Organe. Archiv für Anatomie und Physiologie. 1885;9:519–32.
10. von Frey M. Versuche über den Stoffwechsel des Muskels. Archiv für Physiologie. 1885;9:533–62.
11. Jacobj C. Apparat zur Durchblutung isolirter überlebender Organe. Archiv für Experimentelle Pathologie und Pharmakologie. 1890;26:388–97.
12. Jacobj C. Ein Beitrag zur Technik der künstlichen Durchblutung überlebender Organe. Archiv für Experimentelle Pathologie und Pharmakologie. 1895;31:330–48.
13. Jacobj C. Ein Beitrag zur Methode der Durchblutung isolierter Organe. Centralblatt für Allgemeine Pathologie und Pathologische Anatomie. 1923;33:268–91.
14. Mc LJ. The discovery of heparin. Circulation. 1959;19:75–8.
15. Brukhonenko S. Circulation artificielle du sang dans l'organisme entier d'un chien avec coeur exclu. Journal de Pathologie et de Pathologie Générale. 1929;27:257–72.

16. Brukhonenko S. Appareil pour la circulation artificielle du sang des animaux à sang chaud. J de Physiologie et de Pathologie Générale. 1929;27:12–8.
17. Brukhonenko S, Tchetchuline S. I Expériences avec la tête isolée du chien. J de Physiologie et de Pathologie Générale. 1929;27:31–45.
18. Brukhonenko S, Tchetchuline S. VII Expériences avec la tête isolée du chien. J de Physiologie et de Pathologie Générale. 1929;27:64–79.
19. Alexi-Meskishvili V, Potapov E, Beyer E, Terebinski HRN. A pioneer of the open valve operation. Ann Thorac Surg. 1998;66:1440–3.
20. Gibbon J. Application of a mechanical heart and lung apparatus to cardiac surgery. Minn Med. 1954;37:171–87.
21. Dewall R, Lillehei CW, Hodges P, Long D, Wade J, Cardozo R. Description of the helical reservoir bubble-type pump oxygenator for hemodilution hypothermic perfusions. Dis Chest. 1963;44:113–20.
22. DeWall RA. Origin of the helical reservoir bubble oxygenator heart-lung machine. Perfusion. 2003;18:163–9.
23. DeWall RA, Bentley DJ, Hirose M, Battung V, Najafi H, Roden T. A temperature controlling (omnithermic) disposable bubble oxygenator for total body perfusion. Dis Chest. 1966;49:207–11.
24. Dewall RA, Gott VL, Lillehei CW, Read RC, Varco RL, Warden HE. Total body perfusion for open cardiotomy utilizing the bubble oxygenator; physiologic responses in man. J Thorac Surg. 1956;32:591–603.
25. Kloff WJ. The artificial kidney: a dialyser with a great area. Milestones Nephrol. 1944:121–34.
26. Clowes GH Jr, Neville WE, Hopkins A, Anzola J, Simeone FA. Factors contributing to success or failure in the use of a pump oxygenator for complete by-pass of the heart and lung, experimental and clinical. Surgery. 1954;36:557–79.
27. Kammermeyer K. Silicone rubber as a selective barrier. Ind Eng Chem. 1957;49:1685–6.
28. Kolobow T, Stool EW, Weathersby PK, Pierce J, Hayano F, Suaudeau J. Superior blood compatibility of silicone rubber free of silica filler in the membrane lung. Trans Am Soc Artif Inter Organs. 1974;20A:269–76.
29. Dalton HJ, Rycus PT, Conrad SA. Update on extracorporeal life support 2004. Semin Perinatol. 2005;29:24–33.
30. Fuhrman BP, Dalton HJ. Progress in pediatric extracorporeal membrane oxygenation. Crit Care Clin. 1992;8:191–202.
31. Sievert AN, Shackelford AG, McCall MM. Trends and emerging technologies in extracorporeal life support: results of the 2006 ECLS survey. J Extra Corpor Technol. 2009;41:73–8.
32. Skiens WE, Lipps BJ, Clark ME, McLain EA. Hollow fiber membrane oxygenator. J Biomed Mater Res. 1971;5:135–48.
33. Tsuji T, Suma K, Tanishita K, et al. Development and clinical evaluation of hollow fiber membrane oxygenator. Trans Am Soc Artif Inter Organs. 1981;27:280–4.
34. Suma K, Tsuji T, Takeuchi Y, et al. Clinical performance of microporous polypropylene hollow-fiber oxygenator. Ann Thorac Surg. 1981;32:558–62.
35. Lautier A, Sargentini JC, Norre JL, Touchot B. Low pressure drop microporous hollow fiber membrane oxygenator. Life Support Syst. 1985;3:89–91.
36. Guan Y, Su X, McCoach R, Wise R, Kunselman A, Undar A. Evaluation of Quadrox-i adult hollow fiber oxygenator with integrated arterial filter. J Extra Corpor Technol. 2010;42:134–8.
37. Combes A, Bacchetta M, Brodie D, Muller T, Pellegrino V. Extracorporeal membrane oxygenation for respiratory failure in adults. Curr Opin Crit Care. 2012;18:99–104.
38. Dalton HJ, Reeder R, Garcia-Filion P, et al. Factors associated with bleeding and thrombosis in children receiving extracorporeal membrane oxygenation. Am J Respir Crit Care Med. 2017;196:762–71.
39. Abrams D, Combes A, Brodie D. Extracorporeal membrane oxygenation in cardiopulmonary disease in adults. J Am Coll Cardiol. 2014;63:2769–78.
40. Andrews AF, Roloff DW, Bartlett RH. Use of extracorporeal membrane oxygenators in persistent pulmonary hypertension of the newborn. Clin Perinatol. 1984;11:729–35.
41. Lou S, MacLaren G, Best D, Delzoppo C, Butt W. Hemolysis in pediatric patients receiving centrifugal-pump extracorporeal membrane oxygenation: prevalence, risk factors, and outcomes. Crit Care Med. 2014;42:1213–20.
42. Annich GM. Extracorporeal life support: the precarious balance of hemostasis. J Thromb Haemost: JTH. 2015;13(Suppl 1):S336–42.
43. Werho DK, Pasquali SK, Yu S, et al. Hemorrhagic complications in pediatric cardiac patients on extracorporeal membrane oxygenation: an analysis of the Extracorporeal Life Support Organization Registry. Pediatr Crit Care Med. 2015;16:276–88.
44. Bartlett RH, Andrews AF, Toomasian JM, Haiduc NJ, Gazzaniga AB. Extracorporeal membrane oxygenation for newborn respiratory failure: forty-five cases. Surgery. 1982;92:425–33.
45. Hill JD. Acute pulmonary failure: treatment with extracorporeal oxygenation. Med Instrum. 1977;11:198–201.
46. Zapol WM, Snider MT, Hill JD, et al. Extracorporeal membrane oxygenation in severe acute respiratory failure. A randomized prospective study. JAMA. 1979;242:2193–6.
47. Peek GJ, Clemens F, Elbourne D, et al. CESAR: conventional ventilatory support vs extracorporeal membrane oxygenation for severe adult respiratory failure. BMC Health Serv Res. 2006;6:163.
48. Park PK, Dalton HJ, Bartlett RH. Point: efficacy of extracorporeal membrane oxygenation in 2009 influenza A (H1N1): sufficient evidence? Chest. 2010;138:776–8.
49. Dalton HJ. Extracorporeal life support: moving at the speed of light. Respir Care. 2011;56:1445–53; discussion 1453–6.
50. Joffe AR, Lequier L, Robertson CM. Pediatric outcomes after extracorporeal membrane oxygenation for cardiac disease and for cardiac arrest: a review. ASAIO J. 2012;58:297–310.
51. Papazian L, Herridge M. Outcomes and risk stratification for severe ARDS treated with ECMO. Intensive Care Med. 2013;39:1857–60.
52. Gow KW, Lao OB, Leong T, Fortenberry JD. Extracorporeal life support for adults with malignancy and respiratory or cardiac failure: the Extracorporeal Life Support experience. Am J Surg. 2010;199:669–75.
53. Biscotti M, Lee A, Basner RC, et al. Hybrid configurations via percutaneous access for extracorporeal membrane oxygenation: a single-center experience. ASAIO J. 2014;60:635–42.
54. Agerstrand CL, Bacchetta MD, Brodie D. ECMO for adult respiratory failure: current use and evolving applications. ASAIO J. 2014;60:255–62.
55. Gow KW, Wulkan ML, Heiss KF, et al. Extracorporeal membrane oxygenation for support of children after hematopoietic stem cell transplantation: the Extracorporeal Life Support Organization experience. J Pediatr Surg. 2006;41:662–7.
56. Bourquin JP, Thornley I, Neuberg D, et al. Favorable outcome of allogeneic hematopoietic stem cell transplantation for relapsed or refractory acute promyelocytic leukemia in childhood. Bone Marrow Transplant. 2004;34:795–8.
57. Rosenzweig EB, Brodie D, Abrams DC, Agerstrand CL, Bacchetta M. Extracorporeal membrane oxygenation as a novel bridging strategy for acute right heart failure in group 1 pulmonary arterial hypertension. ASAIO J. 2014;60:129–33.
58. Mercurio MR. The EXTEND system for extrauterine support of extremely premature neonates: opportunity and caution. Pediatr Res. 2018;84:795–6.
59. Whitman GJ. Extracorporeal membrane oxygenation for the treatment of postcardiotomy shock. J Thorac Cardiovasc Surg. 2017;153:95–101.

Simulating ECMO: Rationale and Genesis

2

Louis Patrick Halamek

Learning Objectives

1. List the limitations of didactic lectures and water drills and the advantages of using simulation and feedback/debriefing for training in the management of patients on ECMO.
2. Describe the value of scenarios that include the simultaneous malfunction of the ECMO circuit and decompensation of the patient.
3. List the three types of cues that create realism during simulation of ECMO.
4. State how debriefing ECMO scenarios may differ from debriefing other types of simulated clinical events.

Rationale for Simulating ECMO

Extracorporeal membrane oxygenation (ECMO) was first used in pediatric patients with severe cardiorespiratory failure in the 1970s [1–3]. As anyone who has cared for a patient on ECMO knows, while it is a lifesaving therapy for many, it can also be life threatening. The complexity of ECMO technology and the tenuous hold on life that characterize patients on ECMO collude to demand rapid and correct responses to any significant perturbation in equipment functionality or patient physiology. This makes ECMO the classic low-frequency, high-risk activity that is ideally suited to the use of simulation-based training for skill acquisition in order to reduce the risk of potentially devastating events.

Indeed, the necessity that healthcare professionals caring for patients on ECMO be able to manage not only routine interventions but also unpredictable emergencies calls for proficiency in a wide range of cognitive, technical, and behavioral skills [4]. Cognitive skills involve the storage and recall of content knowledge as well as decision-making; these skills can be especially challenging when healthcare professionals must operate under the intense time pressure that is associated with an ECMO emergency. Technical skills include the techniques used to not only care for the patient but also those used to manipulate the ECMO circuit to maintain it in working order and repair or replace failing components. Finally, successful management of the patient on ECMO requires the use of behavioral skills such as effective communication; behavioral skills are important in many clinical domains such as neonatal resuscitation (Fig. 2.1). These three skill sets form the basis of the learning objectives that serve as the core of simulation-based training in ECMO (Table 2.1).

Historically, competence in the care of patients on ECMO has been achieved by (a) attendance at didactic lectures used to communicate such information as the physiology of ECMO and the management of anticoagulation coupled with (b) "water drills" where trainees are required to manipulate a liquid-filled ECMO circuit in order to address a problem with the function of that circuit. Listening to a lecture is one means of content knowledge acquisition, although arguably self-study followed by interactive discussion with a knowledgeable healthcare professional is a superior method for adult learners. Water drills allow the practice of important technical skills and do require the recall and application of certain content knowledge as well as decision-making skills. However, water drills alone fail to include a key element: the patient. When a problem with the ECMO circuit arises, it is the risk to and/or decompensation of the patient attached to that circuit that drives healthcare professionals to react. Without a patient and the resultant sense of time pressure, neither lectures nor water drills create sufficient realism to fully prepare trainees to effectively and safely manage patients on ECMO.

L. P. Halamek (✉)
Division of Neonatal and Developmental Medicine, Department of Pediatrics, Stanford University, Palo Alto, CA, USA
e-mail: halamek@stanford.edu

L. C. Johnston, L. Su (eds.), *Comprehensive Healthcare Simulation: ECMO Simulation*, Comprehensive Healthcare Simulation,
https://doi.org/10.1007/978-3-030-53844-6_2

Know your environment.
Knows all aspects of environment; thoroughly checks all equipment to ensure that it is present and in working order prior to delivery; confirms readiness of environment with members of team; does not hesitate to ask questions of others in the environment when the need arises.

Anticipate and plan for problems.
Appears thoroughly prepared for the delivery; inquires as to why the presence of the pediatric team is requested at the delivery; inquires about gestational age, presence of meconium; recognizes prior to the delivery whether all of the appropriate personnel are present and actively ensures that the team is complete by the time the baby is born; explicitly assigns the roles of the team members prior to delivery (conducts a briefing); asks questions indicating an in-depth understanding of potential problems and subsequent consequences of the evolving case; does not appear surprised by predictable situations; effectively deals with changing circumstances.

Assume a leadership role.
Team members appear calm; the leader is clearly identified prior to the delivery; leader helps to facilitate coordination of all of the activities of the team; the leader is actively engaged in the situation and calmly inspires confidence among team members.

Communicate effectively.
Problems are clearly communicated to the team; team members speak clearly, succinctly, and in even tones; important communications can easily be heard by the other members of the neonatal team; intended recipients of commands are clearly identified; "repeat -backs"/"closed loop" communications occur at all times; team members listen to others, clarify ambiguous communications and encourage cooperation.

Distribute workload and delegate responsibility optimally.
Specific tasksare clearly assigned to specific team members; the skills of all team members are utilized well; overtaxed team members are assisted/relieved when necessary; an appropriate level of supervision is always provided.

Allocate attention wisely.
Does not become distracted; cognizant of details yet adequately monitors patient's overall condition; prioritizes demands for attention well; avoids fixation errors.

Utilize all available information.
Recognizes emergency situations instantly; recognizes all disease states requiring intervention in the delivery room; able to quickly assimilate all pertinent data (including historical data) in formulating a diagnosis and logical plan of care; interprets physical findings accurately; repeats physical examination when fin dings are equivocal; frequently reassesses patient status; immediately recognizes changes in patient condition and revises plan of care accordingly.

Utilize all available resources.
Readily solicits and incorporates the expertise of others without prompti ng; reacts to equipment or personnel failures by quickly identifying and implementing alternative solutions.

Recognize limitations and call for help early enough.
Immediately recognizes when at his/her limits in medical knowledge and technical and behavioral skills; recognizes situations where additional help will be required and requests such assistance early (before it is actually needed).

Maintain professional behavior.
Maintains composure at all times; does not engage in any unnecessary conversation; language and approach are always professional; consistently demonstrates a caring attitude toward patients and families; recognizes and responds to all nonverbal and verbal cues; readily accepts advice and encourages input from other team members; generates a positive atmosphere while supervising and teaching; non-judgmental; non-defensive.

Fig. 2.1 Key behavioral skills referenced in the NeoSim program @ CAPE

Table 2.1 ECMO SIM @ CAPE Comprehensive Learning Objectives

Cognitive
Know the indicators of failing intensive care
Understand the pathophysiologies that cause a patient to require ECMO support
Know the clinical criteria for initiating ECMO
Know the differences between VA and VV ECMO
Know the indications for VA ECMO
Know the indications for VV ECMO
Know in which cases ECMO is clearly indicated, optional or should not be offered
Know what medical/surgical services to contact in order to initiate ECMO
Understand the physiology of ECMO
Know what equipment and supplies are required to initiate ECMO
Understand the function of each component of the ECMO circuit
Know the indications for initiating and weaning from ECMO
Technical
Be able to perform ECMO procedures including but not limited to:
Circuit priming
Safety inspection of circuit
Preparation for cannulation
Adjustment of pump flow
Adjustment of sweep gas flow
Infusion and withdrawal of fluids
Adjustment of water bath temperature
(Complete) circuit change-out
Circuit component change-out
Preparation for decannulation
Be able to perform patient care procedures on ECMO:
Intubation
Suctioning
Chest compressions
Repositioning on bed, change of linens, etc.
Behavioral
Anticipate and plan for emergencies
Be able to effectively troubleshoot problems when under intense time pressure
Assume the leadership role during an emergency
Know how to communicate effectively in a crisis
Distribute the workload of attending to both patient and circuit simultaneously
Allocate attention wisely
Utilize all available information
Utilize all available resources
Call for help early enough
Maintain professional behavior

The realistic simulation of ECMO requires both a circuit and a patient where perturbations in circuit function (eventually) affect the patient or changes in patient physiology create problems with the circuit. When individuals and teams are presented with realistic visual, auditory, and tactile cues that indicate a possible, evolving, or immediate problem, they must employ not only their cognitive and technical skills but also their behavioral skills in order to successfully resolve the situation. Simulation-based training, when performed appropriately, effectively elicits all three skill sets and thereby overcomes the limitations associated with the use of lectures and water drills to prepare teams to care for real patients.

Genesis of ECMO Simulation

The use of ECMO in the neonatal population has been slowly decreasing for a number of years, due to improved prenatal care and the introduction of postnatal therapies such as high-frequency oscillatory ventilation (HFOV) and inhaled nitric oxide (INO) that have proven effective in managing the cardiopulmonary failure associated with neonatal diseases such as meconium aspiration, pulmonary hypertension, and sepsis [5–7]. Fewer patients requiring ECMO means fewer encounters with real ECMO situations and therefore less experience for healthcare professionals in the management of those situations. This is an especially acute problem for physicians in training programs who, despite the lack of actual clinical experience, must nevertheless develop the skills necessary to save lives when faced with real ECMO emergencies.

The world's first simulation-based training program in ECMO management was conducted at the Center for Advanced Pediatric and Perinatal Education (CAPE, http://cape.stanford.edu) at Stanford University in 2003 (Fig. 2.2) [8, 9]. The ECMO Sim© program was developed in response to a need to provide highly realistic and effective learning opportunities for post-residency fellows in neonatal-perinatal medicine and is one of a suite of programs, along with NeoSim© (management of difficult neonatal resuscitation situations) and CounselSim© (conduct of challenging prenatal and end-of-life discussions) that are offered at CAPE to address critical skill acquisition and maintenance needs in high stress, high consequence clinical situations. Although developed with neonatologists, ECMO specialists, perfusionists, and neonatal intensive care unit (NICU) nurses in mind, ECMO Sim© also effectively serves as a template for pediatric and adult ECMO training programs. Given the investment in time, effort, technology, and supplies necessary to conduct simulated ECMO scenarios, it is wise to allow as many disciplines as possible to benefit from this activity.

Core Developmental Strategies

All simulation-based training programs at CAPE start with identification of the trainees, including their range of clinical experience. Once the trainees are identified, a list of learning objectives that are tailored to their specific needs is generated. Each learning objective is then characterized by the cognitive, technical, and behavioral skills necessary to

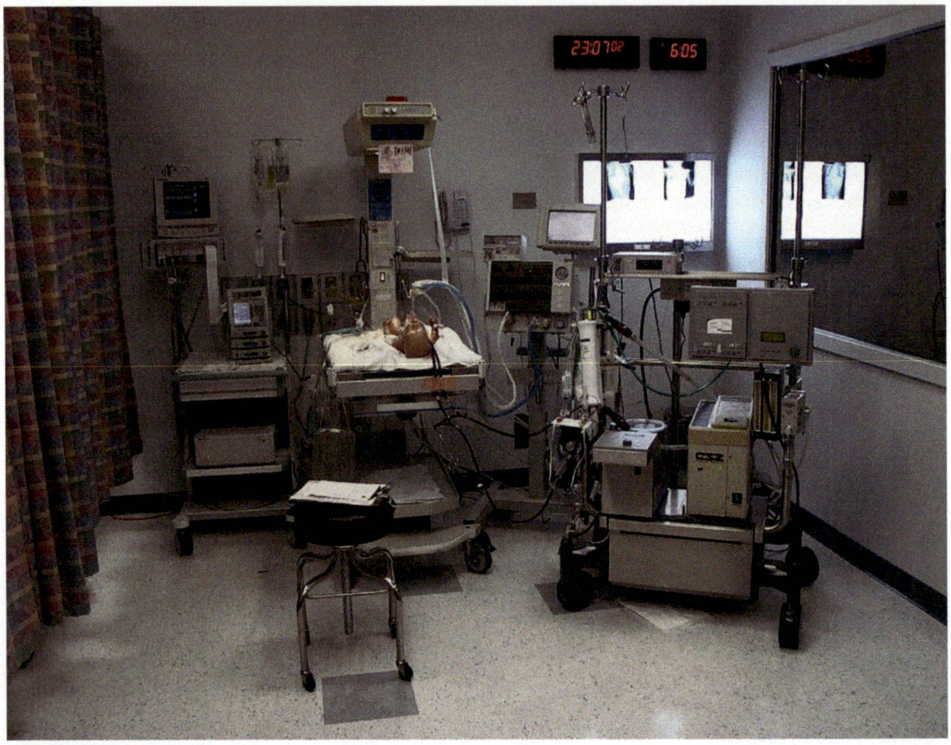

Fig. 2.2 ECMO Sim @ CAPE

achieve that objective. Once the appropriate learning objectives and skill sets are determined, a scenario is designed to achieve those learning objectives. Writing a scenario requires that key visual, auditory, and tactile cues are embedded within it in order that those experiencing the scenario can achieve the same mental model of the clinical situation that the writer of the scenario possesses. It also mandates that all scenarios should be thoroughly trialed/piloted by the instructor team prior to being deployed for trainees; this reduces the risk of unanticipated malfunction of technologies and misinterpretation of cues resulting in a "scenario gone astray" when conducted with trainees.

Pre-program preparation is an absolute must for both the instructor team and the trainees. The complexity of a full-scale ECMO scenario involving both a simulated patient and a functional ECMO circuit requires significant time for set-up. Even when using a patient simulator/manikin that has already been "cannulated" (ECMO cannula already in place in the simulated patient), it still requires time to prime the circuit and the simulated patient, connect the patient to the circuit, ensure that all is in normal working order, and then test the ways in which problems with the patient and the circuit will be generated. At CAPE, 8 hours is typically set aside for this process.

Weeks before arrival, trainees are informed of the date, starting time, and duration of the program. They are provided with a schedule of the day's events but are not informed of the details of the scenarios that will be conducted. Prior to their arrival at CAPE, all trainees will have participated in didactic sessions describing ECMO and in water drills. Thus they are expected to possess the content knowledge and technical skills necessary to function during ECMO Sim© scenarios. Upon arrival to the program, the trainees are familiarized to the training room, including the patient, circuit, and all equipment and supplies. Any questions regarding content knowledge are answered during this time, and any requests to practice manipulating the circuit are facilitated. This is then followed by a series of simulated clinical ECMO scenarios in which individual trainees diagnose and treat the patient and/or circuit issues that become manifest. At a minimum, the trainees consist of the physician responsible for ECMO management and the ECMO specialist managing the circuit; additional trainees may include a perfusionist, NICU nurse, and/or respiratory therapist. Some roles may be filled by members of the instructor team who function to provide important information and/or key cues to the trainees in order to improve the realism of the scenarios. Upon conclusion of each scenario, all of the trainees (primary and secondary responders to the scenario as well as those who simply observed) are debriefed.

Lessons Learned

Since the first ECMO Sim© program at CAPE in 2003, a number of valuable lessons have been learned regarding conducting simulated ECMO scenarios (Table 2.2):

Table 2.2 Lessons learned

Scenario development and conduct
1. A simulated patient should be connected to the circuit to enhance realism and add complexity
2. Incorporate key visual, auditory, and tactile cues to engender realistic performance
3. Include as many ECMO team members (either as responders or as assistants) as possible in complex scenarios
4. Multiple relatively brief scenarios may be conducted when the learning objectives are focused on discrete technical skills
5. Patient history and clinical course to date can be standardized across many or all simulated scenarios, increasing the time available for hands-on activity
6. When conducting multi-scenario training programs, start with a relatively uncomplicated situation to allow trainees to become familiar with how cues will be presented
Debriefing
1. ECMO scenarios that are focused primarily on technical skill acquisition and are of relatively short duration can be reviewed using feedback with trainees gathered around the circuit
2. ECMO scenarios that require the display of multiple skills by trainees may be best reviewed using formal debriefing techniques
3. The CAPE model of debriefing focuses on the actions of the individual, how those actions contribute to the performance of the team, and ultimately how team performance influences the care of the patient; this model is useful when debriefing complex simulated ECMO scenarios
4. Technical performance debriefings, not critical incident stress debriefings, are used to debrief simulated ECMO scenarios

The addition of a simulated patient to the ECMO circuit adds a tremendous amount of realism to scenarios. In an actual ECMO emergency, a problem that prevents the circuit from functioning will also prevent adequate gas exchange (and potentially cardiac output, if the patient is on veno-arterial ECMO); this situation causes the patient's vital signs to decompensate. Healthcare professionals responsible for the patient need to effectively address both the malfunctioning circuit and the decompensating patient *simultaneously*. A fall in patient heart rate and SpO_2 creates a very realistic sense of time pressure that simply is not present during water drills. In order to address both the problem and its consequences, healthcare professionals must use their content knowledge to recognize and diagnose the underlying root cause, employ critical decision-making to formulate a solution, apply technical skills to manipulate the circuit, and exercise key behavioral skills such as distributing workload appropriately.

The goal of any comprehensive simulated clinical scenario is to engender the same behavior in the simulated scenario that the trainees would exhibit in a real situation; that will facilitate an understanding of both their strengths and the tactics needed to replicate them as well as their weaknesses and the tactics necessary to avoid them in the future. One of the ways in which to enhance the ability of trainees to do what they would do in a real-life situation is to embed key visual, auditory, and tactile cues into the unfolding simulated scenario. When trainees see, hear, and touch what they would when caring for a real patient, it becomes much easier for them to "buy into" the scenario and do what they would do in real life. One of the most effective visual cues is the use of simulated blood in the circuit. This can be accomplished by the addition of red food coloring to the liquid-filled circuit. This cue not only prompts trainees to don gloves when manipulating the circuit but also makes problems such leaks in the tubing as visible as they would be in real life.

Key roles in simulated ECMO scenarios include a nurse to attend to the patient, an ECMO specialist to manage the circuit, and a physician who is responsible for responding to any problems with the patient or circuit. While a typical scenario focuses on calling the physician to respond to a problem (while the nurse and specialist may function as assistants who know the details of the scenario and help it unfold in a realistic manner), ECMO simulation provides a tremendous opportunity for multidisciplinary team training. When it is desirable to involve more than just the physician as a trainee, the scenario can begin with a change-of-shift handoff between teams followed by evolution of the problem.

Many of the learning objectives associated with ECMO involve troubleshooting a problem with the circuit followed by application of technical skills while working under time pressure. By their nature, some of these problems are relatively uncomplicated and are capable of being solved relatively quickly; therefore, it is possible that some scenarios may last only a few minutes, followed by debriefings that are of a similar duration. Other scenarios may involve multiple system failures or include learning objectives that are primarily behavioral in origin; these typically require a longer period of time to unfold and also require more extensive discussion during debriefing. Because many scenarios are focused on solving a single, discrete problem with the circuit through the application of a particular technical skill, it is possible to conduct a relatively large number of scenarios in a typical training program. During ECMO Sim© at CAPE, approximately 12–15 scenarios are conducted in the course of a day-long program (Table 2.3). The choice of specific scenarios for any one ECMO Sim© program is driven by the learning objectives that are tailored to meet the specific needs of the trainees.

A patient on ECMO may have a very complex and detailed history. The relevance of all of the elements of that history to a particular ECMO scenario may be very limited, however. For example, a response to a raceway rupture does not depend on the patient's history but rather on a rapid replacement of either the raceway tubing or the entire circuit (if a primed circuit is already available). When conducting a large number of scenarios in the course of a single training program, it is unwise to require trainees to spend significant time with historical details as they enter each scenario. A strategy for allowing trainees to quickly assimilate the historical information relevant to each scenario is to standardize that information across multiple scenarios (Fig. 2.3). Similarly, the course to date on ECMO can be standardized from scenario to scenario (Fig. 2.4). There is very little reason to vary the number of hours on ECMO, circuit parameters, and patient vital signs for each scenario.

Table 2.3 ECMO SIM @ CAPE scenario master list

Cannulation dilemmas
Speak with parents over phone/person re: risks/benefits
Parents refuse ECMO for patient with trisomy 21 over phone as patient arrests
Parents at bedside when US tech finds a bilateral grade II IVH
Parents at bedside when US tech finds a unilateral grade IV IVH
Need for CPR and "crash" cannulation
Surgeon unable to place cannula
ECMO daily dilemmas
Low SvO2 on VA ECMO – need to increase pump flow
Low SvO2 on VV ECMO – need to optimize pump flow
Low SvO2 – O2 tubing disconnected
Low SvO2 – bridge incompletely clamped
Low SvO2 – low hematocrit
Low SvO2 – patient hyperactive, in need of sedation
Pump cutting out – hypovolemia
Pump cutting out – bleeding from cannula insertion site
Pump cutting out – pneumothorax
Pump cutting out – pneumopericardium
Pump cutting out/cycling down – pressure limit set too low
Pump cutting out/cycling down – hypervolemia
High post-oxy pressure – patient in pain and hypertensive
High post-oxy pressure– patient seizing and hypertensive
High pre-oxy pressure – clotted oxygenator
High pre-oxy pressure – partially closed pressure transducer stopcock
Patient hyperthermic – water bath temp too high
Patient hyperthermic – patient febrile
Patient hypothermic – water bath temp too low
Patient hypothermic – sepsis
Pulmonary hemorrhage
Gastrointestinal hemorrhage
Bleeding from cannulation site
Wet membrane
Pump stops – bladder box alarm/low volume
Pump stops – needs to be re-set
Pump stops – needs to be replaced
Power failure – disconnected power cord
Power failure – blown fuse
Cardiac stun on VV ECMO
Cardiac arrest on VV ECMO
Air in bladder
Air in circuit – venous cannula side port open to atmosphere
Air in circuit – loose stopcock
Leak in bridge
Leak elsewhere in circuit
Raceway rupture
Circuit change – routine
Circuit change with patient decompensation
Transport dilemmas
Transporting patient on ECMO to cardiac catheterization lab
Decannulation dilemmas
Inadvertent decannulation

When the initial scenario(s) in a multi-scenario program involves a small number of learning objectives that are relatively simple, it allows trainees to quickly assimilate important information such as how key cues will be presented during the scenarios. The complexity of the simulated clinical situation can then increase with each succeeding scenario, presenting greater and greater challenges to the trainees, without the need to spend valuable time unnecessarily reviewing clinical documentation.

A *debriefing* is defined as an interactive discussion of events that have already occurred; information flows between the leader(s) of the debriefing and the members of the team as well as among the members of the team. More information on debriefing for ECMO simulation will be covered in Chap. 15. The flow of information during *feedback*, however, is one way; discussion is limited. While less interactive, feedback nevertheless can facilitate learning. For example, the acquisition and maintenance of a technical skill does not require formal debriefing; rather, feedback from an instructor experienced in that skill delivered to a trainee who is practicing that skill is typically sufficient to enable acquisition of that skill.

As mentioned previously, many ECMO scenarios are focused on learning objectives that are primarily technical in nature and may be solved relatively quickly by a single trainee. In these instances, the common dictum that debriefings require 2–3 times the length of the scenario does not apply. Upon the conclusion of such a scenario, those trainees who participated in it (as well as those who may have simply been observers) assemble around the circuit for a quick, to-the-point discussion that is predominantly characterized by feedback. Gathering the trainees at the circuit allows for additional hands-on practice, if indicated, before starting the next scenario.

Scenarios that involve multiple technical interventions, focus primarily on behavioral skills, or require trainees to display a combination of cognitive, technical, and behavioral skills usually require more extensive discussion; this is when formal debriefings are utilized. These can be held in an environment different than the one in which the scenario took place to avoid distractions, unless instructors feel that it is important to use the ECMO circuit to illustrate key points or provide trainees with an opportunity to practice procedures on the ECMO circuit during the debriefing. Such debriefings may involve playback of video of the scenario to refresh trainees' recall of events and clearly illustrate particular learning objectives.

The method used by the team at CAPE for debriefing is quite different than the methods that have been described to date in the healthcare literature. Most of these previously published methods use a very similar approach to those listed here [10–19]:

Fig. 2.3 Patient history

Pertinent History: 4-day old 40-week estimated gestational age 3-kg neonate with severe meconium aspiration syndrome, respiratory failure and sepsis, now on hour 88 of V-A ECMO; uneventful course thus far

Vital Sign Range (last 16 hours):
- heart rate = 120-136
- systolic blood pressure = 45-53
- diastolic blood pressure = 29-40
- mean arterial pressure = 37-45
- central venous pressure = 5-9
- respiratory rate = 22-34
- temperature = 36.6-37.2

Current Circuit Settings/Data
pump flow = 300 ml/min
sweep gases = FiO2 = 50%, 0.4 lpm;CO2 = 0 lpm
pre-oxygenator pressure = 81 mm Hg
post-oxygenator pressure = 78 mm Hg
SaO2 = 96%
H2O temperature = 37.4*C
SvO2 = 72%

Current Ventilator Settings:
FiO2 = 21%
PIP = 20 cm H2O
PEEP = 5 cm H2O
IMV = 20
Tinsp = 0.5 seconds

ECMO FLOW SHEET (V-A)

TIME	ECMO H	PUMP FLOW	WATER TEM	SWEEP FLO	SWEEP FIO	PRE-OXY B	POSY-OXY B	SVO2	SAO2	BLOOD GASES						LABS		
										MIXED VEN		ARTERIAL		POST-OXY		PLT	HCT	FIBRINOGEN
										O2	PH	O2	PH	O2	PH			
										CO2	HCO3	CO2	HCO3	CO2	HCO3			
100	72	300	37.4	0.4	0.5	92	82	70	96									
800	73	300	37.4	0.4	0.5	84	71	71	96	39	7.37	62	7.46	430	7.52	211	45	242
900	74	300	37.4	0.4	0.5	86	74	72	95	53	22	41	28	32	36			
1000	75	300	37.4	0.4	0.5	80	68	71	94									
1100	76	300	37.4	0.4	0.5	82	72	70	96									
1200	77	300	37.4	0.4	0.5	83	72	70	95	40	7.36	72	7.45	399	7.51			
1300	78	300	37.3	0.4	0.5	90	79	72	93	50	23	42	29	33	34			
1400	79	300	37.3	0.4	0.5	81	69	70	92									
1500	80	300	37.4	0.4	0.5	78	70	68	96									
1600	81	300	37.4	0.4	0.5	77	68	70	97	41	7.38	68	7.47	437	7.49	178	42	223
1700	82	300	37.4	0.4	0.5	81	74	72	94	52	27	44	31	35	35			
1800	83	300	37.3	0.4	0.5	83	73	73	91									
1900	84	300	37.3	0.4	0.5	86	75	72	93									
2000	85	300	37.3	0.4	0.5	83	81	74	95									
2100	86	300	37.4	0.4	0.5	80	69	71	95									
2200	87	300	37.4	0.4	0.5	81	78	72	96									
2300																		
2400																		
100																		
200																		
300																		
400																		
500																		
600																		

Fig. 2.4 ECMO course to date

1. An individual trained in debriefing who is not a member of the team leads the discussion.
2. The discussion typically includes reaction, description, analysis, and summary phases.
3. Patient outcome is not routinely emphasized, especially if it is felt to potentially produce negative reactions in trainees.

In contrast, the CAPE debriefing model focuses on the actions of the individual, how those actions contribute to the performance of the team, and ultimately how team performance influences the care of the patient. Team members must understand how actions beneficial to the patient can be replicated and how actions that were nonproductive or harmful can be avoided. The type of debriefing conducted at CAPE aligns very closely with debriefing methods used in other industries where the risk to human life is high [20–31]. The guiding strategies and specific tactics that facilitate delivery of this model of debriefing are listed in Figs. 2.5 and 2.6, respectively.

Fig. 2.5 ECMO Sim @ CAPE. Effective Human and System Performance Debriefings: Guiding Strategies

Effective Human and System Performance Debriefings: Guiding Strategies

1) Instructors should set a professional, business-like, matter-of-fact tone for the debriefing and maintain that tone whether the performance of the learners was exemplary or highly flawed.
2) The role of the instructor in a debriefing is to facilitate, rather than dominate, discussion among learners.
3) Debriefings should be focused on:
    a) the actions of the individual learner
    b) how those actions contributed to the performance of the team
    c) how team performance influenced patient outcome
    d) developing strategies for
        i) replicating actions that facilitate successful human and system performance
        ii) avoiding those actions that are ineffective or harmful.

Fig. 2.6 ECMO Sim @ CAPE. Effective Human and System Performance Debriefing: Specific Tactics

Effective Human and System Performance Debriefings: Specific Tactics

Debriefing Basics

1) Preparing learners: Clearly communicate expectations.
2) Initiating debriefings: "What happened in 10 words or less?"
3) Sequencing debriefings: Chronological order is easiest to follow.
4) Pacing debriefings: Maintain awareness of time remaining for debriefing.
5) Terminating debriefings: "Any final questions/comments?"

Facilitating Discussion

6) Asking questions, avoiding statements: Target a question-to-statement ratio of 3:1.
7) Using silence: Wait approximately 10-15 seconds for a response.

Encouraging Self-assessment

8) De-emphasizing instructor viewpoint: Limit use of first-person pronouns.
9) Avoiding qualitative statements: Draw performance assessment from learners.
10) Minimizing personal anecdotes: Emphasize learner (not instructor) experiences.
11) Eschewing hindsight bias: Debrief as if experiencing the event for the first time.

Asking Questions

12) Formulating pertinent questions: Create lists of debriefing points from four sources -
    a. primary: learning objectives upon which the scenario is based
    b. secondary: unexpected events during the scenario
    c. tertiary: concerns raised during the debriefing
    d. quaternary: hypothetical situations
13) Listening for "red flags": Recognize phrases that indicate a need to drill down.
14) Drilling down to root causes: Use a series of four questions -
    a. What happened/what did you notice (at that point in the scenario)?
    b. What circumstances led to that?
    c. What happened to the patient as a result?
    d. What can be done to:
        i. facilitate the recurrence of that positive event?
        ii. prevent that negative event from happening again?

Maintaining Focus

15) Deconstructing defensiveness: Limit use of second person pronouns.
16) Dealing with emotion: It is not necessary to assume all trainees need to ventilate.
17) Deciding when to intervene: Interject only when necessary -
    a. inability to recognize performance gaps
    b. talking over one another
    c. lack of gravitas
    d. inappropriate laughter
    e. harsh criticism

Special Debriefing Circumstances

18) Debriefing with video: Scroll to segments of interest and pause playback for discussion.
19) Debriefing novices and experts: Employ the same strategies regardless of experience.
20) Debriefing real clinical events: Formal process is required.

Debriefings during ECMO Sim© are technical performance debriefings that are used to assess human and system performance; they are not critical incident stress debriefings conducted to provide emotional/psychological support.

Human and System Performance Assessment During ECMO Simulation

When evaluating human performance during any activity, it is important to ensure that the type of skill being evaluated is clearly identified, and the appropriate evaluation tool for that skill is utilized. For example, the evaluation of technical skills used in resolving ECMO emergencies cannot be adequately evaluated with a written or computer-based examination. The ability to carry out a technical skill such as removal of air from the circuit requires that trainees actually stop the pump, manipulate the tubing to move the air to a location where it can be removed, and then use a syringe to pull the air from the circuit. Trainees should never be allowed to simply talk about what they would do in a particular simulated situation but rather must actually demonstrate the requisite skills while working under realistic time pressure.

Conducting simulated ECMO scenarios in the actual clinical environment creates the opportunity to assess not only the human beings working within the environment but also the systems and subsystems that comprise that environment (e.g., electronic health record, phone and paging technologies, etc.). Obviously, if the training program is focused solely on technical skill acquisition and not inclusive of team behavioral skills or elements of the surrounding physical environment, the utility of conducting such a program in the actual clinical environment is limited.

Program Assessment

Each simulation program that is conducted should be formally evaluated by trainees and instructors. This evaluation should be comprehensive, covering all aspects of the program including but not limited to equipment, supplies, the physical space in which the scenarios are conducted, the patient simulators, ECMO circuits, scenarios, debriefings, and instructor teams. Trainees should be asked to focus on elements of the program that did not work well (at least from their perspective) in order that these can be improved the next time that the program is run. Instructors, too, should critique the entire program, paying special attention to any apparent weaknesses. The ability of the debriefings to achieve the learning objectives is a key criterion; it is often worthwhile for instructors to record their own debriefings and critique them, either individually or as a group, once the program is complete.

More will be said about human, system, and program assessment in later chapters in this text.

Looking to the Future (The Future Is Now)

With the development of more effective therapies over time, the use of ECMO is steadily decreasing across patient populations, making the need for better training and assessment tools and methods increasingly acute. No longer is it possible for those charged with caring for patients on ECMO to be able to rapidly acquire sufficient expertise through patient care alone. The need to simulate ECMO with a level of fidelity that allows a healthcare professional to be *certified*, not just trained, in the care of ECMO patients is now a reality. Certification implies that performance during simulation is predictive of performance in real life. Achieving such a goal will require technical innovations such as the development of new materials that accurately simulate human tissues and the use of augmented and virtual reality-based technologies to overcome the limitations in physical patient simulators that will undoubtedly persist; only then can invasive procedures be practiced to proficiency. It will require debriefing strategies focused on objective outcomes similar to those used in other industries where the risk to human life is high. Finally, evidence-based markers of individual and team performance capable of predicting execution of their responsibilities during real-life events must be developed.

Summary

ECMO is the classic low-frequency, high-risk activity that is ideally suited to the use of simulation-based training. Simulated clinical scenarios allow the practice of the cognitive, technical, and behavioral skills that are necessary for the safe and effective care of patients on ECMO. By physically linking a patient simulator with a circuit, highly realistic, complex, and challenging scenarios can be conducted for all members of the ECMO team. Simulation-based training in managing the patient on ECMO facilitates both the acquisition and maintenance of necessary skills and will become increasingly important as the frequency ECMO diminishes in response to newer and less invasive therapies.

References

1. Bartlett RH, Gazzaniga AB, Jeffries MR, Huxtable RF, Haidue NJ, Fong SW. Extracorporeal membrane oxygenation (ECMO) cardiopulmonary support in infancy. Trans Am Soc Artif Intern Organs. 1976;22:80–93.
2. Bartlett RH, Gazzaniga AB, Fong SW, Jeffries MR, Roohk HV, Haidue NJ. Extracorporeal membrane oxygenator support for car-

diopulmonary failure. Experience in 28 cases. J Thorac Cardiovasc Surg. 1977;73(3):375–86.
3. Bartlett RH, Gazzinga AB, Huxtable RF, Schippers HC, O'Connor MJ, Jefferies MR. Extracorporeal circulation (ECMO) in neonatal respiratory failure. J Thorac Cardiovasc Surg. 1977;74(6):826–33.
4. Halamek LP. Teaching versus learning and the role of simulation-based training in pediatrics. J Pediatr. 2007;151(4):329–30.
5. Barrington KJ, Finer N, Pennaforte T, Altit G. Nitric oxide for respiratory failure in infants born at or near term. Cochrane Database Syst Rev. 2017;1:CD000399. https://doi.org/10.1002/14651858.CD000399.
6. Barrington KJ, Finer N, Pennaforte T. Inhaled nitric oxide for respiratory failure in preterm infants. Cochrane Database Syst Rev. 2017;1:CD000509. https://doi.org/10.1002/14651858.CD000509.
7. Froese AB, Kinsella JP. High-frequency oscillatory ventilation: lessons from the neonatal/pediatric experience. Crit Care Med. 2005;33(3 Suppl):S115–21.
8. Anderson JM, Murphy AA, Boyle BB, Yaeger KA, Halamek L. Simulating extracorporeal membrane oxygenation (ECMO) emergencies to improve human performance, Part I: methodologic and technologic innovations. Simul Healthc. 2006;1:220–7.
9. Anderson JM, Murphy AA, Boyle BB, Yaeger KA, Halamek L. Simulating extracorporeal membrane oxygenation (ECMO) emergencies, Part II: qualitative and quantitative assessment and validation. Simul Healthc. 2006;1:228–32.
10. Jaye P, Thomas L, Reedy G. 'The Diamond': a structure for simulation debrief. Clin Teach. 2015;12(3):171–5.
11. Garden AL, Le Fevre DM, Waddington HL, Weller JM. Debriefing after simulation-based non-technical skill training in healthcare: a systematic review of effective practice. Anaesth Intensive Care. 2015;43(3):300–8.
12. Kolbe M, Weiss M, Grote G, et al. TeamGAINS: a tool for structured debriefings for simulation-based team trainings. BMJ Qual Saf. 2013;22(7):541–53.
13. Cheng A, Palaganas J, Eppich W, Rudolph J, Robinson T, Grant V. Co-debriefing for simulation-based education: a primer for facilitators. Simul Healthc. 2015;10(2):69–75.
14. Dreifuerst KT. The essentials of debriefing in simulation learning: a concept analysis. Nurs Educ Perspect. 2009;30(2):109–14.
15. Dreifuerst KT. Using debriefing for meaningful learning to foster development of clinical reasoning in simulation. J Nurs Educ. 2012;51(6):326–33.
16. Zigmont JJ, Kappus LJ, Sudikoff SN. The 3D model of debriefing: defusing, discovering, and deepening. Semin Perinatol. 2011;35(2):52–8.
17. Eppich W, Cheng A. Promoting Excellence and Reflective Learning in Simulation (PEARLS): development and rationale for a blended approach to health care simulation debriefing. Simul Healthc. 2015;10(2):106–15.
18. Gardner R. Introduction to debriefing. Semin Perinatol. 2013;37(3):166–74.
19. Rudolph JW, Simon R, Raemer DB, Eppich WJ. Debriefing as formative assessment: closing performance gaps in medical education. Acad Emerg Med. 2008;15(11):1010–6.
20. Salas E, Klein C, King H, et al. Debriefing medical teams: 12 evidence-based best practices and tips. Jt Comm J Qual Patient Saf. 2008;34(9):518–27.
21. Dismukes RK, Gaba DM, Howard SK. So many roads: facilitated debriefing in healthcare. Simul Healthc. 2006;1(1):23–5.
22. Henricksen JW, Altenburg C, Reeder RW. Operationalizing healthcare simulation psychological safety: a descriptive analysis of an intervention. Simul Healthc. 2017;12(5):289–97.
23. Bartone PT, Adler AB. Event-oriented debriefing following military operations: what every leader should know. U.S. Army Medical Research Unit – Europe, Unit 29218, APO AE 091021995:1–9.
24. Lauber JK, Foushee HC. Guidelines for line-oriented flight training. NASA Conference Publication 2184. 1981;I:1–41.
25. McDonnell LK. Facilitation techniques as predictors of crew participation in LOFT debriefings. NASA Contractor Report 196701. 1996:1–36.
26. McDonnell LK, Jobe KK, Dismukes RK. Facilitating LOS debriefings. NASA Technical Memorandum 112192. 1997:1–37.
27. Dismukes RK, Jobe KK, McDonnell LK. LOFT debriefings: an analysis of instructor techniques and crew participation. NASA Technical Memorandum 112192. 1997:1–85.
28. Hysong SJ, Galarza L, Holland AW. A review of training methods and instructional techniques: implications for behavioral skills training in U.S. astronauts. NASA Technical Publications 2007-213726. 2007.
29. Sawyer TL, Deering S. Adaptation of the US Army's after-action review for simulation debriefing in healthcare. Simul Healthc. 2013;8(6):388–97.
30. McGreevy JM, Otten TD. Briefing and debriefing in the operating room using fighter pilot crew resource management. J Am Coll Surg. 2007;205(1):169–76.
31. Tompkins M. Facilitating a critical incident stress debriefing. In: Dismukes RK, Smith GM, editors. Facilitation and debriefing in aviation training and operations. Burlington: Ashgate Publishing Company; 2000. p. 93–105.

Part II

Educational Theory Behind ECMO Simulation

The Critical Role of Simulation in ECMO Education

3

Lindsay C. Johnston, Dianne Lee, and Christie J. Bruno

Abbreviations

ALT	Adult learning theory
ECMO	Extracorporeal membrane oxygenation
ELSO	Extracorporeal life support organization

Learning Objectives

1. Describe the utility of ECMO simulation, specifically with regards to adult learning theory and varying learning styles.
2. Discuss the role of an institutional ECMO simulation program as part of an overarching ECMO educational curriculum.
3. Describe the potential role for simulation in the evaluation of ECMO providers, for both formative and summative assessment.

Introduction

Extracorporeal membrane oxygenation (ECMO) is a very specialized treatment modality reserved for the most critically ill patients, and providers need to possess specific knowledge, as well as technical and interpersonal skills, to reduce potential morbidity and mortality. To acquire the requisite knowledge and skills, robust educational curricula are necessary for initial and ongoing ECMO provider training. Originating in high-risk industries such as the military, aviation, and nuclear power [1], simulation has rapidly gained popularity in medical education. ECMO simulation has quickly gained acceptance as a mainstay in the training of ECMO providers [2], but to date, there continues to be significant variability in the simulation training offered globally. There is a growing desire to standardize this aspect of ECMO education and potential utilization for competency assessment, as a way to help assure that patients receive the highest quality care.

This chapter will review the evolution of simulation in healthcare education, including its underpinnings in adult learning theory, as well as applicability to individuals with different learning preferences. Next, ECMO simulation will be discussed specifically, including the role of simulation in an ECMO educational curriculum. Finally, the current ELSO guidelines for simulation training of ECMO providers will be reviewed. The potential role of simulation for the evaluation of ECMO providers, both for formative and summative assessment, will be described.

Simulation in Medical Education

Adult Learning Theory

Given that medical education (including simulation-based methodologies) is intended for adult learners, it is imperative that educators have a thorough understanding of how to best develop educational sessions and curricula targeted toward this population. Adult learning theory (ALT) consists of a number of individual theories that describe how adults learn optimally in different environments and situations. Although none of the learning theories is individually comprehensive, astute educators can apply elements of each relevant theory in order to optimize the learning environment (Table 3.1).

L. C. Johnston (✉) · D. Lee · C. J. Bruno
Department of Pediatrics, Yale University School of Medicine, New Haven, CT, USA
e-mail: Lindsay.Johnston@Yale.Edu

L. C. Johnston, L. Su (eds.), *Comprehensive Healthcare Simulation: ECMO Simulation*, Comprehensive Healthcare Simulation,
https://doi.org/10.1007/978-3-030-53844-6_3

Table 3.1 Adult learning theories adress various aspects of the learning process. Several theories most relevant to simulation-based education are included [3]

Learning theory	Description	Application to adult learning
Behaviorism	Behavior results from a particular stimulus in the environment Behavior is likely to continue if rewarded or reinforced, and likely to disappear if not reinforced or rewarded Learning is a change in observable behavior, not internal mental processes or emotions	Role of feedback, reinforcement, learning objectives, and behavior modification is important Learning progresses from basic to higher level skills when learners are required to demonstrate competency at certain levels before moving on
Humanism	Learning is about growth and development of the person in a self-directed manner Individuals are free to make choices and determine their own behavior	Adults may thrive when they are able to participate actively and make decisions about their learning
Social cognitive	Learning occurs in a social community Behavior is shaped by modeling and observing others in a social environment/context	Adults learners are shaped by observing and modeling others their environment Examples include mentorship or on-the-job training
Constructivism	Knowledge is constructed from experience that is situation specific, and relevant	Learning is the creation and exchange of relevant and viable meanings from relevant experiences and social contexts
Cognitivism	Learning is a mental process that incorporates patterns, feelings, and prior knowledge to create new information This information is stored and able to be retrieved from memory	Adult learners have generally achieved abstract hypothetical reasoning in cognitive development They are able to process, store, and retrieve information into and from memory

Although this chapter is not intended to serve as an all-encompassing review of ALT, some of the most relevant theories that can be applied to ECMO education will be described in further detail.

Andragogy

Malcolm S. Knowles defined the concept of *andragogy*, the science of teaching adults, and contrasted this with *pedagogy*, the science of teaching children [4]. In pedagogy, learning is instructor-centric and assumes that the children have little relevant previous knowledge. In contrast, andragogy supports the ability of adults to learn in a self-directed and learner-centric manner by incorporating previous knowledge and experience into the learning experience. Andragogy makes six assumptions of adult learners that are grounded by humanistic principles, which are found in Box 3.1.

Box 3.1 Andragogy: Assumptions About Adult Learners [4]

- Self-concept: learners are self-directed and independently make choices about their learning.
- Personal experience: learners accumulate a reservoir of experiences to reference and use as a resource for learning.
- Readiness to learn: learners see value in their education and are ready to learn developmental tasks and social roles of adult life.
- Problem-centered: learners seek practical, problem-centered applications to help address challenges in their lives.
- Motivation: internal motivators, such as quality of life, job satisfaction, and self-esteem, are more potent drivers of learning than external motivations, such as money or promotion.
- Relevance: learners need to understand the reason for learning new knowledge and how they will apply it in the context of real-life situations.

Social Learning Theories

The social learning theories acknowledge that social factors influence how learning occurs [5]. Albert Bandura and Lev Vygotsky were key developers of social learning theory, which emphasizes that people learn knowledge, rules, skills, strategies, beliefs, and attitudes from each other through observation, imitation, or modeling. Additionally, behavior is shaped by the environment and the social context in which it occurs through a set of shared concepts and practices, also known as a *learning community*.

Bandura described four key processes that must occur for effective learning to take place [6, 7]:

- (1) Attention (learning requires focus and attention on the behavior being modeled); (2) Retention (the learner stores the learned observation into memory for recall in similar situations); (3) Reproduction (the learner replicates the behavior); and (4) Motivation (the learner demonstrates a willingness to perform the behavior).

In ECMO education, social learning theories are relevant specifically to the development of effective team behaviors, including leadership, communication, and conflict resolution. For example, a simulation educator may be faced with a large group of learners. They may choose to divide the learners into two groups, Group 1 watching the simulation remotely as observers, while Group 2 actively takes part in the simulation. The educator can assign a specific area of the simulation for each observer to watch (Attention), in addition to providing a checklist for each observer to record their observations (Retention). After the scenario, the two groups switch places, and the initial observation group now performs the simulation scenario (Reproduction). The educator may note in the debriefing how Group 1 (the original observation group) was subsequently able to learn from their observations to avoid some errors made by Group 2 (the performing group) while replicating positive actions (Motivation).

Constructivism

Constructivists define learning as actively creating relevant meaning from experiences, rather than learning through observation [8]. Additionally, learning occurs in context and is situation specific, also known as situated cognition.

Cognitivism

According to cognitivism theory, the human mind is metaphorically like a computer, where information is inputted in from the environment, processed, and stored into memory, and output is demonstrated by learned behavior [8]. David Ausubel (1967) described meaningful learning as connecting new concepts to existing knowledge already present in a person's cognitive structure [9]. Meaningful learning is in contrast to rote learning, which is quickly forgotten, as it does not relate to a person's existing cognitive structure. He described the use of *advance organizers*, which are relevant introductory materials, in order to bridge the gap between existing knowledge and new knowledge that the learner needs to acquire [3, 9]. Additionally, Bloom's taxonomy of cognitive outcomes, which is frequently used in curriculum development, classifies levels of learning into a hierarchy [10]. Learning begins with knowledge and remembering facts or concepts. The next stage of learning is comprehension, followed by application, analysis, evaluation, and creation, which is the highest level of cognitive outcome.

Transformative

Jack Mezirow (1991) first described the transformative learning process as learning that "involves an enhanced level of awareness of the context of one's beliefs and feelings, a critique of their assumptions and particular premises, an assessment of alternative perspectives, a decision to negate an old perspective in favor of a new one or to make a synthesis of old and new, an ability to take action based upon the new perspective, and a desire to fit the new perspective into the broader context of one's life" [11, 12].

Hence, the transformational learning theory highlights the importance of thinking, reflecting, questioning, and examining one's assumptions and beliefs, as this evaluative process can transform into significant meaningful changes in an individual's perceptions about themselves and their environment. Reflection allows for activation of a learner's prior experiences to elicit knowledge gaps, cognitive errors, and variations in thought processes to either create new knowledge or correct flaws in existing mental models. Through this process, learners can solidify new knowledge in a meaningful and permanent manner for use in future decision-making.

Experiential

Philosopher and educator John Dewey described learning as a lifelong process of applying and adapting new situations to previous experiences in an experiential manner [13]. Additionally, theorist David Kolb focused on the role of personal experience in the learning process. Kolb's cycle of experiential learning states that learning occurs through a "cycle of experience," where the learner actively tests and reflects on his or her experiences in the process of creating new knowledge [14]. Kolb's learning cycle consists of four steps: (1) a concrete experience, (2) observation and reflection, (3) formation of abstract concepts and generalizations, and (4) active experimentation of these abstract conceptualizations in new situations that govern future behavior and decision-making. This cycle can be entered at any point, and learners may continue through the cycle many times as they work to establish an understanding of a concept. The concrete experience can be a clinical encounter, or one created by the educator to provide an opportunity for learning purposes, such as a simulation scenario. It is only through intensive reflection and analysis that learners are fully able to apply personal experience and evaluate their own existing understanding in order to adapt, create, and use novel information for future behavior and decision-making.

Procedural Skills Training

In addition to learning cognitive knowledge, learning theorists provide insight on how to optimize procedural skills training, which is frequently required in ECMO education. Grounded in behavioralist theories, procedural skills training begins with learning basic skills and must demonstrate competency before progressing to higher-level skills. As noted previously, learned behaviors are likely to continue if reinforced and likely to disappear in the absence of reinforcing stimuli. Research on skill acquisition has found that learners uniformly demonstrate improved performance when they are given tasks with well-defined learning objectives, motivated to improve, provided with immediate formative feedback, and have ample opportunities to repeat the process and make gradual refinements in their performance [15].

According to the work of Anders Ericsson, a learner can achieve "expertise" through *deliberate practice*, "a regimen of effortful activities designed to optimize improvement" which involves "training focused on improving particular tasks" [16]. Deliberate practice requires a learner's full concentration. Ericsson described performing everyday tasks to a satisfactory level that will eventually become automated and quicker, due to bypassing one's control of intentional cognitive adjustments. Examples of this include tasks such as tying shoelaces or driving a car. Once automaticity (where intentional cognitive adjustments are bypassed) and effortless execution of a psychomotor skill occur, additional experience will not refine or improve the skill. Therefore, accumulated experience will not relate to higher level expert performance. Expert performers, however, continue to counteract automaticity by remaining in the cognitive phase and intentionally and frequently refining behaviors and knowledge, setting new goals and higher performance standards in order to exceed their current level of performance. By remaining in the cognitive phase, these expert performers avoid *arrested development,* which occurs when regular engagement of deliberate practice is terminated and becomes automated.

Simulation in medical education incorporates and utilizes various portions of all of the learning theories discussed. Application of the ALT for simulation and medical education will be discussed in the next section.

Simulation in Medical Education

Simulation is a type of training which is "used to replace or amplify real experiences with guided experiences that evoke or replicate substantial aspects of the real world in a fully interactive manner" for learning purposes [17]. Simulation is frequently applied in high-risk industries such as aviation [18, 19], military [20], mining [21], and nuclear power [22] to significantly improve in safety outcomes. The release of the report *To Err is Human* by the Institute of Medicine in 2000 highlighted the vast number of preventable medical errors, resulting in a movement to improve national standards of healthcare safety and quality [23]. Simulation was recommended as an important learning tool to improve patient safety in healthcare. Simulation training in medicine began with low technology task trainers for procedural skills training. Subsequent advances in technology led to high-technology patient simulators ranging from newborn to adult manikins with realistic airway anatomy and chest movements, auscultatable breath and heart sounds, palpable pulses, and realistic vocalizations and movements in order to replicate real patients for training purposes [24]. These simulators revolutionized medical education by allowing for the creation of a realistic simulation environment which could be standardized and repeated for all learners.

Effective medical simulation-based training incorporates relevant ALT principles to promote knowledge acquisition, as well as the development and retention of clinical skills (cognitive, technical, and behavioral) [25–34]. Simulation effectively allows learners to apply knowledge and practice critical decision-making under stress, concepts of crisis resource management, effective communication, and team behaviors in an environment of psychological safety [35]. Simulation technology also creates numerous opportunities to incorporate technical and procedural skills into a curriculum. Additionally, a unique benefit of simulation is the ability to recreate rare or high stakes clinical scenarios to target specific learning objectives. Learners are able to practice simulation scenarios repeatedly for cognitive or procedural skills acquisition or maintenance without the risk of harm to patients. Simulation also provides learners with the opportunity for intra- and interprofessional collaboration to build communication and teamwork skills. Simulation in medical education also allows learners to transfer acquired knowledge and skills into real clinical practice, which is classified as the highest level of training program outcome by the Kirkpatrick hierarchy [36]. The repetition of clinical scenarios provides learners with the opportunity for the refinement of cognitive and procedural skills over time to continue advancing professional development.

Debriefing the simulation experience is one of the most important aspects of the entire simulation experience for learning to occur. The simulation experience can be discussed in a bidirectional and reflective nature between participants and simulation instructor(s), and timely feedback can be provided. During debriefing, topics frequently discussed include performance strengths of participants, identification of knowledge gaps and areas for improvement, and correction of flawed mental models so learners can store newly created or corrected knowledge into their memory for future recall and application. Specific debriefing models are discussed further in Chap. 15.

Overall, simulation can be viewed as an active application of Kolb's experiential learning cycle, discussed previously in this chapter. The simulation session is the concrete experience. Through debriefing (reflective observation), the learner creates a new understanding of the situation experienced in the simulation (abstract conceptualization), and the learner can then apply and test the new knowledge in the clinical setting or during future simulation-based sessions (active experimentation).

In summary, it is critical that medical educators apply relevant ALT concepts to maximize the relevance and effectiveness of their instruction for adult learners in medical education. Simulation-based education incorporates various ALT and is a powerful tool for learners seeking to improve clinical decision-making and knowledge, procedural and technical skills, team behaviors, leadership skills, and communication skills.

Simulation as Part of an Overarching ECMO Educational Curriculum

Creation of Goals and Objectives Based on Institutional Needs

Essential to the creation of a simulation-based ECMO educational curriculum is a clear delineation of goals and objectives. Stated goals should broadly detail what a learner should be able to successfully complete at the end of an educational session. Learning objectives should detail more specific points such as the intended learners, what the learners are expected to accomplish (as well as how well they should perform), the expected time frame, and how the end result will be assessed. Performing a needs assessment prior to the creation of goals and objectives is crucial in structuring the goals and objectives of a given educational session and can assist in selection of the optimal educational method to achieve these goals [37]. The topic of curriculum development is discussed more thoroughly in the dedicated chapter in this text.

Incorporating simulation as part of an ECMO educational curriculum can be essential in allowing learners to cultivate and optimize the technical and behavioral skills necessary to function effectively as a leader and/or member of an ECMO team. In planning an ECMO educational curriculum, it is important to understand the specific needs of the particular institution which will inform the training and allow educators to understand which learning needs are best met by simulation as opposed to other educational offerings, such as readings or didactics. For example, a program's goal may be to start an ECMO program, expand an existing program to incorporate ECPR, improve understanding of a new type of equipment, or optimize interprofessional teamwork. After conducting a needs assessment, simulation educators will better understand how to meet the unique needs of the institution and can develop specific simulation scenarios to target particular objectives. Additionally, in order to share best practices, it may be helpful for programs to learn from others who have gone through similar challenges previously. When building a new ECMO program (or ECMO simulation program), interviewing individuals or polling focus groups from experienced institutions may help to identify key factors for success as well as potential pitfalls to be avoided [38]. As an example, the creation of a novel ECMO simulation curriculum was critical in the development of a successful ECMO transport program in the country of Poland, as it allowed for creation of procedural processes, elimination of early errors, and optimization in identifying and transporting patients for ECMO therapy [39, 40]. These materials may be subsequently shared and adapted for use by other educators.

Use of Simulation for Low-Frequency, High-Risk Events and Review of Rare Cases

Given that ECMO management is applied for the most critically unstable patients, it is fraught with risk of patient morbidity or mortality. ECMO complications, while potentially severe, are relatively low frequency, and individual providers may not have the opportunity to clinically manage many potential emergencies. Therefore, simulation may be utilized for review of difficult clinical ECMO cases (potentially with adverse patient outcomes), allowing for identification of potential latent safety threats, knowledge gaps, suboptimal technical skills, or challenges in teamwork and communication. In creating a simulation for an adverse ECMO event, such as an accidental decannulation, pump failure, or air entrainment, it is first necessary to review the circumstances of the actual clinical event to understand contributing factors. Subsequently, a similar simulation scenario could be created and implemented for the ECMO team members with the goal of enhancing knowledge among the entire team and improving future patient care.

Use of Simulation for Implementation of Programmatic Changes

ECMO simulation scenarios can be essential in educating ECMO teams on programmatic changes. These could include changes in equipment [such as type of pump (roller-head versus centrifugal) or catheter utilized], management strategies, workflow, communication frameworks, or guidelines/protocols. In these instances, having an opportunity to practice the technical and behavioral skills required for utilizing novel equipment or strategies, to interact with other members of the interprofessional team, or to solidify new knowledge or a novel workflow can help to smooth the learning curve and optimize ECMO clinical care.

Creation of Goals and Objectives Based on Learner Population

In developing ECMO simulation scenarios, it is important to consider the level of experience of the participants, as learning objectives may differ significantly for novice versus experienced ECMO providers. Novice providers may focus on aspects such as patient selection criteria, circuit component review, technical sequence of the cannulation process, and routine management of a patient on ECMO [38]. For experienced ECMO providers, learning objectives may include topics related to ECMO complications and challenges, such as pump failure, oxygenator failure, or air embolism [41]. Novice providers typically focus on basic workflow and technical/behavioral skills, while more experienced provider can focus on advanced medical concepts, technical/behavioral skills, as well as application of crisis resource management strategies [42]. This ability to titrate the level of difficulty of the case based upon a learner's or teams' level of experience is known as adjusting the "signal to noise ratio" [43]. This involves a concept known as "cognitive load" [44], which states that an individual only has a finite amount of working capacity to think and solve problems. It takes an increased amount of capacity to deal with new or unfamiliar circumstances, so novice learners often do best with simple cases without added complexities. For experienced providers, who have mastered basic concepts, less working capacity is required to address medical management. These individuals may benefit from the difficulty of the scenario being increased, for example, through the inclusion of additional challenges, such as the presence of a distraught family member, conflict with another team member, or additional medical complexities. Simulation educators can indicate potential adaptations to the scenario for learners of varying experience levels in the written template, and these can be utilized to optimize training for specific individuals or groups. More information can be found on this topic in Chap. 4.

Additionally, having a successful ECMO cannulation and run requires the cooperation of numerous members of the multidisciplinary and interprofessional team. Therefore, ECMO simulations that incorporate all members of the actual ECMO team are able to most closely simulate real clinical ECMO experiences. Goals and objectives written for an interprofessional team will vary significantly from those intended for use in a uniprofessional group. Additional information on interprofessional teamwork and communication is found in Chap. 10.

Matching Goals to Instructional Methods

Even though simulation is a powerful educational tool, it is not optimally suited to address all educational objectives and, as such, is only part of an ECMO program's educational arsenal. It is important to match goals and objectives with appropriate educational methods. There are three types of objectives: knowledge (cognitive, what the learner should know), skills (psychomotor, what the learner should do/ how they should behave), and attitudinal (affective, what the learner should value) [37]. Cognitive objectives may be best approached using methods such as assigned readings, didactic lectures, or programmed learning. For example, reading on a topic or attending a lecture may allow learners to gain basic understanding of ECMO physiology. Interactive games or computer modules could allow for review of ECMO physiology or the structure of the ECMO circuit. Attitudinal objectives can be addressed using role modeling, facilitated reflection, or group discussion about experiences. Finally, technical or behavioral objectives are optimally approached using more active learning strategies such as simulation, role-play, or incorporation of standardized patients [37]. Simulation is optimally effective when used to target objectives such as critical decision-making, especially during times of stress, interprofessional interactions/communication, and technical skills. By effectively organizing the ECMO educational curriculum, with other educational methods utilized prior to participation in ECMO simulation, participants are able to apply learned knowledge to the simulated scenarios. More information on curriculum development for ECMO simulation can be located in Chap. 6.

How to Incorporate Procedural/Technical Skills training into an ECMO Program

Effective management of ECMO patients requires providers to develop competency in a number of procedural or technical skills. Numerous authors have described implementation of a step-wise procedural training paradigm for varying learner groups, such as providers learning neonatal resuscitation [45] or pediatric advanced life support [46], as well as individuals working in ECMO teams [47]. In these models, baseline knowledge should ideally be attained prior to opportunities for hands-on practice of skills.

These examples follow an evidence-based educational paradigm for procedural skills acquisition and maintenance, learn-see-practice-prove-do-maintain (LSPPDM), which has been developed to enhance psychomotor training [48]. This model is applicable to ECMO education and could be applied in an ECMO simulation program. In the "learn" phase, participants gain requisite knowledge through reading, didactics, or modules. They may be assessed through computer modules or other examination techniques. They will next "see" an expert perform the procedural skill and are given the opportunity to "practice" these skills in a simulated environment. The learner is then required to "prove" that they can successfully perform the procedure by achieving a passing score on an observational assessment tool. After this assessment, they will typically be permitted to perform ("do") the procedure clinically (with appropriate supervision in place). Maintenance or refresher training is also employed as a critical part of skill maintenance ("maintain").

There are many possibilities for incorporating LSPPDM into procedural training for ECMO education. Providers may need to perform thoracentesis or pericardiocentesis on an ECMO patient with a tension pneumothorax or pericardial effusion, in order to allow for adequate venous drainage and circuit flow. Understanding the critical procedural steps and demonstrating the ability to complete them in a simulated environment are desirable before a provider performs them on a critically ill, heparinized ECMO patient, as optimal skill and precision will likely result in improved patient outcomes. Additionally, other procedures that are important to practice given their high stakes and potentially dangerous nature include changing out the ECMO circuit (or a circuit component), removing air from the circuit, and coming off of bypass during an emergency situation.

One of the challenges with skills training in medical simulation is overreliance on suspension of disbelief and lack of authenticity in simulating real-life practice. This is a particular problem for ECMO simulation, and numerous providers have attempted to develop new systems to more effectively mimic real-life clinical experience. This is discussed in greater detail in Chap. 7. As an example, an international group is working on a prototype ECMO simulator that improves realism substantially, allowing for alterations in pressure parameters, hemorrhage, line chatter, air bubble noise, and changes in "blood" color [49]. With the emergence of more advanced ECMO simulators, the effectiveness of ECMO simulation for skills training will continue to be enhanced.

Benefits of Simulation on Cognition

Critical Thinking Under Stress

One of the major benefits of inclusion of simulation in an ECMO educational curriculum is providing individuals the opportunity to practice making critical decisions under stress. Emergencies on ECMO, including patient complications, such as pericardial tamponade, tension pneumothorax, or massive hemorrhage, as well as circuit complications, such as arterial air embolus, accidental decannulation, or power failure, occur rarely [50]. However, these situations have high rates of morbidity and mortality, so prompt recognition and correct interventions are essential. Novice ECMO providers may learn of the various emergencies during self-study or didactic lecture and may be able to recognize the issue on a cognitive assessment test. However, it requires a very different skillset to gather information from a patient's vital signs and physical exam, circuit pressures and monitoring, and laboratory/diagnostic studies, arrive at the proper conclusion, and implement the appropriate intervention while also dealing with stress associated with the situation.

Indeed, reinforcing the specific *patterns* of information that indicate an emergency situation is critical. Simulation provides an opportunity to standardize exposure among all providers, which would never be possible if educators needed to rely on clinical encounters alone. It is important to note that creating scenarios anew presents the significant challenge of ensuring that the data presented to the participants is realistic and that the simulated patient responds appropriately to the interventions provided. Educators may consider writing scenarios based upon a specific clinical case that presented challenges to the managing team. The available vital signs, circuit pressures, and labs/diagnostic studies from clinical cases are all available after de-identification, and educators can be confident that these values have a high degree of realism and fidelity. Another option is to utilize the concept of "mirror patients" [51]. In this model, educators base a scenario on an existing patient in the unit and simulate that patient's development of a clinical complication. In this case, the participating providers will be familiar with the history of the mirror patient and will be able to use the concept of transfer to consider how they would respond to an emergency situation in this individual.

Benefits of ECMO Simulation on IPE Teamwork

Interprofessional

ECMO care is delivered by an interprofessional team of providers [52], rather than an individual person. Some of the specialists involved in the care of patients on ECMO include physicians and surgeons (both faculty and trainees), practitioners (such as physician assistants and advanced practice nurses), nurses, respiratory therapists, and specialists monitoring the ECMO circuit (perfusionists or individuals with other specialized training). Depending on the particular objectives of a case, additional ancillary staff, such as individuals working in the blood bank or pharmacy, may benefit from participation.

The ECMO team can actually be conceptualized as a team of teams, consisting of the team caring for the patient and the team monitoring the circuit. During an emergency situation, high-level skills in communication, teamwork, and leadership are required to coordinate knowledge sharing among the group and enable timely delivery of the medical interventions [53]. Educators can provide specific opportunities to practice communication and team behaviors through the inclusion of "standardized participants" or "confederates" [54] to introduce challenges. Specific team challenges might include a medical error (such as an erroneous medication dose through failure to utilize closed-loop communication), an aggressive team member, or having a conversation about withdrawal of support with a family member. ECMO simulation training has been utilized for team members taking on a supervisory role in ECMO clinical practice. By focusing on the importance of interprofessional practice, individual skills, communication, and hands off were all noted to improve [55]. Additionally, numerous authors have published on the benefits of using simulation training for the interprofessional team, relating to team confidence and morale, knowledge base, and quality of care provided [2, 56–60].

Current ELSO guidelines for Simulation Training

The extracorporeal life support organization (ELSO) is the leading international organization that provides recommendations on standards for ECMO training and experience [61, 62], which are discussed in depth in Chap. 12. ELSO provides guidance on the requisite topics that should be covered in an ECMO provider course. New ECMO specialists typically first participate in didactic lectures covering an array of topics. Essential technical skills are rehearsed and perfected through "water drills," which utilize a water-filled circuit. Animal laboratories had previously been utilized to allow novice providers to experience ECMO physiology in a living organism. However, this is being phased out in favor of high-technology simulation-based training [63].

Currently, individual centers are permitted significant discretion in developing their own educational curricula based upon their local environment and perceived needs, which are likely impacted by the center's clinical volume, program maturity, and experience of team members [64, 65]. Continuing education is required and needs to be documented thoroughly. ECMO specialists are required to successfully complete written examinations annually and water drills biannually. However, there is no current regulation of the timing or frequency of educational sessions, including use of simulation-based training. Additionally, there is not a formal system for certification of ECMO providers. Hence, this flexibility contributes significantly to lack of standardization across ECMO centers and may lead to variability in the quality of care provided.

As noted above, simulation has quickly gained popularity for the training of medical teams and providers. However, there is limited data available regarding the use of ECMO simulation across the global community of ECMO providers. Weems et al. surveyed ELSO centers in the United States in 2012 to assess the role of simulation in ECMO education [63]. At this time, approximately half of centers had an ECMO simulation program in place, and approximately 50% of the remainder were in the process of developing a program. There is no current data to describe the role of ECMO simulation outside North America.

Potential Role for Simulation in Assessment of ECMO Providers

In addition to value in knowledge acquisition and retention, critical decision-making, and optimization of communication and team behaviors, simulation provides an opportunity to assess providers and/or teams in a standardized manner. Currently, the responsibility for credentialing of ECMO providers lies with the individual institution, with centers requiring varying training, clinical exposure, and successful completion of written or performance-based assessments. While there are challenges that exist in using simulation to assess ECMO care, there are certainly positive aspects to this type of evaluation. Most importantly, there is a desire to ensure that all ECMO providers are able to meet minimum performance standards and decrease variability in care delivered across ECMO centers.

Formative feedback can be provided to improve performance after participation in simulation-based scenarios through several methods. First, trained facilitators lead debriefings using any of a number of specific frameworks

[66–69]. For adult learners, who are able to relate new concepts to previous learning, skilled facilitators can assist in filling of knowledge gaps, improvement in technical performance, and optimization of teamwork/communication skills. Discussion about performance can be enhanced through review of video clips of the team's performance during the scenario. This permits objective assessment of various aspects of the case and can provide a new perspective to enhance learning. Scenario authors can also outline particular interventions that are deemed necessary for "successful" management of the case. These often include critical actions checklists, which outline specific interventions that should be implemented in a proper sequence. Some of these interventions may lend themselves to inclusion of a time-based goal, with *successful* completion only occurring within a limited time frame.

Similar methods may be utilized for summative, or high-stakes, assessment. Several authors have described the local implementation of ECMO simulation in the credentialing process [70–73]. There is significant interest among some members of the global community to have ELSO develop a method for summative evaluation and assessment of ECMO providers to permit formal credentialing. Some of the challenges that exist in the development of these standards include (1) availability of trained simulation educators to conduct assessments; (2) standardized performance assessment tools that have been rigorously evaluated for sources of validity; (3) similar expectations for performance across the global ECMO community; (4) varying modes of ECMO support available; (5) varying types of ECMO equipment utilized across centers; (6) varying patient population, ranging from neonatal to pediatric to adult; (7) logistical challenges, including scheduling for assessments, determining location of assessments (local, regional, or national options), and addressing costs associated with assessment; and (8) consequences to centers and providers who are not able to successfully complete the assessment. Despite these challenges, however, there remains enthusiasm about this project, and it appears likely that some sort of ECMO provider credentialing will be developed in the future. Further information on the use of simulation for the certification/credentialing of ECMO providers can be found in Chap. 16.

Conclusion

In summary, there is a natural application of simulation for the training of ECMO providers based upon key concepts in ALT, including the foundational work by Knowles and Kolb. Just as simulation has been applied in many other high-risk fields, its use in medical training has resulted in significant benefits for patients. ECMO simulation gives providers an optimal environment to focus on critical decision-making under pressure, practice of procedural/technical skills, and optimization of communication strategies across the interprofessional team. However, simulation is just one part of an ECMO educational curriculum, and educators will need to employ other instructional methods to ensure that strategies are employed that most appropriately align with the goals and objectives. Assessment of ECMO providers remains a topic of significant interest, and it is highly likely that a formal system for credentialing ECMO providers will be developed.

References

1. Gaba DM, DeAnda A. A comprehensive anesthesia simulation environment: re-creating the operating room for research and training. Anesthesiology. 1988;69(3):387–94.
2. Anderson JM, Boyle KB, Muprhy AA, Yaeger KA, Leflore J, Halamek LP. Simulating extracorporeal membrane oxygenation emergencies to improve human performance: part I: methodologic and technologic innovations. Simul Healthc. 2006;1:220–7.
3. Merriam SB, Bierema LL. Adult learning, linking theory and practice. San Francisco: Wiley; 2013.
4. Knowles MS. The modern practice of adult education: from pedagogy to andragogy. 2nd ed. New York: Cambridge Books; 1980.
5. Durning SJ, Artino AR. Situativity theory: a perspective on how participants and the environment can interact: AMEE guide no. 52. Med Teach. 2011;33:188–99.
6. Bandura A. Social learning theory. Englewood Cliffs: Prentice-Hall; 1977.
7. Bandura A. Social foundations of thought and action: a social cognitive theory. Englewood Cliffs: Prentice-Hall; 1986.
8. Merriam SB, Caffarella RS, Baumgartner LM. Learning in adulthood: a comprehensive guide. 3rd ed. San Francisco: Jossey-Bass; 2007.
9. Ausubel DP. A subsumption theory of meaningful verbal learning and retention. J Gen Psychol. 1962;66:213–24.
10. Anderson LW, Krathwhol DR, et al., editors. A taxonomy for learning, teaching and assessing: a revision of Bloom's taxonomy of educational objectives. New York: Longman; 2001.
11. Merriam SB, Bierema LL. Adult learning: linking theory and practice. San Francisco: Wiley, Incorporated; 2013. p. 84.
12. Mezirow J. Transformative dimensions of adult learning. San Francisco: Jossey-Bass; 1991.
13. Dewey J. Experience and education. New York: Simon and Schuster; 1938.
14. Kolb DA. Experiential learning. Prentice Hall: Upper Saddle River; 1984.
15. Ericsson KA, Krampe RT, Tesch-Romer C. The role of deliberate practice in the acquisition of expert performance. Psychol Rev. 1993;100:363–406.
16. Ericsson KA. Deliberate practice and acquisition of expert performance: a general overview. Acad Emerg Med. 2008;15(11):988–94.
17. Gaba DM. The future vision of simulation in health care. Qual Saf Health Care. 2004;13(suppl 1):i2–10.
18. Boeing Commercial Aircraft Group. Statistical study of commercial jet aircraft incidents in worldwide operations. 1994.
19. Sexton JB, Thomas EJ, Helmreich RL. Error, stress, and teamwork in medicine and aviation: cross sectional surveys. BMJ. 2000;320:754–9.

20. Alonso A, Baker D, Day R, et al. Reducing medical error in the military health system: how can team training help? Hum Resour Manag Rev. 2006;16:396–415.
21. Anon. Report by the International Committee of Experts on the Lassing mine accident. Commissioned by: Dr H. Farnleitner Federal Minister for Economic Affairs. ec.europa.eu/employment_social/health_safety/docs/lassing_report_en.pdf. Accessed 25 July 2008.
22. Jervis MW. Models and simulation in nuclear power station design and operation. In: Lewins J, Becker M, editors. Advances in nuclear science and technology, vol. 17. Boston: Springer; 1986.
23. Kohn LT, Corrigan JM, Donaldson MS, editors. To err is human: building a safer health system. Institute of Medicine (US) Committee on Quality of Health Care in America. Washington, DC: National Academies Press; 2000. PMID: 25077248.
24. Alinier G. A typology of educationally focused medical simulation tools. Med Teach. 2007;29(8):e243–50.
25. Epstein CD, Hovancsek MT, Dolan PL, et al. Lights! camera! action!: video projects in the classroom. J Nurs Educ. 2003;42:558–61.
26. Wikström BM. Nursing education at an art gallery. J Nurs Scholarsh. 2000;32:197–9.
27. Fried MP, Gallagher AG, Satava RM. Training to proficiency: aircraft to OR. Arch Otolaryngol Head Neck Surg. 2004;130:1145–6.
28. Seymour NE, Gallagher AG, Roman SA, et al. Virtual reality training improves operating room performance: results of a randomized, double-blinded study. Ann Surg. 2002;236:458–63.
29. Kayes AB, Kayes DC, Kolb DA. Developing teams using the Kolb team learning experience. Simul Gaming. 2005;36:355–63.
30. Anderson JM, Murphy AA, Boyle KB, et al. Simulating extracorporeal membrane oxygenation emergencies to improve human performance. Part II: assessment of technical and behavioral skills. Simul Healthc. 2006;1:228–32.
31. Crofts JF, Bartlett C, Ellis D, et al. Management of shoulder dystocia: skill retention 6 and 12 months after training. Obstet Gynecol. 2007;110:1069–74.
32. Wayne DB, Butter J, Siddall VJ, et al. Simulation-based training of internal medicine residents in advanced cardiac life support protocols: a randomized trial. Teach Learn Med. 2005;17:210–6.
33. Lammers RL. Learning and retention rates after training in posterior epistaxis management. Acad Emerg Med. 2008;15:1181–9.
34. Sinha P, Hogle NJ, Fowler DL. Do the laparoscopic skills of trainees deteriorate over time? Surg Endosc. 2008;22:2018–25.
35. Anderson AM, Warren KB. Using simulation to enhance the acquisition and retention of clinical skills in neonatology. Semin Perinatol. 2011;35(2):59–67.
36. Kirkpatrick DL. Evaluating Training Programs. 2nd ed. San Francisco: Berrett-Koehler; 1998.
37. Kern DE, Thomas PA, Hughes MT. Curriculum development for medical education: a six-step approach. 2nd ed. Baltimore: The Johns Hopkins University Press; 2009.
38. Johnston L, Williams SB, Ades A. Education for ECMO providers: using education science to bridge the gap between clinical and educational expertise. Semin Perinatol. 2018;42:138–46.
39. Puslecki M, Ligowski M, Dabrowski M, Stefaniak S, Ladzinska M, Ladzinski P, Pawlak A, Zielinski M, Dabrowska A, Artynska A, Gezela M, Sobczynski P, Szarpak L, Perek B, Jemeility M. BEST life-"bringing ECMO simulation to life"-how medical simulation improved a regional ECMO program. Artif Organs. 2018:1–10.
40. Puslecki M, Ligowski M, Dabrowski M, Stefaniak S, Ladzinska M, Pawlak A, Zielinski M, Szarpak L, Perek B, Jemielity M. Development of regional extracorporeal life support system: the importance of innovative simulation training. Am J Emerg Med. 2018:1–8.
41. Di Nardo M, David P, Stoppa F, Lorusso R, Raponi M, Amodeo A, Cecchetti C, Guner Y, Taccone FS. The introduction of a high-fidelity simulation program for training pediatric critical care personnel reduces the times to manage extracorporeal membrane oxygenation emergencies and improves teamwork. J Thorac Dis. 2018;1(6):3409–17.
42. Lucas A, Edwards M. Development of crisis resource management skills: a literature review. Clin Simul Nurs. 2017;13(8):347–58.
43. Kieser R, Reynisson P, Mulligan TJ. Definition of signal-to-noise ratio and its critical role in split-beam measurements. ICES J Mar Sci. 2005;62:123–30.
44. Sweller J. Cognitive load theory, learning difficulty, and instructional design. Learn Instr. 1994;4:295–312.
45. Sawyer T, Ades A, Ernst K, Colby C. Simulation and the neonatal resuscitation program 7th edition curriculum. NeoReviews. 2016;17(8):e447–53.
46. Donoghue A, Nishisaki A, Sutton R, Hales R, Boulet J. Reliability and validity of a scoring instrument for clinical performance during Pediatric Advanced Life Support simulation scenarios. Resuscitation. 2010;81:331–6.
47. Raffaeli G, Ghiradello S, Vanzati M, Baracetti C, Canesi F, Conigliaro F, Gentilino V, Macchini F, Fumagalli M, Ciralli F, Pesenti N, Passera S, Neri S, Franzini S, Leva E, Plevani L, Mosca F, Cavallaro G. Start a neonatal extranorporeal membrane oxygenation program: a multistep team training. Front Pediatr. 2018;6(151):1–9.
48. Sawyer T, White M, Zaveri P, Chang T, Ades A, French H, Anderson J, Auerbach M, Johnston L, Kessler D. Learn, see, practice, prove, do, maintain: an evidence-based pedagogical framework for procedural skill training in medicine. Acad Med. 2015;90(8):1025–33.
49. Alinier G, Fawzy Hassan I, Alsalemi A, Al Disi M, Ait Hssain A, Labib A, Alhomsi Y, Bensaali F, Amira A, Saif Ibrahim A. Addressing the challenges of ECMO simulation. Perfusion. 2018;33(7):568–76.
50. Brogan TV, Lequier L, Lorusso R, MacLauren G, Peek G. Extracorporeal life support: the ELSO red book. 5th ed. Ann Arbor: Extracorporeal Life Support Organization; 2017.
51. Harwayne-Gidansky I, Culver K, Cavanaugh S, Panesar R. Using mirror patients to enhance patient safety. Simul Healthc. 2019;14(3):195–200.
52. Interprofessional Education Collaborative Expert Panel. Core competencies for interprofessional collaborative practice: report of an expert panel. Washington, DC: Interprofessional Education Collaborative; 2011.
53. Deering S, Johnston LC, Colacchio K. Multidisciplinary teamwork and communication training. Semin Perinatol. 2011;35(2):89–96.
54. Adler MD, Overly FL, Nadkarni VM, Davidson J, Gottesman R, Bank I, Marohn K, Sudikoff S, Grant VJ, Cheng A. An approach to confederate training within the context of simulation-based research. Simul Healthc. 2016;11(5):357–62.
55. Fouilloux V, Gran C, Guervilly C, Breaud J, El Louali F, Rostini P. Impact of education and training course for ECMO patients based on high-fidelity simulation: a pilot study dedicated to ICU nurses. Perfusion. 2018:1–6.
56. Allan CK, Thiagarajan RR, Becke D, et al. Simulation-based training delivered directly to the pediatric cardiac intensive care unit engenders preparedness, comfort, and anxiety among multidisciplinary resuscitation teams. J Thorac Cardiovasc Surg. 2010;140:646–52.
57. Anderson JM, Murphy AA, Boyle KB, Yaeger KA, Halamek LP. Simulating extracorporeal membrane oxygenation emergencies to improve human performance. Part II: assessment of technical and behavioral skills. Simul Healthc. 2006;1:228–32.
58. Su L, Spaeder MC, Jones MB, et al. Implementation of an extracorporeal cardiopulmonary resuscitation simulation program reduces extracorporeal cardiopulmonary resuscitation times in real patients. Pediatr Crit Care Med. 2014;15:856–60.
59. Burton KS, Pendergrass TL, Byczkowski TL, et al. Impact of simulation-based extracorporeal membrane oxygenation training in

the simulation laboratory and clinical environment. Simul Healthc. 2011;6(5):284–91.
60. Brazzi L, Lissoni A, Panigada M, et al. Simulation-based training of extracorporeal membrane oxygenation during H1N1 influenza pandemic: the Italian experience. Simul Healthc. 2012;7(1):32–4.
61. Extracorporeal Life Support Organization. ELSO guidelines for training and continuing education of ECMO specialists, version 1.5. 2010: 1–9. https://www.elso.org/Portals/0/IGD/Archive/FileManager/97000963d6cusersshyerdocumentselsoguidelinesfortraiingandcontinuingeducationofecmospecialists.pdf. Accessed 17 Oct 2017.
62. Short BL, Williams L. ECMO specialist training manual. 3rd ed. Ann Arbor: Extracorporeal Life Support Organization; 2010.
63. Weems MF, Friedlich PS, Nelson LP, et al. The role of extracorporeal membrane oxygenation simulation training at extracorporeal life support organization centers in the United States. Simul Healthc. 2017;12(4):233–9.
64. Ogino MT, Chuo J, Short BL. ECMO administrative and training issues, and sustaining quality. In: Annich GM, Lynch WR, MacLauren G, Wilson JM, Bartlett RH, et al., editors. ECMO extracorporeal support in critical care. 4th ed. Ann Arbor: Extracorporeal Life Support Organization; 2012. p. 479–97.
65. Extracorporeal Life Support Organization. ELSO guidelines for ECMO centers, version 1.8. Last updated March 2014. https://www.elso.org/Portals/0/IGD/Archive/FileManager/faf3f6a3c7cusersshyerdocumentselsoguidelinesecmocentersv1.8.pdf. Accessed 17 Oct 2017.
66. Rudolph JW, Simon R, Dufresne RL, Raemer DB. There's no such thing as "nonjudgmental" debriefing: a theory and method for debriefing with good judgment. Simul Healthc. 2006;1(1):49–55. PMID: 19088574.
67. Eppich W, Cheng A. Promoting Excellence and Reflective Learning in Simulation (PEARLS): development and rationale for a blended approach to health care simulation debriefing. Simul Healthc. 2015;10(2):106–15.
68. Phrampus PE, O'Donnell JM. Debriefing using a structured and supported approach. In: Levine AI, DeMaria S, Schwartz AD, Sim AJ, editors. The comprehensive textbook of healthcare simulation. New York: Springer; 2013.
69. Zigmont JJ, Kappus LJ, Sudikoff SN. The 3D model of debriefing: defusing, discovering, and deepening. Semin Perinatol. 2011;35(2):52–8.
70. Muratore S, Beilman G, John R, Brunsvold M. Extracorporeal membrane oxygenation credentialing: where do we stand? Am J Surg. 2015;210:655–60.
71. Steadman R, Burden A, Huang Y, Gaba D, Cooper J. Practice improvements based on participation in simulation for the maintenance of certification in anesthesiology program. Anesthesiology. 2015;122(5):1154–69.
72. Chan S, Figueroa M, Spentzas T, Powell A, Holloway R, Shah S. Prospective assessment of novice learners in a simulation- based extracorporeal membrane oxygenation (ECMO) education program. Pediatr Cardiol. 2013;34(3):543–52. https://doi.org/10.1007/s00246-012-0490-6.
73. Braga M, Tyler M, Rhoads J, et al. Effect of just-in-time simulation training on provider performance and patient outcomes for clinical procedures: a systematic review. BMJ Simul Technol Enhanc Learn. 2015;1(3):94–102.

A Conceptual Framework for Development of a Simulation-Enhanced ECMO Training Program: Use of a Zone-Based Framework

4

Catherine K. Allan and Jill Zalieckas

Learning Objectives

1. Describe the three microteams involved in the care of ECMO patients, and identify the specific training needs for each microteam and the ECMO team as a whole.
2. Apply the SIMZone framework to choose the optimal instructional design and/or debriefing methodology for the intended learner or group of learners.
3. Design simulations that address both individual technical skill gaps and team learning objectives that optimize intrinsic, extrinsic, and germane load for the specific learner.

Introduction

Extracorporeal membrane oxygenation (ECMO) is a high-risk, high-complexity but low-frequency therapy. Successful deployment and maintenance of ECMO requires the coordinated efforts of a team of practitioners with diverse and specific skillsets beyond that required for standard resuscitation. While the intensive care unit team must be adept in the application of standard resuscitation algorithms, additional required skills of the team include preparation (often emergent) and operation of the ECMO circuit, as well as surgical cannulation. Additional challenges in the care of the ECMO patient stem from the highly complex nature of the ECMO team, comprised of several microteams – surgical, perfusion, and ICU – which must work seamlessly to complete individual but highly interrelated tasks. A program of training to prepare teams to provide high quality and safe ECMO care, therefore, must include components that address a broad variety of technical, cognitive, and teamwork skills, often across providers with a wide range of experience from relative novice to expert. In this chapter, we present a conceptual framework for the design of simulation-enhanced curricula to prepare teams to achieve high performance in the care of ECMO patients.

The factors described above make ECMO training an ideal target for the use of simulation as a training tool. Indeed, simulation has been successfully applied to address surgical cannulation skills [1], technical and cognitive skills related to ECPR and management of ECMO emergencies [2, 3], teamwork skills [4], and circuit management and competency assessment. A recent survey of centers contributing the Extracorporeal Life Support Registry in Europe and North America found that (46%) of respondents was using some form of simulation in training their teams for ECMO [5]. Despite the widespread adoption, however, there are no standardized curricula and no recommended approach to integration of simulation within an ECMO training program. Here we describe an approach to creation of simulation-enhanced ECMO training curricula that considers required technical and cognitive skills across various levels of learners. We describe a modular curriculum that pairs the right methodology with the right learner at the optimal phase of their professional development.

C. K. Allan (✉)
Department of Cardiology, Boston Children's Hospital and Department of Pediatrics, Harvard Medical School, Boston, MA, USA

SIMPeds, Boston Children's Hospital Simulator Program, Boston Children's Hospital and Harvard Medical School, Boston, MA, USA
e-mail: Catherine.allan@cardio.chboston.org

J. Zalieckas
Department of Surgery, Boston Children's Hospital, Boston, MA, USA

Department of Surgery, Harvard Medical School, Boston, MA, USA

L. C. Johnston, L. Su (eds.), *Comprehensive Healthcare Simulation: ECMO Simulation*, Comprehensive Healthcare Simulation,
https://doi.org/10.1007/978-3-030-53844-6_4

Zone-Based Framework for Simulation-Enhanced Training

Roussin and Weinstock [6] have described a framework for classification of simulation-based training activities that link appropriate simulation methodologies and instructional or debriefing strategies with type of learning objectives and level of learners. Zone 0 activities include those with automated feedback which are typically task-oriented, such as laparoscopic surgical trainers with automated feedback. Screen-based ECMO simulators, such as the MSE screen-based ECMO simulator for adult ECMO, fall into this category [7]. In-person instruction or facilitation is not required for these exercises. Zone 1 activities focus on goals and objectives related to clinical proficiency. These activities frequently involve a single discipline of care providers and are led by an instructor who is expert in the content. Instructional techniques may include the use of "pause principle" to give timely feedback and corrections and help novice learners stay on course. In this technique, the instructor pauses the simulation briefly to offer feedback or clarify actions of learners and then quickly resumes the simulation. This strategy allows instructors to understand how learners are applying critical thinking to scenarios. Zone 2 simulations, often involving more than one discipline, also focus on goals related to clinical proficiency, but involve more nuanced clinical scenarios, uninterrupted simulation action, and debriefing at the end of the event as opposed to use of "pause principle." Some types of learner distractions may also be introduced in Zone 2 simulations. Zone 3 activities, typically described as "team training," focus on understanding the underlying beliefs, assumptions, and cognitive rules that govern behaviors among team members – so-called double loop learning [8] – rather than on instruction in specific clinical or teamwork concepts. For example, a double loop learning approach might seek to understand why staff might not speak up with concerns during a crisis situation, rather than simply instructing clinicians to speak up. Understanding barriers to a specific behavior enables learning and change by giving participants specific skills to overcome those barriers. Zone 3 activities are geared toward team and system development. Zone 3 simulations involve a full native multidisciplinary team, complex scenarios, realistic distractors (parent presence, alarms, interruptions through pages and phone calls), and run uninterrupted. These design elements are critical to create an environment that will allow expert learners to fully engage in the simulation experience that supports deep conversations about team behaviors. Debriefing for Zone 3 simulations is a facilitated conversation among expert clinicians designed to understand the "whys" behind behavior.

Overall Framework for Simulation-Enhanced ECMO Training

Required competencies for ECMO care can be divided into major categories: cannulation and initiation of ECMO, daily routine care, and management of ECMO emergencies. Within each of these three broad categories are a set of required psychomotor and critical thinking skills as well as requirements of team-based practice, with varying requirements depending on the individual provider roles – surgical team, ECMO specialists/perfusionist, and intensive care unit team/resuscitation team (Table 4.1). A comprehensive ECMO training program will cover all of these skills using

Table 4.1 Psychomotor, cognitive, and teamwork skills required for members of the ECMO team

	Learners		
Learning category	ECMO specialists	Surgeons/proceduralist	ICU team
Psychomotor skills			
Surgical cannulation		xX	
Percutaneous cannulation		xX	
ECMO circuit assembly	X		
Initiation of flows	X		
Membrane/component changes	X		
Air removal	X		
CPR			xX
Cognitive skills/critical thinking			
Monitoring CPR quality			xX
Initiation of flows	xX	xX	xX
Troubleshooting ECMO emergencies	xX	xX	xX
Teamwork behaviors			
Directed communication	X	X	xX
Closed loop communication	X	X	X
Speaking up	X	X	X
Role clarity	X	X	X
Global assessment	X	X	X

curricular design that is appropriate to the level of the learner, potentially ranging from novice to expert, a daunting task even for those most experienced in instructional design. Application of a clear instructional framework provides an effective rubric to ensure quality and relevance of the curriculum. The SIMZones framework is particularly well-suited to this task, as it provides comprehensive guidance for all design elements, including development of learning objectives, design of simulation scenarios (both case development and technical aspects of simulation), and debriefing goals and methodology.

Attention to the knowledge base and prior experience of the learner is of particular importance to the design of individual curricular elements. Cognitive load theory describes the way in which learners process and incorporate new knowledge into existing frameworks by describing the relationship between working memory and learning [9]. Long-term memory has limitless capacity; however, working memory can retain only 5–7 elements and can actively process only 2–4 elements simultaneously, and these elements are lost rapidly if not immediately "refreshed." For effective storage in long-term memory and accessibility for later retrieval and application, new elements must be organized into frameworks or "schema" [9]. In general, a greater degree of scaffolding will be required for novice learners to create these schema.

Cognitive load can be broken down into three types of load. *Intrinsic load* describes the complexity of the learning task itself (i.e., diagnosis of ECMO circuit emergencies). The more complex the information or task presented, the higher the intrinsic cognitive load. *Extrinsic (extraneous) load* is the work imposed by the learning environment itself, including both the manner in which information is presented and external factors such as noise and other distractions. Extrinsic load is of particular relevance in the creation of simulation-based educational offerings, where distractors can readily be dialed up or down depending on the level of the learner. *Germane load* describes the cognitive effort required to process and organize elements into effective schema. Attention to management of germane load is of particular importance when teaching complex topics that require integration of data from multiple sources, such as diagnosis of ECMO emergencies. In simulation-based teaching and learning exercises, content and learning environment can be carefully manipulated to help faculty create the optimal learning experience. The SIMZones architecture provides concrete guidance on management of all three elements of cognitive load.

In general, novice learners will be more challenged by curricular design elements that impose greater extrinsic load. Conversely, oversimplification may lead to disengagement and poor learning outcomes for more experienced learners, a principle known as the "expertise reversal effect [10]." In order to optimize cognitive load for learners of all expertise, individual curricular elements relevant to each psychomotor, cognitive, or team-based skills can be designed that build through the SIMZones framework from Zone 1 to Zone 3 to accommodate all levels of learners and to aid in transitioning learners from novice to expert. The remainder of this chapter will provide concrete guidance on the creation of a modular ECMO curriculum from which elements relevant to the individual learner or learner group can be selected to meet specific program's training requirements. Table 4.2 provides an example of such a modular curriculum.

Development of Psychomotor Skills

Fitts and Posner described a series of 3 levels of motor skill acquisition: cognition, integration, and automation [11]. During level I skill acquisition and cognition, the learner builds an understanding of the procedure that includes elements such as how to physically manipulate a device and how to complete the individual tasks that comprise the steps of a procedure. Level II describes the learner who can perform the procedure step by step and begin to connect all the individual steps of the task, but for whom the procedure as a whole remains unrefined. In level 3, the learner gains automation, picking up fluidity, efficiency, accuracy, and speed. Design of simulation-based curricula for acquisition of psychomotor skills using the SIMZones framework supports the learner in transitioning through these phases of skills acquisition. In Zone 1 activities, learners receive side-by-side coaching from an expert instructor through the individual steps of a skill. The flipped classroom approach can be used to support Zone 1 learning, through use of video demonstrations or provision of guides with detailed step-by-step written instructions from a detailed task analysis. As learners master the individual task steps and gain the ability to sequence them, Zone 2 activities support the ability of the learner to connect the individual steps of the procedure into a whole. In Zone 2 skills, session learners work through a task largely uninterrupted and receive feedback from an expert primarily at the end of the procedure, though as learners transition from Zone I to Zone II experiences some ongoing "real-time" feedback may be beneficial. Zone 2 experiences allow for deliberate practice – focused practice of tasks with clear performance goals combined with expert feedback [12] – and, as such, provide learners a way to move from Level II of skill acquisition (integration) to the automation seen in Level III. In addition to automation, successful learners must also develop the ability to diagnose and

Table 4.2 Zone-based modular curriculum elements for training of surgeons, perfusionists, and intensive care unit team members

	Zone 1	Zone 2	Zone 3
Surgical training – cannulation			
Learning objectives	Positioning/draping Identification of landmarks Procedural steps	Fluency of procedural steps Management of limited cognitive distractions	Management of cognitive distractions during ECPR Application of teamwork principles
Technical design	en lay task trainer on low fidelity manikin	en lay task trainer ongoing vital sign changes	en lay task trainer full multidisciplinary team circuit integrated with manikin with ability to manipulate circuit pressures and flows
Debriefing/ facilitation	Side-by-side coaching	Pause principle and post-simulation debriefing Expert surgeon	Post-simulation multidisciplinary debriefing focusing on team elements Facilitator focusing on double loop learning
Perfusion			
Learning objectives	Circuit assembly Initiation of flows Component changes	Recognition and management of circuit emergencies	Management of cognitive distractions during circuit preparation, establishment of flows, and management of circuit emergencies Application of teamwork principles
Technical design	Wet lab drills	Circuit integrated with manikin with ability to manipulate circuit pressures and flows May be multidisciplinary with ICU team	Full multidisciplinary team Circuit integrated with manikin with ability to manipulate circuit pressures and flows
Debriefing/ facilitation	Side-by-side coaching	Post-simulation debrief by content expert Focus on integration of data to correctly diagnose circuit emergencies	Post-simulation multidisciplinary debriefing focusing on team elements Facilitator focusing on double loop learning
Intensive care team			
Learning objectives	Basic circuit physiology	Diagnosis and management of circuit emergencies	Management of team elements during cannulation and ECPR events Management of cognitive load during circuit emergencies
Technical design	Tabletop exercises/ chalkboard exercises (Table 4.3)	Circuit integrated with manikin with ability to manipulate circuit pressures and flows, patient vital signs ICU team and perfusion team together	Full multidisciplinary team Circuit integrated with manikin with ability to manipulate circuit pressures and flows, patient vital signs
Debriefing/ facilitation	Side-by-side coaching/ instruction by content expert	Post-simulation debrief by content expert Focus on integration of data to correctly diagnose circuit emergencies	Post-simulation multidisciplinary debriefing focusing on team elements Facilitator focusing on double loop learning

respond to problems that come up during a procedure, a hallmark of procedural competency [13]. Zone 2 activities can be varied to introduce technical challenges that learners may face in real-life settings. Introduction of Zone 3 activities can help learners build toward competency, as they are asked to apply technical skills in fully contextualized settings, processing a barrage of clinical data, noise, and team interactions while executing the skill.

Cannulation Skills Training Surgeons required to cannulate patients for ECMO in the urgent or emergent setting may bring a broad range of expertise, from novice to seasoned expert. The learning goals for these individuals will vary significantly, and the design of the cannulation curriculum must address the needs of the specific learner. Table 4.2 summarizes elements of a cannulation curriculum across all three zones. Zone 1 activities support novice learners in development of individual tasks that make up the complete skill and include elements such as patient positioning, identification of landmarks, incision, tissue dissection, vessel isolation, cannula selection, insertion (including correct depth), cannula securement, and connection to ECMO circuit. The use of realistic en lay trainers as part of a structured Zone 1/Zone 2 curricula has been demonstrated to lead to sustained improvement in time to cannulation, global rating scores of surgical proficiency, and a composite ECMO cannulation score addressing procedure-specific competencies all in the simulated setting [1]. The proceduralist must be able to accomplish this within the context of time pressure due to critical clinical status of the patient, a potentially noisy and chaotic environment, and ongoing patient resuscitation, including potentially CPR. Thus, once a trainee has demonstrated competency in the basic skills of cannulation in a controlled setting, Zone 2 offerings can begin to introduce distractors that increase cognitive load [14], such as alarm noises, multiple team members, and even CPR, though the focus of these simulations remains on procedural competency. Finally, Zone 3 activities, such as full team ECPR exercises, allow surgeons to apply procedural skills while simultaneously integrating patient data, making time-sensitive decisions, demonstrating team work skills, as well as recognizing and managing complications that are required for full proficiency.

ECMO Circuit Skills Training Similar to surgical cannulation for ECMO, preparation and management of the ECMO circuit require a high degree of technical proficiency as well as the ability to apply these technical skills under time pressure and as part of a complex interdisciplinary team. The SIMZones framework can be utilized to develop a curriculum for ECMO specialists from novice to expert. Low fidelity exercises that introduce the components of an ECMO circuit, including location of pressure monitors, and basic circuit physiology are useful for the new specialist. For instance, Hospital for Sick Children (Toronto, Ontario, CA) utilizes photographs of individual ECMO circuit components for this early phase of training. Specialists are asked to "assemble" the pieces in order on a table, and deliberate practice is readily incorporated into this exercise. Once confident with the ordering of circuit components, wet labs can be added in to allow specialists to train on circuit assembly and priming. Initial attempts at this exercise fall firmly in Zone 1 territory, with side-by-side coaching from an experienced specialist, but as learners gain experience, circuit assembly happens independently with instructor feedback at the end. Contextualized training (Zone 2), such as during a full team cannulation scenario, is next incorporated so that specialists gain experience at circuit assembly and priming under urgent or emergent conditions. The emphasis in these exercises is still on the technical aspects of circuit preparation. Similarly, management of circuit emergencies can be introduced first in isolated skills sessions with side-by-side coaching from experts (Zone 1) followed by practice during fully contextualized scenarios (Zone 2) in which specialists must integrate data from circuit and patient monitors to diagnose and treat circuit emergencies. Zone 3 activities, such as full team ECPR scenarios, allow the ECMO specialist to apply the technical skills of circuit preparation, circuit connection, team work skills during cannulation, and integration of patient, and circuit data necessary for proficient circuit management.

Development of Cognitive Skills

ECMO emergencies are low-frequency, high-risk events that require rapid integration of complex physiologic data from both the patient and the ECMO circuit to correctly diagnose the problem followed by rapid implantation of an appropriate treatment plan. The cognitive load, therefore, associated with diagnosis of ECMO emergencies is high. The list of possible ECMO emergencies is extensive, and learners can be easily overwhelmed. Cognitive load is reduced when novice learners are presented with schema, or cognitive frameworks, that help them to organize these data for storage in, and later retrieval from, long-term memory. For instance, the majority of ECMO emergencies can fit into one of three categories: decreased venous return to the pump, pump/ oxygenator failure, or increased afterload on the pump. While multiple diagnoses fit into each of these categories, there are certain patterns that unify the category. For example, problems of decreased venous return (e.g., hypovolemia, inadequate venous cannula size, obstructed venous cannula) almost all manifest as more negative pre-membrane pressures and eventually decreased flows for the same revolutions per minute (RPMs) on a centrifugal pump. When confronted with these findings, a learner can quickly narrow down the list of potential problems to those involving decreased venous return. Other physiologic monitoring parameters can then be used to find the specific diagnosis. For instance, decreased patient central venous pressure (CVP) will point toward a diagnosis of hypovolemia, whereas an increased patient central venous pressure points toward a venous cannula issue such as cannula malposition, cannula under sizing, or thrombus.

The SIMZones framework can be used to bring practitioners from novice to competent with respect to management of ECMO emergencies, particularly when cognitive frameworks related to diagnosis of ECMO emergencies are made explicit in early curricular elements and reinforced in more advanced exercises. For example, following an introduction to physiology of ECMO complications through didactic teaching, trainees may engage in a "chalkboard" exercise in which they are asked to complete a complication matrix (Table 4.3). In this exercise, learners must categorize specific complications as venous, arterial, mixed, or pump problems. Learners then complete the matrix by indicating the direction of change for relevant patient or pump physiologic parameters. This exercise reinforces patterns to aid learners in integrating clinical data at the bedside to make an accurate diagnosis and prepares learners to participate in subsequent simulation exercises.

Patterns for ECMO complications introduced through didactic and chalkboard exercises are reinforced through Zone 1/2 simulation exercises. For instance, simple simulations can be conducted for single or multidisciplinary groups in which circuit pressures and patient vital signs are altered to represent specific ECMO emergencies. The team is then asked to work through the changes to identify the nature of the emergency. For novice groups, the "pause principle" style of simulation can be applied, allowing the instructor to pause at key moments to guide participants, provide real-time feedback, or ask questions to tease out cognitive processes as a way to assess team or individual understanding of the event. As learners progress, simulations can progress into

Table 4.3 ECMO complications framework

	CVP	Venous pressure	Pre-membrane pressure	Post-membrane pressure	Delta P	Flow	ABP
Hypovolemia	↓	↓	No change (late ↓ with ↓ flows)	No change (late ↓ with ↓ flows)	No change	↓	↓
Sepsis	↓	↓	No change	No change	No change	↑	↓
Obstructed venous cannula	↑	↓	↓ (late ↓ with ↓ flows)	↓ (late ↓ with ↓ flows)	No change	↓	↓
Undersized venous cannula	↑	↓	↓ (late ↓ with ↓ flows)	↓ (late ↓ with ↓ flows)	No change	↓	↓
Oxygenator failure	No change	No change	↑	No change then ↓	↑	No change or slight ↓	No change
Seizure	↑	Late ↓	↑	↑	No change	↓	↑ (late ↓)
Agitation	↑	Late ↓	↑	↑	No change	↓	↑ (late ↓)
High patient SVR	↑	Late ↓	↑	↑	No change	↓	↓[a]
Undersized arterial cannula	↑	No change	↑	↑	No change	↓	↓
Obstructed arterial cannula	↑	No change	↑	↑	No change	↓	↓
Tamponade	↑	Late ↓	↑	↑	No change	↓	↓
Tension pneumothorax	↑	Late ↓	↑	↑	No change	↓	↓

This table summarizes patient and ECMO circuit physiologic changes for ECMO complications when using a centrifugal pump. Novices can be asked to fill in the elements of a "blank table" as an exercise to reinforce the physiologic manifestations of various ECMO complications

CVP central venous pressure, *Delta P* change in pressure, *ABP* arterial blood pressure, *SVR* systemic vascular resistance

[a]In a high patient SVR state, particularly at initiation of flows in a patient with no native ejection, high SVR will impede flows enough resulting in decreased BP

Zone 2, in which simulations run uninterrupted. Real-time changes in circuit pressures and patient vital signs on the background of a plausible clinical story prompt learners to integrate multiple sources of data to make a diagnosis. Ongoing real-time adjustments to displayed patient and pump data are made to reflect realistic physiologic responses to learner interventions. For instance, in a scenario with decreased flows and high pre- and post-membrane pressures related to patient hypertension in the context of a centrifugal pump, appropriate interventions to address hypertension (reduction in vasopressor/inotropic support, additional of vasodilator, optimization of sedation) will manifest as decreased patient blood pressure, decrease pre- and post-membrane pressures, and increased ECMO flows for the same RPMs. Debriefing of these Zone 2 scenarios focuses on understanding learner's cognitive processes – how they came to a diagnosis and decided upon interventions. These debriefings also serve as an opportunity to reinforce the ECMO complications framework.

As learners progress in their proficiency related to ECMO complications, Zone 3 simulations can be introduced in which learners are asked to navigate teamwork elements while managing ECMO emergencies. In this situation, elements such as parent presence or increased background noise or other distractors can be added to increased cognitive load.

Development of Teamwork Skills

Successful ECMO cannulation and management of ECMO complications requires effective communication and coordination among a large, complex multidisciplinary team. Simulation can be an effective tool to introduce and hone these teamwork skills. For nascent teams without previous introduction to teamwork concepts, teamwork principles may be introduced through Zone 2 simulations, after which team members reflect on and receive direct feedback from an expert facilitator regarding team function in the areas of communication, role clarity, global assessment/avoidance of errors of fixation, and anticipation of resource needs [15, 16]. More experienced teams will benefit from Zone 3 simulations that involve full native multidisciplinary teams, complex case scenarios, and distractors typical of the real clinical environment (code bells, pagers, parent presence, etc.) resulting in an experience that forces expert practitioners to manage a high cognitive load as they would in a real-life

ECMO cannulation event, particularly during ECPR. Zone 3 simulations are typically highly realistic in order to enhance provider engagement. The use of realistic cannulation trainers [1] as well as equipment and supplies identical to those used in actual patient care will enhance engagement of surgeons and ICU/ECMO providers, respectively.

Debriefing for Zone 3 ECMO courses acknowledges that participants are typically highly experienced and proficient in the required clinical skills; the debriefing draws on specific examples of team behavior from the simulation to explore generalizable teamwork concepts, including reflecting on barriers to effective teamwork and solutions to these challenges. The debriefer acts as a facilitator of the conversation.

Several specific teamwork concepts are highly relevant to ECMO emergencies. First, during an ECMO event, three separate microteams [17] (ICU, perfusion, and surgery) make up the full ECMO team. Each microteam must engage in separate but highly interdependent tasks. Communication must take place both within and across microteams to ensure that all team members are able to effectively anticipate and problem-solve. For example, if the surgeon has encountered unexpected bleeding, communication of this allows the ICU team to anticipate need for blood products. If performance gaps related to communication across microteams are observed during a simulation, debriefing might encourage teams to reflect on the challenges to such communication. Using methods such as advocacy-inquiry [18], debriefers can encourage team members to move beyond what happened in the simulation to search for the "why" behind their behaviors.

A second important teamwork theme in ECMO events is avoidance of task fixation and maintenance of global perspective, particularly for the event manager. ECMO cannulation and management of ECMO emergencies are highly task dependent areas of resuscitation, with major tasks including surgical cannulation and preparation and troubleshooting of the ECMO circuit. The event manager must maintain an awareness of how these tasks are proceeding while continuing to orchestrate an effective resuscitation of the patient, a job that imposes a greater cognitive load than resuscitation according to standard Pediatric Advanced Life Support (PALS) Guidelines. Thus, when errors of fixation occur during simulation, debriefing allows an opportunity for team members to explore why fixation occurs and how it can be avoided. More on teams and relevant team science is covered in Chap. 11.

Summary

Training teams to competency to manage patients on ECMO presents a uniquely complex challenge to curriculum design. The team must achieve proficiency in several unique but interdependent complex psychomotor skills, including circuit preparation and management, surgical cannulation, and patient resuscitation. The ECMO team is similarly complex, composed of three separate microteams – intensive care unit/resuscitation team, surgical team, and perfusion/ECMO specialist team. Finally, providers must acquire high level teamwork skills that promote effective communication and coordination both within and among the three microteams. An effective curriculum will build upon individual and teams' existing knowledge and skills, identifying important performance gaps to be addressed; thus, optimal ECMO training is not best addressed through a "one size fits all" curricular approach. This chapter has presented a framework that accounts for training needs of novice to expert across the three microteams and for the team as a whole, with the possibility that learners might enter the progression at the point most appropriate to their existing knowledge and skills.

References

1. Allan CK, Pigula F, Bacha EA, Emani S, Fynn-Thompson F, Thiagarajan RR, et al. An extracorporeal membrane oxygenation cannulation curriculum featuring a novel integrated skills trainer leads to improved performance among pediatric cardiac surgery trainees. Simul Healthc. 2013;8(4):221–8.
2. Whitmore SP, Gunnerson KJ, Haft JW, Lynch WR, VanDyck T, Hebert C, et al. Simulation training enables emergency medicine providers to rapidly and safely initiate extracorporeal cardiopulmonary resuscitation (ECPR) in a simulated cardiac arrest scenario. Resuscitation. 2019;138:68–73.
3. Di Nardo M, David P, Stoppa F, Lorusso R, Raponi M, Amodeo A, et al. The introduction of a high-fidelity simulation program for training pediatric critical care personnel reduces the times to manage extracorporeal membrane oxygenation emergencies and improves teamwork. J Thorac Dis. 2018;10(6):3409–17.
4. Allan CK, Thiagarajan RR, Beke D, Imprescia A, Kappus LJ, Garden A, et al. Simulation-based training delivered directly to the pediatric cardiac intensive care unit engenders preparedness, comfort, and decreased anxiety among multidisciplinary resuscitation teams. J Thorac Cardiovasc Surg. 2010;140(3):646–52.
5. Weems MF, Friedlich PS, Nelson LP, Rake AJ, Klee L, Stein JE, et al. The role of extracorporeal membrane oxygenation simulation training at extracorporeal life support organization centers in the United States. Simul Healthc. 2017;12(4):233–9.
6. Roussin CJ, Weinstock P. SimZones: an organizational innovation for simulation programs and centers. Acad Med. 2017;92(8):1114–20.
7. Adult ECMO Simulator [webpage]. MSE (Australia). 2009. Available from: http://www.ecmosimulation.com/index.html.
8. Argyris C. Teaching smart people how to learn. Harv Bus Rev. 1991;69:99–109.
9. van Merrienboer JJ, Sweller J. Cognitive load theory in health professional education: design principles and strategies. Med Educ. 2010;44(1):85–93.
10. Sweller J, Ayres P, Kalyuga S, Chandler P. The expertise reversal effect. Faculty of Education – Papers. Educ Psychol. 2011;38:23–31.
11. Fitts PM, Posner MI. Human performance. Oxford, UK: Brooks/Cole; 1967.
12. Ericsson KA, Krampe RT, Tesch-Römer C. The role of deliberate practice in the acquisition of expert performance. Psychol Rev. 1993;100(3):363–406.

13. Dreyfus SE, Dreyfus H. A five-stage model of the mental activities involved in directed skill acquisition. Distribution. 1980:22.
14. Mancinetti M, Guttormsen S, Berendonk C. Cognitive load in internal medicine: what every clinical teacher should know about cognitive load theory. Eur J Intern Med. 2019;60:4–8.
15. Howard SK, Gaba DM, Fish KJ, Yang G, Sarnquist FH. Anesthesia crisis resource management training: teaching anesthesiologists to handle critical incidents. Aviat Space Environ Med. 1992;63(9):763–70.
16. Salas E, Sims DE, Burke CS. Is there a "big five" in teamwork? Small Group Res. 2005;36(5):555–99.
17. Roussin C, Maclean T, Rudolph J. The safety in unsafe teams: a multilevel approach to team psychological safety. J Manag. 2016;42(6):1409–33.
18. Rudolph J, Simon R, Dufresne R, Raemer D. There's no such thing as "nonjudgmental" debriefing: a theory and method for debriefing with good judgment. Simul Healthc. 2006;1:49–55.

Brain-Based Learning

5

David L. Rodgers and Roberta L. Hales

Learning Objectives

1. State the role of learning theory in the development of ECMO simulation.
2. List at least five learning theories commonly used with healthcare provider simulation.
3. Define brain-based learning.
4. Differentiate brain-compatible versus brain-antagonistic learning.

Introduction

A theory is a set of explanatory assumptions, meaning a primary function is to provide prediction [1, 2]. An understanding of learning theory informs educational practices and allows educators and curriculum designers to create programs with an expectation for outcomes.

While there are many education and learning theories cited in the healthcare literature on simulation and debriefing, five theories dominate the healthcare literature on simulation and debriefing: experiential learning theory [3–22], constructivism [7, 13, 19, 23–31], adult learning theory [4, 7, 13, 20, 22, 32–36], self-efficacy theory [9, 13, 19, 37–41], and social learning theory [13, 19, 37, 39, 41–43].

Experiential Learning Theory – Progressing from John Dewey [44] to Kurt Lewin [45] and on to David Kolb [46], experiential learning theory (ELT) is the process of learning by having an experience, reflecting on that experience, and revising behaviors based on the reflective insights gained from that experience. The experience can then be repeated permitting new understandings to be employed followed again by reflection and revision, creating an ongoing cycle of learning. Most learning does not happen in the experience phase of this cycle; it occurs in the reflective phase. Reflection allows for a transformation in thinking that generates new ideas and concepts on how the experience should be managed. Referencing the work of Donald Schön, it is this *reflection on action* that occurs after the experience where learners can gain the greatest understanding of how to revise their behaviors and earlier mental concepts [47]. Experiential learning theory does not equate with "hands-on-learning." While *reflection in action* or reflection in the moment may take place during a hands-on-learning session and can change behaviors, without dedicated reflection on action during a simulation debriefing, it might not consistently be classified as an ELT-based simulation.

- Example of ELT being applied to an education program – An interprofessional ECMO team participates in a simulation of a neonatal patient where air developed in the ECMO circuit. The team successfully managed this experience, but there were delays in recognizing and communicating the complication. During the debriefing, team members reflected on their experience and noted some communication behaviors that could be improved. Their discussion created new ideas on the importance of speaking up when a problem is recognized. The team then had another simulation experience with a different complication, but the learning from the first simulation was generalized to the new situation as seen with improved communication behaviors.

Another example of the experiential learning cycle in simulation can be seen in Ericsson's depiction of deliberate

D. L. Rodgers (✉)
Clinical Simulation Center, Penn State Health Milton S. Hershey Medical Center, Hershey, PA, USA
e-mail: drodgers1@pennstatehealth.psu.edu

R. L. Hales
Center for Simulation, Advanced Education and Innovation, The Children's Hospital of Philadelphia, Philadelphia, PA, USA

L. C. Johnston, L. Su (eds.), *Comprehensive Healthcare Simulation: ECMO Simulation*, Comprehensive Healthcare Simulation,
https://doi.org/10.1007/978-3-030-53844-6_5

practice [48]. Here, learners have specific focused experiences, followed by reflection on action, often augmented with feedback, to determine revisions required to improve the performance. The ongoing cycle creates a stepwise improvement that continues to build toward higher levels of proficiency with each revision.

Constructivism – Based on foundational work by John Dewey [44], Jean Piaget [49], and Jerome Bruner [50], constructivism states that people have prior experiences upon which new knowledge, skills, or attitudes must be built. While some groups may have shared experiences, individual members may have unique interpretations of these experiences. For this reason, constructivism becomes a very personal individualized learning experience. Noted educational psychologist David Ausubel once said, "If I had to reduce all of educational psychology to just one principle, I would say this: The most important single factor influencing learning is what the learner already knows. Ascertain this and teach him accordingly" [51] (p. vi).

One constructivist concept that has been mentioned in the healthcare simulation literature is the Zone of Proximal Development (ZPD) [52]. Introduced by Lev Vygotsky [53], a learner enters the ZPD at the point their own experiences and the range of their knowledge, skills, and attitudes reach their limits. The educator must now provide scaffolding to help bridge the learner's current capabilities to new potentials. Just like building a brick wall one layer at a time, new knowledge must be constructed on the previous layers.

- Example of constructivism being applied to an education program – An ECMO simulation educator has designed an intricate scenario based on a pump malfunction. During the simulation, the educator observed considerable confusion among the learners around the pump operations. During debriefing, some learners indicated this was not the ECMO pump they were used to using, while other learners expressed some fear in dealing with the pump because they felt their understanding of how it worked was not adequate. While reflecting on the problems encountered, the educator discovered while some learners had experience with ECMO, the different device proved to be problematic as the experience with the different pump could not be translated to these learners' clinical setting. Compounding the situation, the educator also realized some fundamental education about pump failure was missing from their curriculum, making other learners unprepared for the scenario. In both cases, constructivist concepts were ignored by introducing a simulation scenario for which most learners were not prepared to manage properly. This was a situation where the ZPD was bypassed by presenting a case that was too far from the learners' baseline knowledge and skill set.

Adult Learning Theory – Adult learning theory (ALT) has evolved from the work of Eduard Lindeman [54] in the early twentieth century and has progressed through the following 100 years. Most citations in the simulation education literature focus on the work of Malcolm Knowles [55], who himself was heavily influenced by Lindeman's ideas. The basic premise of ALT is that adults learn differently than children and as a result need to be taught differently. Much of educational theory that is commonly referenced in the simulation literature was first developed with children in mind in elementary education; hence the term pedagogy features the prefix "ped" indicating its pediatric focus. Knowles and his colleagues emphasized a difference between pedagogy and what they termed andragogy in the way adults learn.

Knowles generated primary assumptions that serve as the underpinnings for ALT:

- Adults have an established concept of self which leads them to choose what to learn and how. (Autonomy)
- Adults have their own personal experiences that must be integrated into teaching and learning new knowledge, skills, or attitudes. (Experiences)
- Adults have an innate readiness to learn to help them achieve goals. (Readiness)
- Adults have a problem-centered focus with an emphasis on immediate application of the learning to help solve problems. (Problem-centered focus)
- Adult motivation migrates from external (extrinsic) motivators to internal (intrinsic) motivators. (Motivation)
- Adults are relevancy orientated and needing to know why they need to learn and what benefits it will provide. (Relevancy)
- Adults expect a respectful learning environment, both with regard to themselves and to others. (Respect)

Since Knowles' original works in the 1960s, there have been many other adult education concepts and theories introduced, but the simulation literature is primarily reflective of Knowles' work.

- Example of ALT being applied to an education program – An ECMO educator conducts a survey followed by some select interviews of key staff to help determine continuing education priorities for the upcoming year. The educator designs a series of simulations that addresses the top concerns (relevancy). The simulations (problem-centered focus) are presented in a safe learning environment where the stated goal is for learning and experimentation for learners to push beyond their baseline (respect). As the year progresses, the educator works with NICU leadership to post key quality indicators that show the simulations have helped improve performance (motivation).

Self-Efficacy Theory – Self-efficacy theory is frequently embedded in other learning theories including social cognitive theory and social learning theory. Albert Bandura [56] defined this theory as "the belief in one's capabilities to organize and execute the courses of action required to manage prospective situations" [57] (p. 2). Simulation lends itself well to this learning theory as it provides a platform for learners to progress to a level of confidence in their own abilities to take on the task in the real world.

- Example of self-efficacy theory being applied to an education program – As part of orientation to the NICU, the educator designed a series of simulations that each gets progressively more difficult. As new staff members begin the simulation series, they build confidence in their abilities. Debriefings are conducted in a manner where staff feel free to discuss their concerns and remaining limitations in their abilities. The debriefings show that all the learners are learning together and they can see their progress. Because the simulations were designed to allow learners a series of successes, not only is their ability to perform NICU patient care improved, they also have the confidence to enact this care effectively.

Social Learning Theory – Simply stated, social learning theory is when people learn from each other. This could be through observation, imitation, or modeling. Bandura was a key developer of this theory [58]. Vygotsky [53] also contributed to this theory as he proposed much of learning is accomplished through interactions with other.

Bandura described four processes that must be in place for effective modeling: attention (attending to observing the behavior being modeled), retention (embedding the observation into memory), reproduction (replicating the behavior), and motivation (willingness to perform the behavior).

Social learning theory is central to the concept of communities of practice, which are groups that form around activity domains that have a shared set of concepts and practices and involve members with varied abilities [59]. Study groups, which are common in healthcare education, are a version of social learning.

- Example of social learning theory being applied to an education program – A simulation educator is faced with too large a group to be accommodated in a single ECMO transport simulation scenario. The educator decides to have half of the group watch remotely while the other half does the simulation. The educator assigns each observer a specific area of the simulation to watch (Attention) and gives each a checklist for them to record their observations (Retention). After the scenario, the two groups switch places, and the observation group now runs the scenario (Reproduction). The educator notes in the debriefing how the original observation group was able to avoid some errors made by the first group while replicating positive actions (Motivation).

A fuller description of these theories has been provided by other authors [2, 60].

While each of these theories is distinct, there are several overlapping shared concepts. One common point most of these theories have is their origins in psychology. As Wenger pointed out, "Learning has traditionally been the province of *psychological* theories" [59] (p. 216, emphasis in original). This chapter will focus on a relatively newer learning theory that has been evolving since the late twentieth century that shifts from a psychological perspective to a biological viewpoint.

Brain-Based Learning

As neuroscience technology developed, understanding of how the brain functions in memory, recall, and learning has greatly increased. Spurred on by pioneering work by such researchers as Paul MacLean [61] and Nobel Laureate Gerald Edleman [62], investigations into the physiological workings of the brain and how the brain learns have evolved into a new field of educational theory study termed brain-based learning (BBL), also called neuroeducation or educational neuroscience.

First brought to attention by Leslie Hart [63], brain-based learning examines the biology of learning. As James Zull explained, "The main message is that *learning is change*. It is change in ourselves, because it is change in the brain. Thus the art of teaching must be the art of changing the brain" [64] (p. xiv, emphasis in original). Eric Jenson added, BBL is "learning in accordance with the way the brain is naturally designed to learn" [65] (p. 6). With a firm grounding in neuroscience, some educators have been stronger in their emphasis, as David Sousa stated, "no longer is teaching just an art form, it is a science" [66] (p. 35).

The idea that the brain is not a fixed structure but one that is able to grow and create new connections has had a steadily increasing body of evidence. Termed brain plasticity or neuroplasticity, this concept is fundamental to brain-based learning.

In healthcare simulation, brain-based learning has only recently become a topic [36, 67]. However, it is highly applicable to healthcare simulation. Central to its role in education is the concept of brain *compatible* versus brain *antagonistic* practices [68]. Brain antagonistic teaching practices impede learning because they inhibit processes in the way the brain learns. Examples of these brain antagonistic practices include high negative stress, too much information over too short a period of time, inadequate time to process new information, lack of relevance or application, teaching a class to learners who are not physically prepared to learn, and boring or disengaging lessons.

- Example – The NICU educator needs to make sure all staff that attend births as part of the NICU response team are updated on their newborn resuscitation skills. In order to cover the night shift nursing staff, the educator arranges to come in at 7 AM so the night shift can attend after completing their 12 hour shift. Because of an upcoming accreditation visit, the educator has been told to make sure everybody gets through the program and that each of them passes a test that demonstrates competency. The educator has secured a series of videos that demonstrate resuscitation practices; however, the video series is old and uses antiquated equipment and supplies that are no longer current in practice. The educator plans to conclude the program with a skills station focused on a newborn resuscitation. When the accreditation team visits a few weeks later and ask these nurses about resuscitation practices, staff members have difficulty responding with correct actions.
- Analysis: This educator employed several brain *antagonistic* practices:
  - Capacity to learn – The staff were exhausted at the end of a long shift. Their brains were well below optimal learning capacity.
  - Stress – The staff was told they must pass a test, which created negative stress.
  - Engagement – The videos were a one-way transmission and learning methods did not encourage engagement, especially considering how tired the learners were.
  - Relevance – The age of the videos and the outdated equipment and supplies reduced the perception of application for the skills.

On the other hand, brain *compatible* teaching takes advantage of how the brain learns best. Using the same scenario as above, this educator has taken a different approach to learning:

- Revised Example – The educator works with unit management to schedule needed training for the night shift staff that does not require them to stay late after their shift is completed. The education program will now occur during their normal shift time. While there is a required test, the educator devises a program that will allow learners to build successes and prepare them for the final skills evaluation. Combining elements from experiential learning and adult learning theories, the program includes interactive lessons that are directly related to the staff's work world and use equipment, supplies, and practices that are current in the system. Teaching cases were based on actual patient care episodes in the unit.
- Analysis: This educator has now employed several brain compatible practices:
  - Capacity to learn – Respectful of the staff's biologic working habits, the learners attend these sessions at times that are part of their regular routine.
  - Stress – The educator designed a series of exercises to prepare the learners for the final skills evaluation. The educational plan included opportunities for the learners to build confidence as they practiced skills essential to passing the evaluation.
  - Engagement – The education sessions were interactive and engaged learners in a series of experiences that helped them to apply the content more effectively. Because the learning experiences were based on the skills needed for the final evaluation, the shift from learning to evaluation was much more subtle.
  - Relevance – Equipment, supplies, and practices were current with what learners were used to in everyday practice. The use of real cases added to this relevance.

As noted in this example, brain-based learning does not necessarily need to stand on its own as an exclusive learning theory. It can be integrated with other theories, but done so in a way that respects the tenets of BBL.

While there are many authors and researchers who have written about brain-based learning, one research team organized concepts in a manner that is particularly conducive and applicable to simulation-based learning. In their 1991 book *Making Connections: Teaching and the Human Brain*, Renata Nummela Caine and Geoffrey Caine presented three elements to support brain compatible learning [69]. Since its publication, *Making Connections* has become one of the most cited books on the topic in the general education literature. As with much of the education literature that has been adapted in health professions education, Caine and Caine's work had a focus on elementary and secondary education (although they do provide some adult education examples). However, since the concepts are based in human biology – specifically the biology of the brain – extrapolation to health professions education is reasonable.

Caine and Caine introduced three core elements that serve as the base components in their approach to brain-based learning: orchestrated immersion into complex activities, relaxed alertness, and active processing.

Orchestrated immersion into complex activities combines purposeful planning of educational activities with stimulating multisensory experiences. Purposeful planning in health professions education means having a goal, objectives, and purpose. Educators typically use structured curriculum planning processes such as the Dick, Carey, and Carey model [70] or the Kern six-step model [71] to identify the problem for which education is the solution, perform learner and task analysis, create instructional goals, write learning objectives, develop instructional materials, and conduct learner and program evaluation. But while this structure is vital, the need for spontaneity for both learners and teachers is also paramount.

Simulation provides the opportunity for this level of immersion. One of the most common, repeated themes in simulation is the "suspension of disbelief;" the ability to create a learning environment so real, learners respond with actions and emotions as they would in a real-world situation. Simulation scenarios also need to reflect real, relevant problems so that learners see the application or create decision-making processes that can be applied to other situations in their work world.

Interprofessional education (IPE) is another area where this immersion becomes valuable. Caine and Caine discuss the power of groups. Realizing the "human brain is a social brain" [69] (p. 125), the interaction between interprofessional or transprofessional[1] group members is vital to the learning process. Consistent with the concept that IPE is learning with, from, and about each other, the immersive experiences should provide for equal learning opportunities across the group membership.

Relaxed alertness is the idea that learners must be activated, meaning they are alert, engaged, and challenged but not threatened. Harkening back to early brain theories developed by Paul MacLean, brain biology has evolved over many millennia. As part of that evolution, humans have different pathways for processing information, encoding information to memory, retrieving information from memory, and making decisions. Moving from a high level of positive activation (good stress or eustress) to a state of threat (bad stress or distress) changes the way humans manage information as they learn [68, 69].

In healthcare simulation, it may manifest in this example:

> The medical center's air and ground critical care transport team that supports inter-facility ECMO transports is scheduled to complete a training program in neonatal ECMO care. They have been told they must pass the test or their jobs will be at risk. The instructor is overbearing, harsh in his criticisms, and using teaching techniques that one might, at best, call behavioristic. The learners are under tremendous negative stress and fear as they respond to the critiques of the instructor and try to shape their behaviors to meet his demands. The learners' actions eventually are molded to meet the instructor's requirement for passing the test.

So, what happened with their learning? On the surface, it appears they learned since they were able to muster enough knowledge and skill to pass the test requirements. However, the true test of learning will be in demonstrating learned behaviors during a neonatal ECMO transport. This is where some problems may arise.

In simplistic terms, this is what happened: the amount of negative stress and fear activated learning pathways in their brains that triggered what amounted to a survival mechanism, the classic fight-or-flight response. In this case, the survival situation was to get out of this class with an acceptable passing score. The portion of the brain used to process this information is very good at managing short-term decision-making but suffers when it comes to encoding to long-term memory. The means by which learning was validated was an immediate post-course test. However, the information quickly degrades from the short-term working memory used for the scenario, and in a matter of days (maybe even hours), the information is no longer available for retrieval. The problem with this process will manifest itself later when there is a need to apply the information to a real clinical scenario. Without adequate encoding to long-term memory, the information is just not there.

To effectively store information in long-term memory, other pathways are required for encoding – pathways that are bypassed in high negative stress and fearful situations. Leslie Hart calls this "downshifting" [63] (p. 121). Hart used examples such as witnessing a crime or being involved in a car crash. These threatening situations allowed the brain to function well to get out of immediate danger, but when called upon for details later, the detailed memories as witness or victim were not clear. In an educational context, many people experience this same phenomenon when cramming for a test. They may get through the survival situation of passing the test, but long-term memory encoding is impaired.

Threat also limits experimentation and risk taking by learners. In a threatening or fearful environment, the learner will not take control of their own learning; they will relegate themselves to a passive participant responding to the demands of the instructor. The safe learning environment commonly referenced in simulation-based learning is an example of a counter strategy to mitigate threat. With threat neutralized, learners are able to process information more effectively to long-term memory, feel free to take risks through experimentation, and have greater motivation to learn.

Caine and Caine call the optimal learning environment "high challenge and low threat" [69] (p. 143). Knowing that failure is an opportunity to learn, learners will be motivated to push themselves through scenarios that they might not otherwise tackle. A common healthcare simulation strategy is briefing prior to the simulation where learners are advised of the safe learning environment. This briefing leads to

[1]Transprofessional education includes non-healthcare providers including patient, family, and community who join with the interprofessional and interdisciplinary health team members to extend the learning group.

reduced anxiety and fear of the situation [72]. One manifestation of this approach is the concept of the *Basic Assumption* which advocates that instructors view their learners as being intelligent individuals who care about doing their best and want to improve [73].

Another area of focus for reducing distress and fear is democratizing the learning environment. Similar to the patient safety push for removing the clinical hierarchy in practice, this same flattening of the hierarchy in learning situations creates an environment where everyone is equal in their roles as learners, including the instructors who assume a position as a co-learner as they facilitate the learning opportunity.

Techniques for debriefing and feedback must also take into account the safe learning environment and respect for learners.

Debriefing must be done in a collaborative, respectful manner that fosters a sense of trust and sharing between learners and facilitators. Among the debriefing techniques that can be employed that follows a BBL approach is the "Debriefing with Good Judgment" model [74]. This model respects the learner's perspective as the facilitator probes for the source of actions. Rather than just provide direction for behavior changes as in a behavioristic model, the facilitator goes back to the roots of learner's understanding to identify misperceptions, misinterpretations, or knowledge gaps that triggered questionable actions. Realigning these understandings to the needs of the simulation will create a more lasting change and help guide future behavior.

As with debriefing, feedback requires the same attitudinal approach from the facilitator and can refer back to principles of adult learning. To fully engage the learner in brain compatible feedback, the feedback should be two way between learner and instructor. Feedback becomes a conversation rather than directive orders. One feedback technique that can be used is commonly referred to as Pendleton Rules [75].

Similar to the Plus/Delta technique [76], the Pendleton feedback methodology engages the learner in a discussion that first reviews what went well (the Plus of the Plus/Delta model) and what could be changed (the Delta of the Plus/Delta model). Where it differs from the Plus/Delta model is in the intentionality of how the conversation progresses. In a process of taking turns, the learner first states what went well, which is then followed by the facilitator affirming the learner's perspective and adding additional information. Moving on to the next phase of the conversation, the learner again takes the lead by stating what could be changed or done differently. This is followed by the facilitator affirming the learner's viewpoints and adding additional observations. Allowing the learner to self-reflect or critique his or her own experience helps to build higher-order metacognitive capabilities that can be used to analyze self-performance well beyond the simulation session.

Building on the original Pendleton model, some modifications will make this better aligned with brain-based learning:

- Prior to starting the feedback session, determine if the learner is ready for feedback. If the learner is upset with his or her performance or has other emotional responses that will impede the effectiveness of the feedback, it will be better to wait until those subside.
- If there are other learners in the group, they must also be engaged. Inserting an additional step in the turn-taking process to include opportunity from other learners or observers after the primary learner allows for this level of engagement. Additionally, the other learners or observers are performing evaluation which, when looking at Bloom's taxonomy of the cognitive domain [77], demonstrates a high level cognitive function.
- Working together, the learner and facilitator develop a plan to further advance the learner. This may include referring the learner to an article or video, working with another individual in the simulation center on task training, or getting additional feedback in the workplace.

Active Processing is, as Caine and Caine describe, the opportunity for the learner "to make sense of the experience" [69] (p. 156). In simulation practice, this process is typically referred to as reflection and manifests itself in the debriefing. This is the inward examination of how learners view their knowledge, skills, and attitudes and how they shape their understandings based on new information. This step is frequently an essential component in experiential learning cycles such as Kolb's depiction of the Lewian learning cycle [46]. Caine and Caine also reference experiential learning as they described John Dewey's "learning loop."

Active processing is a deliberate act that connects learners' prior experiences with those of the present experience. It allows each learner to make connections and extend understanding (similar to constructivism). Caine and Caine supplied one line that succinctly captures the goal: "It is the path to understanding, rather than simply to memory" [69] (p. 156).

However, healthcare simulation-based education has a limitation in the way active processing is applied. In simulation-based education, active processing is often a specific part of a longitudinal process – a simulation experience followed by an immediate post-simulation debriefing with very little follow-up after the debriefing. This time frame limits what active processing can be done.

Active processing needs to be a continuing process that is not relegated to a designated time and which becomes part of the learner's routine, both after simulation sessions and beyond. As an example, educators John O'Donnell and Joseph Goode integrated a continuing process of reflection in their nurse anesthesia program that first included a standard debriefing using the structured and supported debriefing model after a simulation experience, but was followed by an email communications several days later asking learners for their thoughts (reflections) on how the simulation experience was influencing their clinical learning and practice [78, 79]. Similar to the reflective activity of journaling, the goal was to stimulate thought in the learners beyond the simulation and help to relate it to real clinical events while also integrating the continuing reflective process into daily practice. The ability to develop reflective habits without a facilitator guiding the reflection is indicative of Schön's reflective practitioner [47].

Conclusion

Brain-based learning does not operate in isolation. As seen through the examples and discussion of this chapter, BBL is a foundational theory upon which other situation appropriate learning theories can be applied. These theories working with BBL can create the best opportunities for learners to learn – the ability to know or do something new or different – and can be enhanced by using the right learning theories, adding a level of prediction to outcomes that is more precise than trial and error.

References

1. Brookfield SD. The power of critical theory: liberating adult learning and teaching. San Fransicso: Jossey-Bass; 2005.
2. Kaufman DM, Mann KV. Teaching and learning in medical education: how theory can inform practice. In: Swanwick T, editor. Understanding medical education: evidence, theory, and practice. Oxford, UK: Wiley-Blackwell; 2010. p. 16–36.
3. Alinier G, Hunt WB, Gordon R. Determining the value of simulation in nurse education: study design and initial results. Nurse Educ Pract. 2004;4(3):200–7.
4. Anderson JM, Warren JB. Using simulation to enhance the acquisition and retention of clinical skills in neonatology. Semin Perinatol. 2011;35(2):59–67.
5. Auerbach M, Kessler D, Foltin JC. Repetitive pediatric simulation resuscitation training. Pediatr Emerg Care. 2011;27(1):29–31.
6. Buykx P, Kinsman L, Cooper S, McConnell-Henry T, Cant R, Endacott R, et al. FIRST2ACT: educating nurses to identify patient deterioration – a theory-based model for best practice simulation education. Nurse Educ Today. 2011;31(7):687–93.
7. Chauvin SW. Applying educational theory to simulation-based training and assessment in surgery. Surg Clin North Am. 2015;95(4):695–715.
8. Dreifuerst KT. The essentials of debriefing in simulation learning: a concept analysis. Nurs Educ Perspect. 2009;30(2):109–14.
9. Edward K, Hercelinskyj J, Warelow P, Munro I. Simulation to practice: developing nursing skills in mental health – an Australian perspective. Int Electron J Health Educ. 2007;10:60–4.
10. Fey MK, Jenkins LS. Debriefing practices in nursing education programs: results from a national study. Nurs Educ Perspect. 2015;36(6):361–6.
11. Gardner R. Introduction to debriefing. Semin Perinatol. 2013;37(3):166–74.
12. Hoadley TA. Learning advanced cardiac life support: a comparison study of the effects of low-and high-fidelity simulation. Nurs Educ Perspect. 2009;30(2):91–5.
13. Kaakinen J, Arwood E. Systematic review of nursing simulation literature for use of learning theory. Int J Nurs Educ Scholarsh. 2009;6(1):1–20.
14. Lasater K. High-fidelity simulation and the development of clinical judgment: Students' experiences. J Nurs Educ. 2007;46(6):269–76.
15. Lavoie P, Pepin J, Cossette S. Development of a post-simulation debriefing intervention to prepare nurses and nursing students to care for deteriorating patients. Nurse Educ Pract. 2015;15(3):181–91.
16. Lederman L. Debriefing: toward a systematic assessment of theory and practice. Simul Gaming. 1992;23:145–60.
17. Lederman LC. Debriefing: a critical reexamination of the postexperience analytic process with implications for its effective use. Simul Gaming. 1984;15(4):415–31.
18. Mayville ML. Debriefing: the essential step in simulation. Newborn Infant Nurs Rev. 2011;11(1):35–9.
19. Rourke L, Schmidt M, Garga N. Theory-based research of high fidelity simulation use in nursing education: a review of the literature. Int J Nurs Educ Scholarsh. 2010;7(1):1–14.
20. Zigmont JJ, Kappus LJ, Sudikoff SN. Theoretical foundations of learning through simulation. Semin Perinatol. 2011;35(2):47–51.
21. Rothgeb MK. Creating a nursing simulation laboratory: a literature review. J Nurs Educ. 2008;47(11):489–94.
22. French HM, Hales RL. Neonatology faculty development using simulation. Semin Perinatol. 2016;40(7):455–65.
23. Dreifuerst K. Using debriefing for meaningful learning to foster development of clinical reasoning in simulation. J Nurs Educ. 2012;51(6):326–33.
24. Hallmark BF. Faculty development in simulation education. Nurs Clin North Am. 2015;50(2):389–97.
25. Kolbe M, Grande B, Spahn DR. Briefing and debriefing during simulation-based training and beyond: content, structure, attitude and setting. Best Pract Res Clin Anaesthesiol. 2015;29(1):87–96.
26. Kriz WC. A systemic-constructivist approach to the facilitation and debriefing of simulations and games. Simul Gaming. 2010;41(5):663–80.
27. Kuiper R, Heinrich C, Matthias A, Graham MJ, Bell-Kotwall L. Debriefing with the OPT model of clinical reasoning during high fidelity patient simulation. Int J Nurs Educ Scholarsh. 2008;5(1):1–14.
28. Neill MA, Wotton K. High-fidelity simulation debriefing in nursing education: a literature review. Clin Simul Nurs. 2011;7(5):e161–e8.
29. Palmer MH, Kowlowitz V, Campbell J, Carr C, Dillon R, Durham CF, et al. Using clinical simulations in geriatric nursing continuing education. Nurs Outlook. 2008;56(4):159–66.
30. Parker BC, Myrick F. A critical examination of high-fidelity human patient simulation within the context of nursing pedagogy. Nurse Educ Today. 2009;29(3):322–9.
31. Reilly A, Spratt C. The perceptions of undergraduate student nurses of high-fidelity simulation-based learning: a case report from the University of Tasmania. Nurse Educ Today. 2007;27(6):542–50.
32. Campbell M, Themessl-Huber M, Mole L, Scarlett V. Using simulation to prepare students for interprofessional work in the community. J Nurs Educ. 2007;46(7):340.
33. Feingold CE, Calaluce M, Kallen MA. Computerized patient model and simulated clinical experiences: evaluation with baccalaureate nursing students. J Nurs Educ. 2004;43(4):156–63.
34. Rutherford-Hemming T. Simulation methodology in nursing education and adult learning theory. Adult Learn. 2012;23(3):129–37.
35. Fewster-Thuente L, Batteson TJ. Kolb's experiential learning theory as a theoretical underpinning for interprofessional education. J Allied Health. 2018;47(1):3–8.

36. Clapper TC. Beyond Knowles: what those conducting simulation need to know about adult learning theory. Clin Simul Nurs. 2010;6(1):e7–e14.
37. Goldenberg D, Andrusyszyn MA, Iwasiw C. The effect of classroom simulation on nursing students' self-efficacy related to health teaching. J Nurs Educ. 2005;44(7):310–4.
38. LeFlore JL, Anderson M. Effectiveness of 2 methods to teach and evaluate new content to neonatal transport personnel using high-fidelity simulation. J Perinat Neonatal Nurs. 2008;22(4):319–28.
39. Rhodes ML, Curran C. Use of the human patient simulator to teach clinical judgment skills in a baccalaureate nursing program. Comput Inform Nurs. 2005;23(5):256–62.
40. Schoening AM, Sittner BJ, Todd MJ. Simulated clinical experience: nursing students' perceptions and the educators' role. Nurse Educ. 2006;31(6):253–8.
41. Wayman KI, Yaeger KA, Sharek PJ, Trotter S, Wise L, Flora JA, et al. Simulation-based medical error disclosure training for pediatric healthcare professionals. J Healthc Qual. 2007;29(4):12–9.
42. Berragan L. Simulation: an effective pedagogical approach for nursing? Nurse Educ Today. 2011;31(7):660–3.
43. Clapper TC. Cooperative-based learning and the zone of proximal development. Simul Gaming. 2015;46(2):148–58.
44. Dewey J. Experience and education. New York: Simon & Schuster; 1938.
45. Lewin K. Field theory in social science: selected theoretical papers. 1st ed. New York: Harper; 1951.
46. Kolb DA. Experiential learning: experience as the source of learning and development. 2nd ed. Englewood Cliffs: Prentice-Hall; 1984.
47. Schön DA. The reflective practitioner: how professionals think in action. New York: Basic Books; 1983.
48. Ericsson KA. Deliberate practice and the acquisition and maintenance of expert performance in medicine and related domains. Acad Med. 2004;79(10):S70–81.
49. Paiget J. The construction of reality in the child. Abingdon: Routledge; 1954.
50. Bruner J. Toward a theory of instruction. Boston: Harvard University Press; 1966.
51. Ausubel DP. Educational psychology: a cognitive view. New York: Holt, Rinehart and Winston; 1968.
52. Kneebone RL, Scott W, Darzi A, Horrocks M. Simulation and clinical practice: strengthening the relationship. Med Educ. 2004;38(10):1095–102.
53. Vygotsky LS. Mind in society: the development of higher psychological processes (A. R. Luria, M. Lopez-Morillas & M. Cole [with J. V. Wertsch], Trans.). Cambridge, MA: Harvard University Press; 1978.
54. Lindeman E. The meaning of adult education. New York: New Republic; 1926.
55. Knowles MS, Holton EF, Swanson RA. The adult learner: the definitive classic in adult education and human resource development. 5th ed. Woburn: Butterworth-Heineman; 1998.
56. Bandura A. Self efficacy: toward a unifying theory of behavioral change. Psychol Rev. 1977;84:191–215.
57. Bandura A. Self efficacy in changing societies. New York: Cambridge University Press; 1995.
58. Bandura A. Social learning theory. New York: General Learning Press; 1977.
59. Wenger E. A social theory of learning. In: Illeris K, editor. Contemporary theories of learning: learning theorists – in their own words. London: Routledge; 2009. p. 209–18.
60. Morrison JB, Deckers C. Common theories in healthcare simulation. In: Palaganas JC, Maxworthy JC, Epps CA, Mancini ME, editors. Defining excellence in simulation porgrams. Philadelphia: Wolters Kluwer; 2015. p. 496–508.
61. MacLean PD. A triune concept of the brain and behavior. In: Boag TJ, Campbell D, editors. The Hincks memorial lectures. Toronto: University of Toronto Press; 1973. p. 6–66.
62. Edelman GM. Bright air, brilliant fire: on the matter of the mind. New York: Basic Books; 1992.
63. Hart LA. How the brain works: a new understanding of human learning, emotion, and thinking. New York: Basic Books; 1975.
64. Zull JE. The art of changing the brain: enriching the practice of teaching by exploring the biology of learning. Sterling: Stylus Publishing; 2002.
65. Jensen E. Brain-based learning. Thousand Oaks: Corwin Press; 2000.
66. Sousa DA. Is the fuss about brain research justified? Educ Week. 1998;18(16):35.
67. Rodgers DL. The biological basis of learning: Neuroeducation through simulation. Simul Gaming. 2015;46(2):175–86.
68. Hart LA. Human brain and human learning. London: Longman; 1983.
69. Caine R, Caine G. Making connections: teaching and the human brain. Menlo Park: Addison-Wesley; 1994.
70. Dick W, Carey L, Carey JO. The systematic design of instruction. 8th ed. Bostom: Pearson; 2015.
71. Thomas PA, Kern DE, Hughes MT, Chen BY, editors. Curriclum development for medical education: a six-step approach. 3rd ed. Baltimore: Johns Hopkins University Press; 2016.
72. Tyerman J, Luctkar-Flude M, Graham L, Coffey S, Olsen-Lynch E. Pre-simulation preparation and briefing practices for healthcare professionals and students: a systematic review protocol. JBI Database System Rev Implement Rep. 2016;14(8):80–9.
73. Rudolph JW, Simon R, Raemer DB, Eppich WJ. Debriefing as formative assessment: closing performance gaps in medical education. Acad Emerg Med. 2008;15(11):1010–6.
74. Rudolph JW, Simon R, Dufresne RL, Raemer DB. There's no such thing as "nonjudgmental" debriefing: a theory and method for debriefing with good judgment. Simul Healthc. 2006;1(1):49–55.
75. Pendleton D, Schofield T, Tate P, Havelock P. The consultation: an approach to learning and teaching. Oxford: Oxford University Press; 1984.
76. Fanning RM, Gaba DM. The role of debriefing in simulation-based learning. Simul Healthc. 2007;2(2):115–25.
77. Bloom B, Engelhart M, Furst EJ, Hill W, Krathwohl D. Taxonomy of educational objectives, handbook I: the cognitive domain. New York: David McKay Co. Inc.; 1956.
78. Goode JS Jr. Action, practice and reflection: Dewey's pragmatist philosophy and the current healthcare simulation movement. In: Bluhm R, editor. Knowing and acting in medicine. London: Rowan and Littlefield; 2016.
79. Phrampus PE, O'Donnell JM. Debriefing: using a structured and supported approach. In: Levine AL, Bryson EO, DeMaria S, Schwartz AD, editors. The comprehensive textbook of healthcare simulation. New York: Springer; 2013.

Designing an ECMO Simulation Curriculum

6

Miheer Sane and Mary E. McBride

Learning Objectives

1. Apply the six-step model for curriculum development to create an ECMO simulation curriculum.
2. Assess the different learners involved in an ECMO curriculum, the current state of their established trainings, and how simulation education can improve this training.
3. Compare and contrast resources involved in a simulation curriculum including fidelity, technology, cost, and environmental-specifics and select-appropriate resources for particular goals and objectives.
4. Assess how ECPR simulation can be applied at individual centers to both develop familiarity and uncover latent safety threats.
5. Construct simulation cases of ECMO complications with a physiologic conceptual framework based on preload, contractility, and afterload.

Introduction

The initiation and maintenance of extracorporeal membrane oxygenation (ECMO) support is a complex process that tests all aspects of providers' abilities including knowledge, technical skills, and interprofessional teamwork and communication. ECMO complications account for up to 25% of patient mortality [1]. Even in highly experienced centers, ECMO is an overall low-frequency intervention with significant risks. As supported by reduced time to cannulation [2] and reduced time to initiation of the ECMO circuit to restore circulation, [3] an ECMO simulation curriculum has the potential to improve patient outcomes. Through simulation, providers can practice in a risk-free setting to develop mastery, maintain competency, and advance toward a higher level of performance. The use of simulation has grown rapidly, but successful use of this modality requires thoughtful design and appropriate curriculum development.

M. Sane
Department of Pediatrics, Hospital-Based Medicine, Ann & Robert H Lurie Children's Hospital of Chicago, Chicago, IL, USA

M. E. McBride (✉)
Divisions of Cardiology and Critical Care Medicine, Department of Pediatrics and Medical Education, Ann & Robert H Lurie Children's Hospital of Chicago, Chicago, IL, USA
e-mail: mmcbride@luriechildrens.org

Curriculum Development

An established approach to curriculum development for medical education is the six-step model by Thomas and Kern et al. [4]. This model can also be applied to ECMO simulation curriculum development. The six steps include (a) problem identification and general needs assessment, (b) a targeted needs assessment, (c) goals and objectives, (d) educational strategies, (e) implementation, and (f) evaluation and feedback. Details on each of the six steps and examples of application to an ECMO simulation curriculum are provided in Table 6.1.

The process starts with (a) problem identification and a general needs assessment. The problem first needs to be clearly defined, perhaps initially based on the institution's specific issues, but then expanded to a more global scale. This can be accomplished by review of current relevant published literature to assess what has already been described, what is known or has previously been developed that can be applied to this specific institution, and what advancements have been made [4]. These findings would then help guide the (b) targeted needs assessment, which is specific to the institution and learners at that institution. This step of the process may require questionnaires or surveys to initially gather data from learners and begin involvement of specific stakeholders. The targeted needs assessment may test the learners' knowledge,

L. C. Johnston, L. Su (eds.), *Comprehensive Healthcare Simulation: ECMO Simulation*, Comprehensive Healthcare Simulation,
https://doi.org/10.1007/978-3-030-53844-6_6

Table 6.1 Application of a six-step approach to an ECMO simulation curriculum

Kern's six-step approach	Details	ECMO curriculum examples
1. Problem identification and general needs assessment	Clear definition of the problem and how it is currently being addressed General needs assessment describes the current approach to the problem and how that differs from the ideal approach	Problem- improve ECMO training Review of the current ECMO training requirements and current simulation curricula
2. Targeted needs assessment	Survey stakeholders: Define specific skills and knowledge of these learners Identify and define gaps Institution and learner specific	Stake holders: Medical providers: physicians, nurses, pharmacists, respiratory therapists Surgical providers- physicians, OR nursing and staff ECMO specialists (institution-specific) Administration for finances and needed resources Assess what needs improvement, learning styles, and practicalities for delivery of the training Will differ for programs with an already established ECMO curriculum and those establishing a new curriculum
3. Goals and objectives	Critical step as it guides all further development and evaluation of the curriculum Goals may initially be broad but then should be broken down into specific measurable objectives Objectives may also be organized and built in a sequential order to help guide development from novice to expert	Sample broad goal: improve surgical provider proficiency in cannulation Sample sequential measurable objectives: Know the appropriate cannulation approach in various patients measured by pre and post written test Demonstrate competency of the technical aspects of cannulation measured by expert generated checklist with use of a task trainer for cannulation practice and testing Demonstrate efficient time to cannulation during simulated extracorporeal cardiopulmonary resuscitation (ECPR) measured by time to cannulation during immersive simulation with ongoing active CPR
4. Educational strategies	Tailored to achieve specific goals and objectives both from the perspective of content and methodology Environment can also be manipulated based on learner level May incorporate other modalities where appropriate: classroom didactics, "flipped classrooms", computer based e-learning, and serious games	Sample strategies: Novice- work with lower fidelity models or small group discussions in a sterile environment to allow focus to simply understand the various cannulation strategies Intermediate- task trainers for practicing cannulation Expert- immersive in situ simulation with ongoing CPR that naturally comes with more stress and noise
5. Implementation	Most successful if well-planned and with pre-identified resources Piloting a simulation case is imperative	Once ECMO cases are developed, pilot the cases and get feedback from stakeholders and figure how best to incorporate into an already existent ECMO curriculum if present
6. Evaluation and feedback	Assessment of the learner: achievement, satisfaction, accreditation Assessment of the curriculum: determining if the goals and objectives of the curriculum have been met Blueprinting Assessment tools Continuous feedback of the program	Provide formative feedback to providers after ECMO simulations Consider developing an ECMO certification with use of a rigorously constructed assessment tool

skill, and comfort to identify and define gaps. Stakeholders to survey could include members of the medical team including physicians, pharmacists, nursing, respiratory therapists, ECMO specialists, the surgical team, and administration for resources of protected time, finances, and space.

Developing appropriate goals and objectives (c) is a critical step as it guides all further development and evaluation of the curriculum. Learning objectives are statements that define the goals of the curriculum; they must be specific and measurable to guide the rest of the process. Johnston et al. discuss that objectives should describe the intended learner, what will be accomplished, how it should be performed, over what timeframe, and how the outcome will be assessed [5]. Regarding educational strategies (d), although we are discussing an ECMO simulation curriculum, it should be noted that simulation is just one of many educational modalities. Tailoring the objective to an appropriate educational strategy is useful, as not all objectives will be best achieved through simulation and some may not justify the higher costs, time, space, and other limitations associated with the use of simulation. Other educational methods may include traditional lectures and "flipped classrooms" where the learners develop knowledge on particular topics prior to class and can apply that knowledge using problem-based learning (PBL) or case-based discussions, computer-based programs and e-learning, and "serious games" [5].

Implementation of the curriculum (e) will be most successful if it is well-planned and resources are identified beforehand, during the targeted needs assessment. Even a well-designed curriculum may have difficulty with implementation if not adequately planned, with buy in from stakeholders, and a shared mental model regarding its need. Piloting a simulation curriculum is also imperative. In implementation, thoroughly vetted cases may not run or be perceived by learners as previously planned on paper. It is important to run the case on the patient simulator as written, assessing if physical exam findings and vital signs displayed on the patient monitor accurately depict the intended scenario. A few knowledgeable participants, who are blinded to the content of the case, can then practice the case in the same way a learner will. Feedback can be obtained on the realism, flow, and content of the case to then assist in any adjustments needed [4].

For (f) evaluation and feedback, each step throughout the curriculum development process affects the assessment approach. Well-designed assessments depend on learning objectives that, as noted above, are specific and measurable. Learning objectives evolve into assessment content (i.e., test questions or checklists) by a process called blueprinting. The blueprinting process is an itemized plan of the assessment process to assure that all aspects of the curriculum that need to be evaluated are done so properly. Coderre et al. provide a detailed guide on the blueprinting process [6]. Also, more detail on evaluation designs and methods can be found in Chapter 7 of "Curriculum Development for Medical Education" [4]. In deciding what assessment tool to use, the educator must decide if they will use a tool already found in the literature or create one de novo. In either case, one must have a strong understanding of reliability and validity in order to use a tool properly. The higher the stakes of the assessment, the more rigor is required in assuring reliability and validity of the data obtained via the tool(s). Should an assessment tool be created for certification, it must be constructed rigorously from a psychometric perspective. Data obtained from a rigorous assessment process allows for accurate decisions to be made about the learner (competent or not; certified or not) and the educational program (effective or not). More about the controversies in certification will be covered in Chap. 16.

Components of an ECMO Simulation Curriculum

An ECMO curriculum can be conceptualized in its parts. In addition to the cases themselves, which will be discussed for the remainder of this chapter, other components include (I) the learners, (II) the physical setting, and (III) debriefing and reflection.

(I) Learners can consist of ECMO specialists, medical providers, bedside nurses, pharmacists, respiratory therapists, and surgical providers. An ECMO specialist is defined as "the technical specialist trained to manage the ECMO system and the clinical needs of the patient on ECMO under the direction and supervision of a certified ECMO- trained physician" [7]. At this time, ECMO specialists have the most structured education, relative to other providers, so in designing an ECMO curriculum it is helpful to review what is already established for their training. See Chap. 12 for details on the current training recommendations for ECMO specialists. Briefly, ELSO details recommendations on didactic lectures, water drills, animal laboratory practice, working circuit practice of ECMO emergencies, bedside precepting, summative assessment, and ongoing maintenance of certification requirements [7]. While simulation training has not previously been an explicit recommendation for ECMO specialist training, its role is expanding. The 5th edition of the ELSO Red Book introduces the role of high-fidelity simulation to develop specialists' hands-on skills and practice of emergencies [8]. A recent survey of current ELSO sites reflects this change, with only 7% of sites still using the animal laboratory practice and, instead, substituting this with simulation. Nearly 50% of programs are now including simulation in their training of ECMO specialists [9]. There is also literature to support the use of simulation for not only learning but assessment of ECMO specialists. Work by Fehr et al. demonstrated the feasibility of a psychometrically sound curriculum for ECMO specialists [10].

Currently, there are no standardized requirements for medical or surgical providers [7]. A survey of ELSO sites reflects this with 66% of medical intensivists and 90% of surgeons having no specific required ECMO training [9]. It is assumed that provider competency with ECMO was established through their specialty training, but without a specific assessment, it is unknown if gaps exist. Another potential gap seems to be the training for a bedside nurse with a patient on ECMO. There is a dynamic interplay between the bedside nurse and the ECMO specialist in the management of the patient on ECMO. Training of bedside nurses could focus on improving and standardizing knowledge of ECMO complications and how the circuit affects their patient management. Some examples of areas to focus on include the significant impact of anticoagulation on the nursing care of the patient and the importance of closely monitoring an ECMO patient's neurologic status. The ECMO specialist is responsible for the circuit and the bedside nurse for the patient; however, the two are intimately related. Simulation can provide an avenue to build the teamwork needed for this dyad to function optimally. Simulations have been developed specifically for the medical team [11–13], surgical providers [2], ECMO specialists [10], and the entire team to practice teamwork and behavioral skills together [3, 14, 15]. In designing an ECMO curriculum, it remains an important consideration if learners should complete simulations together as a team, individually, or some combination of both, as these practices develop different skills.

(II) Physical factors to consider include the patient simulator and the environment. Learner "suspension of disbelief" is essential for success of simulation education [11]. By simulating reality as much as possible, facilitators increase the chances that participants will provide management as actively and seriously as they would in resuscitating a real patient, which can aid formative feedback, and can improve transfer of what is learned to real practice. Multiple high-fidelity simulators have been developed to allow practice of cannulation [2] and resuscitation of air embolism and hypovolemia [12]. A model of cardiac tamponade has been developed to simulate the enlarging heart through an open chest [16]. As technology improves, one must balance the use of high-cost and resource-intensive models when necessary with use of less costly, less technological, or lower fidelity education strategies when appropriate for a particular objective. Additionally, the physical environment is a factor that can be adjusted as needed to achieve goals. Initial stages can occur in a calmer, controlled, artificial setting like a simulation laboratory or a classroom. As learners advance, the environment may progress to an in situ environment (e.g., a patient room in the intensive care unit) where these real emergencies will happen with all of the added personnel, stress, and noise. This should be complemented by use of the actual equipment, including drawing up medications from the code cart, operating the defibrillator, getting blood from blood bank, etc. Anderson et al. noted that human performance degrades with significant stress, so it is important to recreate and practice in that stressful environment if possible [11]. Additionally, in situ simulation provides an opportunity to assess for latent safety threats within the system [2]. Such safety threats can be identified and potentially resolved in the simulated environment.

(III) Lastly, multiple sources in the literature underscore that debriefing and feedback are the most important part of simulation from a learning perspective [17–19]. This is supported by Kolb's description of experiential learning. Sawyer et al. describe that "experience alone does not lead to learning but rather deliberate reflection on that learning" is necessary [19]. Both debriefing and feedback have their roles in simulation education. Debriefing is an interactive conversation between all participants and the facilitator. Feedback is more directed from the facilitator to the participants to correct specific actions or thought processes. Debriefing will be further discussed in Chap. 15.

Extracorporeal Cardiopulmonary Resuscitation

While the clinical events that call for ECMO are complex and stressful, this stress and complexity is heightened when cannulating during active cardiopulmonary resuscitation, a process called extracorporeal cardiopulmonary resuscitation or ECPR. ECPR involves the orchestration of the surgical team cannulating the patient, the medical team resuscitating the patient, and the ECMO team dispatching and priming the circuit for ECMO initiation after cannulation. A simulation case in this context allows for individual parties to further develop their own skills, but this resource-intense simulation also allows for a focus on teamwork, communication, and assessment of latent safety threats. In order to uncover these threats, it is important to use the actual space, equipment, personnel, and process that will be employed for an actual patient. Su et al. have demonstrated the complexity of ECPR by creating a master checklist of over 90 tasks that are specifically assigned to 16 roles and, through this process, suggested the alluring possibility of reducing time to ECMO initiation for patients who require this intervention [3]. See Fig. 6.1 for a sample ECPR simulation case.

Physiologic Framework for ECMO Complications

In designing a framework for ECMO complications, thinking of the ECMO circuit as an extension of the patient allows us to apply the same essential physiologic principle of oxygen delivery. Underlying any shock state is the imbalance of oxygen delivery and oxygen consumption, a system of supply and demand. ECMO, as well as less invasive therapies, serves to reestablish this balance. The delivery of oxygen (DO_2) is dependent on the oxygen content in arterial blood (CaO_2) and cardiac output (CO). The oxygen content of arterial blood (CaO_2) depends largely on hemoglobin, and the amount of hemoglobin that is saturated with oxygen. Cardiac output (CO) can be broken down into heart rate and stroke volume; furthermore, stroke volume is influenced by preload,

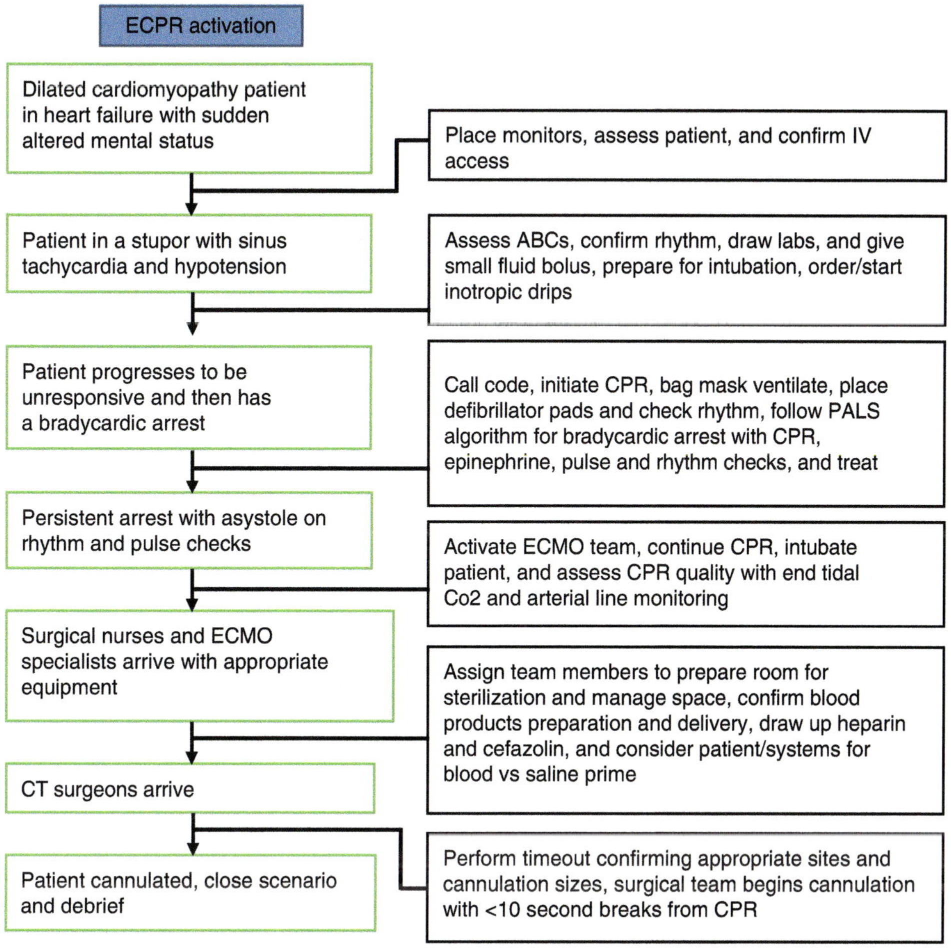

Fig. 6.1 Case 1: ECPR activation

Table 6.2 Physiologic model of ECMO circuit complications

Preload	ECMO pump (contractility)	Afterload
Hypovolemia	Power failure	Pressors
Hemorrhage	Air entrapment	Agitation
Tension pneumothorax	Thrombus within the circuit	Generalized seizures
Pericardial tamponade	Oxygenator failure	Intracranial hypertension
Venous cannula issue Malposition, kink Size Need for a second cannula, i.e., Glenn	Cannula dislodgement	Renal thrombosis Arterial cannula issue Malposition, kink Size Mechanical obstruction

contractility, and afterload. The complications of ECMO can be organized into categories of preload, contractility, and afterload and, more specifically, preload to the ECMO circuit, flow of the ECMO circuit itself (the equivalent of contractility), and afterload against the ECMO circuit as blood returns to the patient (Table 6.2). The key to diagnosis and efficient intervention is recognizing changes in monitoring, including changes and trends in vital signs, the patient's physical exam, and ECMO pump pressures. Different complications can have typical patterns of change with regard to these monitored data points.

ECMO Preload

The ECMO circuit is sensitive to preload [20, 21]. Adequate venous drainage from the patient to the ECMO circuit requires a large bore cannula to maximize flow, but too large of a cannula can collapse a compliant vein. With decreased venous return to the circuit, "chatter" or shaking of the venous cannula can develop. Causes of decreased preload to the ECMO circuit can include hypovolemia or hemorrhage. Hemorrhage is an important complication for patients requiring ECMO. Due to exposure of blood to the artificial surface of tubing and the oxygenator, along with the potential for native cardiopulmonary stasis with patients on ECMO, patients are at high risk for thrombosis and therefore require anticoagulation [20, 21]. This creates a difficult balance, as patients are therefore more prone to hemorrhage. Hemorrhage accounts for nearly 30–40% of all complications in patients

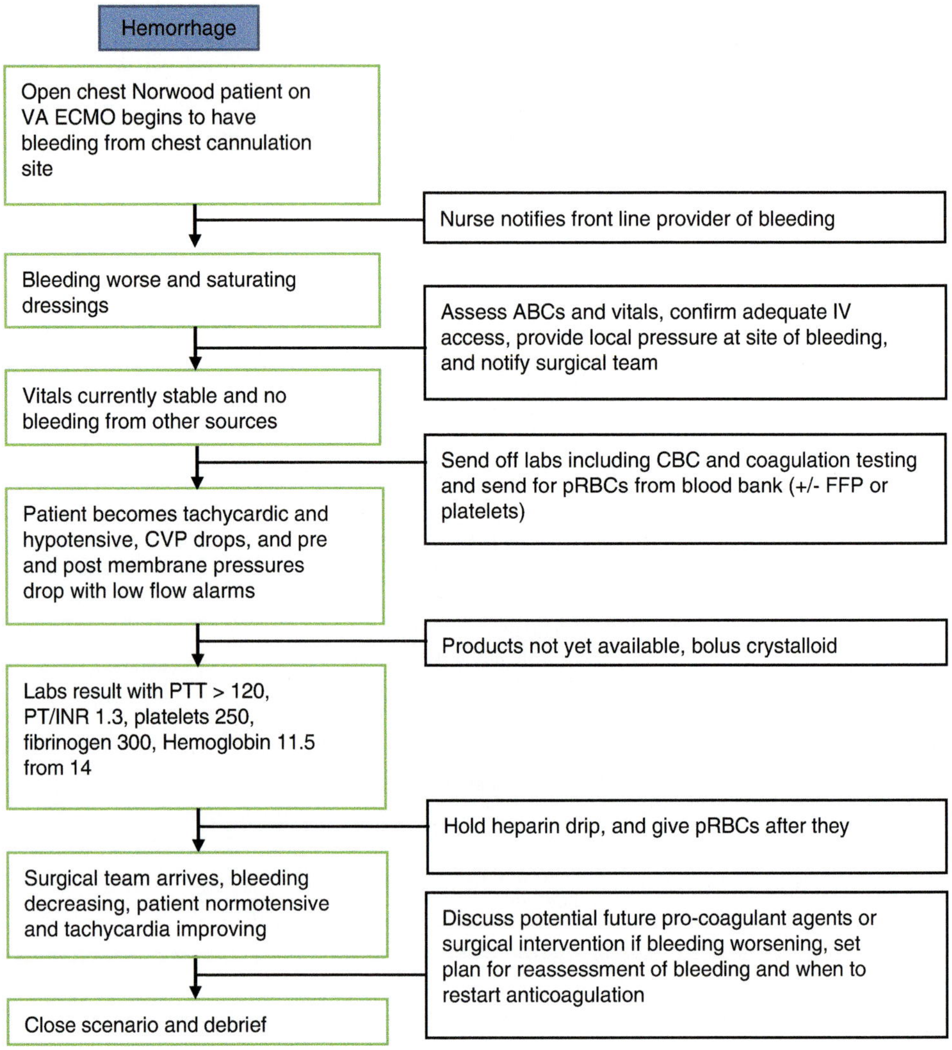

Fig. 6.2 Case 2: Hemorrhage (preload)

of all ages on ECMO from a respiratory etiology and 50% of all complications in patients of all ages on ECMO from cardiac etiologies [22]. The sources of hemorrhage include the cannulation site, potential surgical sites, pulmonary hemorrhage, gastrointestinal bleeding, and cerebral hemorrhage [22]. Simulation cases with hemorrhage could focus on replacing blood products to support hemodynamics and the potential need for replacement of other factors in the coagulation system as well as the potential need for surgical exploration. With hemorrhage being the most common complication, our sample preload case focuses on hemorrhage (Fig. 6.2).

Conditions that increase intrathoracic pressure, including tension pneumothorax and cardiac tamponade, can also inhibit venous return into the thoracic cavity and subsequently into the ECMO circuit. Cardiac tamponade accounts for 5% of patient complications while on ECMO [23]. Simulation cases with these etiologies should focus on early diagnostics based on vital sign changes and physical exam, x-ray, and/or echocardiogram as appropriate and intervention with needle decompression, pericardiocentesis, and chest tube or pericardial drain placement as appropriate. In all ECMO preload-related settings, the venous pressures on the circuit will drop, and overall flow will decrease. In the setting of increased intrathoracic pressures, as occurs with tension pneumothorax or cardiac tamponade, the central venous pressure will increase, while the venous pressures on the pump will decrease (become more negative) as will the overall flow of the circuit. The venous cannula itself can also contribute to issues with venous return. As mentioned, since the flow is very size dependent, too small of a cannula will limit total ECMO flow, as will kinking or thrombosis of the venous cannula. Cannulation of the veins can also result in aneurysm or venous tears [21].

ECMO Pump "Contractility"

Etiologies that affect the pump itself include overall power failure, air entrapment, thrombus within the circuit, oxygenator failure, and cannula dislodgement. Pump failure is an uncommon but concerning event accounting for ~1% of complications. Simulation cases of pump failure can focus on assuring that there is an additional energy source should the pump lose connection to a power supply. This is institutionally specific but may include battery backup or having the circuit plugged into an outlet supported by a backup generator. If these measures fail or are not feasible, manual cranking of the pump is possible [21]. Manual cranking should be practiced so in the event of this rare but catastrophic event, providers are familiar with how to operate this device.

As mentioned, ECMO requires a tight balance of anticoagulation. Thrombi tend to form in areas of turbulence like the oxygenator or tubing connection points [21]. Clots in the ECMO circuit are the most common mechanical complication during an ECMO run. They can affect any part of the circuit and, if significantly large, could inhibit flow and require changing out components or the entire circuit [21]. When exchanging parts of the ECMO circuit, a key focus in simulation cases should be on clamping of the circuit. While there may be institutional preferences, the mnemonic of VBA (venous, bridge, arterial) refers to clamping of the venous cannula, unclamping the bridge, and then clamping the arterial cannula. This should occur in all cases except when an air embolus is detected on the arterial side, as will be discussed below [20].

Air embolism accounts for 4% of all complications [22]. Air emboli can occur because of the negative pressure exerted on the venous drainage as well as positive pressure exerted post pump into the oxygenator [20]. Some centers no longer use a bladder; however, if a bladder is still used, it can help with prevention of cavitation and air embolism. Some centers also utilize air bubble detectors [20]. Air embolism can less commonly be caused by supersaturation of blood with oxygen that can then lead to oxygen dissolving out of solution and causing air bubbles. Due to this, the post-membrane partial pressure of oxygen should remain below 600 mmHg [20]. Simulation cases of air embolism can present different challenges depending on where the air is present. Venous air may be managed, while the patient remains on ECMO support; if more significant, it may require the patient coming off the ECMO circuit and removing the air or, rarely, replacing the whole circuit. Arterial air requires clamping on the arterial side of the circuit immediately after that air is noted to prevent air entry to the patient's circulation. The patient is then placed in the Trendelenburg position so if any air does get to the patient, the likelihood of it going toward the cerebral circulation and causing a stroke is reduced. Key steps are early recognition of air bubbles in the tubing and clamping at appropriate sites. For more advanced learners, the simulation could even progress to an air embolism reaching the cerebral circulation requiring management of a cerebrovascular injury. An example of an air embolism case is seen in Fig. 6.3.

Membrane oxygenator failure accounts for 6–10% of ELSO complications and is more common in adults, as the second most common mechanical complication in this population [20, 22]. For simulations involving membrane oxygenator failure, initial evidence should be noted based on blood gases showing rising CO_2 levels and decreasing O_2 levels. A key learning point is that this is the only situation where the difference between the pre- and post-oxygenator pressure is increased. The appropriate management would be to exchange the oxygenator.

ECMO Afterload

The ECMO circuit is sensitive to sources of increased afterload [20, 21]. Centrifugal pumps, which are now more commonly used than roller pumps, are particularly afterload sensitive as their flow is variable depending on venous and arterial pressures. A rise in systemic vascular resistance (SVR) can decrease centrifugal pump flow [20, 21]. Anything that increases a patient's SVR would result in increased afterload to the ECMO circuit. As Table 6.2 describes, these causes include excess of endogenous catecholamines, use of vasopressors, generalized seizures resulting in hypertension, increased intracranial pressure, agitation, renal thrombosis, or other causes of activation of the renin-angiotensin-aldosterone pathway. If not due to the patient, mechanics of the arterial cannula itself can also cause an increased afterload on the circuit. Seizures from various etiologies account for 3% of ECMO complications [22]. A significant issue with ECMO, as described above, is balance of coagulation and risk of hemorrhage. Cerebral hemorrhage results in nearly 5–6% of all complications and up to 11% of complications in neonates [22]. Cerebral hemorrhage resulting in secondary seizures could be an example of a simulation case for practicing management of increased afterload impacting ECMO flow, as seen in Fig. 6.4, requiring initial management of the seizures with antiepileptic medications which will also reduce afterload. One would then expect providers to consider a differential diagnosis regarding the etiology of the seizures including hemorrhagic or ischemic cerebrovascular accident.

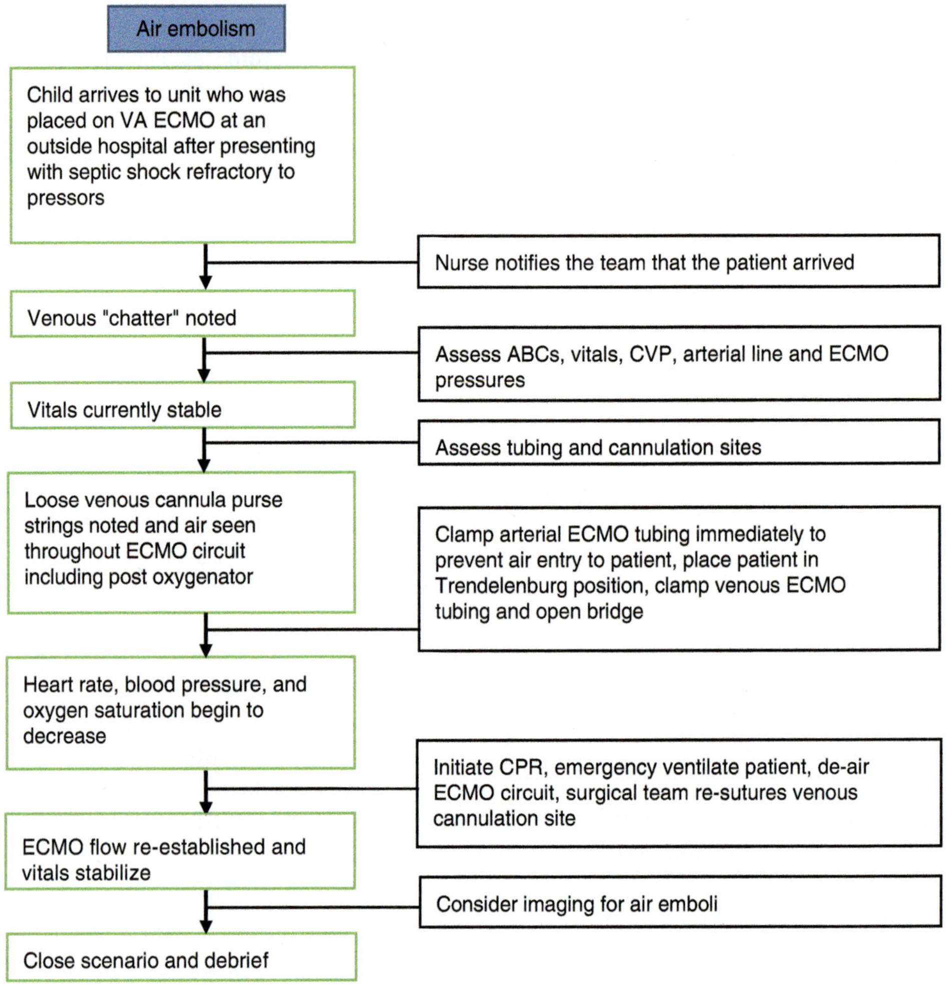

Fig. 6.3 Case 3: Air embolism (contractility)

Considerations

Further considerations in designing an ECMO simulation curriculum should focus on maintenance of knowledge and skills. This includes maintenance of competency for individuals, as well as assessment, updating, and maintenance of the curriculum itself. For individuals, it is not yet clear at what interval simulation sessions should be repeated to prevent degradation of skill. A few studies give insight into this, but this remains a gap in the current literature. Chan et al. created an ECMO simulation program with an initial training course and then reevaluated trainees 6 months later [13]. They found that at 6 months follow-up, trainees had lower scores for knowledge, ability, and confidence than they did in their initial post-assessment surveys [13]. This suggests that repeated education should occur at least 6 months after initial training but likely at an earlier interval. Allan et al. found that in cardiac surgery trainees, after initial training on cannulation with a high fidelity model, the statistically and clinically significant improvement noted in decreasing cannulation time, performance on a global rating scale with established validity evidence, and composite cannulation score was sustained after 3 months follow-up [2]. Cardiopulmonary resuscitation education data demonstrates skill decline 6–9 months after initial training [24]. While more research is needed, together this suggests that repeating training 3–6 months after initial training may be appropriate. It is not yet known if training sessions would need to continue at this frequency or if, as learners progress through a curriculum, the interval between sessions could be increased without skill and knowledge decay.

The last consideration is how ECMO simulation should fit within the larger ECMO education program, understanding that simulation is only one educational strategy. There are various types of learners as well as educational methodologies, and by having multiple modalities, we can hope to best educate all types of learners. Simulation provides an excellent method for learners who prefer doing, and subsequently reflecting on that task, and allows a safe environment for practicing teamwork. Incorporating simulation with other sessions, such as a flipped classroom or small group problem-solving sessions for gaining initial fundamental knowledge,

Fig. 6.4 Case 4: Seizure (afterload)

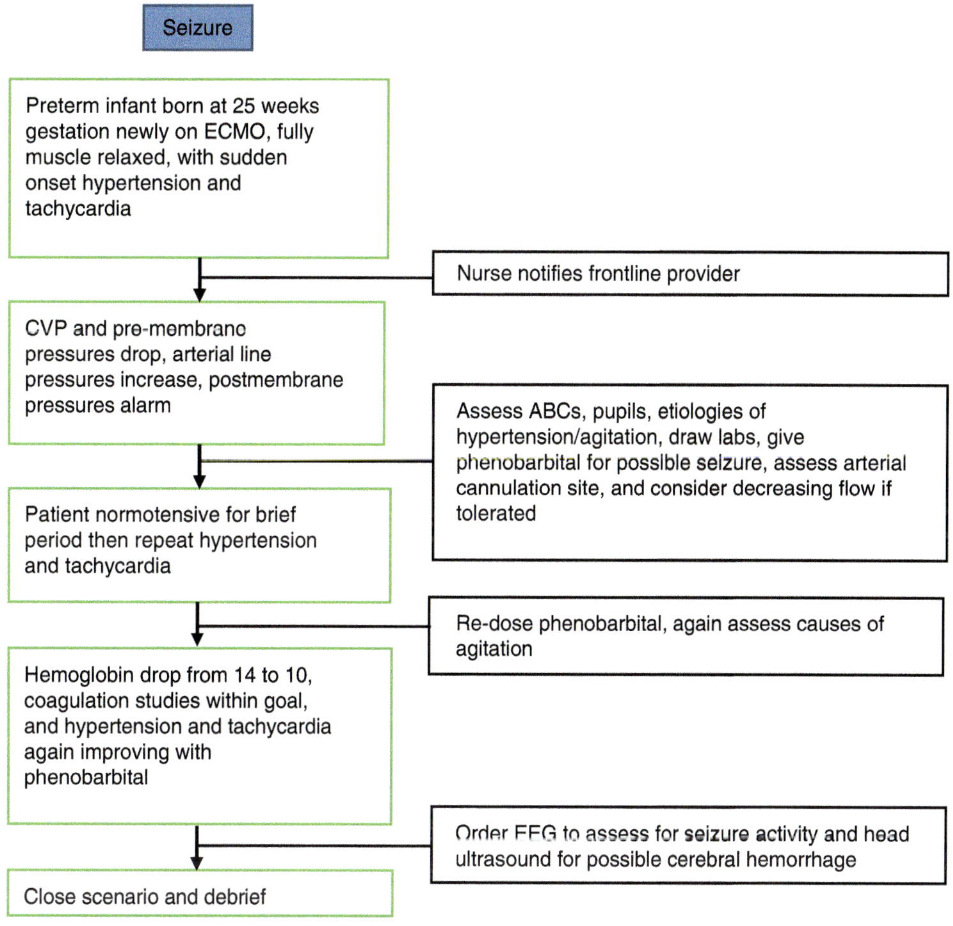

can be helpful. As technology advances, virtual reality and computer-based "serious games" may be available in the future. The best strategy will likely be integration of multiple education strategies together, matching each with where they best suit specific goals and objectives [5].

Conclusions

ECMO remains a high-risk, low-frequency intervention, and ECMO simulation allows providers to safely gain and reinforce knowledge and to practice technical skills and teamwork with the overall goal of learning, transferring that learning to clinical practice and, ultimately, improving patient outcomes. Using the six-step model for curriculum development, learners can be guided from novice to expert performance. The use of a physiologic model for development of ECMO simulation cases by incorporating principles of preload, afterload, and contractility offers a conceptual framework to aid learners in their assessment of the patient on ECMO. Further work is still needed on determining the frequency of simulation sessions to avoid decay and aid in retention of what is learned. In concert with developing a simulation curriculum is the need for development of assessment tools with the principles of validity in mind. Through collaboration of multiple programs and experts, a standardized curriculum and assessment process that generates valid data can be created to train all ECMO providers, including medical providers, surgical providers, and ECMO specialists, in hopes of standardizing care and ultimately decreasing patient morbidity and mortality.

References

1. Zwischenberger JB, Steinhorn R, Bartlett RH, editors. Extracorporeal cardiopulmonary support in critical care. 2nd ed. Ann Arbor: Extracorporeal Life Support Organization (ELSO); 2000.
2. Allan CK, Pigula F, Bacha EA, Emani S, Fynn-Thompson F, Thiagarajan RR, et al. An extracorporeal membrane oxygenation cannulation curriculum featuring a novel integrated skills trainer leads to improved performance among pediatric cardiac surgery trainees. Simul Healthc. 2013;8(4):221–8.
3. Su L, Spaeder MC, Jones MB, Sinha P, Nath DS, Jain PN, et al. Implementation of an extracorporeal cardiopulmonary resuscitation simulation program reduces extracorporeal cardiopulmonary resuscitation times in real patients. Pediatr Crit Care Med. 2014;15(9):856–60.

4. Thomas PA, Kern DE, Hughes MT, Che BY. Curriculum development for medical education a six-step approach. 3rd ed. Baltimore: The Johns Hopkins University Press; 2016.
5. Johnston L, Williams SB, Ades A. Education for ECMO providers: using education science to bridge the gap between clinical and educational expertise. Semin Perinatol. 2018;42(2):138–46.
6. Coderre S, Woloschuk W, McLaughlin K. Twelve tips for blueprinting. Med Teach. 2009;31(4):322–4.
7. Organization ELS. ELSO guidelines for training and continuing education of ECMO specialists 2010 [Version 1.5]. Available from: https://www.elso.org/Portals/0/IGD/Archive/FileManager/97000963d6cusersshyerdocumentselsoguidelinesfortrainingandcontinuingeducationofecmospecialists.pdf.
8. Ogino M, Froehlich CD, Moore EA. Chapter 67. Education and training. In: Brogan T, Lequier L, Lorusso R, editors. Extracorporeal life support: the ELSO red book. 5th ed. Ann Arbor: Extracorporeal Life Support Organization; 2017.
9. Weems MF, Friedlich PS, Nelson LP, Rake AJ, Klee L, Stein JE, et al. The role of extracorporeal membrane oxygenation simulation training at extracorporeal life support organization Centers in the United States. Simul Healthc. 2017;12(4):233–9.
10. Fehr JJ, Shepard M, McBride ME, Mehegan M, Reddy K, Murray DJ, et al. Simulation-based assessment of ECMO clinical specialists. Simul Healthc. 2016;11(3):194–9.
11. Anderson JM, Boyle KB, Murphy AA, Yaeger KA, LeFlore J, Halamek LP. Simulating extracorporeal membrane oxygenation emergencies to improve human performance. Part I: methodologic and technologic innovations. Simul Healthc. 2006;1(4):220–7.
12. Anderson JM, Murphy AA, Boyle KB, Yaeger KA, Halamek LP. Simulating extracorporeal membrane oxygenation emergencies to improve human performance. Part II: assessment of technical and behavioral skills. Simul Healthc. 2006;1(4):228–32.
13. Chan SY, Figueroa M, Spentzas T, Powell A, Holloway R, Shah S. Prospective assessment of novice learners in a simulation-based extracorporeal membrane oxygenation (ECMO) education program. Pediatr Cardiol. 2013;34(3):543–52.
14. Allan CK, Thiagarajan RR, Beke D, Imprescia A, Kappus LJ, Garden A, et al. Simulation-based training delivered directly to the pediatric cardiac intensive care unit engenders preparedness, comfort, and decreased anxiety among multidisciplinary resuscitation teams. J Thorac Cardiovasc Surg. 2010;140(3):646–52.
15. Sanchez-Glanville C, Brindle ME, Spence T, Blackwood J, Drews T, Menzies S, et al. Evaluating the introduction of extracorporeal life support technology to a tertiary-care pediatric institution: smoothing the learning curve through interprofessional simulation training. J Pediatr Surg. 2015;50(5):798–804.
16. Atamanyuk I, Ghez O, Saeed I, Lane M, Hall J, Jackson T, et al. Impact of an open-chest extracorporeal membrane oxygenation model for in situ simulated team training: a pilot study. Interact Cardiovasc Thorac Surg. 2014;18(1):17–20; discussion.
17. Gaba DM, Fish KJ, Howard SK, Burden AR, Gaba DM. Crisis management in anesthesiology. 2nd ed. Philadelphia: Elsevier/Saunders; 2015. xxii, 409 pages.
18. Issenberg SB, McGaghie WC, Petrusa ER, Lee Gordon D, Scalese RJ. Features and uses of high-fidelity medical simulations that lead to effective learning: a BEME systematic review. Med Teach. 2005;27(1):10–28.
19. Sawyer T, Eppich W, Brett-Fleegler M, Grant V, Cheng A. More than one way to debrief: a critical review of healthcare simulation debriefing methods. Simul Healthc. 2016;11(3):209–17.
20. Allen S, Holena D, McCunn M, Kohl B, Sarani B. A review of the fundamental principles and evidence base in the use of extracorporeal membrane oxygenation (ECMO) in critically ill adult patients. J Intensive Care Med. 2011;26(1):13–26.
21. Butt W, Heard M, Peek GJ. Clinical management of the extracorporeal membrane oxygenation circuit. Pediatr Crit Care Med. 2013;14(5 Suppl 1):S13–9.
22. Thiagarajan RR, Barbaro RP, Rycus PT, McMullan DM, Conrad SA, Fortenberry JD, et al. Extracorporeal life support organization registry international report 2016. ASAIO J. 2017;63(1):60–7.
23. Barbaro RP, Paden ML, Guner YS, Raman L, Ryerson LM, Alexander P, et al. Pediatric extracorporeal life support organization registry international report 2016. ASAIO J. 2017;63(4):456–63.
24. Chamberlain D, Smith A, Woollard M, Colquhoun M, Handley AJ, Leaves S, et al. Trials of teaching methods in basic life support (3): comparison of simulated CPR performance after first training and at 6 months, with a note on the value of re-training. Resuscitation. 2002;53(2):179–87.

Part III

Technology for ECMO Simulation

Innovations and Options for ECMO Simulation

7

Peggy Han, Michael-Alice Moga, Katie Fitzpatrick, Steven Brediger, and Catherine K. Allan

Learning Objectives

- Recognize that varying levels of physical resemblance and functional task alignment can be combined to meet the needs of learners in an ECMO simulation.
- Identify the three types of learning objectives for ECMO simulation: clinical, team training and process development/refinement.
- List the components required for a successful ECMO simulation, including clear learning objectives, equipment, personnel and space.

Introduction

When it comes to ECMO simulation, a phrase from poet Robert Browning takes on a new meaning: is it true that "less is more," [1] or is more really more? Increasingly, the field of medical simulation recognizes that the degree of realism is integral in effectively imparting knowledge and acquiring vital skills. In this chapter, we present a practical user's guide to implementing ECMO simulation by first describing the range of realism that can be used within ECMO simulation and then showing the importance of matching the degree of realism to the learning objectives and the specific needs of the learner. ECMO simulation can be simple or complex, but must be focused as a tool to achieve specific educational objectives. Here, we introduce a framework upon which to design scenarios for use in ECMO simulation, discuss in detail the elements needed to execute an ECMO simulation, and give examples to illustrate how to put the framework to use.

Importantly, Diekmann, Gaba, and Rall emphasize that realism matters only in the context of learner engagement [2]. Simulation is a social practice that blends the physical, conceptual, and emotional/experiential modes of reality [3]. The key to a successful simulation lies in the buy-in of participants. No matter how realistic the physical characteristics of a simulator may be, the intended educational objectives will not be effectively met without the willingness of participants to suspend disbelief and engage in the experience. Additionally, learner engagement is enhanced through the creation of scenarios that attend to conceptual and emotional aspects of realism. Assuming a context of learner engagement and the existence of learning objectives that appropriately address institutional needs, we hope to illustrate how ECMO skills can be effectively taught using varying degrees of realism across the spectrum of ECMO programs.

P. Han
Division of Pediatric Critical Care Medicine, Department of Pediatrics, Stanford University School of Medicine, Palo Alto, CA, USA

M.-A. Moga (✉)
Division of Cardiac Critical Care, Department of Critical Care Medicine, The Hospital for Sick Children, The Labatt Family Heart Center, Toronto, ON, Canada

Department of Critical Care Medicine, University of Toronto, The Hospital for Sick Children, Toronto, ON, Canada
e-mail: michael-alice.moga@sickkids.ca

K. Fitzpatrick
Boston Children's Hospital, Simpeds (Simulation Program), Boston, MA, USA

S. Brediger
ECMO Program/Respiratory Care Department, Boston Children's Hospital, Boston, MA, USA

C. K. Allan (✉)
Cardiac Intensive Care Unit, Simulator Program, Boston Children's Hospital, Department of Cardiology, Boston, MA, USA
e-mail: catherine.allan@cardio.chboston.org

L. C. Johnston, L. Su (eds.), *Comprehensive Healthcare Simulation: ECMO Simulation*, Comprehensive Healthcare Simulation,
https://doi.org/10.1007/978-3-030-53844-6_7

Definitions

The term *fidelity* is typically used to describe the degree of realism of a simulator and can be categorized based on how the simulator appears and what it does [4]. However, there is little consensus in the simulation literature, both in healthcare and many other fields, regarding the definition of fidelity [4–8]. More recently, the focus within simulation has turned to utilizing technology and physical platforms to best fulfill specific educational objectives [9–11]. As ECMO simulation demands both elements of realism and ability to complete tasks to augment experiential learning, for the purposes of this work, we adopted definitions proposed by Hamstra et al. (2014), which focus on physical resemblance and functional task alignment, rather than utilizing the traditional term *fidelity* [12].

Physical resemblance refers to aspects of the simulator that make it life-like, including tactile, visual, and auditory features designed to mimic reality [12]. The desired degree of physical resemblance depends on a number of factors, including the context in which the simulator is used, the kind of task for which the learner is being trained, the stages of learning involved, learner abilities and capabilities, task difficulty, and the effects of various instructional features [13].

Functional task alignment refers to matching of the simulator's functional properties with the requirements of the physical task performed in simulation [12]. For healthcare simulation, closely aligning the clinical task with the simulation task is important for the learner to master the intended learning objectives of the simulation, so that learning transfer to the clinical setting can occur related to this specific objective. As an example, an educator may utilize a model with rubber tubing embedded in an inert plastic block for placement of arterial and venous cannulae in a cannulation scenario. While the plastic block bears little physical resemblance to a human patient, when draped and prepped by learners in the typical manner, the model becomes actionable enough for the surgeon to properly execute a cannulation. That is, he or she will need to perform all of the steps of cannulation. This degree of functional task alignment allows the surgeon to engage in the simulation with the objective of meeting learning objectives related to teamwork during ECMO cannulation. Thus, the configurations of the simulator are adapted to make the physical task performed in simulation meaningful, and ideally, these skills will be transferable to the clinical setting. Contrast this to a simulation for which the learning objective is explicitly to teach surgical skills required to cannulate a patient for ECMO. In this situation, a high degree of functional task alignment is required as in the previous example. However, in this latter example, the physical resemblance must also be greater to insure learning transfer – the trainer might require accurate anatomic landmarks, tissue layers including skin, fascia, and muscle, and vessels that are collapsible.

Underlying these definitions is an emphasis on learning objectives, which will vary depending on the needs of the institution and individuals. The learning objectives for ECMO simulation can be grossly divided into three categories: clinical objectives, team training objectives, and process development. Clinical objectives describe the medical knowledge and associated skills that must be highlighted, understood, and practiced in an ECMO simulation. Clinical learning objectives will vary according to provider specialty. For instance, learning objectives for an ECMO specialist or perfusionist in charge of preparing and running the ECMO circuit may be related to pump assembly, initiation of flows, and physical manipulation of the pump to manage pump-related emergencies, among others. On the other hand, learning objectives for the bedside medical team might include integration of physiologic data from both the patient and the pump to diagnose and manage ECMO emergencies. Team training objectives address how teams work together most effectively, particularly for high-risk, low-frequency events such as ECMO emergencies. The emphasis for team training lies in the utilization and mastery of various tools and strategies for effective communication and team behavior. Lastly, objectives addressing process development refer to testing unit-based or hospital systems around ECMO deployment, transport, staffing, and other quality improvement measures that are important to facilitate smooth ECMO runs.

In Table 7.1, we illustrate how a conceptual framework combining physical resemblance and functional task alignment can be applied to meet specific learning goals related to ECMO care. While the example in the table is specific to the ECMO specialist, the concepts can be applied to various categories of learners (ICU fellow, ICU nurse, pediatric surgeon, transport physician, etc.), medical teams (using objectives that target specific crisis resource management principles), and systems (using objectives that address specific operational questions including how to improve personnel, environmental, and safety factors influencing an ECMO run).

Combining the various degrees of physical resemblance and functional task alignment to create ECMO scenarios can provide a wide variety of possibilities for training and education. The key is to choose the combination that best suits the identified learning objectives and matches the learners' capability and institutional needs.

Foundational Knowledge and Skills Acquired Through Low Physical Resemblance, Low Functional Task Alignment Simulation

Low physical resemblance, low functional task alignment simulation options have particular value for novice learners, for whom cognitive load must be carefully managed [14–16]. These simulations allow learners to develop cognitive skills before layering on complex psychomotor skills, which

Table 7.1 Example curriculum for training a novice ECMO specialist or medical team member

		Degree of physical resemblance		
		Low	Medium	High
Functional Task Alignment	Simple	*Objective*: Identify circuit components *Tool:*" ECMO in an envelope"-photos of individual circuit components and labels *Activity:* Label photos	*Objective*: Identify circuit components *Tool:* "ECMO in a bag"-dry circuit components laid on a table *Activity*: Label components on a table	*Objective*: Identify individual circuit components *Tool:* "ECMO in space"-wet, assembled ECMO circuit +/− mannikin *Activity*: Label individual components with sticky notes
	Intermediate	*Objective*: Arrange circuit components in order, identify monitoring points *Tool:* "ECMO in an envelope" *Activity:* Arrange components in correct order, label pressure and flow monitoring points	*Objective*: Correctly assemble ECMO circuit from component parts *Tool:* "ECMO in a bag" *Activity*: Arrange components in correct order; state their function	*Objective:* Assemble and prime ECMO circuit for elective ECMO cannulation *Tool:* "ECMO in space" *Activity:* Assemble and prime teaching circuit for future sim
	Complex	*Objective*: Articulate differential diagnosis for changes in pressure and flow *Tool:* "ECMO in an envelope" *Activity:* Tabletop exercise. Denote monitoring changes on assembled ECMO in an envelope; Note diagnosis and required intervention	*Objective:* Hand off lines to surgeon and initiate ECMO flows *Tool:* Pre-cannulated manikin + ECMO lines *Activity:* Demonstrate sterile handoff, initiation of flows with pressure and air monitoring	*Objective:* Effective communication and safe establishment of flows in setting of ECPR *Tool:* Wet circuit, multidisciplinary team, manikin *Activity*: Multidisciplinary ECPR simulation including CPR, cannulation and establishment of flows

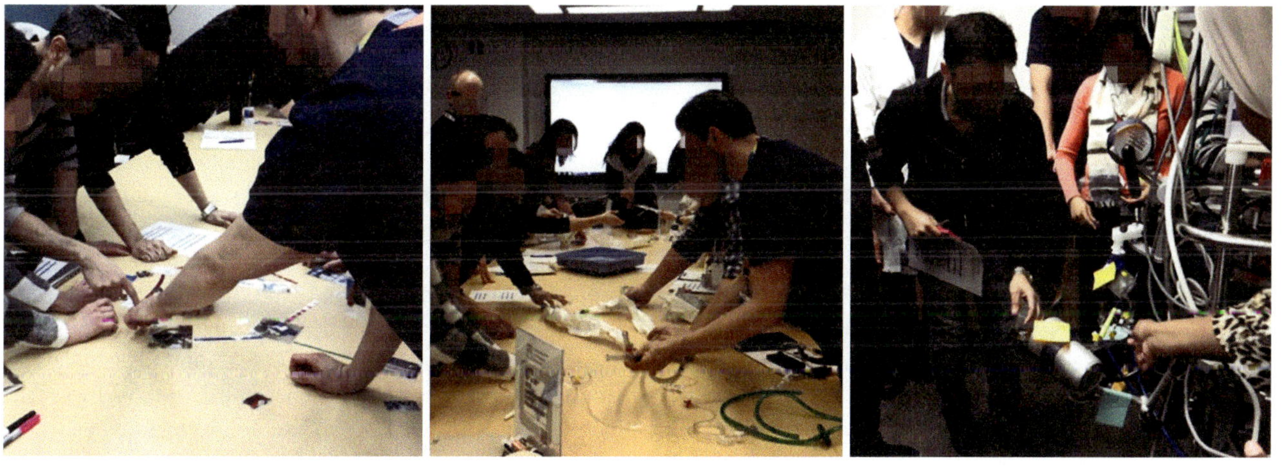

Fig. 7.1 ECMO in an envelope, ECMO in a bag and 3D ECMO

may overload a novice learner. "ECMO in an envelope" is an example of a transportable, economical simulation activity that bears very little physical resemblance to a fully assembled ECMO circuit. However, it has been used as an important foundational exercise at the Hospital for Sick Children in Toronto for training a wide variety of learners (fellows, ECMO specialists, staff physicians) of varying skill levels (Michael-Alice Moga, personal communication). In this simple tabletop simulation, learners arrange pictures of ECMO circuit components in the correct orientation, effectively building a 2D ECMO circuit. Often, this task is done individually as a flipped classroom activity prior to an ECMO workshop; learners send the instructors a picture of the assembled circuit to demonstrate completion of the pre-learning activity. This serves as a catalyst to in-classroom exercises, shown in Fig. 7.1, in which learners work in groups to assemble circuits with greater degrees of physical resemblance (such as "ECMO in a bag," which incorporates real components) culminating in assembly of a dry 3D circuit that can be converted into a functional, wet circuit in motion (4D ECMO-"ECMO in motion"). These simple, 2D, static ECMO simulators can be used in concert with varying levels of functional task alignment spanning from labeling circuit components to identification of areas of pressure/flow measurement to facilitating a full tabletop exercise in which learners are given a series of flow/pressure alterations on the circuit and expected to identify the underlying cause. Successful use of these tools to identify the steps to intervene in specific ECMO emergencies reflects a high degree of understanding of ECMO physiology. When applied as the first steps in a sequence of exercises, "ECMO in an envelope" allows the learner to master a cognitive task before layering on psychomotor skills. The tabletop exercises described can also be used to facilitate "just in time" training for clinician teams (nurse, physician, ECMO specialist, RT) prior to caring for an actual ECMO patient [17].

Development of Psychomotor and Critical Thinking Skills

ECMO teams must become facile with management of a patient and the circuit during both "routine" ECMO care and crisis situations, including circuit emergencies. Teams must learn to simultaneously integrate multiple, evolving data streams from the ECMO circuit and the patient to diagnose and remedy ECMO emergencies. Centers have multiple options for moderate physical resemblance ECMO circuits, ranging from complete, commercially available packages with fully integrated circuit, manikin, and monitors to DIY options utilizing basic equipment and standard manikins.

Commercially available ECMO simulation software including products by Eigenflow, Califia, Nijmegen, Innovative ECMO Concepts, Chalice Medical, and Ulco Technologies [18–22] can cost anywhere from $20,000 to as much as $100,000 for advanced systems that can also simulate cardiopulmonary bypass. These simulators allow for realistic, real-time changes in circuit pressures and blood flow rates according to a number of preprogramed ECMO simulation scenarios which utilize hydraulic simulators interfaced with a computer running associated real-time computerized models. ECMO simulation trainers have been separately developed to allow for practice in dissecting and placement of ECMO cannulae and can be overlaid on top of a manikin. These simulation trainers are sold by 3-Dmed, MenTone Educational, Creaplast, and The Chamberlain Group [23–26]. It must be noted that this equipment cannot be substituted for expert facilitators, well-designed ECMO scenarios and targeted learning objectives. Even the deluxe package including a commercially integrated system, built-in library of ECMO scenarios, and the capability for high physical resemblance, real-time changes in circuit pressures and flow rates does not guarantee a high impact training session, as the focus should remain on the alignment of the simulated task with the needs of the learner. Furthermore, these commercially available devices are often expensive and do not take the place of facilitated experiential learning that is the hallmark of simulation.

Low-cost alternatives to these simulators can be created using readily available ECMO supplies and additions from any local hardware store. Intermediate physical resemblance can be created using expired cannulae, dry circuits, tubing, and oxygenators. In this category, the capacity to change vital signs in real time may exist if a high-technology manikin or software is utilized. The changes in the ECMO circuit pressures and blood flow rates can be stated aloud by the facilitator, but the ECMO simulator may not have the capacity to provide real-time feedback to clinical interventions. Complex physical resemblance requires a functioning ECMO circuit with the ability to manipulate flows and pressures (see below). Learners must then respond to real-time changes, integrating data from the ECMO circuit and patient physiologic monitoring. Direct feedback is then provided on interventions through both the circuit and the patient monitor controlled by the simulation facilitator.

Development of Surgical Cannulation Skills

Allan et al. describe the use of an integrated ECMO cannulation trainer in training of pediatric cardiothoracic surgical residents and fellows in technical aspects of infant neck cannulation. This en lay trainer, fashioned out of widely available materials, is created by embedding siliconized tubing representing artery and vein in a hydrogel matrix. "Skin" is fashioned from liquid rubber paints applied over the hydrogel matrix. This technical innovation allows novice surgical trainees to carry out all the individual steps required for neck cannulation. The use of this trainer as part of a curriculum including expert feedback can lead to sustained improvements of cannulation time and other markers of proficiency [27]. The degree of physical resemblance of this model is adequate to teach novices the individual steps of cannulation. However, our anecdotal experience with this model was that the physical resemblance was not high enough to be a valuable tool for more experienced learners. Therefore, subsequent generations of the model have added in features such as more tissue-like materials and addition of fascia and muscle layers requiring more nuanced dissection techniques.

ECMO Team Development and Crisis Management

For expert clinicians and practitioners well-versed in ECMO physiology, ECMO simulation offers an opportunity to hone teamwork skills and evaluate systems. Optimal team engagement and suspension of disbelief during such simulations relies on the team working in an environment of complex functional task alignment. In these activities, using an actual

Fig. 7.2 Framework to coordinate ECMO simulation logistics

1) Weeks to months prior to simulation
   - o Establish session objectives: individual, team and/or systems training
   - o Write and revise scenario, consult subject matter experts as needed
   - o Construct equipment checklist
     - o Reserve manikin or other equipment (if required)
     - o Clarify if special (cameras, etc) equipment needed
   - o Determine space requirements for simulation and debrief: classroom, in situ, learning lab, other
     - o Reserve room (if needed)
     - o If conducting in situ simulation, consider reserving backup space
   - o Construct facilitator checklist and invite facilitators
   - o Invite participants
2) Days prior to simulation
   - o Verify equipment is in working order
   - o Verify facilitators still available and distribute scenario for review
   - o Assemble equipment if needed
   - o Verify participants available. Alert participants of any concurrent research being conducted
3) Day of simulation
   - o Before: set the stage (assemble physical environment, equipment, etc)
   - o During
     - o Pre-brief
     - o Run simulation
     - o Debrief
     - o Gather feedback from participants
   - o After
     - o Reset simulation space
     - o Debrief facilitators and combine session notes/observations
     - o Create lessons learned for distribution and cataloguing
     - o Download any data from devices/mannikins
4) Days after simulation:
   - o Analyze video and/or other session data
   - o Refine scenario
   - o Distribute lessons learned and recommendations to participants and stakeholders

ECMO circuit with ability to manipulate both the circuit (see below) and vital signs in real-time to respond to team interventions is critical. In addition, both team engagement and ability to effectively evaluate systems of care may be optimal when simulations are carried out at the point of care utilizing the same equipment and technology available to providers during clinical activities.

Logistics of ECMO Simulation: A User's Guide

The logistics of executing a well-run ECMO simulation session can initially seem overwhelming, particularly when planning a session with a high degree of complexity. With adequate planning and coordination, even relatively novice teams can set themselves up for success through preparation, anticipation of needs, and brainstorming what can go wrong. It is important for simulation teams to learn from each session, refining preparation and execution in an iterative process to improve the efficiency and efficacy of future simulations. Once the learner group and objectives have been identified, when approaching an ECMO simulation session it is helpful to break down required elements into equipment (what), personnel (who), and space (where). An example of a checklist (Fig. 7.2) is included to provide readers with a basic framework from which to create personalized logistic aids.

Equipment

Equipment needs are largely dependent on the desired level of fidelity and whether the session is focused solely on the circuit, or if training will also incorporate care of the patient (i.e., a simulation manikin). In general, we find it helpful to train using the same equipment that is utilized in patient care to ease translation of the training exercise into care for real patients. For a "How To" guide on assembly of an ECMO circuit for simulation, please refer to the dedicated chapter in this book (Chap. 46). Beyond the circuit itself, one must consider appropriate equipment to support circuit-related functions and interventions including clamps, syringes, volume, pressure gauges, and flow meters. For scenarios incorporating patient care, teams should include appropriate manikins, monitoring devices, medical information (X-rays, laboratory results, etc.), and medical supplies/task trainers to support anticipated interventions by learners. At an extreme, scenarios involving surgical intervention and/or simultaneous patient resuscitation require a long list of necessary equipment. It is often helpful to keep a supply checklist for these types of situations, refining the list with each iteration of the session to ensure completeness.

Table 7.2 provides a brief list of equipment required to simulate a live ECMO circuit, including the components needed for a complex physical resemblance scenario. Additional medical supplies that are helpful to run ECMO simulations of varying degrees of physical resemblance are provided in Table 7.3.

Table 7.2 Equipment list to simulate a live ECMO circuit

Circuit components	Circuit pressures and flow
ECMO cannulae	Flow meter
Reservoir bag to which ECMO cannulae would attach with an open end to attach to ECMO circuit tubing (one that comes with the circuit or a 1 liter bag)	Working pressure gauges
ECMO circuit tubing	2 large tubing pinch clamps ("C-clamps," Fig. 7.3)
ECMO pump	4 regular tubing clamps
ECMO oxygenator	Three-way stop cock (ideally on venous side) to introduce an air embolus if desired
Gas source	

Table 7.3 Sample equipment checklist for ECMO simulation

Monitoring	Clinical information	Additional medical supplies
Situation monitoring: Computer to control vital sign changes Monitor to display vital sign changes *Patient monitoring:* NIRS EKG Saturation probe ETCO2 Arterial line BP cuff Temperature probe Pressure transducers (arterial line, CVL)	Pertinent laboratory results X-ray and echocardiography/ ultrasound images	*Basic supplies:* Code cart Intravenous fluid bags Vascular access supplies (e.g., PIV, IO, CVL) Arterial lines Ventilator + tubing ETT Chest tubes IV pumps Medications Blood components *OR Supplies:* Surgical cart/OR cart OR table or room Bovie Surgical lights/ headlamps surgical instruments *Specialty equipment:* Rapid transfuser Warmer

Technical Innovations for Simulation of ECMO Emergencies

As noted above, scenarios with complex task resemblance require the ability for the team to integrate physiologic data from both the ECMO circuit and patient monitoring devices, to respond in real time to changes, and to anticipate the results of these interventions. An ECMO circuit integrated with a manikin, both of which can be manipulated by the facilitator, enables these scenarios. Details of creating an ECMO circuit integrated with a manikin are addressed in Chap. 46. Manipulation of the circuit to replicate various ECMO emergencies can be achieved by causing either impedance to circuit venous return or increasing resistance to arterial flow through the application and adjustment of C-clamps (Fig. 7.3) to the arterial and venous limb obscured from participants. In other terms, decreased pump preload simulates low venous return states, such as hypovolemia, too small or malpositioned venous cannula, venous cannula/venous limb kink, or occlusive clot. Increased pump afterload simulates high systemic vascular resistance states, such as patient agitation, vasopressors that cause systemic vasoconstriction, patient movement impeding flow through the arterial cannula or causing

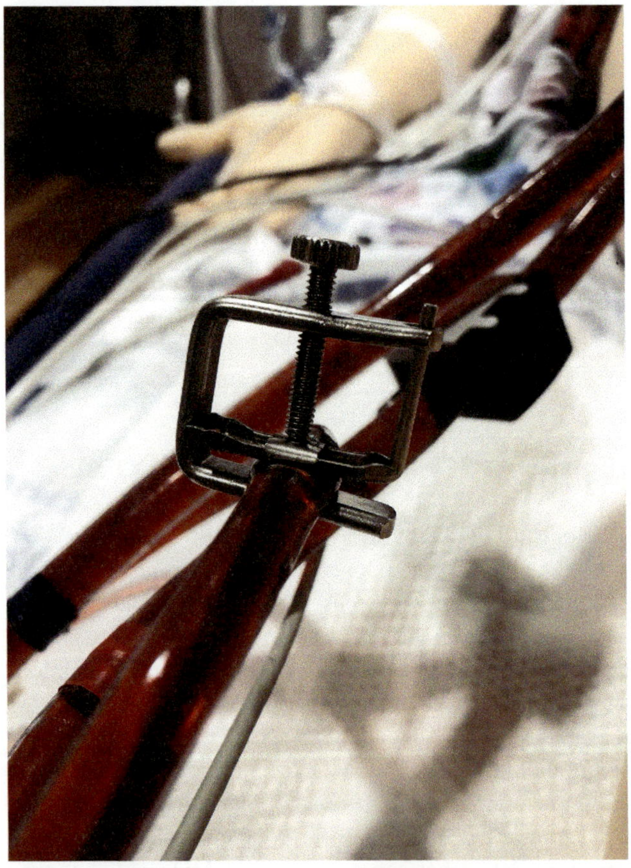

Fig. 7.3 Tubing closure pinch clamp AKA "C-clamp"

arterial cannula malposition, arterial cannula kink or occlusive clot, or too small arterial cannula. After the C-clamps are placed loosely on the arterial and venous limbs, ECMO flows are increased to a level approximately 300 ml above the flows desired for the scenario. The venous or arterial clamp is then tightened until circuit pressure monitors represent the desired baseline pressures. Note that flow will be somewhat decreased from the starting point (and thereby closer to physiologic range). Pressure alarms can then be set according to usual clinical practice. As the scenario progresses, the C-clamp on the arterial or venous side may be tightened to produce the desired physiologic changes for simulation of the emergency and loosened again in response to appropriate learner interventions. These exercises may be performed as circuit-specific drills designed for an individual learner to respond to the physiologic change or in a multidisciplinary simulation. For expert clinicians and practitioners who are well versed in ECMO physiology, a scenario with complex physical resemblance and simple functional task alignment might be better suited, as the emphasis of the scenario may be team training, communication, and/or systems improvement.

Personnel

The most realistic manikin and state-of-the-art, high-tech simulator will not be able to save a simulation from understaffing and poorly trained facilitators. Conversely, a well-prepared cadre of expert facilitators can transform a low-tech, low-fidelity scenario into a dynamic, fulfilling experience. When determining the human resources needed to adequately support an ECMO simulation, one must ensure adequate numbers, skillsets, and knowledge to meet the needs of each given scenario. Facilitators are often medical staff and can represent any number of backgrounds (medicine, surgery, nursing, perfusion, ECMO specialists) with additional expertise in ECMO, simulation, and debriefing. As a group, they should be able to ensure medical integrity of the scenario as it unfolds, whether or not learners follow the anticipated actions. Most importantly, the facilitator group should be able to support a fruitful, rigorous debriefing to support the objectives of a given scenario. In many centers, facilitators are supported by simulation technicians, who have expertise in simulation equipment, setup, and operation. The technician frees the medical facilitator to contribute to the session in other important ways, such as observing trainee actions or recording specific events. In programs without access to technicians, facilitators must often assume those responsibilities, as well.

The "right" number of facilitators in an ECMO simulation depends on the goals of the session, which informs the number of tasks to be accomplished, as well as the skillsets of potential facilitators. Whenever possible, it is best to have a facilitator complement that mirrors that of participants. This often aids in debriefing role-specific performance. Depending on the objectives of the simulation, specific observers and subject matter experts without specific ECMO expertise (e.g., blood bank, process analysis, EMR analysts) may be needed. To ensure adequate human resources are available to support a simulation, it is helpful to create a task list to determine how many, and which type, of facilitators are required. Specific tasks can then be assigned during the scenario (e.g., observe surgical technique, examine communication patterns). However, too many facilitators can cloud the learning space, result in task confusion, and even impede learner actions.

Space

Where to hold an ECMO simulation depends on the type of activity, space availability, and the goals of the session. Tabletop exercises can be conducted in almost space with a flat surface, whereas more complex simulations have different space requirements and can come with unique challenges. Dedicated simulation laboratories offer a standardized, reservable space in which a simulation can be setup and run without affecting, or being affected by, patient flow. These spaces often include specialized technology (cameras, control rooms, microphones) and access to dedicated debriefing rooms that can enhance the simulation experience for learners and aid in post-hoc analysis. These spaces are often useful for assessing and practicing individual and team tasks. In contrast, in situ simulations occurring within the clinical space offer unique challenges and benefits. While ongoing patient care can complicate space availability and result in crowded setup and take down, in situ simulation offers a powerful means by which to test systems and processes and allow teams to practice in their "natural environment."

Conclusion

ECMO simulation can be accessible to all learners and all institutions, regardless of size or budget. Clinical, team-based, and process development objectives can be met across all spectrums of physical resemblance and physical tasks. While simulators that provide feedback to stimulate all senses are often considered necessary to execute ECMO simulation, we describe a range of physical resemblance that can be effective in meeting universal learning objectives regarding ECMO physiology. Importantly, there are low-cost, effective training options available, especially as ECMO is being implemented to rescue patients in resource-limited settings. As long as ECMO simulation is focused on specific learning objectives that are relevant to the learners and the institution, ECMO simulation is worthwhile, can be low cost, and is an effective way to train individuals, teams, and test systems.

References

1. Browning R, Roberts A, Karlin D. The major works, Pbk. edn. Oxford: Oxford University Press; 2009.
2. Dieckmann P, Gaba D, Rall M. Deepening the theoretical foundations of patient simulation as social practice. Simul Healthc. 2007;2(3):183–93.
3. Rudolph JW, Simon R, Raemer DB. Which reality matters? Questions on the path to high engagement in healthcare simulation. Simul Healthc. 2007;2(3):161–3.
4. Allen JA, Buffardi LC, Hays RT. The relationship of simulator fidelity to task and performance variables. Alexandria; 1991.
5. Alessi SM. Fidelity in the design of instructional simulations. J Comput Based Instruct. 1988;15(2):40–7.
6. Kneebone R. Evaluating clinical simulations for learning procedural skills: a theory-based approach. Acad Med. 2005;80(6):549–53.
7. Rehmann AJ, Mitman RD, Reynolds MC: A handbook of flight simulation fidelity requirements for human factors research; 1995.
8. Sharma S, Boet S, Kitto S, Reeves S. Interprofessional simulated learning: the need for 'sociological fidelity. J Interprof Care. 2011;25(2):81–3.
9. McGaghie WC, Issenberg SB, Petrusa ER, Scalese RJ. A critical review of simulation-based medical education research: 2003-2009. Med Educ. 2010;44(1):50–63.
10. Issenberg SB, McGaghie WC, Petrusa ER, Lee Gordon D, Scalese RJ. Features and uses of high-fidelity medical simulations that lead to effective learning: a BEME systematic review. Med Teach. 2005;27(1):10–28.
11. Cook DA, Erwin PJ, Triola MM. Computerized virtual patients in health professions education: a systematic review and meta-analysis. Acad Med. 2010;85(10):1589–602.
12. Hamstra SJ, Brydges R, Hatala R, Zendejas B, Cook DA. Reconsidering fidelity in simulation-based training. Acad Med. 2014;89(3):387–92.
13. Hays RT: Simulator fidelity: a concept paper; 1980.
14. Fraser KL, Ayres P, Sweller J. Cognitive Load Theory for the Design of Medical Simulations. Simul Healthc: J Soc Simul Healthc. 2015;10(5):295–307.
15. van Merrienboer JJ, Sweller J. Cognitive load theory in health professional education: design principles and strategies. Med Educ. 2010;44(1):85–93.
16. Sweller N, Hayes BK. More than one kind of inference: re-examining what's learned in feature inference and classification. Q J Exp Psychol. 2010;63(8):1568–89.
17. Aggarwal R. Just-in-time simulation-based training. BMJ quality & safety. 2017;26(11):866–8.
18. EigenFlow 2 Plus., http://curtisliferesearch.com/product/eigenflowplus-ecmo/.
19. Califia, https://www.biomedsimulation.com/products/.
20. Nijmegen ECMO Simulator, www.ecmosim.com.
21. Education & Training., https://www.innovativeecmo.com/services/ecmo-education/?gclid=CjwKCAiA4t_iBRApEiwAn-vt-5YMF-w33rM3AHPCXtQRqpvHXO5CdAJkJCezIhPuZw8eQC-CieewPGCRoC1cgQAvD_BwE.
22. Parallel Simulator, https://www.chalicemedical.com/products/parallel-simulator/.
23. ECMO Simulation Kit., https://www.3-dmed.com/catalog/ecmo-simulation-kit.
24. ECMO Professional Simulator., https://www.mentone-educational.com.au/simulation/surgical-simulation/ecmo-professional-simulator.
25. ECMO simulator for femoral-jugular or femoro-femoral cannulation, http://www.medicalexpo.com/prod/creaplast-101182.html#product-item_787462.
26. ECMO Simulation with Perfusion Beating Heart Trainer., https://www.thecgroup.com/ecmo-simulation-with-perfusion-beating-heart-trainer/.
27. Allan CK, Pigula F, Bacha EA, Emani S, Fynn-Thompson F, Thiagarajan RR, Imprescia A, Hayes G, Weinstock P. An extracorporeal membrane oxygenation cannulation curriculum featuring a novel integrated skills trainer leads to improved performance among pediatric cardiac surgery trainees. Simul Healthc J Soc Simul Healthc. 2013;8(4):221–8.

Physiologic Modeling

8

Tim Antonius

Learning Objectives

1. Describe basic concepts of physiological modeling and how these can be applied to ECMO education and simulation.
2. Discuss what types of problems physiologic models can be used to solve in ECMO simulation.
3. Identify potential barriers and challenges to the development and use of a physiologic model-driven ECMO simulator.

Overview of the Chapter

Introduction to Physiological Modeling

In this introduction, the basic concepts of physiologic modeling are discussed using examples of models from subsystems of the body and ECMO systems.

Physiologic Modeling in ECMO Simulation

In this section, we discuss how modeling can be used in ECMO simulation. We discuss the necessary prerequisites, potential challenges, as well as the pros and cons of the use of modeling in ECMO simulation.

Full Model-Driven and Hybrid ECMO Simulation

In this section, different ways models can be used in ECMO simulation will be discussed, including full model-driven systems (where all systems are modeled) versus a hybrid system (where only parts of the physiology are modeled) to aid the instructor.

Explanatory Models in ECMO Simulation

Physiologic models can be used to explain difficult physiological and pathophysiological phenomena. The use of screen-based ECMO simulation using models which explain ECMO physiology will be demonstrated.

Current Available Models for Use in ECMO Simulation

In this section, an overview of the current available (open source) models for use in ECMO simulation will be discussed, including examples of when and how they can be applied for ECMO training.

Future of Physiological Modeling

This section will address what's on the horizon regarding physiological modeling, including a broader scope outside of ECMO simulation. Patient-specific or device-specific models will be addressed, including elaboration on the use of models in predicting physiological or pathophysiological responses and how to use these models in training and clinical practice.

T. Antonius (✉)
Division of Neonatology, Department of Pediatrics, Radboudumc Amalia Children's Hospital, Nijmegen, The Netherlands
e-mail: tim.antonius@radboudumc.nl

L. C. Johnston, L. Su (eds.), *Comprehensive Healthcare Simulation: ECMO Simulation*, Comprehensive Healthcare Simulation,
https://doi.org/10.1007/978-3-030-53844-6_8

Introduction to Physiological Modeling

A model is a representation of a system using general rules and definitions. We generally construct models to describe, understand, explain, and make predictions on the behavior of systems, where a "system" can be defined as a collection of interacting objects [1]. Physiological modeling is a type of modeling where a conceptual model of a physiological process is translated into a mathematical model or physical model. A *conceptual* model is typically a more general, abstract, and qualitative model, where a *mathematical* model is a description of a system represents using mathematical language and concepts. A *physical* model is a system represented by a tangible, real-world object.

The complexity of these models is always a trade-off between simplicity and accuracy, and while added complexity usually improves accuracy, it can make the model more difficult to build and understand. As the human body is an incredibly complex system of interacting systems where only a limited number of conceptual models are available, constructing a solid mathematical or physical model which can be used in ECMO simulation is an enormous challenge.

To understand how a model (mathematical of physical) is constructed, we first have to introduce some basic terminology. We have already defined a system as a collection of interacting objects. A system interacts with its environment through variables and signals (time-dependent variables). A variable from the environment which influences the evolution of a system is called an *independent* or *input* variable. The signal from a system, or *output* variable, is a *dependent* variable [1]. It can be helpful to visualize a system using a block diagram (Fig. 8.1).

When it is not possible or feasible to experiment on, or utilize a real system because of patient safety concerns, we can develop a model of that system. This may be a physical model, where the system is a tangible, real-world object the user can interact with, such as an anatomical model of a lung used for airway and respiratory management training. In this example, the independent variable could be the applied airway pressure, and the output variable (dependent variable) could be the expansion of the lungs. The properties of the system (such as compliance of the balloons used to model the lungs) have significant impact on the behavior of the system. However, physical models have their limitations, including expense or difficulty in construction, or challenges in adaptation to suit the needs of varying scenarios. The advantages of physical models, when of appropriate fidelity to the real system, include the ability for the user to interact with the materials with an intuitive and hands-on feel. A physical model also offers the possibility of interaction with real-world medical devices, improving the realism of the experience.

When it is not feasible to use a physical model, a mathematical model can be constructed to represent the relationships between system variables. An ideal mathematical model contains a lot of information about the system. Additionally, an interface is required to input variables into the model and present output variables to the user. For example, if the applied airway pressure is measured and this pressure is used as the independent input variable, the computational model calculates the volume change depending on the airway pressure and the system properties. The model output could be a screen-based representation of the lung or translated into an electrical signal driving a linear attenuator (motor) which drives the thoracic excursions of a real manikin.

One major advantage of using a mathematical model is the ability to adapt to numerous input variables. It is also quite easy to adapt the systemic properties, making the model suitable for simulating a range of different scenarios. It is also possible to model more complex states, where multiple input variables combine to alter the baseline state of the model, resulting in changes in multiple output variables.

Physiological Modeling in ECMO Simulation

ECMO simulation can be approached in several different ways. The typical format utilizes a manikin that appears to be connected to an ECMO circuit, and vital signs are displayed on a bedside monitor. The instructor can change the vital signs, activity, and physical exam findings of the manikin, as well as alter the baseline state of ECMO system to simulate different clinical scenarios. Changes in vital signs and circuit pressures can either be scripted or adjusted *on the fly* by the instructor using a screen-based interface.

This classic form of ECMO simulation may be challenging for the instructor, as it is difficult to keep track of all

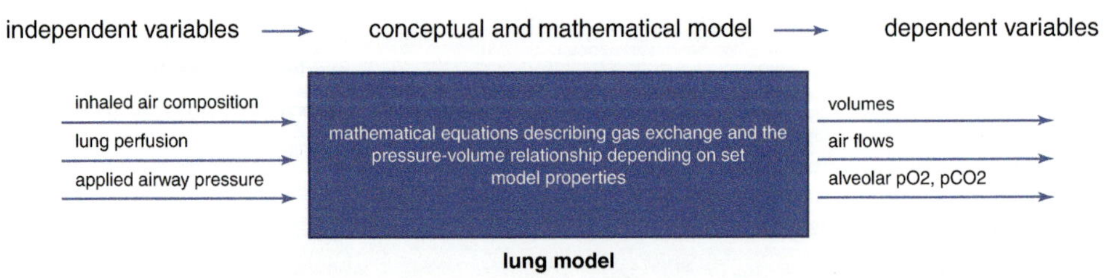

Fig. 8.1 Example of a general block diagram of a lung model

interventions the learners have provided and titrate the manikin's response in a realistic manner. Let us consider a typical VA-ECMO simulation incident where there is an emergency with an abrupt decrease in venous drainage. In response, the team alters the ventilator settings, provides a volume bolus, and attempts to increase the ECMO flow simultaneously. The instructor will need to consider the summative impact of all of these changes and determine how the vital signs and circuit pressures will be affected. This is a typical multi-input, multi-output problem. Since there are so many variables to consider, scripting is almost impossible. For this reason, there has been great interest in the potential ability of a computational model to adapt to numerous types of input variables over a broad range, as this may be a solution for this common type of problem facing the instructor in ECMO simulation.

At the beginning of this chapter, characteristics of dependent and independent variables were described, and the mathematics describing the relation between these variables were noted to be key components of a system. In order to utilize computational modeling for ECMO simulation, one must first consider its requirements. What should the model be able to do? More elaborate requirements necessitate an increased level of complexity of the model utilized. The requirements depend on the type of simulator, the simulation environment, and the learning objectives. The requirements of a model used to solve the multi-input, multi-output problem of the instructor described above will be significantly more complex than requirements of a model of a screen-based ECMO simulator. A screen-based ECMO simulator does not need an interface with the manikin, ventilator, nor the ECMO machine to present the output variables to the users.

As an illustration of this concept, the requirements of a model used to solve the multi-input, multi-output problem of the instructor described above (volume bolus, ventilator settings and ECMO flow change) will be considered.

To solve this problem, numerous pieces of information must be contemplated. First to consider are the vital signs of the simulated ECMO patient, including the common values of heart rate, blood pressure, and oxygen saturation. These will serve as the dependent variables of the new model. More advanced (and more complicated) models might incorporate additional values, such as central venous pressure, end tidal carbon dioxide levels, and blood gas composition, as part of the requirements, but for the current example, only heart rate, blood pressure, and oxygen saturation will be considered. The next priority is to determine which organ systems need to be modeled to provide these dependent variables. For this example, the model will need to incorporate the cardiovascular system, the pulmonary system, oxygen transport, baroreflex, and the ECMO circuit. The next step is to determine the required complexity. For instance, the ECMO system might be represented by a simple model where all blood is saturated to 100% and a fixed partial oxygen pressure is maintained. The patient's lung model can be a single compartment model with variable resistance and compliance. It might be sufficient to model the heart as a two-chamber pump where the contractility can be adjusted. These choices will be driven primarily by the learning objectives and the level of sophistication of the learners. Next, the required independent variables are determined, as these will need to be inserted into the model. In the current example, the independent variables include the ECMO flow, the applied airway pressure and FiO2, as well as net gain or loss in the patient's overall blood volume. Finally, the parameters of the model, which describe the relationship between the independent and dependent variables, must be identified. Examples of potential parameters include factors such as contractility, baroreflex sensitivity, lung compliance, and blood volume. One can imagine that adding additional requirements will increase the complexity of the model very quickly.

Finding an appropriate balance between the requirements and the necessary complexity of the model is the greatest challenge of using mathematical models in ECMO simulation. It is also most likely the largest potential drawback. As additional requirements are included, the models become increasingly complex and difficult to build and manipulate.

Another important aspect of using computational models in simulation is the way the independent variables are inserted into the model. In the previous example, it was determined that ECMO flow, applied airway pressure, and patient volume status would be considered. This requires consideration of how this information is inserted into the model. Computational models handle continuous high-resolution data much more effectively than fragmented, low-resolution data. As such, there will be a need to measure the actual ECMO flow and airway pressure of the ECMO machine and mechanical ventilator used in the simulation setup, which requires reliable sensors and an interface to transmit the data from the sensors into the model. Some data can be handled by the simulation operator, however. For example, if the learners transfuse 500 ml of blood, the simulation operator can insert this information into the model using an interface on the simulator.

Full Model-Driven and Hybrid ECMO Simulation

In the previous section, the example provided represented a computational model where only parts of the physiology were modeled to solve the multi-input, multi-output problem. In this situation, it was noted that increasing the requirements of the model quickly increased its complexity. When we only model parts of the physiology on ECMO, for example, only the relationship between ECMO flow and blood pressure, and manually adjust or script the other output variables like blood gas composition, the term hybrid ECMO simulation will be utilized.

Using a different type of model, a full model-driven ECMO simulation, the role of the instructor/simulator technician changes. Whereas in a typical ECMO simulation the operator needs to change the vital signs, manikin exam and behaviors, and simulated settings of the ECMO circuit on-the-fly or using scripts, in full model-driven simulation this is not necessary. In full model-driven simulation, the condition of the patient is set using predefined settings; all responses of the simulator are determined by the model, depending on the interventions provided by the candidates. The instructor or technician can adapt the model properties to the scenario if needed. This type of ECMO simulation generally requires an extensive model and an array of sensors interfacing with the simulator and measuring the independent variables to be inserted into the model. It also requires significantly more computational power than hybrid models. At this time, no full model-driven ECMO simulator is available.

A hybrid ECMO simulation uses a computational model for calculation of some of the dependent variables. As an example of a hybrid model, one might simulate the occurrence of an air embolus in the ECMO circuit. The learning objective is to manage the patient while removing air from the system. A hybrid model connecting the heart rate, blood pressure, and oxygen saturation to the measured ECMO flow will allow for realistic changes while the ECMO flow fluctuates during the deairing process. Other more sophisticated uses of hybrid models are also possible. A simple hybrid model of the ECMO artificial lung can calculate the pre- and post-oxygenator pressures and oxygen and carbon dioxide transfer across the lung, depending on the measured flow. The operator needs to set the resistance of the lung and the diffusion coefficients. Using an external display, the pressures and measured oxygen saturation levels can be interfaced to the candidates. Using this method, the instructor does not have to tamper with the ECMO machine using external hardware to simulate ECMO membrane failure. A good example of a hybrid ECMO simulator is the parallel simulator from Chalice Medical where several dependent parameters as blood pressure, heart rate, and O_2 saturation can be calculated from an independent variable (ECMO flow) using a very basic linear model.

A more elaborate simulator using mathematical modeling is Califia perfusion simulator system (Biomed Simulation, Inc., San Diego, CA) where several dependent variables like blood pressure, heart rate, and blood gas composition can be calculated using a mathematical model.

Explanatory Models in ECMO Simulation

An explanatory model is a representation of relevant physiologic processes that provides insight into the relationships between therapeutic interventions and monitored variables and their dependency on incidents and pathologies [2]. This educational technology facilitates understanding, reasoning, and communication in the clinical environment.

An explanatory model for ECMO is a screen-based form of a full model-driven ECMO simulator, but the graphic representation is carefully constructed to facilitate learning. The learner can play with selected interventions like changing the systemic and pulmonary vascular resistance, cardiac contractility, or ventilator settings in different ECMO modalities. Changing the ECMO settings or properties, such as gas flow, blood flow, or lung resistance, and assessing impact on other facets of the model can give students the opportunity to grasp complex physiology in a more intuitive way.

The ECMOjo software [3] can be seen as a very early form of an explanatory model. In this software package, the learner can manage ECMO events and emergencies using a screen-based representation of an infant on ECMO without the need for an instructor. It uses a gaming engine to teach learners how to handle ECMO events and gives feedback on performance. Although this software is not actively maintained, it is still available for download at http://ecmojo.sourceforge.net.

Figure 8.2 shows unpublished work from Antonius and van Meurs detailing an explanatory model of the pathophysiology of neonatal ECMO. This software uses a very elaborate mathematical model of the neonatal physiology on ECMO based on previous work on a congenital heart disease called transposition of the great arteries. On the left side of the screen, the user can adjust the independent variables of the model. The middle pane shows a graphical representation of the circulation and gives feedback on volumes, pressures, and oxygen saturation. The right panel displays the dependent variables of the model.

Explanatory models hold a great promise in improving understanding and reasoning in the clinical environment and could be applied in other situations, such as facilitation of case discussions.

Current Available Models for Use in ECMO Simulation

Currently, there is no complete physiological model of a patient on ECMO which is available for use in ECMO simulation. The fact that the models must run in real time severely limits the use of some of the available computational models of an ECMO system. Also, interfacing the models with cur-

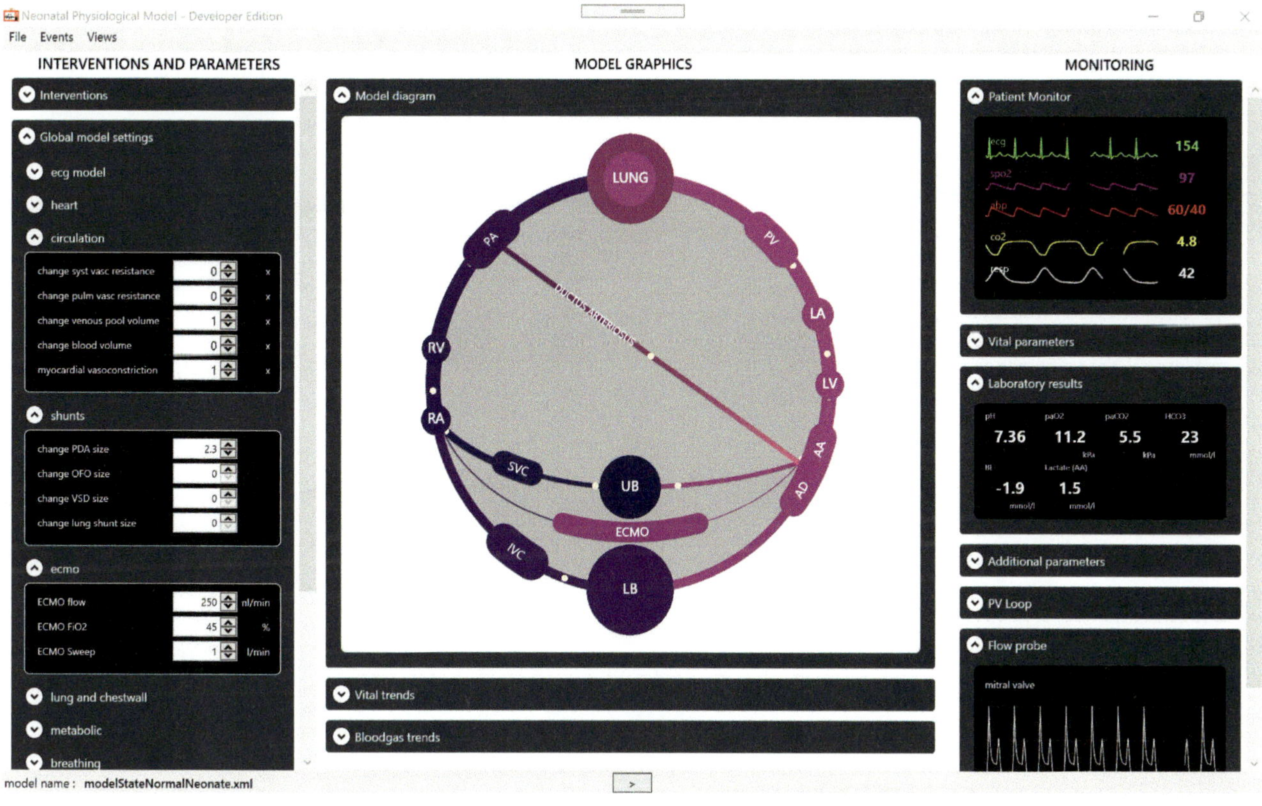

Fig. 8.2 ECMO explanatory model by Antonius and van Meurs

rently available ECMO simulators has numerous challenges and is not feasible at this time.

However, several available computational models may be useful to educators. BioGears offers an open-source, comprehensive, extensible human physiology engine which can be adapted to run in real time [4]. Another company, Kitware, has based a Pulse Physiology Engine on the BioGears engine [5]. The Physiome project hosts a vast array of computational models ranging from cardiovascular to acid base [6]. Physiolibary is a free open-source library designed for modeling human physiology using Modelica [7]. None of these open-source models currently incorporate an ECMO system (pump and oxygenator), but it would be possible to make these extensions in the future.

Future of Physiological Modeling

The use of computational models in ECMO simulation and in clinical practice is still very limited. However, large worldwide initiatives like Physiome [6] and the Virtual Physiological Human aim to develop next-generation computer models of human physiology ranging from molecular to organ and full body scale [8]. These next-generation computational models will make it possible to develop new therapies and diagnostic tools, improve medical devices, and trial the impact of new drugs. Using these next-generation models, educators will be able to run patient-specific simulations, facilitate case discussions, and make predictions on how a patient will respond to specific interventions (both individually and in combination). Although the aim of these initiatives is not focused on education, the field of ECMO simulation can still benefit from this work.

Conclusion

Model-driven ECMO simulators have the potential to greatly enhance simulations by solving the multi-input multi-output problem. They can relieve the cognitive load of the instructors and operators and provide the candidates with a more realistic experience than in the typical ECMO simulation scenario. However, the use of model-driven ECMO simulators is still challenging in this setting due to the issues of interfacing with the real-world devices and the complexity of the models which need to run in real time. Screen-based or mixed-reality full model-driven ECMO simulators do not require the interface with a manikin or ECMO device and, thus, are easier to create. Finally, explanatory models hold a great promise in improving understanding and reasoning in the clinical environment. Significant improvements in physiological modeling are anticipated to continue in the future and will likely be applicable to improving the accuracy and fidelity of ECMO simulation.

References

1. van Meurs W. Modeling and simulation in biomedical engineering: applications in cardiorespiratory physiology. 1st ed: McGraw-Hill Education; 2011.
2. van Meurs WWL, Antonius TAJ. Explanatory models in neonatal intensive care: a tutorial. Adv Simul. New York; 2018;3:27.
3. ECMOjo [Internet]. Honolulu: Telehealth Research Institute, John A. Burns School of Medicine (JABSOM) of the University of Hawaii. Available from: http://ecmojo.sourceforge.net/.
4. Biogears [Internet]. Applied Research Associates, Inc. Available from: https://www.biomedsimulation.com/.
5. Pulse Physiology engine. [Internet]. Kitware, Inc. Available from: https://physiology.kitware.com/.
6. Physiome [Internet]. International Union of Physiological Sciences. Available from: http://physiomeproject.org/.
7. Physiolibrary [Internet]. Marek Mateják, Charles University in Prague. Available from: http://www.physiolibrary.org/.
8. Virtual Physiological Human. VPH Institute. Available from: https://www.vph-institute.org/.

Immersive Technologies in ECMO Simulation

9

Jack Pottle and Jenny Zhou

Learning Objectives

1. Provide an overview of the immersive technologies (AR, VR and MR).
2. Discuss uses of VR in healthcare.
3. Define the utility and evidence base of VR simulation.
4. Outline future directions of VR simulation applied to ECMO.

Introduction

As healthcare systems around the world struggle with growing demands and limited budgets, pressure is increasing to deliver more simulation, at reduced cost, while demonstrating outcomes. Over the last 20 years, the impact of physical simulation has been proven in multiple fields. Within healthcare, there is now substantial evidence for the benefits of simulation in surgical, medical, and nursing fields. It has been shown to improve the confidence and competence of healthcare professionals, improve performance, and enhance patient care and outcomes [1].

Simulation covers a vast range of activities, and it is important to focus on the learning objectives of any simulation-based activity to determine the optimal modality with which to approach it. Though the bulk of simulation over the past two decades has involved the use of physical manikins, equipment, and actors, there has been a rapid increase in the ability of immersive technologies to deliver proven simulation techniques using novel technology. The immersive technologies include augmented reality (AR), mixed reality (MR), and virtual reality (VR), and this chapter examines their use across healthcare and potential in medical training. These modalities are particularly pertinent to the training of ECMO providers.

ECMO simulation has a number of challenges in common with standard simulation. These include the financial burden (hardware, reusables, running costs), equipment difficulties, scheduling conflicts, space limitations, and the substantial demands on faculty time, to name but a few [2]. The difficulties associated with ECMO simulation are compounded by a number of factors. Technical issues include the lack of suitable manikins for ECMO, the difficulty accurately simulating circuit/patient interactions, and even technical issues such as the color of blood in different circuits and make it very difficult to simulate clinically accurate ECMO scenarios with a high degree of fidelity [2].

Additionally, staffing difficulties common to any type of simulation are compounded in ECMO, due to the potential desire to train with the native interprofessional care team. In this setting, it is preferable to have expert staff members from each discipline, such as a physician, a perfusionist or ECMO specialist, and a nurse, available to facilitate the simulation. Though staff required are frequently not compensated for their time, they are often taken out of clinical practice to act as role players, increasing the hidden costs of simulation [3]. Financial constraints are perhaps the most pertinent issue with ECMO simulation. Though costs vary widely between institutions, the cost of ECMO simulation is frequently considerably to be higher than for non-ECMO scenarios. One-off costs specific to ECMO include the potential purchase and modification of manikins not designed for this particular use. Ongoing costs are frequently attributed to consumable products, such as oxygenator, bladder, tubing, cannulae, etc., all of which can significantly increase the cost relative to standard simulation [4].

J. Pottle (✉) · J. Zhou
Oxford Medical Simulation, London, UK
e-mail: jack@oxfordmedicalsimulation.com

L. C. Johnston, L. Su (eds.), *Comprehensive Healthcare Simulation: ECMO Simulation*, Comprehensive Healthcare Simulation,
https://doi.org/10.1007/978-3-030-53844-6_9

Considering all these factors, the opportunities leveraged by the immersive technologies are particularly relevant to ECMO simulation.

Definitions

Note the language around immersive technologies is constantly evolving, but the definitions below give a practical overview. These definitions are explained in more detail, with examples, in later paragraphs.

Immersive Technology: Immersive technology is an umbrella term for technologies including VR, AR, and MR.

Virtual Reality: Virtual reality (VR) is the use of software to create an immersive simulated environment. Unlike traditional user interfaces, VR places the user inside an experience where they are able to engage with the environment in a way that feels real.

Augmented Reality: Augmented reality (AR) is the integration of digital information and objects with the user's real environment. Unlike virtual reality, which creates a totally artificial environment, augmented reality uses the existing environment and overlays new information on top of it.

Mixed Reality: Mixed reality (MR) also involves the integration of digital information and objects with the user's physical environment. However, unlike AR – where the objects are overlaid on the real world – in MR the real and digital objects coexist and interact in real time.

Fidelity: Fidelity is a measure of how much an environment, object, or situation "feels real."

Presence: Presence is the feeling of *being there* in an immersive environment. It can be produced by the combination of immersion, engagement, and interactivity that causes the user to suspend disbelief and act as they would in the real world.

Gamification: Gamification is the application of typical elements of game playing (e.g., point scoring, competition with others, rules of play) to other areas of activity, generally to encourage engagement.

Haptics: The use of technology that simulates the senses of touch and motion that would be felt by a user interacting directly with physical objects.

Voice control: The ability to use one's voice to interact as one would in real life with a digital character or object.

Single-player: A virtual scenario where there is only one learner (player) is in the virtual environment at one time. There may be other computer-generated characters in the scenario, but the learner is the only autonomous player.

Multiplayer: A virtual scenario where more than one learner (player) is in the scenario at one time. This allows multiple individuals to interact in a virtual environment.

Immersive Technologies

As noted above, the immersive technologies include augmented reality (AR), mixed reality (MR), and virtual reality (VR). The reality-virtuality continuum described by Milgram et al. is useful to conceptualize thinking around the various formats available [5] (Fig. 9.1).

The core concepts of immersive technologies have been established for decades, though have evolved over time. It is only in the last 5 years that they have become available at a price point that has allowed them to become widely available. On one end of the continuum is reality, and on the other end is virtuality. Virtuality refers to a constructed "near" reality that is completely simulated through the use of software. It is possible to mix different aspects of reality and virtuality to produce different kinds of realities, and AR, MR, and VR describe different portions of this continuum.

Augmented Reality (AR)

Augmented reality overlays digital items onto reality. Users commonly experience AR using handheld devices such as smartphones and tablets. These have cameras to capture and display reality on screen, and the picture can be overlaid with computer-generated items (Fig. 9.2).

Augmented reality is also available via head-mounted displays, such as Google Glass or Microsoft Hololens (Fig. 9.3). With these headsets, the user can still see the real world through a visor and digital material superimposed on top of this, much like a head-up display.

Mixed Reality (MR)

Mixed reality is similar to augmented reality in that the user still wears a headset allowing them to see the real world and digital objects, but in MR these digital objects can interact with the real world (Fig. 9.4).

For example, a learner could be in a simulation center participating in a physical ECMO simulation while wearing a headset. In augmented reality, the patient's vital sign monitoring parameters could be displayed as a head-up display

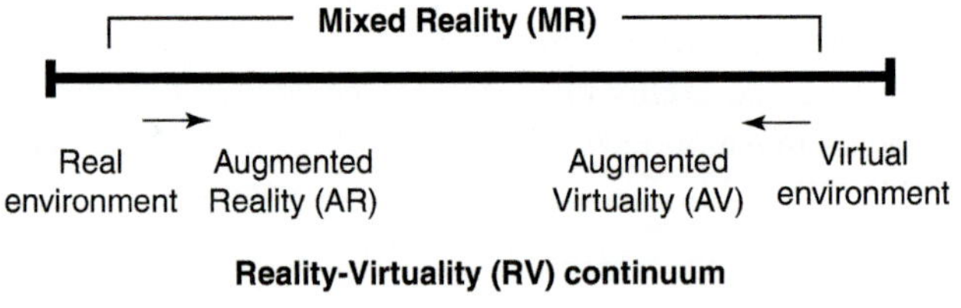

Fig. 9.1 Milgram and Kishino's mixed reality on the reality-virtuality continuum. (Used with permission of [5])

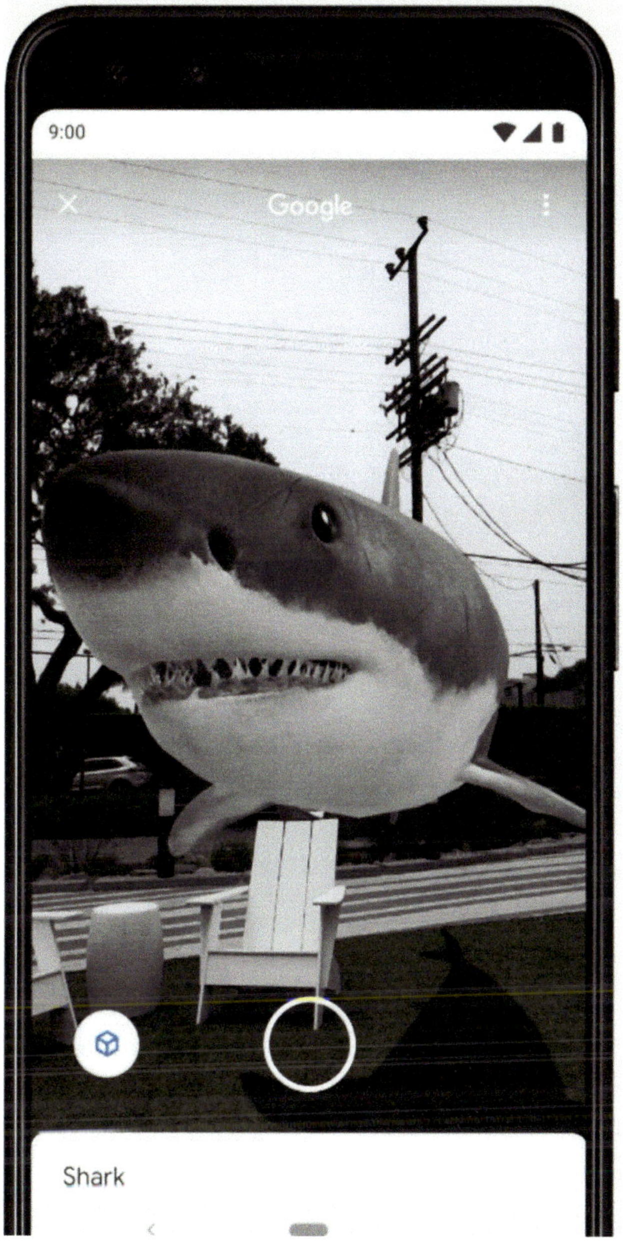

Fig. 9.2 Augmented reality is used to overlay images, such as this shark, onto views of the real world. (Used with permission from Google)

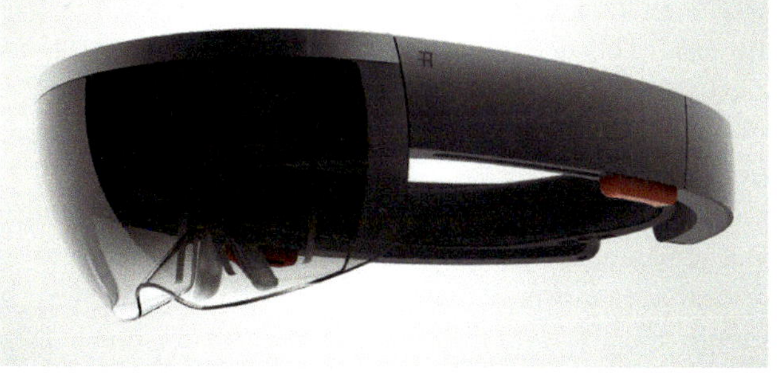

Fig. 9.3 Microsoft Hololens. (Used with permission from Microsoft)

when the learner looks in a certain direction. No matter what occurred in that location, the monitor would always be seen when the user looked there.

However, in MR – though the monitor would look fundamentally the same as in AR – it would be obscured if anyone moved "in front of" the virtual monitor, as if in real life. In other words in MR, the digital monitor would appear to be integrated in the real world, whereas in AR it is overlaid.

Augmented and mixed reality theoretically allow the user to be in a real environment – such as a simulation center with a real ECMO machine and ECMO team – while virtual patients are overlaid on it. A part task trainer could be integrated with the augmented world to allow learners to insert lines and work with their real team, while all participants could see the virtual patient and virtual vital signs projected onto their AR or MR headsets.

While it is an exciting prospect, the technology available to date – the most advanced of which are Microsoft Hololens and Magic Leap at the time of writing – is relatively heavy and can only overlay digital objects on a small part of the user's vision. These limitations in the hardware and complexities in software creation have made the user experience in AR and MR suboptimal, particularly for situations such as ECMO. As a seamless user experience is vital in order to allow the learner to forget about the technology and focus on the simulated clinical problem, application of AR and MR in simulation is currently limited.

Virtual Reality (VR)

In contrast to AR and MR, in virtual reality (VR) the user is completely immersed in the virtual environment and cannot see the real world at all. This immersive visual input is combined with 3D audio to create a complete sense of presence in a virtual environment.

Whereas in AR and MR the learner needs to be in a clinically realistic setting such as a simulation center, VR has the unique capability of allowing experiential learning to happen in any setting; in putting on the headset, the learner is cognitively transported to a different world [6]. In addition, with multiplayer functionality in VR, scenarios can have many disparate learners interacting in one virtual scenario. This allows remote training of many individuals in a common environment.

While AR, MR, and VR are therefore all part of the immersive technologies spectrum, they are pragmatically different technologies suitable for different needs. As with any simulation, deciding on the learning objectives and then choosing the appropriate technology with which to tackle them is the best approach, rather than being led by the technology itself.

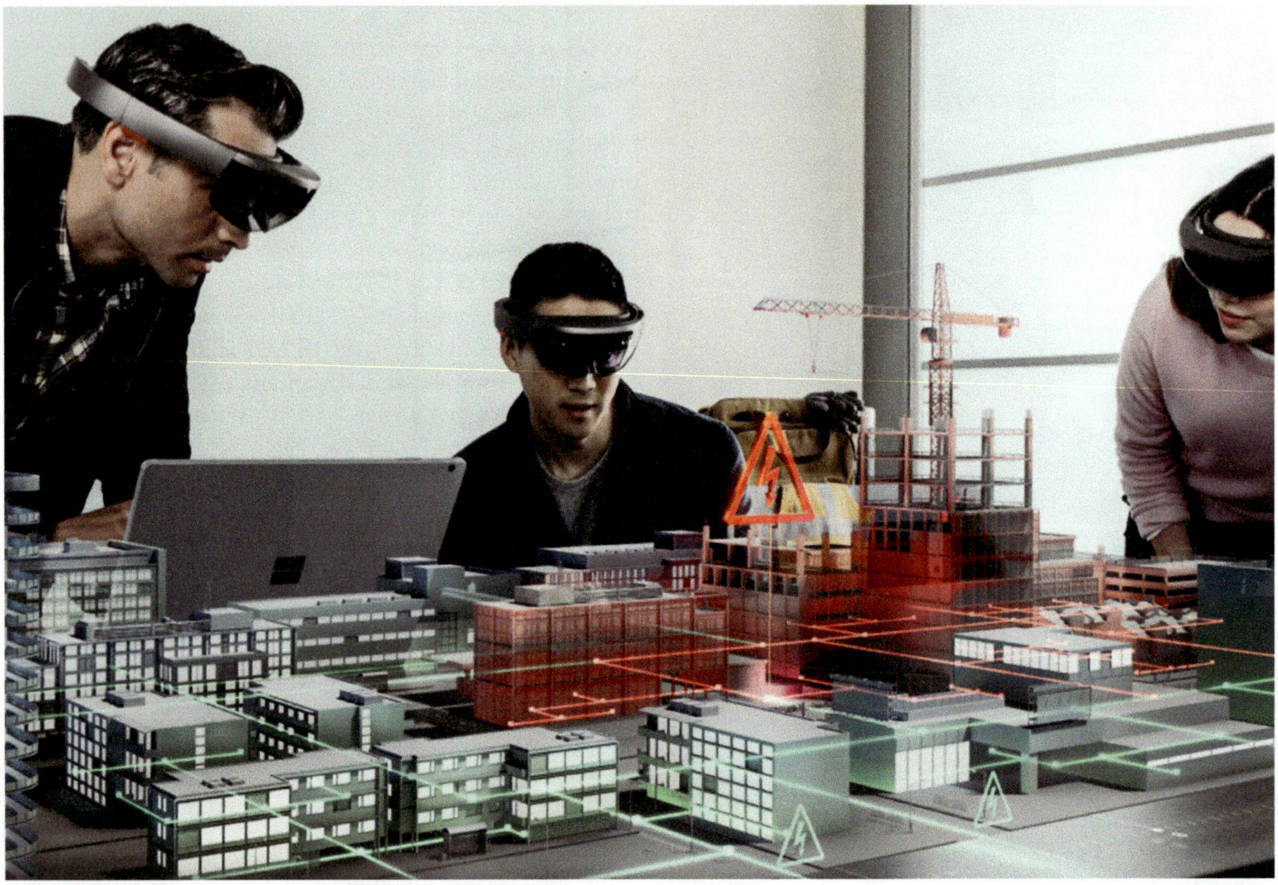

Fig. 9.4 Representation of mixed reality in action. (Used with permission from Microsoft)

Note that in the past screen-based simulation on computers was frequently referred to as virtual reality. This was partly driven by marketing, with screen-based products taking advantage of the hype around VR, and partly due to genuine uncertainty in how to label novel technology. However, there is now an understanding that the value of virtual reality simulations comes from immersion and the sense of presence that they produce (see section "Evidence"). As such, virtual reality now generally refers only to immersive virtual reality carried out in headsets rather than computer-based simulation.

This lack of clarity of definitions has made literature surveys difficult – with much of the "virtual reality" literature from 2000 to 2015 years being screen based – but we will refer to virtual reality only in terms of headset-based VR for this chapter.

The Psychology of VR Design

To understand the potential of VR, it is beneficial to appreciate factors that underlie its effectiveness. We will next focus on presence, immersion, and fidelity all of which play into the design of VR experiences.

Presence is the feeling VR can create for the user of *being there*. It is this feeling of being there that ensures scenarios in the virtual world are memorized in the same way as real events, ensuring VR produces true experiential learning.

Immersion is the ability of a technology to produce presence. It is influenced by software design and the hardware used. For example, a low-quality headset such as Google cardboard will offer lower immersion than a high-quality headset such as Oculus Rift. Generally, the more immersive a virtual environment is, the better the learning in it [7].

Fidelity, a concept widely discussed in the physical simulation literature, is also vital. We consider fidelity to be "feeling real." This definition deliberately disentangles the term fidelity from technology, as a scenario that feels real can be produced using low-tech solutions provided the conditions are correct.

In VR, fidelity is influenced by a large number of factors. The graphics, animations, the character modeling, vocals, clinical scenario itself, and the user interface (the way a learner interacts with the environment) all play a role. This does not necessarily mean that all interactions should try to exactly replicate real life, rather that the user interface should be matched to the learning objectives. For example, if VR was being used to teach how to insert a VV line in VR, then haptic gloves simulating the feel of a needle going through the tissues would be ideal. However, if the objective includes simulating the decision-making principals around ECMO, then a menu-driven system may work just as well, if not better. This is similar to functional task alignment as described by Adams [8]: there needs to be a functional fidelity to the scenario that matches the learning goals. Importantly, more is not always better. Paradoxically, more technology can decrease fidelity if it does not work seamlessness enough to be forgotten.

Immersive Technologies in Healthcare

Now that we have an understanding of the Immersive technologies, the key elements to their design and how they affect us as users, we will examine some of their use cases. In healthcare, the uses of the immersive technologies are frequently split into categories, including therapeutic (direct to patients), clinical (to facilitate care), and educational (to teach or train either patients or clinicians).

Therapeutic Uses

Virtual reality has a unique power to make users believe they are in a different environment. This dissonance produced between the real and virtual world has been used in multiple ways clinically with excellent results. For example, VR can be used to control pain [9–11] and to distract patients undergoing painful procedures such as dressing changes [12]. In physical rehabilitation, VR headsets can help provide a motivator for movement and provide encouraging feedback in the form of movement in the virtual environment [13, 14]. VR can be used to facilitate therapeutic conversations and to facilitate graduated forms of exposure therapy for phobias, eating disorders, and posttraumatic stress disorder (PTSD) [15, 16]. It can also be used as a trigger for emotional states in autism and to trigger memories in dementia [17, 18]. This rapid increase in VR take up is driven by the body of available content and decreasing costs of devices. As such, therapeutic VR is likely to become a mainstream therapy over the coming years.

Clinical Use Cases

AR and MR are used more in the clinical sphere than therapeutic, as clinicians usually need an awareness of their surroundings to perform their role. Usage examples include using AR to overlay outlines of the venous system on a patient's arm to help with IV access [19] or projecting radiological images with other relevant intraoperative information to help aid surgical planning and execution – avenues being pursued by companies such as Proximie and Digital Surgery.

VR has also found clinical uses, such as in recreating scans in 3D to allow surgeons to visualize and navigate anatomy before operating or providing radiologists with a different perspective on a scan [20]. Researchers are also exploring the development of VR content for diagnosing disorders such as autism and dementia [21, 22]. The use of immersive technologies in the clinical sphere is rapidly growing and looks set to continue.

Educational Use Cases

Anatomy teaching was one of the first areas to take up immersive learning, and numerous companies, including Pearson and 3D4Medical, provide immersive anatomical teaching be that in AR, MR, or VR. As such experiences were developed for students, it also became clear that they could help in patient education. VR, particularly 360 video, has been widely used to provide an immersive preview of hospital experiences to help reduce patient anxiety [23–25]. Both of these use cases require minimal interaction in the immersive environment and so are relatively simple to create.

As simulation is inherently interactive, immersive simulation took a little longer to arrive, and it was surgical training that pushed the development of immersive simulation initially. With the growing use of laparoscopic and minimally invasive surgery requiring surgeons to operate while viewing screens, it was no surprise that screen-based and VR simulation increased rapidly in these fields first. A number of companies such as Simbionix, Digital Surgery, Fundamental Surgery, Proximie, and Osso VR now develop training modules in various surgical specialties.

Only within the past few years has there been a growth in the immersive technologies more broadly in medical and nursing training. This is in part because the cost of immersive technology hardware and software development has decreased and also because of the growing recognition that simulation-based education is effective in these areas [26]. While surgical and procedural immersive simulation relies on replicating well-defined, physical interactions, the learning objectives in medical or nursing simulation generally revolve around clinical reasoning, critical thinking, crisis resource management, teamwork, and nontechnical skills.

Simulating a full complex clinical case for doctors and nurses in a way that feels real, involving full virtual teams, patients, environments, and realistic interactions, is complex and requires high development cost. This has therefore largely been carried out by well-funded academic centers with a potential reluctance to share their offerings.

However, commercial companies such as Oxford Medical Simulation, Sim-X, and VES all now produce clinical VR training at scale, dramatically reducing the cost of delivering VR simulation.

Educational use cases for immersive tech are therefore plentiful, but what can they offer and what pitfalls should we be aware of?

Advantages and Disadvantages of the Immersive Technologies in Simulation

The immersive technologies offer a number of advantages over physical simulation. For learners, they are available 24 hours a day, are not tied to large centers, and allow flexible access, helping alleviate scheduling difficulties. They are also repeatable on demand, allowing true deliberate practice over time [26]. If well-designed, VR scenarios can feel even more realistic than manikin-based simulation as the manikin is replaced by an interactive character. In addition, the psychological safety, enjoyable nature, and potential for gamification of VR encourage engagement and autonomous learning.

Next, from an institutional standpoint, immersive technologies allow simulation to be delivered at reduced cost with fewer resources. Such technologies can free up space and faculty time to allow other simulation activities to take place, ensuring optimal use of a center. Any virtual scenario can also be objective and standardized, ensuring consistent quality and adherence to protocols. Additionally, many immersive systems allow the creation of bespoke simulation curricula and can generate large amounts of performance data. This data is valuable for monitoring and encouraging learner engagement, as well as for identifying struggling students who may benefit from further training. Finally, from a global health perspective, this reduction in cost and ease of access allows simulation to be distributed globally, potentially revolutionizing simulation delivery worldwide.

However, there are a number of potential issues with immersive simulation. Firstly, the immersive technologies require hardware, some of which is expensive, as an initial barrier to entry. Additionally there is always a learning curve to any new technology, though the commercially available equipment has limited this as an issue in recent years. Also, immersive technology is not suitable for every possible educational opportunity. As with any simulation, the focus should be on learning objectives and identifying what technology best meets those needs, rather than seeing AR, MR, or VR as a panacea. For example, even though VR is the most advanced immersive technology, we should appreciate that it is not the best way to teach abdominal palpation as there is no need for complex immersion in this situation, just an accurate physical representation of an abdomen to practice on. Likewise, in situ simulation necessitates the real environment to be able to work with real-world layouts and identify real latent threats, so VR is not appropriate. Next, the subtleties of breaking bad news are best taught through expert standardized patients, as the complexities of language processing and facial expressions used cannot accurately be replicated by software yet. Additionally, some of the additional immersive technology required for specific learning objectives, including voice recognition for communication skills and haptics for procedural skills, are still in the process of being developed fully. As such, many of the immersive simulations focus on only a limited number of objectives – either procedural skills or patient communication, for example – rather than integrating all of these into one scenario (Table 9.1).

As mentioned, there are a number of companies producing VR medical simulation. These include Oxford Medical Simulation, Sim-X, and VES, many of whom have large libraries of scenarios. However, they do not necessarily have all the scenarios a center may require and may not be able to instantly customize the scenario to a center's needs. If a center does have highly specific requirements and decides to produce their own VR scenarios, then the cost of production, specialist expertise required, and duration of development are often prohibitive. Finally, one of the primary issues with VR simulation in ECMO is that, as yet, we are not aware of any companies who have actively entered the space of

Table 9.1 Advantages and disadvantages of the immersive technologies for simulation

Advantages	Disadvantages
Available 24 hours a day	Requires specialist hardware
Repeatable	Hardware limitations in AR/MR to date (small visual window, hot)
Standardized	Single player VR removes subtlety of human interaction (multiplayer VR, AR and MR resolve this)
Objective	Only simulate a certain range of scenarios or certain defined learning objectives
Available outside large centers	Can decrease realism if done badly
Can increase realism if done well	High up front development time and technical expertise
No need for faculty (or save faculty time)	
Need minimal space	
Generates performance data automatically (traceable)	
Once built, scenarios can be reused indefinitely	
Decrease cost per simulation	
Enjoyable and easy to gamify	
Increase learner autonomy	

immersive VR for ECMO simulation specifically. However, it is only a matter of time, and an academic-industry partnership is likely to be the most practical approach.

Evidence Behind VR Simulation

While the evidence of immersive technology in ECMO is therefore lacking, there is a large body of literature on VR medical simulation in multiple contexts over the last 20 years. VR literature was initially confined to gaming or technical journals. As the use of virtual environments in medical simulation became more widespread in the 1990s, the term "virtual" and "virtual reality" began to appear in the medical literature. However, it was widely used to refer to screen-based simulation and e-learning. As detailed previously, this differs from immersive VR.

Compared to screen-based learning, the greater immersion provided by VR significantly enhances learning performance in medical simulation. There are numerous lines of evidence to demonstrate that the only presence offered by immersive virtual reality leads to true learning from experience [7, 27]. For example, a study of medical students using a head-mounted display vs. screen-based learning demonstrated significantly higher knowledge gain in the immersive group than the screen-based group [28].

This power has positioned VR as vital teaching tool in multiple fields, including aviation, oil, shipping, and the military [29]. In fact, the aviation industry credits VR-based education as a major contributor to a nearly 50% reduction in human error-related airline crashes since the 1970s [30].

Virtual reality simulation has been widely adopted in surgical training where it has been shown to decrease injury, increase speed of operations, and improve overall outcomes. It has now been adopted by a large number of surgical programs with excellent results [31], and while the medical and nursing fields have been slower to take up virtual reality simulation, there is plenty of evidence out there. For example, VR can be used to train clinicians in complex procedures such as transvenous lead extraction [32], is effective in CPR training [33], and can improve communication skills [34], enhance critical thinking, and improve clinical decision-making [35, 36].

In nursing simulation, VR has also been found to be as effective as physical simulation. In Haerling's 2018 paper, 84 nursing students were randomized to either virtual or physical nursing simulation. There were no significant differences in quantitative measures of learning or performance between participants in the manikin-based and virtual simulation groups, but the VR group was found to be significantly less expensive [37]. As such, VR medical and nursing simulation is likely to continue to expand rapidly over the coming years.

The Future of Immersive Technology in ECMO Simulation

So the immersive technologies have come of age, are now being widely used in medical and nursing simulation, and have a solid evidence base. It is surely only a matter of time before they are applied for ECMO training. Let us consider what that might look like.

Any of the immersive technologies may be suitable for ECMO simulation depending on learning objectives. The importance of the interprofessional team, the complex decision-making, the circuits, and the procedures used indicate that technical, nontechnical, and procedural skills should all be addressed when planning a simulation.

Mixed reality scenarios would allow the team to assemble in an empty room, put on headsets, and have the patient and equipment virtually appear in front of them. This would allow the team to perform together in any number of scenarios without setting up a physical center. This real-time training could also be done in situ, immediately before real ECMO sessions, to ensure optimal performance with the real patient.

Equally, multiplayer VR could be used instead, allowing ECMO teams to practice together wherever they were in the world. An expert perfusionist in Johns Hopkins could be in the same virtual simulation as team learning ECMO in Ghana, providing mentorship and advice during the scenario. Such a VR system could have complete photorealistic fidelity and motion capture to make all virtual characters indistinguishable from real life. It could then potentially use body tracking and machine learning to assess nonverbal communication and provide feedback on this as well.

To cover procedural aspects, haptic gloves could be used to allow the feeling of inserting lines. The system could monitor the users actions to provide them with detailed feedback on their performance, both individually and as a team, and if any of the team were not present on the day, artificially intelligent virtual team members with inbuilt voice recognition could stand in for them.

Scenarios could be instantly created to match real-life situations allowing repetition of serious incidents, or examination of latent threats in a replicated virtual world rather than in situ. Additionally, all of the performance data could be fed into algorithms that not only identify good or poor performance now but also predict performance in future.

If this all sounds a little similar to Minority Report, we can assure you it would not be coming immediately! However, it is all possible with the technologies already available, it just takes time, money, and expertise. It can be expected that ECMO simulationists will soon have another tool in their armory to scale simulation delivery and improve outcomes.

Summary

The immersive technologies are powerful methods of delivering simulation at scale and offer enormous possibilities in ECMO simulation. Though, as yet, companies have not put their resources into building virtual ECMO simulation, it is only a matter of time. As both ECMO and the immersive technologies continue to expand at pace, this promises to be a new and exciting frontier in simulation.

Notes Section The authors disclose that they receive financial support from Oxford Medical Simulation.

References

1. Brydges R, Hatala R, Zendejas B, Erwin PJ, Cook DA. Linking simulation-based educational assessments and patient-related outcomes: a systematic review and meta-analysis. Acad Med. 2015;90(2):246–56.
2. Alinier G, Hassan IF, Alsalemi A, Al Disi M, Ait Hssain A, Labib A, Alhomsi Y, Bensaali F, Amira A, Ibrahim AS. Addressing the challenges of ECMO simulation. Perfusion. 2018;33(7):568–76.
3. McIntosh C, Macario A, Flanagan B, Gaba DM. Simulation: what does it really cost? J Soc Simul Healthc. 2006;1(2):109.
4. Development of an ECMO simulation program: experience at Yale New Haven Hospital [Internet]. Medical Training Magazine; 2012 [cited 2019 Apr 12]. Available from: https://medicalsimulation.training/technology/development-of-an-ecmo-simulation-program-experience-at-yale-new-haven-hospital/.
5. Milgram P, Takemura H, Utsumi A, Kishino F. Augmented reality: a class of displays on the reality-virtuality continuum. Proceedings of telemanipulator and telepresence technologies. 1994. pp. 2351–2334.
6. Bailenson JN. Experience on demand: what virtual reality is, how it works, and what it can do. New York: W.W. Norton; 2018.
7. Repetto C, Serino S, Macedonia M, Riva G. Virtual reality as an embodied tool to enhance episodic memory in elderly. Front Psychol. 2016;7:1839.
8. Adams R, Gilbert G, Buckley L, et al. A method for functional task alignment analysis of an arthrocentesis simulator. Simul Healthc. 2018;13(4):289–94.
9. Dascal J, Reid M, IsHak WW, Spiegel B, Recacho J, Rosen B, Danovitch I. Virtual reality and medical inpatients: a systematic review of randomized, controlled trials. Innov Clin Neurosci. 2017;14(1-2):14–21.
10. Tashjian VC, Mosadeghi S, Howard AR, Lopez M, Dupuy T, Reid M, Martinez B, Ahmed S, Dailey F, Robbins K, Rosen B, Fuller G, Danovitch I, IsHak W, Spiegel B. Virtual reality for management of pain in hospitalized patients: results of a controlled trial. JMIR Ment Health. 2017;4(1):e9.
11. Won AS, Bailey J, Bailenson J, Tataru C, Yoon IA, Golianu B. Immersive virtual reality for pediatric pain. Children (Basel). 2017;4(7):52.
12. Scapin S, Echevarría-Guanilo ME, Boeira Fuculo Junior PR, Gonçalves N, Rocha PK, Coimbra R. Virtual reality in the treatment of burn patients: a systematic review. Burns. 2018;44(6):1403–16.
13. Maggio MG, Russo M, Cuzzola MF, Destro M, La Rosa G, Molonia F, Bramanti P, Lombardo G, De Luca R, Calabrò RS. Virtual reality in multiple sclerosis rehabilitation: a review on cognitive and motor outcomes. J Clin Neurosci. 2019;65:106.
14. Maggio MG, Latella D, Maresca G, Sciarrone F, Manuli A, Naro A, De Luca R, Calabrò RS. Virtual reality and cognitive rehabilitation in people with stroke: an overview. J Neurosci Nurs. 2019;51(2):101–5.
15. Clus D, Larsen ME, Lemey C, Berrouiguet S. The use of virtual reality in patients with eating disorders: systematic review. J Med Internet Res. 2018;20(4):e157.
16. Gonçalves R, Pedrozo AL, Coutinho ES, Figueira I, Ventura P. Efficacy of virtual reality exposure therapy in the treatment of PTSD: a systematic review. PLoS One. 2012;7(12):e48469.
17. Mesa-Gresa P, Gil-Gómez H, Lozano-Quilis JA, Gil-Gómez JA. Effectiveness of virtual reality for children and adolescents with autism spectrum disorder: an evidence-based systematic review. Sensors (Basel). 2018;18(8). pii: E2486.
18. Zucchella C, Sinforiani E, Tamburin S, Federico A, Mantovani E, Bernini S, Casale R, Bartolo M. The multidisciplinary approach to Alzheimer's disease and dementia. A narrative review of non-pharmacological treatment. Front Neurol. 2018;9:1058.
19. Guillon P, Makhloufi M, Baillie S, Roucoulet C, Dolimier E, Masquelier AM. Prospective evaluation of venous access difficulty and a near-infrared vein visualizer at four French haemophilia treatment centres. Haemophilia. 2015;21(1):21–6.
20. Bekele E, Zheng Z, Swanson A, Crittendon J, Warren Z, Sarkar N. Understanding how adolescents with autism respond to facial expressions in virtual reality environments. IEEE Trans Vis Comput Graph. 2013;19(4):711–20.
21. Coutrot A, Schmidt S, Coutrot L, Pittman J, Hong L, Wiener JM, Hölscher C, Dalton RC, Hornberger M, Spiers HJ. Virtual navigation tested on a mobile app is predictive of real-world wayfinding navigation performance. PLoS One. 2019;14(3):e0213272.
22. Cogné M, Taillade M, N'Kaoua B, Tarruella A, Klinger E, Larrue F, Sauzéon H, Joseph PA, Sorita E. The contribution of virtual reality to the diagnosis of spatial navigation disorders and to the study of the role of navigational aids: a systematic literature review. Ann Phys Rehabil Med. 2017;60(3):164–76.
23. Pandrangi VC, Gaston B, Appelbaum NP, Albuquerque FC Jr, Levy MM, Larson RA. The application of virtual reality in patient education. Ann Vasc Surg. 2019. pii: S0890-5096(19)30247-X
24. Bekelis K, Calnan D, Simmons N, MacKenzie TA, Kakoulides G. Effect of an immersive preoperative virtual reality experience on patient reported outcomes: a randomized controlled trial. Ann Surg. 2017;265(6):1068–73.
25. Jimenez YA, Cumming S, Wang W, Stuart K, Thwaites DI, Lewis SJ. Patient education using virtual reality increases knowledge and positive experience for breast cancer patients undergoing radiation therapy. Support Care Cancer. 2018;26(8):2879–88.
26. McGaghie WC, Issenberg SB, Petrusa ER, Scalese RJ. Revisiting 'A critical review of simulation-based medical education research: 2003-2009'. Med Educ. 2016;50(10):986–91.
27. Makowski D, Sperduti M, Nicolas S, Piolino P. "Being there" and remembering it: presence improves memory encoding. Conscious Cogn. 2017;53:194–202.
28. Gutiérrez F, Pierce J, Vergara VM, Coulter R, Saland L, Caudell TP, Goldsmith TE, Alverson DC. The effect of degree of immersion upon learning performance in virtual reality simulations for medical education. Stud Health Technol Inform. 2007;125:155–60.
29. Vozenilek J, Huff JS, Reznek M, Gordon JA. See one, do one, teach one: advanced technology in medical education. Acad Emerg Med. 2004;11(11):1149–54.
30. Levin A. Fewer crashes caused by pilots [Internet]. USA Today 2004 [cited 2019 Apr 12]. Available from: http://usatoday30.usatoday.com/news/nation/2004-03-01-crash_x.htm.

31. Bric JD, Lumbard DC, Frelich MJ, et al. Current state of virtual reality simulation in robotic surgery training: a review. Surg Endosc. 2016;30:2169.
32. Maytin M, Daily TP, Carillo RG. Virtual reality lead extraction as a method for training new physicians: a pilot study. Pacing Clin Electrophysiol. 2015;38(3):319–25.
33. Creutzfeldt J, Hedman L, Felländer-Tsai L. Cardiopulmonary resuscitation training by Avatars: a qualitative study of medical students' experiences using a multiplayer virtual world. JMIR Serious Games. 2016;4(2):e22.
34. Real FJ, DeBlasio D, Beck AF, Ollberding NJ, Davis D, Cruse B, Samaan Z, McLinden D, Klein MD. A virtual reality curriculum for pediatric residents decreases rates of influenza vaccine refusal. Acad Pediatr. 2017;17(4):431–5.
35. Burke SM. Cultivating critical thinking using virtual interactive case studies. J Pediatr Nurs. 2017;33:94–6.
36. Harrington CM, Kavanagh DO, Quinlan JF, Ryan D, Dicker P, O'Keeffe D, Traynor O, Tierney S. Development and evaluation of a trauma decision-making simulator in oculus virtual reality. Am J Surg. 2018;215(1):42–7.
37. Haerling KA. Cost-utility analysis of virtual and mannequin-based simulation. Simul Healthc. 2018;13(1):33–40.

Part IV

Other Topics for ECMO Simulation

Interprofessional Education and ECMO Simulation

10

Summer Elshenawy, Christine D. Franciscovich, Susan B. Williams, and Heather M. French

Learning Objectives

1. Understand the theory behind IPE as an effective educational tool for healthcare team.
2. Discuss the benefits of IPE simulation in crisis resource management.
3. Analyze barriers and challenges of IPE ECMO simulation and methods to overcome them.
4. Reflect upon clinical scenarios in which IPE ECMO simulation may improve quality of care.

Introduction

The complexity of knowledge and skills required to care for patients in intensive care has led to increased specialization and disciplinarity among healthcare providers. This shift toward specialization, while important for deepening knowledge of given medical conditions, has created a healthcare system that is composed of providers from different disciplines educated in separate silos. These disciplines often have unique leadership structures, vocabulary, methods of communication, and approaches toward problem-solving. Interprofessional education seeks to mitigate the effects that educational silos can have on effective interdisciplinary communication and collaboration. The high-risk procedure of initiating, maintaining, discontinuing, and responding to emergencies in extracorporeal membrane oxygenation (ECMO) requires a large and diverse team of healthcare providers to work together to perform a variety of complex interrelated tasks and behaviors. Interprofessional teamwork and communication can be developed and maintained using simulation-based team training. This chapter will provide a practical framework for the development and maintenance of an interprofessional simulation program to support hospital-based ECMO programs.

Theory to Support Interprofessional Education

Interprofessional education (IPE) in healthcare is defined by an educational approach that focuses on teamwork and targets learners of diverse healthcare professions. IPE occurs when learners from more than one profession, such as nursing, respiratory therapy, medicine, and pharmacy learn from and about each other to improve collaboration and quality of patient care [1]. IPE encourages a collaborative approach to learning that prioritizes quality and safety through improved communication and behaviors of the healthcare team. Efforts to promote and adopt IPE are evident on national and global scales. The Center for the Advancement of Interprofessional Education (CAIPE), a global collaborative that supports interprofessional education, provides resources for practical application of IPE in healthcare settings [1, 2]. The increasing emphasis on IPE in healthcare reflects the importance of an educational environment that fosters the development of

S. Elshenawy
Department of Pediatrics, Emory University School of Medicine, Atlanta, GA, USA

C. D. Franciscovich · S. B. Williams
The Children's Hospital of Philadelphia, Philadelphia, PA, USA

H. M. French (✉)
Division of Neonatology, Department of Pediatrics, The Children's Hospital of Philadelphia, Perelman School of Medicine at the University of Pennsylvania, Philadelphia, PA, USA
e-mail: frenchh@email.chop.edu

L. C. Johnston, L. Su (eds.), *Comprehensive Healthcare Simulation: ECMO Simulation*, Comprehensive Healthcare Simulation,
https://doi.org/10.1007/978-3-030-53844-6_10

the healthcare team as a whole and validates individual expertise and roles within that team.

The development of expertise in a given discipline is a process that starts with acquiring and retaining cognitive knowledge as described by Miller's Pyramid (Fig. 10.1) [3]. For single discipline learning, learners first focus on the acquisition and application of cognitive knowledge (Knows, Knows How) followed by integration of that cognitive knowledge with performance behaviors (Shows How, Does). Deeper understanding and application of knowledge occurs through deliberate practice and experience [4]. Once discipline-specific knowledge is acquired, steps must be taken to integrate that provider and their knowledge into the interdisciplinary actions and goals of the healthcare team. Miller's Pyramid can easily be adapted to interprofessional education and teamwork. Teams have the opportunity to integrate discipline-specific skills and knowledge in a team setting where collaboration, mutual support, and trust between team members are essential to reach a common objective. Members of interdisciplinary healthcare teams rely on discipline-specific skills and knowledge while working collaboratively and communicating effectively to solve a common problem [5].

The complexity of care involved in management of patients on ECMO necessitates educational strategies that support effective communication, collaboration, and teamwork among professionals of diverse backgrounds with unique skill sets. Thus, the training of an individual ECMO provider goes beyond the cognitive learning to behavioral learning as seen in Fig. 10.1. ECMO training requires acquisition and maintenance of role-specific technical skills ("knows" and "knows how") as well as sharpening communication, teamwork, and crisis resource management (CRM) as a part of a healthcare team ("shows how" and "does"). Several educational theories provide support for IPE for teams comprised of providers with diverse training backgrounds. Understanding these theories can help educators design training activities that promote interdisciplinary communication and collaboration that reflects the healthcare setting. These theories include andragogy (adult learning theory), transformative learning, and social psychology [6].

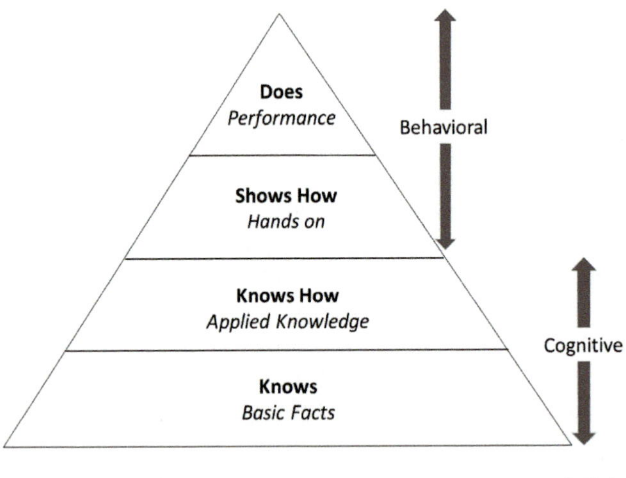

Fig. 10.1 Miller's pyramid. (Adapted from "The assessment of clinical skills/competence/performance" by GE Miller, Academic Medicine, 1990, pp. 63–67)

Andragogy and IPE

Malcolm Knowles developed the concept of andragogy. According to Knowles, the characteristics of the adult learner include self-motivation, learning that is based on past experiences, a readiness to acquire and apply knowledge, and a problem-based orientation to learn [7, 8] (Fig. 10.2). Thus, IPE educators can apply the principles of andragogy to promote practical and experiential learning that supports learners in using prior experiences to contextualize new knowledge and concepts with clear implications in their practice.

The application of each of these concepts is supported in IPE. IPE augments the efforts of self-directed individuals through participation on a team with a common educational goal [2]. Furthermore, prior experience of the learner serves to both inform and shape knowledge acquisition. The combined experience of the interprofessional team deepens the reservoir of experience that the team can build upon to enrich the encounter. Successful healthcare teams must be adept in both technical skills and teamwork and communication. IPE prioritizes team-based skills of the multidisciplinary health-

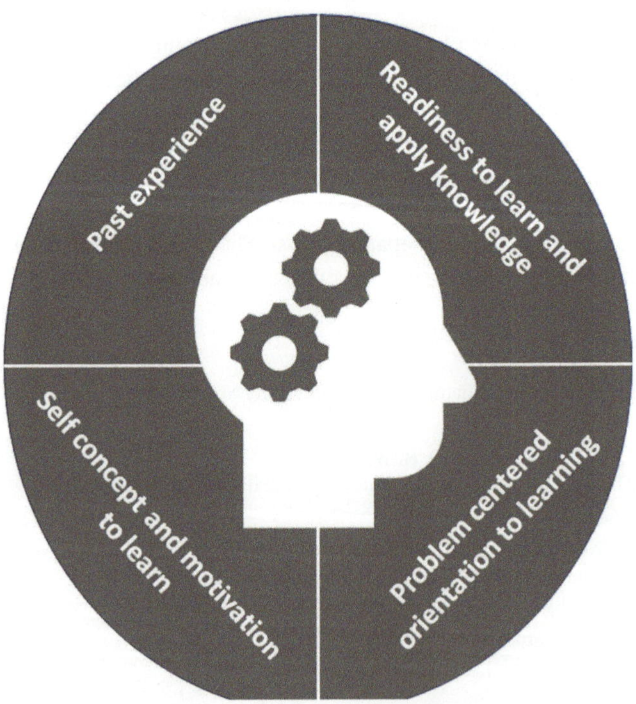

Fig. 10.2 Characteristics of adult learner [7, 8]

care team, like teamwork and communication, which are directly tied to patient outcomes, thereby aligning with the problem-centered orientation of the adult learner.

Transformative Learning and IPE

The process of causing change within, or transforming, one's frame of reference is described in transformative learning theory [9]. Transformative learning theory suggests that individual habits are transformed when a learner reflects on his or her frame of reference with an opportunity to gain a different perspective. By learning from colleagues in other professions, IPE allows learners to gain new perspectives and ideas to solve problems or address challenges. This approach elevates learning beyond the traditional "profession-centric" learning that is employed in formal education and professional licensure [10] and enriches the shared experience of the learners. Transformative learning occurs best in an environment that is safe, open, and trusting allowing for collaboration, reflection, and exploration [11]. Fostering trust and mutual respect among learners with different backgrounds is an important component of transformative learning in IPE. Referring back to Miller's pyramid (Fig. 10.1), transformative learning may be limiting for cognitive acquisition of knowledge but has a clear role in behavioral acquisition and integration for the interdisciplinary team.

Social Psychology and IPE

An actual or perceived hierarchy often exists in healthcare systems. This hierarchy is reinforced by intergroup biases and training silos that exist in each profession [6, 12]. IPE can encourage learners to de-identify exclusively with a specific discipline and realign themselves as a member of a multidisciplinary team. This can occur by repeated exposure to different professional groups in a safe learning environment thereby reducing intergroup bias as participants discover interdependency. IPE encourages collaboration and flattening of traditional medical hierarchies by allowing learners to see strength in unique individual professional identities. This leads to an interprofessional team that works together with complementary efforts to achieve a common goal of quality patient care.

Interprofessional Team Training

Healthcare workers are tasked with providing highly reliable, quality care in the face of increasingly complex health issues. It is widely accepted that interprofessional and collaborative care is critical to promote quality healthcare, improved health outcomes, and an efficient, cost-effective model of healthcare [13]. A growing body of evidence demonstrates that IPE and team training can help different professions learn and develop important team skills that contribute to better patient outcomes [14]. Successful IPE can lead to effective and efficient healthcare teams which move a healthcare organization from one that operates with fragmented professions to a more collaborative culture. IPE is more effective when adult learning theory is applied, educational methods reflect real-world experiences, and respectful interactions occur between learners.

IPE educators can train healthcare workers in the core principles of teamwork and crisis resource management (CRM). An effective, high-functioning healthcare team is one whose members have mutual trust and commitment to one another, a shared understanding of clinical situations, coordination and clarity of roles, conflict management and communication skills, adaptability, and ability to reflect and assess team performance [15]. Team members must take accountability for their actions and understand the demands and challenges of the roles they play within critical situations. The Agency for Healthcare Research and Quality (AHRQ) and the Department of Defense developed and validated TeamSTEPPS (Team Strategies and Tools to Enhance Performance and Patient Safety) [16]. Building on principles of crew resource management from the aviation industry to improve safety with teamwork communication, situation monitoring, and mutual support training programs [17], TeamSTEPPS highlights medical education aimed at training teams to focus on identifying and avoiding communication breakdown and promoting collaboration. CRM relies on effectual leadership and followership, communication, teamwork, resource utilization, and situational awareness [18]. Thus, effective CRM is dependent on interprofessional education and practice.

Interprofessional team training programs described in the literature that aim to improve team performance and patient outcomes include interprofessional workshops, performance feedback using tools such as SBAR (Situation, Background, Assessment, Recommendation), team meetings, and interprofessional simulation training. Since 2001, Gaba has promoted simulation as the ideal educational intervention to teach and practice teamwork and team-based CRM skills [19]. Because of its alignment with adult learning theory, simulation has been shown to be an effective tool for teaching knowledge, skills, and behaviors [20] and is more effective than traditional clinical educational approaches for achieving specific skill acquisition goals [21]. Simulation emphasizes the *learning* environment over the *teaching* environment [22]. Interprofessional simulation team training can provide an opportunity for multidisciplinary team members to work together to learn, practice, refine, and master the cognitive, technical, teamwork, and crisis resource management skills necessary to ensure readiness to provide acute medical care to patients when needed.

IPE simulation helps to increase team member understanding of the difficulties specific to each team role, enhancing both learning about and appreciation for the various roles necessary to provide comprehensive patient care [23]. IPE simulation brings together a team composed of members from various professions and/or disciplines and allows the team to practice management of high stakes clinical emergencies in an environment free from adverse events. However, it is important to note that development of IPE simulations is a complex process and may involve mobilizing staff from different faculties, work settings, and locations. Sustaining IPE can be equally complex and requires supportive institutional policies and managerial commitment, enthusiasm for education, a shared vision of benefits of the educational intervention, and champions responsible for coordinating simulation activities and identifying and addressing barriers to progress [15].

While there are many strengths and opportunities provided by IPE simulation, it is not without its challenges and barriers (Fig. 10.3). Miscommunication and misunderstandings can result from siloed education in both the pre- and post-licensure phase. A long-standing culture of hierarchy within medicine and surgery, whether actual or perceived, can potentiate communication barriers between team members, and the disconnect between professions is cited as a significant barrier to effective team performance and patient safety [24]. Team members with variable personality traits

	Helpful	Harmful
Internal origin	**STRENGTHS** • Aligns with adult learning theory • Mimics clinical emergencies without threat to patient safety • Facilitates broad vision of collaboration, perception and knowledge sharing	**WEAKNESSES** • Significant time, resources, labor needed • Frequency of refresher training for IPE simulations unknown • Off-shift IPE simulation education opportunities limited
External origin	**OPPORTUNITIES** • Develop teamwork & communication skills • Develop sustainable ECMO simulation curriculum • Safer neonatal, cardiac & pediatric ECMO management for improved outcomes	**THREATS** • Financial & administrative commitment to IPE • Limited faculty development resources for IPE educators • Differing licensure & demands for continuing education credit

Fig. 10.3 SWOT analysis of interprofessional simulation for ECMO

and communication styles can lead to bias and unprofessionalism. Practicing respectful communication and mindful conversations in simulation exercises can flatten hierarchical team structures and foster professionalism and collaboration between professions and disciplines. Furthermore, IPE requires significant commitment of personnel, time, and resources from learners and educators alike; this commitment can threaten sustainability if the entire healthcare team is not fully invested.

Interprofessional Simulation for ECMO Teams

ECMO is a high-risk, low-volume therapy for critically ill patients dependent on a team of highly skilled, multidisciplinary professionals working together. Clinical opportunities to maintain necessary clinical and teamwork skills to ensure high quality care of ECMO patients are limited and subject to random chance. A recent survey of 94 ELSO centers reported a wide variation in annual ECMO cases with 54% of centers reporting ≤20 cases per year [25]. The survey also reported an average of 20 ECMO specialists, 8 medical intensivists, and 6 surgeons per ELSO center, which demonstrates the immense potential for variation of the member of the ECMO team. The non-static nature and variability of multidisciplinary team membership highlights the need for frequent opportunities to engage in IPE and team training.

Both routine and emergency management of patients on ECMO requires application of disciplinary content knowledge and technical skills, as well as interdisciplinary behavioral and teamwork skills. The combination of both disciplinary and interdisciplinary performance can be challenging for expert teams under optimal conditions. Thus, the execution of discipline-specific cognition and tasks coordinated within a multidisciplinary team framework with unstable patients and non-static teams makes a high-risk therapy even riskier. Given that technical emergencies on ECMO are associated with a high mortality rate [26, 27], it is essential that ECMO teams prepare for these emergencies using evidence-based educational strategies and deliberate practice.

Traditionally, training for ECMO has relied on didactic education, hands-on water drills, and animal models [22]. This educational approach may overemphasize cognitive skills, underemphasize technical skills, and ignore behavioral skills at the individual level [22, 28]. This approach also underemphasizes the importance and critical nature of interdependent teamwork and communication. Using simulation, it is possible for ECMO team members to learn both technical and nontechnical skills that are essential for the safe initiation, maintenance, and discontinuation of ECMO in an intensive care environment. Building an interprofessional ECMO simulation has significant research-proven benefits but challenges associated with this instructional methodology must be acknowledged (Table 10.1).

Table 10.1 Benefits and barriers of interprofessional ECMO simulation

Benefits	Technical and nontechnical skills training
	Allows for rehearsal of unusual or infrequent critical events/emergencies [29–31]
	Reduces ECMO deployment time in pediatric eCPR [32, 33]
	Improves time to completion of technical skills [22, 29, 34, 35]
	Team behaviors
	Improves behavioral markers of ECMO team performance [22, 29, 34, 36]
	Improves patient care delivery when combined with quality improvement (QI) tools [32, 34]
	Communication
	Improves communication when interruptions, stress levels, and cognitive load are increased [28, 36]
	Improves coordination, documentation, and communication [32, 37]
	Assessment of knowledge and skills
	Long term improvements in team performance and knowledge retention [29]
	Provides opportunity for assessment of initial and ongoing ECMO competency and CME for maintenance of ECMO skills [25, 38]
	Scholarly productivity
	Potential for regional/national collaboration to lead professional continuing education among ECMO institutions [39]
Barriers	Miscommunication
	Siloed pre- and post-licensure education can lead to communication challenges due to discipline-specific language [5]
	Medical hierarchy
	Can lead to anxiety and discourage appropriate communication and safety monitoring [40]
	Resource limitations
	Scheduling complexity and financial cost of simulation equipment, skilled simulation facilitators and debriefers, teaching space (in situ vs other), and learner time [25, 41, 42]
	Lack of realism of available ECMO simulators may promote negative learning [22, 42]
	Licensure requirements
	Different professions have unique requirements for competency training and assessment, creating challenges for the use of universal learning objectives [24]
	No formal/standard ECMO credentialing process exists [25, 39, 43]
	Training frequency
	No guidelines exist on the recommended frequency of IPE ECMO simulation [43]
	No information is known about the degradation of ECMO skills to support recommendations for training frequency [44]

A Practical Guide for Interprofessional ECMO Simulation

Given that ECMO is one of the most complex medical treatments available in the intensive care environment, the training and continuing education required to provide safe ECMO care are considerable. The ELSO Red Book [38] includes a chapter on education and training which acknowledges the challenges associated with the initial training and continuing education of the interprofessional team members who deliver ECMO care. This team, comprised of clinicians, nurses, respiratory therapists, and ECMO specialists, requires both discipline-specific and team-based education. Using Miller's Pyramid (Fig. 10.4), described earlier in this chapter as a framework, the leadership of ECMO centers can develop educational materials, training guidelines, and assessment procedures informed by adult learning theory.

The base of Miller's Pyramid requires all members of the ECMO team to "Know" the physiologic concepts of extracorporeal life support and the pathologic conditions that necessitate ECMO support. Acquiring discipline-specific knowledge is also essential at this stage to understand the "how" and "why" behind task performance for individual roles and responsibilities. The second level of Miller's Pyramid is "Knows How." At this stage, ECMO team members should demonstrate the performance of discrete role-specific tasks, either in isolation or alongside other team members. After skills are mastered, disciplines can be combined into healthcare action teams to practice "Shows How." The "Shows How" of ECMO education is best accomplished using interprofessional simulation training so ECMO team members can demonstrate discipline-specific tasks within an interdependent team structure and practice collaboration, communication, and crisis resource management until competency is established. Group learning and debriefing develop situational awareness and increase overall understanding of ECMO

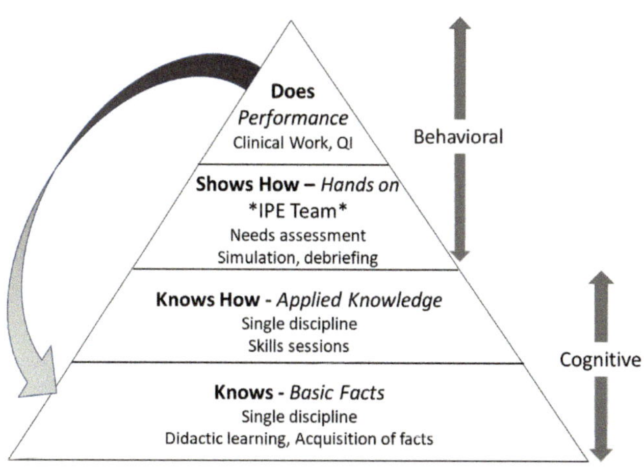

Fig. 10.4 Miller's pyramid for IPE ECMO simulations. (Adapted from "The assessment of clinical skills/competence/performance" by GE Miller, Academic Medicine, 1990, pp. 63–67)

management leading to improved team performance [25]. The top level of Miller's Pyramid or "Does" is the practical application of the educational goals during actual patient care. Continued assessment of clinical performance by measure of clinical outcomes and events should be monitored and measured using quality improvement methodology to inform changes in educational materials, training guidelines, and continuing education opportunities. Skills can then be maintained through refresher training [45].

Knows

Expertise development is a process that starts with acquiring content knowledge and progresses to expert performance through deliberate practice exercises and clinical experience with a multidisciplinary team. Acquisition of knowledge about pathophysiologic conditions that require ECMO, understanding ECMO physiology, and an awareness of the parts of the ECMO circuit is required by all members of the ECMO team. Basic knowledge of ECMO physiology may be acquired through passive methodologies like self-study, didactic lectures, and videos.

There is a role for individual or role-specific training for ECMO providers [25]. Depending on one's role on the ECMO team, additional knowledge may be essential for job performance. Individual healthcare disciplines have ECMO-specific cognitive and technical skills which need to be mastered prior to participation in interprofessional education activities, including simulation. For example, a surgeon needs to have a thorough understanding of neck anatomy to perform ECMO cannulation, but this information is not necessary for an ECMO specialist to perform his/her job.

Knows How

Once an ECMO team member acquires knowledge, the application of that knowledge in a clinical setting is essential to solidify learning. Knowledge application can take on many forms from quizzes and water drills for ECMO specialists to surgical task trainers for neck vessel cannulation for surgeons. Like knowledge acquisition, knowledge application of discrete tasks is often performed in single disciplines. The assessment of knowledge application in a training or actual clinical environment should be performed by content experts within a given discipline to ensure accuracy.

Knowledge application can also occur in a classroom setting through the use of the "flipped classroom" (FC) model [46]. The FC model assigns content for knowledge acquisition by learners prior to the instructional session, thus permitting class time to focus on knowledge application of these learned concepts through small group case discussions or simulations. The content material can be delivered through self-study of textbook chapters or journal articles or through the utilization of technology such as video demonstrations or computer-based interactive "serious games" designed for training rather than entertainment purposes [7]. Used in this manner, a FC model can optimize the effectiveness of a learning session for either a single discipline or for an interprofessional ECMO team. When used with an interprofessional team, class time can be utilized for active discussion of concepts as well as best practices for teamwork and communication.

Shows

Needs Assessment

When beginning to build an IPE simulation program, it is important to involve all key stakeholders in a needs assessment. Key stakeholders include the ECMO leadership team, intensive care unit medical directors, and team leaders of the interprofessional ECMO team (i.e., perfusionists, RNs, RTs). The needs assessment will help identify existing strengths, areas of weakness and threats, and systems issues that can help or hinder ECMO IPE educational efforts. The needs assessment will guide scenario development, create learning objectives, and provide educators with insight on educational needs and opportunities.

Learning Objectives

A diverse IPE simulation development team ensures learning objectives that are applicable to and achievable by each team member. For example, an objective such as successful cannulation of the patient or timely oxygenator exchange may only target the surgeon or ECMO specialist, respectively, and this education can be accomplished in a non-IPE simulation session. A more junior team of providers may not achieve an objective such as ordering correct medications and blood products for cannulation. An achievable learning objective for more junior learners may be to recognize the clinical need for or consideration of ECMO for a given patient/pathophysiology.

For IPE ECMO simulations, learning objectives may focus on communication and collaboration in addition to or in lieu of technical skills. Learning objectives will depend on the goal of the simulation as well as the aforementioned expertise level of ECMO team members. For junior learners, recognition of the need to activate ECMO may be the only learning objective required. Several learning objectives may be necessary if the goal is to simulate a systems process. For example, IPE learning objectives for a cannulation simulation may include team recognition of a patient requiring ECMO cannulation, review of ECMO orders, and demonstration of appropriate bedside and patient preparation. In this cannulation example, the use of IPE learning objectives changes the emphasis from focusing on the technical surgical skills for cannulation to those of systems facilitation and team communication.

Resources for IPE ECMO Simulation

The needs assessment identifies learning objectives which determine optimal time, resources, and setting for development of ECMO simulation sessions and scenarios. The choice of simulation settings, whether it is a simulation lab or an in situ simulation, may be determined by the learning objectives. For full-scale interprofessional team training, the visual, auditory, and tactile clues from the actual clinical environment may be needed to allow for team members to "suspend disbelief." High-functioning teams benefit from realism, and the in situ environment may be needed for optimal team performance [47, 48]. In a cannulation simulation with scenario objectives that target procedural planning for surgeons, including configuration of operating room equipment, ECMO cannulation carts, and patient position, in situ simulation would be preferable. Similarly, if the simulation scenario is to focus on ECMO team communication, technical skills, or ECMO physiology, a simulation lab would suffice.

The equipment necessary for proper operationalization of the ECMO simulation scenario should also be considered. Useful equipment for ECMO simulations is listed in Table 10.2. In a scenario addressing systems issues and ECMO equipment set-up, scenario realism would be optimized if performed in situ with all required personnel and equipment present. The simulation manikin is an essential piece of equipment. There are numerous manikin models available, and choice of simulation manikin will be driven by budgetary constraints as well as learning objectives. A low-technology manikin may be sufficient if objectives are geared toward communication or ECMO physiology independent of clinical changes. However, a high-technology manikin that can be "cannulated" would be beneficial for a full-scale simulation involving experienced members of the interprofessional team to support the increasing degree of realism needed for high-functioning teams.

Table 10.2 Resources for IPE ECMO simulation

Equipment	Personnel	Miscellaneous Considerations
ECMO pump/ console	Simulation educators	Simulation space (lab or in situ)
Manikin (high or low technology)	Skilled debriefers	Debriefing space
Simulated medications, IV fluids, blood products	Multidisciplinary simulation participants	Storage for simulation supplies
Monitors	Simulation specialists	Maintenance of simulation equipment
Surgical equipment	ECMO content expert	Personnel time away from clinical duties
ECMO related supplies (cart/ cannulas)	Simulation actors	Duration of simulation
Ventilator		Experience level/ profession of participants

Scheduling for IPE ECMO Simulation

Timing and frequency of interprofessional ECMO simulations and institutional resources should be considered in conjunction with scenario objectives. Timing of ECMO simulation sessions should address the challenges of ECMO education that include the diversity of ECMO team composition, the non-static nature of teams, and the need for frequent opportunities for providers on different schedules to participate in interprofessional simulation. Lack of off-shift educational opportunities presents alternative challenges and system process issues. For example, ECMO procedures not routinely performed on off-shifts may require additional IPE simulations to provide additional learning opportunities and reinforcement of key concepts to address time-specific challenges and resources. Similarly, if the scenario objectives relate to interprofessional team communication and requires participation from multiple team members, it may be beneficial to offer the simulation during the day shift when more staff are present and available.

The number of learning objectives should match the amount of time scheduled for interprofessional education. Accomplishment of multiple learning objectives in a short period of time is difficult. Additionally, the scenario objectives and team expertise should be considered when scheduling time for simulation and debriefing. For a given simulation and learning objectives, junior learners may require considerably more time for simulation and debriefing compared to an experienced IPE team. A full-scale cannulation scenario with a large multidisciplinary team requires more time for simulation and debriefing. Full-scale scenarios are time, resource, and labor intensive, which will impact the ability to schedule and refresh educational experiences. Another challenge of scheduling IPE ECMO simulations is lack of awareness of the frequency at which refresher sessions should occur. The frequency of education may be dictated by the baseline expertise of the ECMO team, frequency of occurrence of ECMO-related events, and skill deterioration between educational sessions. Research in the area of knowledge and skills deterioration for IPE is limited. However, research supports that the more complicated the patient, the higher the cognitive load on the team and individual team members suggesting the need to train more frequently to decrease cognitive load and improve patient outcomes [49].

Debriefing

Debriefing an IPE ECMO simulation benefits from a multidisciplinary debriefing team consisting of ECMO content experts and skilled debriefers. ECMO teams often have a real or perceived hierarchical structure which can limit participant engagement in debriefing exercises if a debriefer is unfamiliar with a given individual's scope of practice. Similarly, debriefers may feel reluctant to provide feedback about skills or behaviors with which they are not familiar. A multidisciplinary debriefing team can overcome this challenge by offering a breadth of expertise that can facilitate a balanced discussion. Content experts in cannulation or medical management may be necessary to ensure accurate feedback on technical and skills-based team performance. Skilled debriefers can provide feedback on nontechnical skills such as communication, crisis resource management, shared mental modeling, and teamwork. Co-debriefers or content experts from multiple disciplines may assist in eliminating barriers to effective debriefing while maintaining psychological safety. Recognizing the expertise of skilled and experienced clinicians of different disciplines who participated in the simulation exercise enhances the debriefing experience for all participants.

Logistically, it is unlikely that all ECMO team members can be present for every IPE ECMO simulation exercise. However, lessons learned and key concepts can be disseminated to the entire team following scenario debriefing. For example, an email of "lessons learned" that highlights de-identified strengths and weaknesses of team performance and discussed solutions to areas for improvement can be sent to all members of the ECMO team, not just the simulation participants. Any systems issues discovered through simulation exercises must be brought to the appropriate divisional or departmental leadership for further examination and analysis. In addition, quality improvement projects can be identified from these IPE simulation exercises to improve future ECMO patient outcomes.

Does

The clinical application of education and training is the pinnacle of Miller's Pyramid. The base of the pyramid is meant to solidify learning on the individual, single discipline, and interprofessional level to support the ultimate goal of effective team performance to provide high-quality, safe patient care. With this goal in mind, interprofessional team performance in the clinical setting requires frequent review to assess for latent safety threats, knowledge gaps, and systems issues which informs future educational goals. This review can be in the form of clinical event debriefing, quality improvement initiatives, and review of outcomes data. Information that is gathered from clinical performance is brought back to the IPE team for design of didactics, skills training, and simulations. Adverse events in the clinical setting may lead the interprofessional team to apply clinical changes including designing cognitive aids, adjusting protocols, and trialing different equipment or techniques, all of which can then be tested in a simulation setting with an interprofessional team prior to clinical application. Figures 10.5 and 10.6 detail how this iterative cycle may occur in response to patient scenarios. Figure 10.5 is an example of pericardial tamponade which can happen in the setting of a malpositioned ECMO cannula. Figure 10.6 depicts a case of acute hypocarbia caused by delay in weaning the ventilator after ECMO cannulation. As demonstrated by these examples, the

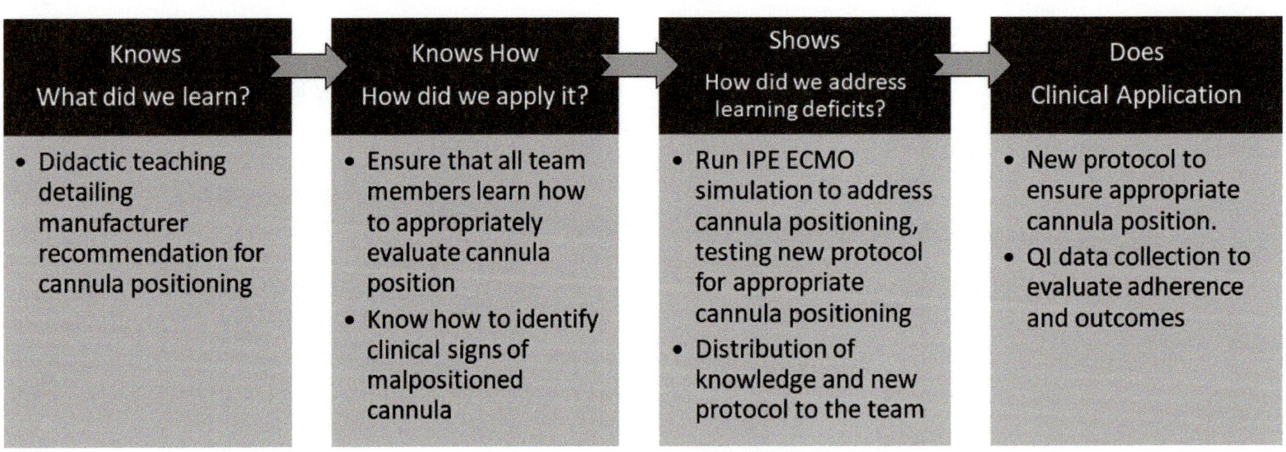

Fig. 10.5 Application of lessons learned – Pericardial tamponade

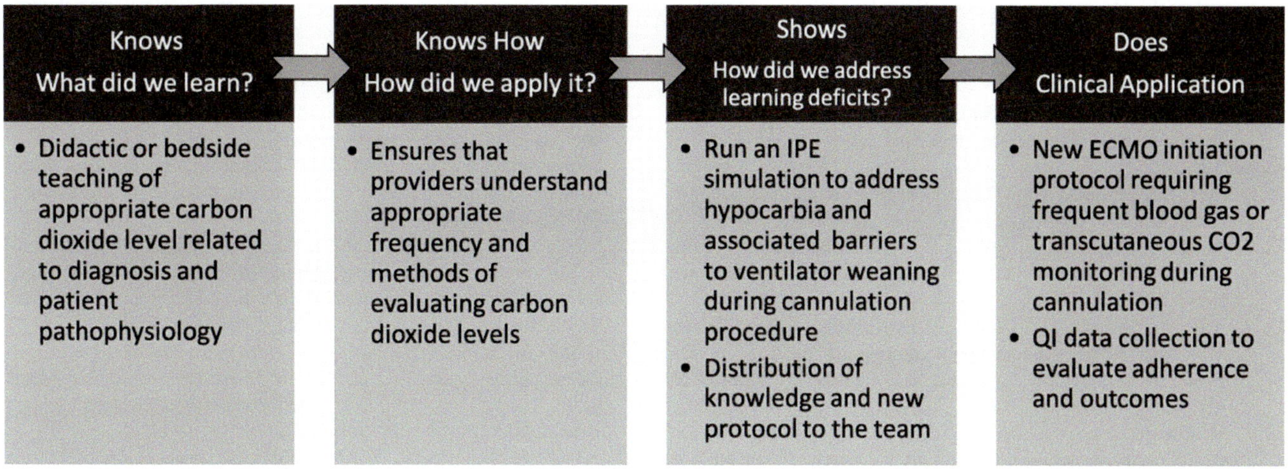

Fig. 10.6 Application of lessons learned – Acute hypocarbia

opportunities for quality improvement of team performance necessitate individual, single-discipline, and team training and are significantly strengthened by an interprofessional educational approach that respects the roles and the expertise of a team that is transparent, open, cohesive, and effective.

Conclusion

When a diverse team of healthcare providers, each with unique skills and insights, partners effectively and collaboratively to care for patients requiring ECMO support, teamwork is strengthened, and patient outcomes improve. The use of IPE to train and maintain technical and nontechnical skills of ECMO teams has many benefits and several barriers. Available research highlights the positive outcomes associated with simulation-based team training for ECMO patients. Thus, institutions should work to overcome barriers of IPE to improve patient care. ECMO IPE should be reinforced often by scheduling frequent simulation sessions to accommodate all ECMO medical professionals in developing their interprofessional teamwork, communication skills, and professionalism. The incorporation of strategies founded in adult learning theory will improve IPE efforts by layering both single-discipline and multidisciplinary educational opportunities to support professional development. After knowledge in ECMO management and emergencies is acquired, opportunities for knowledge application are essential. IPE simulation offers a safe, supportive environment for multidisciplinary teams to practice managing both routine and emergency ECMO procedures. Teamwork, communication, and crisis resource management strategies can be highlighted in debriefing to improve these essential nontechnical skills. Supporting a culture of IPE will help to foster safer ECMO management for all patients and improve ECMO outcomes globally.

References

1. Edwards M. Interprofessional education and medical libraries: partnering for success. Lanham: Rowman & Littlefield Publishers; 2016. Accessed 10/10/2018.
2. Barr HLH. Introducing interprofessional education; 2013.
3. Miller GE. The assessment of clinical skills/competence/performance. Acad Med. 1990;65(9 Suppl):S63–7.
4. Ericsson KA. Deliberate practice and the acquisition and maintenance of expert performance in medicine and related domains. Acad Med. 2004;79(10 Suppl):S70–81.
5. Kilgore RV, Langford RW. Reducing the failure risk of interdisciplinary healthcare teams. Crit Care Nurs Q. 2009;32(2):81–8.
6. Ballard J. Theories underlying interprofesional education. In: Edwards M, editor. Interprofessional education and medical libraries : partnering for success. Lanham: Rowman & Littlefield; 2016. p. 13–31.
7. Johnston L, Williams SB, Ades A. Education for ECMO providers: using education science to bridge the gap between clinical and educational expertise. Semin Perinatol. 2018;42(2):138–46.
8. Knowles MS. Application in continuing education for the health professions: chapter five of "Andragogy in Action". Mobius. 1985;5(2):80–100.
9. Mezirow J. Transformative learing: theory to practics. In: Merriam S, editor. New directions for adult and continuing education. San Fransisco: Jossey Bass; 1997.
10. Pecukonis E, Doyle O, Bliss DL. Reducing barriers to interprofessional training: promoting interprofessional cultural competence. J Interprof Care. 2008;22(4):417–28.
11. J P. Transformative learning in healthcare. PAACE J Lifelong Learn. 2010;19:39–54.
12. Leape LL, Berwick DM. Five years after to err is human: what have we learned? JAMA. 2005;293(19):2384–90.
13. Health HPNNMHRf. Framework for action on interprofessional education & collaborative practice. Geneva: World Health Organization; 2010.

14. Meurling L, Hedman L, Fellander-Tsai L, Wallin CJ. Leaders' and followers' individual experiences during the early phase of simulation-based team training: an exploratory study. BMJ Qual Saf. 2013;22(6):459–67.
15. Lo L, The Canadian Patient Safety Institute. Teamwork and communication in healthcare: a literature review. 2011. Accessed 03/19/2018.
16. Clancy CM, Tornberg DN. TeamSTEPPS: assuring optimal teamwork in clinical settings. Am J Med Qual. 2007;22(3):214–7.
17. Low XM, Horrigan D, Brewster DJ. The effects of team-training in intensive care medicine: a narrative review. J Crit Care. 2018;48:283–9.
18. Cheng A, Donoghue A, Gilfoyle E, Eppich W. Simulation-based crisis resource management training for pediatric critical care medicine: a review for instructors. Pediatr Crit Care Med. 2012;13(2):197–203.
19. Gaba DMHS, Fish KJ, Smith BE, Sowb YA. Simulation-based training in anesthesia crisis resource management (ACRM): a decade of experience. Simul Gaming. 2001;32(2):175–93.
20. Cook DA, Hatala R, Brydges R, et al. Technology-enhanced simulation for health professions education: a systematic review and meta-analysis. JAMA. 2011;306(9):978–88.
21. McGaghie WC, Issenberg SB, Cohen ER, Barsuk JH, Wayne DB. Does simulation-based medical education with deliberate practice yield better results than traditional clinical education? A meta-analytic comparative review of the evidence. Acad Med. 2011;86(6):706–11.
22. Anderson JM, Boyle KB, Murphy AA, Yaeger KA, LeFlore J, Halamek LP. Simulating extracorporeal membrane oxygenation emergencies to improve human performance. Part I: methodologic and technologic innovations. Simul Healthc. 2006;1(4):220–7.
23. McGaghie WC, Issenberg SB, Petrusa ER, Scalese RJ. A critical review of simulation-based medical education research: 2003-2009. Med Educ. 2010;44(1):50–63.
24. Nelson S, White CF, Hodges BD, Tassone M. Interprofessional team training at the prelicensure level: a review of the literature. Acad Med. 2017;92(5):709–16.
25. Weems MF, Friedlich PS, Nelson LP, et al. The role of extracorporeal membrane oxygenation simulation training at extracorporeal life support organization centers in the United States. Simul Healthc. 2017;12(4):233–9.
26. Zwischenberger JBSR, Bartlett RH. Extracorporeal cardiopulmonary support in critical care. Ann Arbor: Extracorporeal Life Support Organization (ELSO); 2000.
27. ECLS registry report international summary. Extracorporeal life support organization; January 2016.
28. Burton KS, Pendergrass TL, Byczkowski TL, et al. Impact of simulation-based extracorporeal membrane oxygenation training in the simulation laboratory and clinical environment. Simul Healthc. 2011;6(5):284–91.
29. Zakhary BM, Kam LM, Kaufman BS, Felner KJ. The utility of high-fidelity simulation for training critical care fellows in the management of extracorporeal membrane oxygenation emergencies: a randomized controlled trial. Crit Care Med. 2017;45(8):1367–73.
30. Nimmo GRWG, Scarth J, Simpson J, Gracie E, Torrance I, Liddell M, Davies C. Critical events simulation for neonatal and paediatric ECMO. J Int Care Soc. 2008;4:160–2.
31. Burkhart HM, Riley JB, Lynch JJ, et al. Simulation-based postcardiotomy extracorporeal membrane oxygenation crisis training for thoracic surgery residents. Ann Thorac Surg. 2013;95(3):901–6.
32. Su L, Spaeder MC, Jones MB, et al. Implementation of an extracorporeal cardiopulmonary resuscitation simulation program reduces extracorporeal cardiopulmonary resuscitation times in real patients. Pediatr Crit Care Med. 2014;15(9):856–60.
33. Sanchez-Glanville C, Brindle ME, Spence T, et al. Evaluating the introduction of extracorporeal life support technology to a tertiary-care pediatric institution: smoothing the learning curve through interprofessional simulation training. J Pediatr Surg. 2015;50(5):798–804.
34. Anderson JM, Murphy AA, Boyle KB, Yaeger KA, Halamek LP. Simulating extracorporeal membrane oxygenation emergencies to improve human performance. Part II: assessment of technical and behavioral skills. Simul Healthc. 2006;1(4):228–32.
35. Allan CK, Pigula F, Bacha EA, et al. An extracorporeal membrane oxygenation cannulation curriculum featuring a novel integrated skills trainer leads to improved performance among pediatric cardiac surgery trainees. Simul Healthc. 2013;8(4):221–8.
36. Allan CK, Thiagarajan RR, Beke D, et al. Simulation-based training delivered directly to the pediatric cardiac intensive care unit engenders preparedness, comfort, and decreased anxiety among multidisciplinary resuscitation teams. J Thorac Cardiovasc Surg. 2010;140(3):646–52.
37. Brum R, Rajani R, Gelandt E, et al. Simulation training for extracorporeal membrane oxygenation. Ann Card Anaesth. 2015;18(2):185–90.
38. Ogino MTFC, Moore EA. Education and training. In: Brogan TVLL, Lorussa R, MacLaren G, Peek G, editors. Extracorporeal life support: the ELSO red book. Ann Arbor: Extracorporeal Life Support Agency; 2017.
39. Johnston L, Oldenburg G. Simulation for neonatal extracorporeal membrane oxygenation teams. Semin Perinatol. 2016;40(7): 421–9.
40. McKee L, Charles K, Dixon-Woods M, Willars J, Martin G. 'New' and distributed leadership in quality and safety in health care, or 'old' and hierarchical? An interview study with strategic stakeholders. J Health Serv Res Policy. 2013;18(2 Suppl):11–9.
41. Muratore S, Beilman G, John R, Brunsvold M. Extracorporeal membrane oxygenation credentialing: where do we stand? Am J Surg. 2015;210(4):655–660 e652.
42. Alinier G, Hassan IF, Alsalemi A, et al. Addressing the challenges of ECMO simulation. Perfusion. 2018;33(7):568–76.
43. Brogan TVLL, Lorusso R, MacLaren G, Peek G. Extracorporeal life support: The ELSO red book, vol. 5. Ann Arbor: Extracorporeal Life Support Organization; 2017.
44. Chan SY, Figueroa M, Spentzas T, Powell A, Holloway R, Shah S. Prospective assessment of novice learners in a simulation-based extracorporeal membrane oxygenation (ECMO) education program. Pediatr Cardiol. 2013;34(3):543–52.
45. Sawyer T, White M, Zaveri P, et al. Learn, see, practice, prove, do, maintain: an evidence-based pedagogical framework for procedural skill training in medicine. Acad Med. 2015;90(8):1025–33.
46. Persky AM, McLaughlin JE. The flipped classroom - from theory to practice in health professional education. Am J Pharm Educ. 2017;81(6):118.
47. Silverman E, Tucker SA, Imsdahl S, et al. Conducting elite performance training. Surg Clin North Am. 2015;95(4):839–54.
48. Randall L. Rethinking faculty development: toward sustaining a community of learners. Senate Forum. 2008;24(1):18–22.
49. Eisen LA, Savel RH. What went right: lessons for the intensivist from the crew of US Airways flight 1549. Chest. 2009;136(3):910–7.

Optimizing ECMO Teams: What Every ECMO Educator Needs to Know About the Latest Advances in Team Science

11

Lillian Su, Seth Kaplan, and Mary J. Waller

Learning Objectives
By the end of the chapter, the reader should:

1. Understand the aspects of ECMO that requires expertise in team science.
2. Know the latest terminology in team science that is applicable to ECMO and ECMO simulation.
3. Be aware of several techniques that can potentially enhance team functioning in ECMO simulations.

ECMO Simulation as the Ultimate Team Sport

The delivery of ECMO to a critically ill patient is the ultimate team sport requiring coordination of teams within teams. There are at least two teams involved: the "ECMO" team caring for the ECMO circuit and the medical team caring for the patient. If there is an issue which requires surgical intervention, a third (surgical) team must also be involved. The three teams share a common goal of providing the best care to the patient to optimize outcomes. However, these teams may have different ideas of how best to obtain this goal. They also may possess different immediate priorities and foci. It is important to establish clear lines of communication when inevitable conflicts arise. Ideally, common issues and the processes used to address them would be clarified outside of the stress of a real clinical event and can be informed by the team science literature. All ECMO simulation educators become de facto educators of healthcare teams, and optimizing the ECMO team's performance is a crucial aspect of that education. This chapter will focus on reviewing the applicable team science literature for techniques and team processes that may be relevant to optimizing an ECMO team's performance.

As described previously in earlier chapters, there are myriad tasks and decisions involved in ECMO management; these can be further complicated by time constraints and the stress of a critically ill and decompensating patient. There may also be competing priorities for each of the bedside providers if a limited number of staff are available. For example, when air enters the circuit, a bedside provider may be asked simultaneously both to draw up epinephrine for the patient and to draw up fluid to use in deairing the circuit. Additionally, in ECPR (ECMO deployed during cardiac arrest), there can be competing priorities of a patient's need for chest compressions and a surgeon's need to establish a stable surgical field. While some of these issues have no clear "right answer" within the existing literature, teams ideally should have discussions about these issues before they arise with a real patient. ECMO simulation can be useful to trigger discussions of how a team would determine priorities in such a setting. This chapter aims to articulate a common language concerning such situations in healthcare teams.

Simulation as a Lab to Study the Human Behavior of Teams

ECMO simulation is an extreme example of the stressful environment surrounding a critically ill patient. As such, it provides a unique opportunity to gain insight into the effects of these extreme conditions and the techniques teams can utilize in maintaining effective communication performance

L. Su (✉)
School of Medicine, Stanford University, Stanford, CA, USA
e-mail: lisu@stanford.edu

S. Kaplan
Department of Psychology, George Mason University, Fairfax, VA, USA

M. J. Waller
Neely School of Business, Texas Christian University, Fort Worth, TX, USA

L. C. Johnston, L. Su (eds.), *Comprehensive Healthcare Simulation: ECMO Simulation*, Comprehensive Healthcare Simulation,
https://doi.org/10.1007/978-3-030-53844-6_11

despite such conditions. These teams must balance the performance of routine and predictable tasks while simultaneously remaining alert to respond to any unexpected, non-routine events [1]. In the psychology and behavioral science literature, this type of team is referred to as a dynamic team that must be trained to adapt to different, changing contexts [2]. Whereas the other chapters in this book focus on many aspects of creating an ideal ECMO simulation to promote learning, this chapter will focus on how we can use ECMO simulation both to [1] inform us as educators about the team processes that affect team performance by studying simulations and also to [2] educate teams on concepts described in this chapter by incorporating these concepts into ECMO education and debriefing ECMO simulations.

Team Science and Relevant Team Processes

Many educators of simulation science in healthcare may be familiar with team science concepts popularized by TeamSTEPPS [3]. This is the Agency for Healthcare Research and Quality's team training program developed with the Department of Defense. Programs like these have helped concepts such as closed loop communication and situational awareness become more familiar to healthcare providers. The origins of this type of work come from the field of team science which has deep roots in psychology [4, 5]. Eight key teamwork dimensions have been identified, including adaptability, shared understanding of the situation, performance monitoring and feedback, leadership, interpersonal relations, coordination, communication, and decision-making. Moreover, they further elaborated the distinction between *task work*, or the task-specific behaviors related to performing the task at hand, and *teamwork*, or the set of behaviors that facilitate the coordinated functioning of the team itself. The word "teamwork" may conjure up images of learning to get along and other behaviors children should have been taught when growing up. Instead, teamwork refers to the enactment of teamwork processes that support effective team performance [5]. These processes need to be studied, learned, and adapted for specific contexts.

Team science has continued to evolve from describing general concepts such as coordination and leadership into even more nuanced areas for research investigation. Team science relevant to ECMO and ECMO simulation must include acknowledgement that different medical contexts demand different teamwork skills, and teams must learn how to adapt to an ever-evolving situation. Here, we explore several different team science concepts – teaming, coordination, leadership, sensemaking – and then discuss several possible techniques to improve team performance, including team reflexivity and training for adaptation.

From Teamwork to Teaming

In her book, *Teaming*, Harvard Professor Amy Edmondson makes a distinction between teamwork and teaming. She defines teaming as "…teamwork on the fly – coordinating and collaborating, across boundaries, without the luxury of stable team structures [6]." Teaming is required when the work is complex and, therefore, unpredictable. For our purposes, we define a team as a group of individuals who assemble together for a specific purpose. In healthcare, we must confront the challenges of teamwork when we work in so many unstable collectives defined as teams that form for a specific ad hoc purpose such as an unexpected cardiac arrest and then disband after the event so that members may attend to their routine work. Teams in healthcare will recognize that such unstable teams are a reality in many facets of their work. As an example, Zhike Lei, a Professor in Organizational Behavior at Pepperdine University, computed, given 80 nurses, 8 residents, and 16 attending physicians and the need to form a team based on immediate availability comprised of 3 nurses, 1 resident, and 1 attending physician, there are over 10.5 million combinations possible [7]. As emphasized by Valentine and Edmondson, there are no constant teams in healthcare; everyone must learn to work with everybody else [8].

Coordination

Research has shown that healthcare teams often fail to perform to appropriate standards, thereby compromising patient outcomes [9]. While informative, this previous research has led to a narrow, and arguably ineffective, paradigm. Specifically, the focus has been on individual task work (skills) and on leaders as the sole managers of such task work. Largely neglected is the fact that team effectiveness requires more than training for individual skills or task leadership. Given the interdependence of all team members' tasks, individuals must learn to coordinate and synchronize their activities with those of other team members. While the leader may facilitate these goals to some extent, team members also must be able to coordinate their behaviors in the absence of explicit direction by the leader, leading to inefficiencies in time management. Further complicating the task of achieving this coordination, members of ECMO may have to coordinate without having the benefit of having previously worked with, or even having met, one other. Team membership stability improves resuscitation outcomes [10], but maintaining this stability may not be realistic. Coordination is thought to be essential to teamwork because different team members routinely perform multiple interdependent tasks simultaneously [11, 12]. Ethnographic research in anesthesia has highlighted that teams coordinate not only through verbal communication but also through their work environment (e.g., precise alignment of team members' bodies, tools, and the patient's body) [13]. This coordination strategy requires that team members possess an intimate knowledge of work roles and procedures to enable smooth team performance in most routine situations. However, during unfamiliar, ill-structured or critical situations, more explicit forms of coordination may be necessary [14].

Human factor research in other high-risk industries indicates that effective teams adapt their coordination strategies to the situational requirements [12]. For example, effective teams exhibit more implicit coordination during routine situations and more explicit coordination during critical situations. Other work indicates that effective teams use routine periods to engage in real-time contingency planning [15]. Most of the research in medical teams has occurred in the operating room setting [16] or in the field of anesthesia [17].

These discussions should include the differences in implicit versus explicit coordination and when each is necessary, as well as the need to vary leadership behaviors according to different contexts [17]. Different medical contexts demand different teamwork skills and continued adaptability of team members in the dynamic context of healthcare.

The Pattern of Team Communication Closely related to the concept of coordination is that of team communication. One critical aspect of communication is in its patterning. In most procedures, healthcare teams can follow standard protocols. Adhering to these protocols often leads to predictable patterns of team communication. For example, in routine surgeries, there often will be an almost rhythmic back-and-forth "volley" between the surgeon and the scrub technician as they coordinate the handing off of surgical instruments and materials.

However, in rarer and more dynamic and unpredictable cases (such as a patient in full cardiac arrest requiring ECMO but with limited venous and arterial access), the team either does not possess such a formulaic protocol or, even if it does, may need to deviate from a protocol depending on what it finds. As a result, team communication can vary dramatically – both within a given (ECMO) scenario and across different scenarios. Evidence from healthcare and other high reliability contexts documents that, despite the complexity and fluidity of non-routine events, some teams continue to exhibit systematic communication patterns [18]. For instance, the team leader (more or less knowingly) may survey each of the other team members at regular intervals as the scenario unfolds. Such consistent patterning may be advisable in predictable and familiar situations. However, in non-routine, dynamic, and potentially catastrophic scenarios (such as where the diagnosis is not yet known), teams are not advised to be so formulaic in their communication. Rather, research suggests that teams need to be more adaptive in these types of cases [12, 15]. This adaptability manifests in a number of ways, such as different people talking to each other as the case unfolds, interactions varying in nature (e.g., the same person is not necessarily always asking questions while the other individual is always responding to questions), and the interactions differing in the number of people participating in them [12].

Team Leadership Although it is widely recognized that leadership in any resuscitation is crucial [19] and is a primary strategy to accomplish team coordination, one size does not fit all. Leaders in resuscitation need to be aware that leadership needs to be task-contingent to respond to specific cooperation requirements at different times in the process [9]. Explicit leadership is defined as leadership that is directive and authoritative. Teams with more experience may in fact not need such explicit direction, as it may affect performance negatively [9]. Descriptive studies in the field of anesthesia have analyzed both high-functioning and low-performing teams and in this domain have demonstrated that higher functioning teams share their leadership while lower performing teams do not [20]. "Shared leadership" is defined by the management of personnel and resources among the individuals on a team. It is thought to be more flexible than a more traditional functional leadership where management and delegation are accomplished by one person [21]. A new area of work on leadership and followership behaviors in adaptive teams focuses on the ability of teams to enact efficient directive leadership during routine situations and quickly switch to adaptive participative leadership during non-routine events [22].

Team Sensemaking

Team sensemaking is described as the processes by which teams manage and coordinate their efforts to explain the situation they are in and to anticipate future situations, typically under uncertain and/or ambiguous conditions [23]. The basic assumption of team sensemaking is that a team establishes a frame or a mental model about the situation based on environmental data. The team then constantly tries to fit new emerging situational information into the frame. If newer data do not fit into a frame, the team "re-frames" and adapts the existing model. Thus, a frame can be seen as a working hypothesis from which emerging information will be evaluated and added. At a certain point, the working hypothesis might not hold true anymore and it has to be reformulated. The basic steps of team sensemaking are:

- "Formulating a frame": a team member announces a frame and others seek information to further identify it (e.g., a team leader surmises aloud that ECMO flows are decreased because of high negative pressures from hypovolemia secondary to third spacing and sepsis).
- Questioning a frame: speaking up if the current frame seems inappropriate (e.g., a team member questions the presumed diagnosis of sepsis because the inflammatory markers were not suspicious for infection, and new information is presented that suggests an alternative diagnosis such as noticing that the patient has decreased mediastinal chest tube output suspicious for new tamponade).
- Reframing: comparing frames (e.g., team discusses the differential diagnosis of high negative pressures and low flow on ECMO and evaluates the evidence for sepsis and third spacing versus cardiac tamponade).
- Elaborating a frame: looking for data that contradicts, confirms, or extends existing frame (e.g., the team considers obtaining a chest x-ray or echo to rule out other causes of high negative pressure including a pneumothorax and pericardial effusion) [24]

Team sensemaking must be a collaborative process and therefore is more difficult to accomplish than individual sensemaking. Uitdewilligen and Waller [22] found a significant positive relationship between team-level sensemaking behavior and team decision outcomes in their study of crisis management teams. Such sensemaking requires significant coordination effort from a team, and this effort needs to be learned and practiced. Tschan and colleagues illustrated nicely the benefits of this sort of explicit reasoning ("talking to the room") and showed an increase in diagnostic accuracy [24].

The above concepts – teaming, coordination, leadership, and sensemaking – are just a few of a vast and growing array of team science concepts relevant not only to ECMO teams but to healthcare teams in general. A very nice review of the existing science of healthcare teams was the subject of a dedicated issue of American Psychologist [25]. The next section will address techniques based on team science research that could improve human performance during ECMO, both in the context of simulations and clinical practice.

Solutions to Improve Human Performance in ECMO Teams

The following concepts may provide insight into how ECMO team performance can be optimized and specifically how these insights can be utilized to create opportunities for improved team performance.

Thinking of ECMO as a Multiteam System

An ECMO team can be viewed as a system of teams needing to coordinate actions to achieve a superordinate goal – i.e., as a multiteam system (MTS). As noted previously in this chapter, there is a team tending to the ECMO circuit, a team treating the patient, and potentially a team addressing surgical issues as well. Team science research over the last decade has demonstrated that various systems can be characterized as MTS. This research also has highlighted the formidable challenges that emerge when several teams need to act in a coordinated manner. Luciano and colleagues cite examples such as agencies failing to share information when responding to disasters, military teams being unable to coordinate international, multiagency endeavors, and instances of laboratories failing to act in a cooperative manner when trying to solve major medical questions [26].

Part of what makes MTS so complex is that these systems require collaboration both within and between teams. Team processes transpire, and must be managed, at both levels. For instance, effective leadership must exist within the team attending to the ECMO circuit, within the team attending to the patient, and between (i.e., coordinating) those two teams. This duality can become especially challenging to handle when enacting these team processes at one level interferes, or conflicts with, doing so at the other level. For example, tending to the patient and trying to coordinate that team's actions may serve to restrict attention to the most local circumstances. Other relevant information being discussed in the room – such as that about the readiness of the ECMO circuit – may not receive its due attention, thereby resulting in poorer between-team coordination. Also, this configuration can present challenges because the norms, timelines, and hierarchical structures that exist within each team may conflict and ultimately may need to be resolved when the constituent teams intersect or merge. These negotiations and attempts for teams to "get on the same page" all must happen, of course, within a matter of seconds and as individuals continue to carry out their primary tasks.

Although still in a nascent stage, the science on MTS offers tentative guidance to prevent or manage these challenges, while capitalizing on the benefits that such a system can provide. In particular, studies suggest that constituent teams should have a designated "boundary spanner," who serves as the communication point person for his or her team [27]. These point people transmit information with one another and also share information with their respective teams – both transmitting collective information to the local team and sharing information from the local team with the larger collective. Having designated communicators reduces the likelihood that important information otherwise exchanged between any two members will fail to be shared with the entire team or with the entire set of teams. An important note to this conclusion, though, is that much of the research on the MTS has been conducted on teams that are geographically dispersed or on medical teams operating in different units or during different shifts. ECMO presents a dissimilar scenario in that all teams may be collocated and functioning simultaneously. Still, the research on teams consistently documents the importance of role clarity, including clarity regarding communication structure. Thus, we would still advise hospitals to develop (and train on) protocols where the communication structure is established – rather than negotiating this structure on the fly during real scenarios.

Tool to address multiteam teams: Think about assigning a "boundary spanner" who can cross teams.

Team Reflexivity

Another team process that overlaps with the principles of sensemaking is team reflexivity (TR) [28–30]. TR is defined as a team's ability to collectively reflect on group objectives, strategies (e.g., decision-making), processes (e.g., communication), and outcomes of past and current performance and ultimately adapt accordingly [31]. Through the reflective process, teams recognize discrepancies between actual and desired circumstances and adapt accordingly to reach their goal. TR includes looking back and seeking information (e.g., "Can we summarize what we have done so far?"); evaluating information in order to acquire a deeper understanding about a process, situation, or action (e.g., "Why did this treatment work/ not work?"); and finally looking forward by planning what action(s) to take based on the evaluation made previously (e.g., "What are our next steps then?", "What will we do differently next time?"). Depending on when teams engage in TR, it takes on a different form and vary in scope, thus enabling different outcomes [28]. Teams can reflect either before, during, or after patient care. Especially brief reflective moments during patient care (e.g., situation assessment or a team time out) help a team to assess and evaluate all relevant information during the process. As a result, a team is then able to collectively make the right decisions for further treatments. "10 for 10" which stands for 10 seconds for 10 minute is a concept described in the safety science literature. It recognizes that circumstances which are time urgent can actually benefit from a short pause to reevaluate the overall direction of the resuscitation. It is described by Rall et al. in a Bulletin for the Royal College of Anesthetics in 2008 as "Spend 10 seconds more in data gathering, diagnosing and team planning, and save time and improve safety for the next 10 minutes" [32].

Teams as large as ECMO teams are particularly likely to benefit from implementation for team reflexivity [30]. In one study, large teams only outperformed smaller ones when the larger teams took the time to coordinate using reflexivity. The lesson here is that teams can only access the benefit of more people if they can coordinate to optimize performance.

Psychological Safety

The concept of psychological safety [33] has been popularized by the Aristotle Project [34] which was Google's quest to discover what differentiated great teams from mediocre ones. The usual ingredients thought to be important to a great team such as amount of individual talent, personality traits, certain skills sets, great leadership abilities, familiarity, and social interaction outside of work did not end up predicting great teams. After multiple analyses, only one factor was consistent throughout all the great teams, and that was psychological safety. As defined by Amy Edmonson, a leading researcher on this topic, psychological safety represents "the belief that the work environment is safe for interpersonal risk taking." Edmondson credits professors Edgar Schein and Warren Bennis from the Massachusetts Institute of Technology in the early 1960s with being the first to describe it in their 1965 book [35]. However, she ignited a flurry of interest in the subject with her 1999 article Psychological Safety and Learning Behavior in Work Teams [36].

Psychological safety is commonly misunderstood to be about being "nice." In reality, this concept certainly does not refer to incompetence going unaddressed (See Fig. 11.1). Rather, it empowers members to use their cognitive energy to achieve the primary collective goal (i.e., patient care) instead

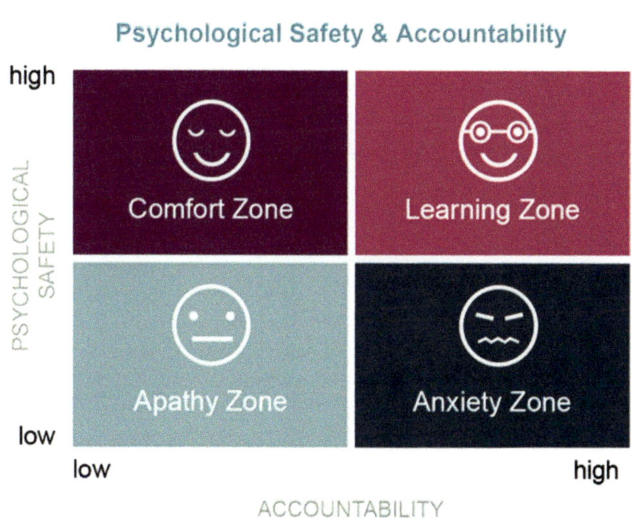

Fig. 11.1 Psychological safety and accountability. (Reproduced with permission of Amy Edmondson, PhD)

of wasting cognitive and emotional resources on concerns about how they will be seen when discussing the situation at hand. In ECMO, an example of low psychological safety would be when the ECMO specialist has a novel idea for reducing risk of air emboli but hesitates to speak up due to concerns of appearing nonsensical to the ECMO surgeon or medical lead.

Some practical tips for leaders who want to create a culture of psychological safety are discussed in Edmondson's book. These include a leader tool kit with the following main categories and its applications to ECMO simulation.

1. Setting the Stage – classifying ECMO as a complex error-prone system and that error is in fact expected but still needs to be managed and understood. Simulation educators could either pre-brief the simulation or start the debriefing explaining this approach.
2. Inviting Participation – The sample question of "Was everything as safe as you would like to have been with your ECMO patient when you were caring for this patient?" will hopefully expose near misses or opportunities for improvement.
3. Responding Productively – This includes a detailed discussion of the modifiable factors that the team believed influenced the outcome and follow-up after the simulation as to how these discussions impacted changes to the system.

Conclusion

Team science research has grown in recent years, and more healthcare providers are being exposed to team training. This chapter is not meant to be all-inclusive but instead to serve as a reference for some of the core concepts in team science that are relevant to ECMO teams and ECMO simulation. As advances in ECMO technology increase in complexity, so too must the ability of ECMO teams increase in order to quickly and accurately coordinate in rapidly changing, complex situations.

References

1. Su L, Spaeder MC, Jones M, Sinha P, Nath D, Jain P, Berger J, Williams L, Shankar V. Implementation of an ECPR simulation program reduces ECPR times in real patients. Pediatr Crit Care Med. 2014;15(9):856–60.
2. Lei Z, Waller M, Hagen J, Kaplan S. Team adaptiveness in dynamic contexts: contextualizing the roles of interaction patterns and in-process planning. Group Org Manag. 2016;41:491–525.
3. TeamSTEPPS 2.0. Content last reviewed November 2018. Agency for Healthcare Research and Quality, Rockville. Available at http://www.ahrq.gov/teamstepps/instructor/index.html.
4. Cannon-Bowers JA, Tannenbaum SI, Salas E, Volpe CE. Defining team competencies and establishing team training requirements. In: Guzzo R, Salas E, Associates, editors. Team effectiveness and decision making in organizations. San Francisco: Jossey-Bass; 1995. p. 333–80.
5. Salas E, Rosen MA, Burke CS, Goodwin GF. The wisdom of collectives in organizations: an update of the teamwork competencies. In: Salas E, Goodwin GF, Burke CS, editors. Team effectiveness in complex organizations. New York: Routledge; 2009. p. 39–82.
6. Edmondson AC. Teaming: How Organizations Learn, Innovate, and Compete in the Knowledge Economy. San Francisco: Jossey-Bass; 2012.
7. Su L. Simulation: a lab of human behavoir and cognition: CIO Applications; 2019.
8. Valentine M, Edmondson AC. Team scaffolds: how minimal team structures support role-based coordination. Organ Sci. 2015;26(2):405–22.
9. Abella BS, Alvarado JP, Myklebust H, Edelson DP, Barry A, O'Hearn N, Vanden Hoek TL, Becker LB. Quality of cardiopulmonary resuscitation during in-hospital cardiac arrest. JAMA. 2005;293:305–10.
10. Nallamoutu BK, Guetterman TC, Harrod M, Kellenberg JE, Lehrich JL, Kronick SL, et al. How do resuscitation teams at top-performing hospitals for in-hospital cardiac arrest succeed? A qualitative study. Circulation. 2018;138:154–63.
11. Entin EE, Serfaty D. Adaptive team coordination. Hum Factors. 1999;41:312–25.
12. Stachowski AA, Kaplan SA, Waller MJ. The benefits of flexible team interaction during crises. J Appl Psychol. 2009;94:1536–43.
13. Hindmarsch J, Pilnick A. Knowing bodies at work: embodiment and ephemeral teamwork in anaesthesia. Organ Stud. 2007;28:1395–416.
14. Manser T. Teamwork and patent safety in dynamic domains of healthcare: a review of the literature. Acta Anaesthesiol Scand. 2009;53:143–51.
15. Lei Z, Waller MJ, Hagan J, Kaplan S. Team adaptiveness in dynamic contexts: contextualizing the roles of interaction patterns and in-process planning. Group Org Manag. 2016;4:491–525.
16. Magnussun MS. Discovering hidden time patterns in behavior: T-patterns and their detection. Behav Methods Instrum Comput. 2000;32:93–110.
17. Künzle B, Zala-Mezö E, Kolbe M, Wacker J, Grote G. Substitutes for leadership in anaesthesia teams and their impact on leadership effectiveness. Eur J Work Organ Psychol. 2010;19:505–31.
18. Su L, Waller M, Kaplan S. Variability in effective interaction patterns in medical trauma teams. In: Lei Z, editor. (Chair), Information-laden processes during complexity and uncertainty: individual and team perspectives. Paper presented at the annual meeting of the Academy of Management. Boston; 2012, Aug.
19. Cooper S, Wakelam A. Leadership of resuscitation teams: "Lighthouse leadership". Resuscitation. 1999;42:27–45.
20. Hunziker S, Kolbe M, Jenni N, Marsch SU. Leadership in different resuscitation situations. Trends Anaesth Crit Care. 2014;4(1):32–6.
21. Zala-Mezo KB, Wacker J, Kolbe M, Sahn G. Leadership in anesthesia teams: the most effective leadership is shared. Qual Saf Health Care. 2010;19:1–6.
22. Uitdewilligen S, Waller MJ. Information sharing and decision making in multidisciplinary crisis management teams. J Organ Behav. 2018; https://doi.org/10.1002/job.2301.
23. Klein G, Wiggins S, Dominguez CO. Team sensemaking. Theor Issues Ergon Sci. 2010;11(4):304–20. https://doi.org/10.1080/14639221003729177.
24. Tschan F, Semmer NK, Gurtner A, Bizzari L, Spychiger M, Breuer M, et al. Explicit reasoning, confirmation bias, and illusory transactive memory: a simulation study of group medical decision making. Small Group Res. 2009;40:271–300.

25. American Psychologist Volume 73, Issue 4 from 2018.
26. Luciano M, DeChurch L, Mathieu J. Multiteam systems: a structural framework and meso-theory of system functioning. J Manag. 2015;44:1065–95.
27. Kapucu N. Interagency communication networks during emergencies: boundary spanners in multiagency coordination. Am Rev Public Adm. 2006;36:207–25.
28. Schmutz JB, Eppich WJ. Promoting learning and patient care through shared reflection: a conceptual framework for team reflexivity in healthcare. Acad Med. 2017;92:1555–63. https://doi.org/10.1097/ACM.0000000000001688.
29. Schmutz JB, Kolbe M, Eppich WJ. Twelve tips for integrating team reflexivity into your simulation-based team training. Med Teach. 2018 https://doi.org/10.1080/014219X.2018.1464135.
30. Schmutz JB, Lei Z, Eppich WJ, Manser T. Reflection in the heat of the moment: the role of in-action team reflexivity in health care emergency teams. J Organ Behav. 2018:1–17. https://doi.org/10.1002/job.2299.
31. West M. Reflexivity, revolution, and innovation in work teams. In: Beyerlein M, Johnson D, editors. Product development teams. Stamford: JAI Press; 2000.
32. Rall RM, Glavin RJ, Flin R. Bullentin of the Royal college of Anaesthetists. Spec Hum Factors Issue. 2008;51:2613–6.
33. Edmondson AC. The fearless organization: creating psychological safety in the workplace for learning, innovation, and growth. Hoboken: Wiley; 2018.
34. Duhigg C. New York Times Magazine, What Google learned from its quest to build the perfect team, 2016, Feb 25.
35. Schein EH, Bennis WG. Personal and organizational change through group methods: the laboratory approach: New York: Wiley; 1965.
36. Edmondson A. Psychological safety and learning behavoir at work. Adm Sci Q. 1999;44(2):350–83.

Part V

Practical Considerations

Current Training Recommendations for ECMO Providers and Specialists

12

Brian C. Bridges and Jennifer C. King

Learning Objectives
Upon completion of this chapter, the reader will be able to:

1. Describe effective ECMO training for the adult learner.
2. Identify the key topics to cover during an ECMO didactic course.
3. Apply the different types of ECMO simulation and common clinical scenarios that should be demonstrated during an ECMO training course.

Introduction

There has been tremendous growth in the number and complexity of patients supported with ECMO. The number of ECMO centers has grown, and the number of adult patients supported with ECMO has greatly expanded since the H1N1 influenza pandemic and the publication of the CESAR trial of ECMO support for adult patients with severe respiratory failure [1]. With the growth of new ECMO centers and the expanding range of patient populations being supported with ECMO, the need for organized instruction and simulation-based training is greater than ever. The Extracorporeal Life Support Organization (ELSO) currently recommends didactic and simulation training as an essential part of education for both new and established ECMO centers [2]. The ability to provide efficient and cost-effective training for ECMO teams, including the use of simulation, has become a major focus for the global ECMO community. In this chapter, we will review the current recommendations for training and simulation required for the provision of safe and reliable ECMO support and discuss newer educational methods that may be applicable for ECMO education.

Adult Learning and ECMO Training

Adult learners possess characteristics that should be considered when designing educational and training sessions. According to Knowles, adults are self-directed and seek out discovery of relevant knowledge independently [3]. With prior training in respiratory therapy, perfusion medicine, or nursing, an ECMO specialists also have a breadth of prior clinical experience to draw upon when acquiring or reinforcing new knowledge and skills [4]. Physicians and advanced practice providers typically prefer an active approach where they can apply prior knowledge, experience, and critical thinking to solve problems [3].

Medical simulation satisfies many adult learning preferences while also allowing for immediate feedback on performance. As an experiential educational modality, simulation follows Kolb's learning cycle whereby adults experience a new problem, followed by a period of reflection where the learner interprets this experience in light of prior knowledge or experiences. Conceptualization follows as the learner formulates new theories which leads to active experimentation [3, 4].

Medical simulation is also able to invoke educational objectives from the cognitive, affective, and psychomotor domains. The emotional state during the learning experience influences retention and activation of knowledge [4]. ECMO is considered a high-risk procedure with some higher volume centers performing only 40–50 runs per year. Both patient and mechanical complications during ECMO are associated with increased mortality [5–8]. Incorporating ECMO simulation into training allows for systematic, purposeful practice while posing no harm to actual patients [7, 9–11].

B. C. Bridges (✉)
Division of Pediatric Critical Care, Department of Pediatrics, Vanderbilt University School of Medicine, Nashville, TN, USA
e-mail: brian.c.bridges@vanderbilt.edu

J. C. King
Department of Pediatrics, Monroe Carell Jr. Children's Hospital at Vanderbilt University, Nashville, TN, USA

L. C. Johnston, L. Su (eds.), *Comprehensive Healthcare Simulation: ECMO Simulation*, Comprehensive Healthcare Simulation,
https://doi.org/10.1007/978-3-030-53844-6_12

ECMO Provider Didactic Course

While ECMO is provided to a variety of patient populations with numerous disease processes, there is a core set of objectives that is essential for every program. Depending on the preferences of a given ECMO center, there may be a single ECMO training course, or alternatively, there may be focused, specific didactic course for physicians caring for patients supported by ECMO and for specialists responsible for the bedside management of the circuit. ELSO has guidelines for the initial training and continuing education of ECMO specialists and recommendations for topics that should be covered during a didactic course [2], and the ELSO Red Book provides recommendations for an introductory course for ECMO providers [12]. Certain considerations should be made when developing an educational curriculum for ECMO providers. While the provision of ECMO support and the circuit design may be relatively similar across different settings and centers, the patients supported by ECMO may be quite different. The focus and design of an ECMO education course will depend on the intended core audience: physician, advanced practice provider, nurse, respiratory therapist, and/or perfusionist. The content will also depend on the center's target patient population, which may vary based upon the age group supported by the ECMO center (neonates, pediatric patients, and/or adult patients), as well as the major indication for ECMO support (respiratory, cardiac, and/or extracorporeal cardiopulmonary resuscitation (ECPR)). The following represents suggested topics for an introductory didactic course for ECMO [2, 12].

- *Introduction*

The introduction typically includes the history and background of ECMO, including how it was developed from cardiopulmonary bypass technology, as well as how these technologies compare and contrast. It will also discuss the background of the ECMO program at the local center.

- *ECMO Circuit and Pump*

While ECMO functions the same regardless of location, circuit, pump types, and configurations vary widely from center to center. Within a single center, more than one circuit and pump type may be used. For centers that provide ECMO to both neonates and larger children and/or adults, a smaller volume circuit and roller head pump may be utilized for neonates, and small children and a larger volume circuit with a centrifugal pump may be used with larger children and adults. It will be important for participants to gain a thorough understanding of the pump configuration(s) utilized in their program.

- *Physiology and ECMO Mechanics*

This is an opportunity to review the physiology behind oxygen content, oxygen consumption, and oxygen delivery. This core topic includes both the key concepts of ECMO blood flow and oxygenation and countercurrent sweep gas to control ventilation. This session may be utilized to introduce the direct cardiac support provided by venoarterial ECMO as opposed to venovenous ECMO.

- *ECMO Criteria and Patient Selection*

It is important to review both the inclusion criteria for ECMO support and the patient populations that can benefit from ECMO as a bridge to recovery or transplantation when end organ recovery is not possible. This is also an opportunity to review the relative and absolute contraindications to ECMO.

- Cannulation

This lecture discusses the process of circuit priming, preparing the patient for cannulation, and initiation of ECMO support. There should be a discussion of the use of proper cannula sizes, the advantages and disadvantages of different sites of cannulation, and percutaneous versus open techniques for cannula placement.

- *Venoarterial ECMO Support*

This session should include the indications for VA ECMO and a review of the physiology. Depending on an institution's patient population, a discussion of the variations of VA ECMO is essential. Such considerations include the importance of providing adequate flow support to the single ventricle patient with a systemic to pulmonary shunt or adequate venous drainage in the single ventricle patient with passive pulmonary blood flow, cannulation strategies to provide adequate flow in the patient with refractory septic shock, and the need for adequate decompression in patients with poor cardiac function and left atrial hypertension. Indications for weaning flow and a clamping trial before decannulation should also be addressed.

- *Venovenous ECMO Support*

This session should highlight the indications for VV support, as well as advantages and disadvantages of VV compared to VA support. It is essential that the participants understand the importance of lung rest during VV support, as well as the etiology and implications of recirculation. It is also important to discuss clinical signs of improving lung function for patients supported with VV ECMO, weaning of support but not flow, and the use of a capping trial before attempting decannulation.

- *ECMO Blood Management and Anticoagulation*

One of the greatest challenges to providing extracorporeal life support is the prevention of circuit thrombosis and patient bleeding. This session should provide a discussion of blood product transfusion criteria for patients supported with ECMO, laboratory parameters, and the use and titration of anticoagulation. There is significant variation among ECMO centers in how anticoagulation laboratory values are obtained and used, and it is important to present an evidence-based practice. A reference on these topics can be found in Chapter 7 of the 5th edition of the ELSO Red Book [13].

- *The Management of Patients Supported on ECMO*

This session includes the essentials of the management of nutrition, fluids, airway/mechanical ventilation, sedation, and infection control for patients supported with ECMO.

- *The Use of Other Extracorporeal Life Support in Conjunction with ECMO*

As the scope and complexity of the patients supported with ECMO increases, it is worthwhile to discuss other organ support modalities that can be used in conjunction with ECMO. This can include the use of continuous renal replacement therapy and plasma exchange performed in line with the ECMO circuit.

- ECMO Emergencies

This lecture focuses on the immediate identification and management of medical emergencies that can occur with patients supported with ECMO (intracranial hemorrhage, cardiac arrest, arrhythmia, pneumothorax, uncontrolled bleeding, and coagulopathy) and the management of emergencies involving the ECMO circuit (circuit disruption, system/alarm failure, introduction of air into the circuit, circuit thrombosis, circuit disseminated intravascular coagulation, and accidental decannulation).

- *Complications and Outcomes*

This session should cover the thrombotic and circuit complications associated with ECMO support and the hemorrhagic and patient-related complications that can occur on ECMO. Categories of patient complications recorded by ELSO include hemorrhagic, neurologic, renal, infectious, metabolic, cardiovascular, pulmonary, and limb. This should include a discussion of survival to decannulation, survival to hospital discharge, and quality of life outcomes for different age groups, support types, and underlying disease.

In addition to the provision of a didactic course to establish a baseline of knowledge for the ECMO provider, some centers require the participants to demonstrate that they have learned the core concepts essential to ECMO support and require that the participants pass a written test and/or successfully complete a simulation-based assessment at the conclusion of the course. Institutional requirements vary, but currently there is no nationally or internationally available certification for ECMO providers. Additional information on the topic of certification of ECMO providers can be found in Chap. 16.

ECMO Simulation Training

Historical Perspective

Historically, ECMO training has relied on didactic training accompanied by hands on "water drills" and animal lab work. This passive learning approach emphasizes cognitive skills with some allowance for refining technical skills, but it fails to take into account real-time changes in the patient's status [8, 10, 14]. While this permits ECMO specialists the opportunity to troubleshoot technical problems that may arise, it does not allow the specialist to practice the interprofessional and behavior skills required in an actual patient emergency [6, 7, 15–17]. ECMO emergencies require the coordinated management of both the patient and the circuit; balancing these two factors requires a unique skill set that must be honed with practice [7, 14, 17]. Furthermore, contemporary patient simulators are capable of providing visual, auditory, and tactile physiologic cues which closely mimics the clinical environment in which ECMO providers practice [4, 14], decreasing the reliance upon the animal lab component.

ECMO is a high-risk, low-frequency form of support [6–8]. Simulation offers a safe environment for participants to practice procedural skills, critical thinking, and the behavioral skills necessary for managing ECMO emergencies. Medical simulation involving ECMO was first described in 2006 [6, 15]; more information is provided on the inception of ECMO simulation in Chap. 2. Since that time, neonatal, pediatric, and adult centers have incorporated simulation into the training and maintenance of competency for ECMO providers. A recent survey of ELSO-affiliated ECMO programs revealed that 46% of ELSO centers report using manikin-based simulation for ECMO training, and an additional 26% were in the process of developing an ECMO simulation program [8].

Considerations

High- Versus Low-Technology Simulation

The equipment available for medical simulation ranges from low-technology partial task trainers and manikins to high-technology manikins capable of speech and physiologic processes. One of the advantages of high-technology simulation is the improved fidelity to an actual patient and creation of a learning environment that resembles the real-life clinical environment [14]. High-technology manikins allow simulation participants to establish vascular access, secure the airway, and assess for respirations, pulses, and heart sounds. Some high-technology manikins also have the capability of demonstrating cyanosis and pupillary responses as well. Whether or not to use low- versus high-technology equipment depends on the particular learning objective of the simulation exercise [4]. For example, if the objective is to learn how to properly secure and dress the cannula site, a task trainer may be adequate. However, if the goal is to simulate a multidisciplinary ECMO deployment as part of ECPR, a high-technology simulation manikin and environment may better meet the particular learning objectives [11]. Incorporation of high-technology ECMO simulation into the training of medical providers and ECMO specialist has been shown to decrease cannulation times [5, 11] and response times to ECMO emergencies [7, 15] and enhance team work and communication skills [6, 7, 10, 17]. Additional work is ongoing in the development of ECMO-specific high-technology simulators [14].

In Situ Versus Simulation Lab

Another consideration is where simulated ECMO scenarios will occur. The equipment and set up for a high-technology simulation may take hours depending on the scenario. Performing simulations in situ allows participants to practice in the environment where they actually provide care for patients, allowing for the identification of latent safety threats or other systems issues [5]. It is important to consider available resources, as there may be no dedicated space for simulation in the clinical environment. Simulation labs offer several advantages including a dedicated space solely for simulation that may allow for the ability to run more than one simulation at a time [8].

Developing Simulation Scenarios

As an educational modality, one of the most important factors to consider when developing scenarios is to ensure that needs of the learners are addressed [4]. This may impact whether the simulation is conducted in an interprofessional versus single professional manner. Simulation can be applied in a multidisciplinary approach in order to facilitate team training, permitting enhancement of communication and team skills [14]. Effective communication and team work are imperative when handling ECMO emergencies as patient outcomes depend on prompt and accurate interventions [6, 7, 14, 17]. Additional information on the use of interprofessional education strategies for ECMO simulation can be found in Chap. 10.

Many topics may be simulated depending on the needs of the ECMO team. Some common scenarios can be found in Table 12.1.

Table 12.1 Example scenarios

Category	Examples
Routine ECMO management	Blood gas interpretation Circuit pressure interpretation and management Determining when to cannulate/decannulate
Circuit emergencies	Oxygenator failure Air entrainment Power failure Accidental decannulation Tubing rupture
Patient emergencies	Hypovolemia Pneumothorax Cardiac tamponade
Teamwork/communication	Code leadership skills Closed loop communication Counseling families on withdrawal of support
Technical skills	Cannulation De-airing circuit Changing a circuit component Changing an entire circuit
Other	Interhospital/interfacility transport

Reproduced with permission of Johnston et al. [14]

Continuing Education of the ECMO Provider

For the experienced ECMO provider, it is still important to remain current on changes in local ECMO care as well as in the field of extracorporeal life support. Per the ELSO guidelines for training and continuing education of ECMO specialists, it is advisable to have formal team meetings for case reviews, updates on ECMO therapy, quality, and review of policies and procedures. While the frequency varies between ECMO centers, many have at least a monthly meeting to review recent cases, ensure quality of care, and review current ECMO literature. ELSO guidelines state that ECMO bedside specialists participate in simulation training throughout the year, at a minimum frequency of once every 6 months [2]. It is advisable that ECMO simulations should occur more frequently for specialists with fewer pump hours and at centers with lower ECMO volumes. There are no existing formal guidelines for recommended frequency of participation in simulation-based training for other members of the medical team. Requirements are typically driven by institutional needs and credentialing guidelines.

Novel Educational Strategies

ECMO specialists must build their cognitive knowledge of various skills related to ECMO management prior to their participation in simulated scenarios and water drills. Traditionally, this material is delivered in the didactic portion of ECMO training programs. In the past decade, there has been a divergence from a teacher-centered educational approach in favor of learner-centered educational modalities. One such educational modality to consider is a "flipped classroom" approach whereby learners are provided "pre-learning" educational materials before a classroom session, during which the information is applied by the learners with the guidance of a facilitator [4, 18]. As active participants, adult learners may prefer this approach to the traditional lecture-based didactic approach as they are able to apply acquired knowledge to patient-based problems or clinical scenarios to further enhance knowledge acquisition and retention and refine problem-solving skills [4, 18].

The ubiquitous nature of portable electronic devices and availability of the Internet have also made it possible to deliver educational content in various formats from low-technology videos and online learning modules to complex computer-based simulation software, such as that used by the American Heart Association as part of Advanced Cardiac Life Support training [4, 18]. Recently, the Neonatal Resuscitation Program incorporated NRP eSim, a screen-based simulation program, into the certification course. Cognitive skills related to NRP algorithms are reinforced, and learners are able to hone their resuscitation skills prior to attending the live portion of the course [19]. In addition to learner preference, online learning increases retention rates compared to traditional classroom methods and may significantly lessen the time required in didactics [20].

Conclusion

ECMO education, including simulation-based training, is essential to providing safe, high-quality ECMO support, in both established and newer centers. While the mechanics and physiology of ECMO support are similar across centers, due to differences in ECMO pump type, circuitry, and patient population, some portion of the training will be driven by local needs assessment. Despite these differences, the need for a standard core curriculum incorporating simulation training remains. ECMO simulation is early in its inception, but it is growing rapidly in utilization and application. Currently, there is no standardized approach to ECMO simulation. Further work is required in order to develop standards to assess knowledge, technical proficiency, and behavioral skills competency. Another important factor to consider is the "dose" of simulation required for initial acquisition of knowledge and skill proficiency as well as the ideal frequency for maintenance of competency. Development of standardized ECMO simulation training will require collaboration between ECMO clinical experts and medical educators with expertise in simulation.

References

1. Thiagarajan RR, Barbaro RP, Rycus PT, et al. Extracorporeal life support organization registry international report 2016. ASAIO J. 2017;63(1):60–7.
2. Organization ELS. ELSO guidelines for training and continuing education of ECMO specialists. ELSO guidelines: center and training guidelines 2010; https://www.elso.org/Portals/0/IGD/Archive/FileManager/97000963d6cusersshyerdocumentselsoguidelinesfortrainingandcontinuingeducationofecmospecialists.pdf. Accessed 29 Oct 2018.
3. Merriam S, Caffarella R, Baumgartner L. Learning in adulthood: a comprehensive guide. 3rd ed. San Francisco: Jossey-Bass; 2007.
4. Palaganas JC, Maxworthy JC, Epps JA, Mancini ME. Defining excellence in simulation programs. 1st ed. Philadelphia: Wolters Kluwer; 2015.
5. Allan CK, Pigula F, Bacha EA, et al. An extracorporeal membrane oxygenation cannulation curriculum featuring a novel integrated skills trainer leads to improved performance among pediatric cardiac surgery trainees. Simul Healthc. 2013;8(4):221–8.
6. Anderson JM, Boyle KB, Murphy AA, Yaeger KA, LeFlore J, Halamek LP. Simulating extracorporeal membrane oxygenation emergencies to improve human performance. Part I: methodologic and technologic innovations. Simul Healthc. 2006;1(4):220–7.
7. Di Nardo M, David P, Stoppa F, et al. The introduction of a high-fidelity simulation program for training pediatric critical care personnel reduces the times to manage extracorporeal membrane oxygenation emergencies and improves teamwork. J Thorac Dis. 2018;10(6):3409–17.
8. Weems MF, Friedlich PS, Nelson LP, et al. The role of extracorporeal membrane oxygenation simulation training at Extracorporeal Life Support Organization Centers in the United States. Simul Healthc. 2017;12(4):233–9.
9. Anderson J, Murphy A, Boyle K, Yaeger K, Halamek L. Simulating extracorporeal membrane oxygenation emergencies to improve human performance. Part II: assessment of technical and behavioral skills. Simul Healthc. 2006;1(4):228–32.
10. Burton KS, Pendergrass TL, Byczkowski TL, et al. Impact of simulation-based extracorporeal membrane oxygenation training in the simulation laboratory and clinical environment. Simul Healthc. 2011;6(5):284–91.
11. Su L, Spaeder MC, Jones MB, et al. Implementation of an extracorporeal cardiopulmonary resuscitation simulation program reduces extracorporeal cardiopulmonary resuscitation times in real patients. Pediatr Crit Care Med. 2014;15(9):856–60.

12. Ogino MT, Froehlich CD, Moore EA. Education and training. In: Brogan TV, Lequier L, Lorusso R, MacLaren G, Peek G, editors. Extracorporeal life support: the ELSO red book. 5th ed. Ann Arbor: Extracorporeal Life Support Organization; 2017. p. 747–63.
13. Bridges BC, Ranucci R, Anticoagulation LLL. Disorders of hemostasis. In: Brogan TV, Lequier L, Lorusso R, Maclaren G, Peek G, editors. Extracorporeal life support: the ELSO red book. 5th ed. Ann Arbor: Extracorporeal Life Support Organization; 2017. p. 93–103.
14. Johnston L, Oldenburg G. Simulation for neonatal extracorporeal membrane oxygenation teams. Semin Perinatol. 2016;40(7):421–9.
15. Anderson JM, Murphy AA, Boyle KB, Yaeger KA, Halamek LP. Simulating extracorporeal membrane oxygenation emergencies to improve human performance. Part II: assessment of technical and behavioral skills. Simul Healthc. 2006;1(4):228–32.
16. Brazzi L, Lissoni A, Panigada M, et al. Simulation-based training of extracorporeal membrane oxygenation during H1N1 influenza pandemic: the Italian experience. Simul Healthc. 2012;7(1):32–4.
17. Brum R, Rajani R, Gelandt E, et al. Simulation training for extracorporeal membrane oxygenation. Ann Card Anaesth. 2015;18(2):185–90.
18. Johnston L, Williams SB, Ades A. Education for ECMO providers: using education science to bridge the gap between clinical and educational expertise. Semin Perinatol. 2018;42(2):138–46.
19. Sawyer T, Ades A, Ernst K, Colby C. Simulation and the neonatal resuscitation program 7th edition curriculum. NeoReviews. 2016;17(8):e447.
20. Means B, Yoyama Y, Murphy R, Bakia M, Jones K. Evaluation of evidence-based practices in online learning: a meta-analysis and review of online learning studies. Dept of Education. Office of Planning, Evaluation;2010.

The Role of Simulation in Starting a New ECMO Program

13

Peggy Han and Catherine K. Allan

Learning Objectives

- Recognize the capacity for simulation to accelerate the start of a new clinical ECMO program, particularly one with a low projected case volume
- Describe how to operationalize a simulation-based ECMO curriculum to a novice group of learners, particularly in the context of partnering with an expert, high-volume ECMO center
- Construct an ECMO curriculum for ECMO training in a new center

Introduction

High stakes industries have long adopted simulation to enhance performance, safety, and quality and have shown significant improvement in practice over the decades [1–4]. In health care, simulation training has become a preferred modality to practice low-frequency, high-acuity events. Extracorporeal Membrane Oxygenation (ECMO) remains a relatively rare procedure, practiced in a handful of centers, with fewer than 23,000 pediatric cases reported in 2018 worldwide [5]. Thus, ECMO training is well-suited to a simulation-based approach in which learners can practice this low-frequency, high-risk care modality at no risk to patients. Manikin-based simulation training occurs in 46% of 94 US Extracorporeal Life Support Organization (ELSO) centers surveyed, with 63% of these centers using simulation for summative assessment and 76% using simulation for multidisciplinary training [6]. ELSO guidelines recommend simulation for ECMO training, but do not recommend a specific frequency of training or standardized curriculum.

While many authors have reported on the utility of ECMO simulation focused on its use within existing clinical ECMO programs [7, 8], ECMO simulation has also been used to aid in the establishment of new ECMO programs [9, 10]. In this chapter, we provide a framework for how to use ECMO simulation to aid in the establishment of a new ECMO program. The use of simulation in this setting allows an institution to accelerate the learning curve for this complex care modality. The education team can thereby address medical training of providers, familiarization with ECMO technology and recognition of circuit-related emergencies, practice communication between multidisciplinary teams, and test systems to ensure appropriate preparedness, all without exposing patients to risk.

Considerations to Start a New ECMO Program

Initiation of a new ECMO program requires a thorough needs assessment to determine training requirements. The needs assessment should address prior experience of team members, perceived training gaps, and concerns related to the system in which the ECMO program will be operationalized. The needs assessment, along with expert opinion, is then used to define specific learning goals for the ECMO simulation program. The learning goals drive decisions regarding inclusion of specific curricular elements, including which elements are most appropriately addressed through simulation and which goals should be addressed using other educational modalities [11]. In an institution where ECMO is new to the majority of providers, the learning goals will

P. Han (✉)
Division of Pediatric Critical Care Medicine, Department of Pediatrics, Stanford University School of Medicine, Palo Alto, CA, USA
e-mail: peggyhan@stanford.edu

C. K. Allan
Department of Cardiology, Boston Children's Hospital and Department of Pediatrics, Harvard Medical School, Boston, MA, USA

SIMPeds, Boston Children's Hospital Simulator Program, Boston Children's Hospital and Harvard Medical School, Boston, MA, USA

L. C. Johnston, L. Su (eds.), *Comprehensive Healthcare Simulation: ECMO Simulation*, Comprehensive Healthcare Simulation, https://doi.org/10.1007/978-3-030-53844-6_13

include mastery of technical skills, development of knowledge and critical thinking skills related to management of ECMO emergencies, and team and system development. The needs of the learners – in this case, clinical staff members - must be at the forefront not only to ensure buy-in and participation, but also to address knowledge gaps and best prepare clinicians who will be caring for live patients on ECMO, regardless of their prior experience.

To optimize curricular development, the intended structure and characteristics of the ECMO program must be understood. For example, projected clinical volume will influence frequency of training events, with more frequent training opportunities required for maintenance of competency when program volume is low and the interval between ECMO patients is longer. Provider roles and ECMO team composition will determine who needs to be trained. Finally, resources available for simulation-based training must be accurately assessed at the outset of the project, including availability of space, equipment, and simulation faculty time as well as availability of frontline staff to participate in simulations. Early leadership support for simulation-based training activities is key, with leaders making a specific commitment to the time and resources required to train a team to be ready to safely deploy and manage ECMO.

Components of Curriculum for a New ECMO Center

Here, we describe our experience with the creation of an ECMO simulation program to support development of a nascent clinical ECMO program with a projected volume of <5 cases per year and the rationale behind each of the decisions behind the program's development. The ECMO simulation program, paired with other educational methodologies, aimed to address the following challenges: (1) A large group of multidisciplinary leaners, most of whom had no ECMO experience, who were required to learn basic ECMO physiology and to develop the knowledge and critical thinking skills to rapidly recognize and manage EMCO emergencies; (2) a large, diverse team of providers, many of whom had never worked together, which needed to develop effective communication and teamwork behaviors to effectively manage this new technology through team-based practice; and (3) systems and processes for patient selection, initiation, and ongoing ECMO management needed to be developed. Inherent in starting a new simulation-based program, additional challenges included management of simulation equipment, coordination of schedules for providers and simulation space, frequency of training, and curriculum development.

Management of patients on ECMO at our institution was projected to involve a diverse team of providers including both pediatric and neonatal intensive care unit (PICU and NICU) nurses and physicians, pediatric surgeons, pediatric cardiac surgeons, respiratory therapists, and perfusionists. Thus, the target audience for the ECMO training program included 127 individuals with varying levels of ECMO expertise. In our training model, health care providers from different backgrounds and disciplines participated in the same longitudinal curriculum; all disciplines were integrated in each educational session to promote camaraderie, to exchange knowledge, and to foster trust. The requirement for large-scale, simultaneous training of providers to develop competency related to complex physiology and technical and teamwork skills presented unique challenges for curriculum design.

Overall Curriculum Design

The overall structure of the ECMO curriculum (Fig. 13.1) was designed to guide participants' learning of basic concepts through hands-on application of psychomotor and critical thinking skills, following the conceptual framework of simple to complex physical resemblance and functional task alignment described in Chap. 7. In the induction phase, all learners participated in didactic sessions that introduced basic ECMO concepts, including physiology of veno-venous (VV) and veno-arterial (VA) ECMO, clinical indications for ECMO, expected outcomes, and possible complications. These traditional didactic sessions provided core information that learners were then asked to apply during subsequent hands-on portions of training. Following this induction phase, the curriculum involved three major components: monthly interdisciplinary conferences for discussion of current controversies in ECMO, circuit labs focusing on learning the components of an ECMO circuit, and high physical resemblance ECMO simulations that focused on identifying and managing ECMO emergencies. Hands-on activities (circuit labs and high-physical resemblance simulations) were

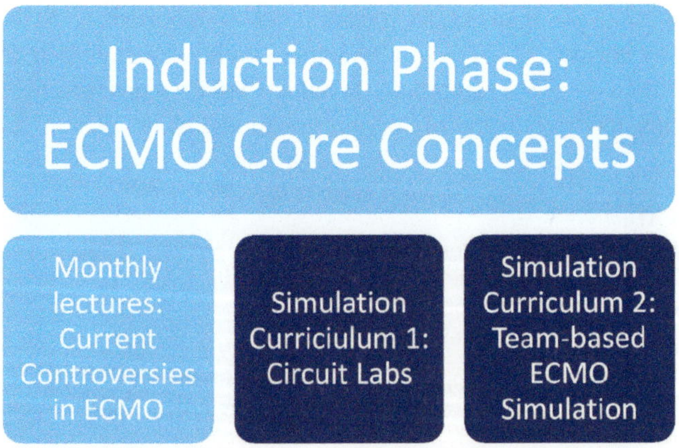

Fig. 13.1 Overall structure of ECMO curriculum combining traditional didactics and simulation

sequenced to (1) reinforce and allow for practice with previously presented content and (2) require learners to apply knowledge to increasingly complex tasks. In our center, a total of 92 simulations focused on ECMO training were performed between March 2016 and December 2016. The clinical ECMO program went live in January 2017 with successful management of two ECMO patients in 2017.

Didactic Sessions and Monthly Lectures

The ECMO curriculum started with traditional lectures presented in two 4 h didactic sessions that introduced the basic concepts of ECMO as described above. Supplementary reading material was provided with review articles on the basics of ECMO prior to each session start. The teaching sessions were attended by 77 health care providers from six disciplines.

Following the introductory sessions in months 1 and 2, a monthly 1 h lecture series was established to present and discuss current concepts in neonatal and pediatric ECMO care. The interdisciplinary conferences were designed to promote discussion of complex management issues in ECMO and in doing so, encourage engagement, promote camaraderie and improve understanding of perspectives from different disciplines. Examples of lecture topics include ethical considerations for length of ECMO run and resource allocation, controversies in patient selection (e.g., polytrauma, stem cell transplant and malignancies, neurologically impaired patients), interpretation and management of anticoagulation challenges, review of ELSO data, pharmacological considerations on ECMO, and nursing and parental concerns. The monthly lecture series has been ongoing since initiation of the training program through present day.

Introduction of Complex Physiology and Hands-On Practice

The progressive design of the ECMO curriculum was created with attention to the principles of cognitive load theory (CLT). CLT describes the relationship between working memory and long-term memory, and provides a framework to think about optimizing the transfer of knowledge from working to long-term memory. Three types of cognitive load have been described: intrinsic, extrinsic, and germane [12]. Intrinsic load describes the complexity of the learning task. Extrinsic load is modified by the manner in which information is presented and elements of the learning environment, such as background noise and other distractors. Germane load describes the cognitive effort required to organize new information into functional schema that can be stored in long-term memory for easy retrieval [12]. To optimize cognitive load for novice learners, concepts related to diagnosis and management of ECMO emergencies were first introduced using a conceptual framework (Fig. 13.2) with the goal of helping learners develop schema on which they could rely when integrating complex data at the bedside. The explicit introduction of conceptual frameworks by experts is an effective means of optimizing germane load for novice learners [13]. The cognitive framework was reinforced by asking learners to engage in nonsimulation educational exercises, such as "chalkboard" exercises in which the team had to work together to complete a table that elaborates expected circuit pressure changes during a comprehensive list of ECMO emergencies (Table 13.1). Hands-on activities in the form of "circuit labs" followed by team-based simulations required learners to apply the concepts introduced through didactics and nonsimulation-based learning exercises.

Design of the Simulation Curriculum: Circuit Labs

Circuit labs focused initially on learning the components of a dry ECMO circuit, with identification of each component of the circuit, articulation of their function, and recognition of the normal and abnormal values of pressure measurements. Subsequently, participants were exposed to increased complexity through the use of facilitated exercises in which learners were asked to diagnose specific ECMO emergences. Using the isolated wet circuit, instructors tightened a clamp on either the venous or arterial limbs of the circuit in order to replicate specific physiologic states and asked participants to describe the expected subsequent changes in pressures and circuit flow rates, as well as what conditions might cause these changes. Additional clinical data, including blood gas measurements and coagulation laboratory data, were also provided to give additional context to changes in pressures and flow and to prompt learners to incorporate these data into considerations of circuit function. Circuit labs followed a specific order that walked learners through a series of cognitive exercises that increased in complexity throughout the session, highlighting deeper understanding of circuit physiology. To ensure engagement and free exchange of ideas and to allow for hands-on learning from all participants, each circuit lab session was limited to 15 people. Depending on available space, circuit labs were conducted either in a conference room setting or in our simulation center.

Design of the Simulation Curriculum: High-Fidelity Simulation

As learners progressed through the training sequence, complexity of simulations was increased, transitioning primarily

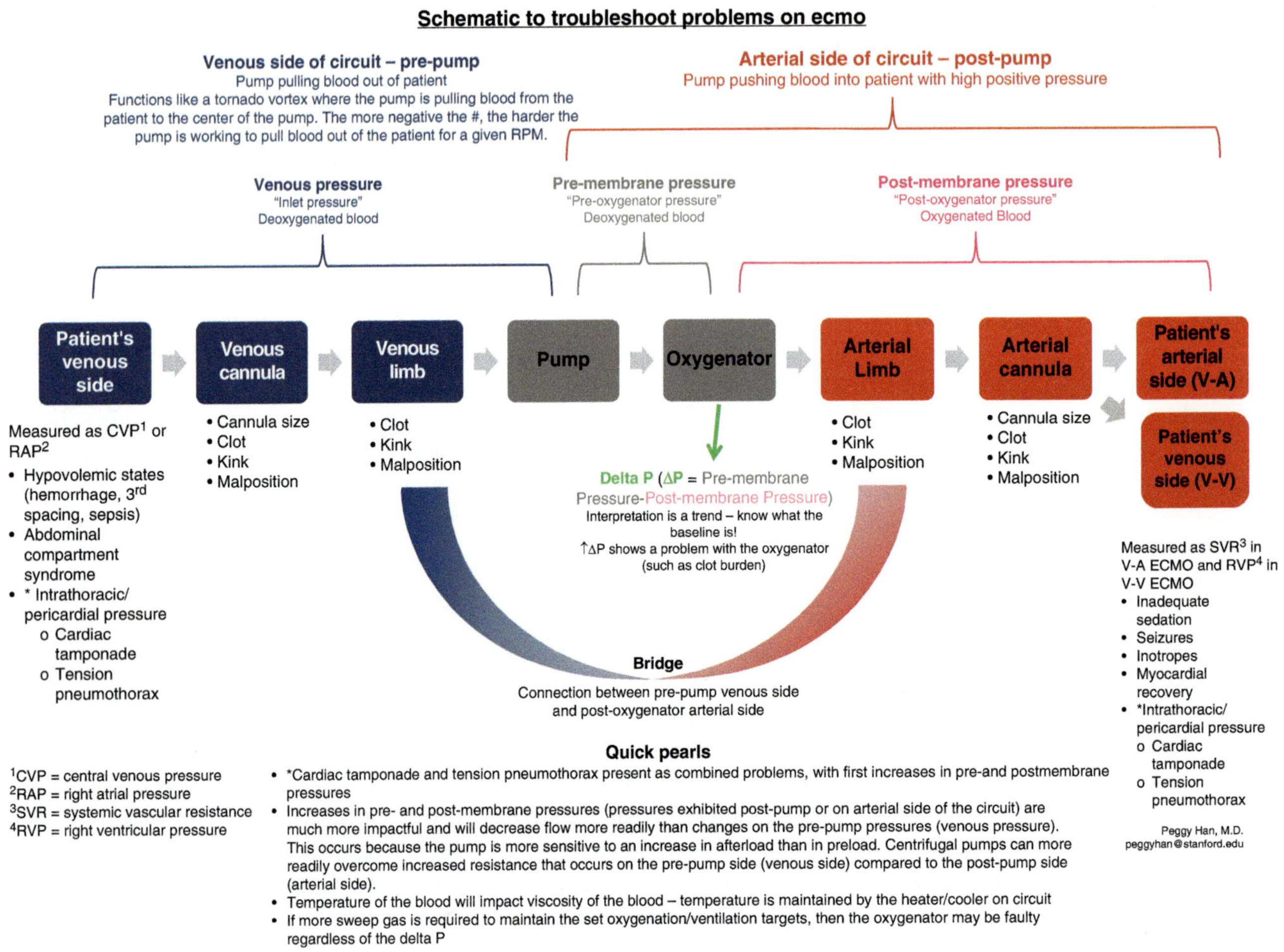

Fig. 13.2 A conceptual framework for understanding changes in pressure and blood flow rate on an ECM circuit and associated ECMO-related problems

from cognitive exercises to ones in which learners were required to integrate data, make a diagnosis, and implement treatment as they would at the bedside, thereby managing increasing cognitive load. After completing and demonstrating understanding of physiologic concepts through circuit labs, learners participated in 2 h sessions in which they were required to work together as a functional team to demonstrate understanding and effective management of two ECMO emergencies. The topics covered in these team-based simulations, summarized in Table 13.2, reflected the conceptual framework that was taught in earlier portions of the curriculum. ECMO emergencies were divided into four categories: venous-side problems, arterial-side problems, combined problems and/or pump failure and problems with gas exchange. These categories allowed our learners to develop a systematic approach to identification and management of various ECMO-related emergencies, pertinent to both V-V and V-A ECMO. Building off of the exercise in the circuit labs where the boundaries of pressure measurements were defined, learners would identify the primary pressure derangement and localize the problem to the corresponding part of the ECMO circuit.

Unlike previous low-fidelity simulations that utilized an isolated ECMO circuit and were often performed remote from the clinical environment (often in a conference room), higher-fidelity simulations were performed either in a patient bed space or in the simulation center. These sessions utilized a manikin with an integrated ECMO circuit, typical patient monitors, and patient monitoring lines as would be expected in the clinical setting. Facilitators made simultaneous adjustments to the ECMO circuit and to the vital signs displayed on physiologic monitors. A centrifugal pump system was used for these simulations. Venous-side problems manifested as decreased blood flow rates as a result of decreased venous return to the pump. This physiologic state was simulated by tightening a clamp on the venous limb of the circuit out of the view of participants. During the simulation, learners were expected to identify the increased negative pressure and decreased blood flow rate on the circuit monitors as well as appropriate changes in patient's vital signs to diagnose a

Table 13.1 Table exercise to associate decreased flow state and circuit pressure changes with ECMO emergencies. Learners are given a blank table and asked to write in how pressures change for a given problem

ECMO circuit pressures chart – diagnosing problems on ECMO					
Problem	ECMO Blood Flow	Venous Pressure "Pre-pump Pressure"	Pre-Membrane Pressure "Post-pump, Pre-oxygenator Pressure"	Post-Membrane Pressure "Post-pump, Post-oxygenator pressure"	Delta P (Pre-membrane pressure – Post-membrane pressure)
Decreased Pump Preload (e.g., Low patient central venous pressure)	*Decreased*	More negative	No change, then slightly decreased with decreased blood flow	No change, then slightly decreased with decreased blood flow	No change
Tension Pneumothorax	*Decreased*	No change, then more negative with decreased blood flow and increase in RPM	Increased	Increased	No change
Cardiac Tamponade	*Decreased*	No change, then more negative with decreased blood flow and increase in RPM	Increased	Increased	No change
Increased Pump Afterload (e.g., Increased patient systemic vascular resistance)	*Decreased*	No change, then less negative with decreased blood flow	Increased	Increased	No change
Oxygenator Membrane Failure	No change to *slightly decreased*	No change	Increased (first)	No change initially, then decreased	Increased (second)
Centrifugal Pump Failure	*Decreased*	No change, then less negative with decreased blood flow	Decreased	Decreased	No change
Small Arterial Cannula (V-A ECMO)	*Never had good flow from time of insertion* (cannot achieve maximum desired flow due to cannula size)	No change	Increased (at time of cannulation)	Increased (at time of cannulation)	No change
Malpositioned Venous Cannula (V-A ECMO)	*Decreased*	More negative	No change, then decreased with decreased blood flow	No change, then decreased with decreased blood flow	No change

Table 13.2 Categorization of ECMO simulations and topics covered in team-based simulation

Decreased Venous Return (Pump Preload)	Pump Failure/ Combined Problems	Increased Pump Afterload (Increased SVR)	Failure of Gas Exchange/ Inappropriate mixing
Hypovolemia (ex: abdominal compartment syndrome, patient hemorrhage)	Air embolus	Residual pressors	Faulty gas source (Ex. Empty O2 tank on transport)
Venous cannula clot	Electrical failure Clot in pump	Too small arterial cannula	Recirculation on V-V ECMO
Sepsis	Cardiac tamponade	Myocardial recovery on V-A ECMO	North-South Syndrome on V-A ECMO
Venous cannula malposition	Tension pneumothorax	Status Epilepticus	Oxygenator Failure
Venous cannula too small		Uncomfortable patient/ Undersedation	
		Arterial cannula malposition	

venous-side problem. Based on knowledge from circuit labs, the team was expected to articulate a differential diagnosis for venous-side problems, identify the specific problem in question, and institute appropriate treatment. Using this process, we were able to introduce a systemic approach to diagnosing ECMO emergencies for a novice group of learners and reinforce the newly developed fund of knowledge related to ECMO physiology and ECMO emergencies. The conceptual framework, dividing problems into venous side, arterial side, mixed problems, or pump failure was used to create a large library of scenarios addressing ECMO-related emergencies. Simulations targeting management of ECMO emergencies were also used to reinforce teamwork principles. Following each simulation, we used a structured debriefing that involved a reactions phase, an opportunity to explore and clarify both medical decision-making and teamwork, as well as a summary of the objectives covered. Debriefing of the first scenario typically focused more on clinical elements, and the second on teamwork principles. Using this format, we were able to provide a hands-on approach to learning about ECMO for a novice team.

A total of 52 team-based ECMO simulations were conducted in an 8 month period. As described above, each session covered two ECMO emergencies and addressed teamwork principles to foster a uniform language for teamwork among a multidisciplinary audience. Each session was attended by an average of 12 learners from multiple disciplines, with a minimum requirement of three simulation sessions per learner prior to the start of the clinical ECMO program.

Operationalizing ECMO Training in a New ECMO Center: Establishment of Superuser Group and Training from Expert Center

To address the challenges of training a large multidisciplinary cohort, most members of which had limited or no ECMO experience, we established a core group of 21 superusers representative of all disciplines who would be responsible for training and serving as a key support for the remainder of personnel on the ECMO team. Following completion of the induction phase of training, these 21 superusers completed an intensive 3-day training with the dual purpose of (1) rapidly acquiring the required ECMO expertise and (2) developing skills to run and debrief multidisciplinary ECMO simulations that would serve as the backbone of training for all personnel. To accomplish this, we partnered with a high-volume ECMO center who had simulation and education expertise. The first portion of the intensive 3-day course focused on building ECMO knowledge among the superuser team, focusing on team management of ECMO cannulations (including during CPR) and development of critical thinking skills to rapidly diagnose and manage ECMO emergencies. The second half taught skills to run and debrief ECMO simulations.

Following this 3-day workshop from an expert center, superusers participated in 12 hands-on circuit labs as described previously. This provided the opportunity to put into practice the previously introduced knowledge and skills and cement knowledge of the ECMO circuit and ECMO physiology. Each superuser participated in at least two of these sessions during a 1-month period immediately after the 3-day workshop. Superusers then participated in 12 team-based, complex ECMO simulations during the subsequent 2-month period, which consisted of 3 h sessions requiring active application of knowledge and skills related to ECMO cannulation as well as the physiologic framework for diagnosing ECMO complications that was introduced during the 3-day intensive training. Formative feedback was given to superusers based on their ability to recognize and articulate the problem at hand, formulate a differential diagnosis, and perform the necessary tasks to improve the clinical situation.

Nine months following the initial 3-day superuser training, the partnering team made a repeat visit to assess superuser progress on ECMO knowledge and skills as well as simulation education skills. During the visit, the superusers ran three ECMO simulations that were then critiqued by the same instructor group. This audit provided feedback to new learners, reinforced confidence that was built while participating in ECMO simulations, and gave encouragement that the superuser group had sufficient understanding of ECMO physiology and debriefing techniques to teach other novice users about ECMO. The 1-day audit also provided additional tools for debriefing and maximizing the learning experience in a simulation.

Dissemination of Simulation Training for Larger Audience

Following the superuser training period, superusers were called on to serve as trainers and peer mentors for the remaining 106 health care providers who required ECMO training. Superuser instructors followed the framework described previously to give their colleagues the same conceptual framework and tools to approach ECMO physiology and ECMO emergencies. Thus, all learners received induction training on basic principles, participated in circuit labs, and applied knowledge in a series of high-fidelity simulations focused on problems incurred on ECMO. This approach proved effective as following a 10-month training period using the aforementioned structured curriculum, providers successfully cared for two patients on V-A ECMO in 2017. The first patient was a 4-year old with acute fulminant myocarditis, who had a 7-day ECMO run. The second was a 1-day old with meconium aspiration syndrome, who had a 5-day ECMO run. Both patients survived to hospital discharge and had returned to their neurologic baseline upon discharge.

Conclusions and Recommendations

Development of a safe and effective new ECMO program requires providers to acquire technical and cognitive skills related to complex ECMO circuit physiology that is outside the scope of everyday Intensive Care Unit practice. We describe a comprehensive simulation-supported training structure designed to bring providers from novice to proficient. The program is designed to optimize cognitive load of learners by building knowledge and skills progressively.

Given the large number of providers with no previous ECMO exposure and limited simulation experience, collaboration with an expert center that could provide both clinical ECMO and simulation expertise was key to launching a large simulation-based curriculum that improved knowledge and familiarity with the technology. The curriculum design incorporated traditional didactics to provide a basic foundation of knowledge and subsequently those concepts were reinforced using ECMO simulation, through both skill-based labs to understand the ECMO circuit components and team-based simulations to identify and troubleshoot ECMO-related emergencies. Early introduction of a conceptual framework that helped learners integrate both patient and circuit data to diagnose and treat ECMO emergencies was key. Additional considerations for programs looking to start a simulation-based ECMO program include frequency and requirements for training, type of training (team based vs. skill based) and the number of learners or practitioners who will care for patients on ECMO.

References

1. de Winter JCF, de Groot S, Mulder M, Wieringa PA, Dankelman J, Mulder JA. Relationships between driving simulator performance and driving test results. Ergonomics. 2009;52:137–53.
2. Pradhan AK, Pollatsek A, Knodler M, Fisher DL. Can younger drivers be trained to scan for information that will reduce their risk in roadway traffic scenarios that are hard to identify as hazardous? Ergonomics. 2009;52:657–73.
3. Jentsch F, Curtis M, Salas E. Simulation in aviation training. University of Central Florida, USA, 2011.
4. McGaghie WC, Issenberg BS, Petrusa ER, Scalese RJ. A critical review of simulation-based medical education research: 2003–2009. Med Educ. 2010;44:50–63.
5. ECLS registry report international summary. Ann Arbor: Extracorporeal Life Support Organization (ELSO); 2018.
6. Weems MF, Friedlich PS, Nelson LP, Rake AJ, Klee L, Stein JE, Stavroudis TA. The role of extracorporeal membrane oxygenation simulation training at extracorporeal life support organization centers in the United States. Simul Healthc. 2017;12(4):233–9.
7. Di Nardo M, Piero D, Stoppa F, et al. The introduction of a high-fidlity simulation program for training pediatric critical care personnel reduces the times to manage extracorporeal membrane oxygenation emergencies and improves teamwork. J Thorac Dis. 2018;10(6):3409–17.
8. Zakhary BM, Kam LM, Kaufman BS, et al. The utility of high-fidelity simulation training for training critical care fellows in management of extracorporeal membrane oxygentation emergenices: a randomized controlled trial. Crit Care Med. 2017;45(8):1367–73.
9. Raffaeli G, Ghirardello S, Vanzati M, et al. Start a neonatal extracorporeal membrane oxygenation program: a multistep team training. Front Pediatr. 2018;6:151.
10. Sanchez-Glanville C, Brindle ME, Spence T, et al. The introduction of extracorporeal life support technology to a tertiary care pediatric institution: smoothing the learning curve through interprofessional simulation training. J Pediatr Surg. 2015;50:798–804.
11. Roussin CJ, Simzones WP. An organizational innovation for simulation programs and centers. Acad Med. 2017;92:1114–20.
12. van Merrienboer JJ, Sweller J. Cognitive load theory in health professional education: design principles and strategies. Med Educ. 2010;44:85–93.
13. Mancinetti M, Guttormsen S, Berendonk C. Cognitive load in internal medicine: what every clinical teacher should know about cognitive load theory. Eur J Intern Med. 2019;60:4–8.

Using Simulation to Develop an ECMO Transport Program

14

Kathleen R. Ryan and Vamsi V. Yarlagadda

Learning Objectives

After reading this chapter, providers will be able to:

1. Discuss how knowledge of the differing backgrounds of target learners is critical in conceptually designing an ECMO transport simulation
2. Incorporate principles of transport medicine as well as ECMO management into an ECMO transport simulation
3. Describe the elements of both an uncomplicated ECMO transport as well as emergency scenarios to be incorporated into ECMO transport simulation

Introduction

The goal of this chapter is to provide readers with a guide to designing a curriculum and executing ECMO simulation as part of the development and ongoing education for an ECMO transport program. The safety of transporting patients supported on ECMO has been well established in the literature for both adult and pediatric populations [1, 2]. It is a high-risk, low-frequency event that requires substantial preparation, and simulation can be vital to safe, successful transports of these critically ill patients, particularly for newly developed programs or when introducing new aspects of care into more established programs.

In the current economic environment, clinicians are increasingly feeling pressure to keep patients in their unit rather than transfer to another institution. This is one reason many more centers are developing ECMO programs [3]. With that said, even with an increased number of hospitals having functioning ECMO programs, there still may be clinical situations that warrant the transfer of a patient who has already been cannulated. As an example, ECMO may be initiated at a referring center for primary cardiac failure and the patient requires transport to a transplant center for evaluation for possible heart transplantation or other cardiac intervention. Similarly, patients cannulated to ECMO for respiratory failure may be candidates for lung transplantation and require transport to an appropriate center for further evaluation and management. Finally, transport may be needed for institutions with limited resources that are unable to maintain a patient on ECMO for a more extended period of time.

ELSO Guidelines Regarding ECMO Transport

Extracorporeal Life Support Organization (ELSO) recommends that ECMO transports are managed by an interprofessional team comprised of ECMO specialists, respiratory therapists, critical care nurses, and physicians [4]. The ultimate team makeup will, in part, be guided by the members of the transport team existing at one's home institution. Most critical care transport teams are made up of a combination of critical care nurses, respiratory therapists, physicians, and emergency medical technicians (EMTs). An ECMO transport will require adaptation of this core group to include individuals skilled in caring for patients on ECMO and ECMO circuits, such as specially trained nurses, respiratory therapists, or perfusionists.

At our institution, which has provided care to patients on ECMO for more than 20 years, we recommend an ECMO transport team consist of at least two providers whose primary focus will be the patient, two providers who will be responsible for managing the ECMO circuit, and a physician lead. The role of the patient-focused providers will

K. R. Ryan (✉) · V. V. Yarlagadda
Division of Pediatric Cardiology, Department of Pediatrics, Lucile Packard Children's Hospital at Stanford, Stanford University Medical Center, Palo Alto, CA, USA
e-mail: kateryan@stanford.edu

L. C. Johnston, L. Su (eds.), *Comprehensive Healthcare Simulation: ECMO Simulation*, Comprehensive Healthcare Simulation,
https://doi.org/10.1007/978-3-030-53844-6_14

vary by institution. For instance, our institution utilizes a respiratory therapist and an RN as transport team members, but other institutions may have two RNs who divide up tasks related to patient care. The two ECMO specialists will likewise divide up tasks related to the ECMO circuit. Having two ECMO providers allows emergency situations due to technical issues with the circuit to be dealt with quickly and efficiently. EMTs should be part of the team but maintain the same role as they would on any critical care transport. One key element to consider is how many total providers can be accommodated on a particular mode of transportation. For instance, critical care ambulances vary in size; this may impact the number of providers capable of being transported safely. Fixed and rotor-wing travel will potentially require further paring of the team. At a minimum, a bedside nurse, a trained ECMO specialist and a physician are recommended by ELSO [4]. Given the scope of ECMO transport simulation, this chapter will focus solely on ground transport. However, once a ground transport team is successfully trained, the same concepts can be applied to other modes of transportation with particular attention placed on physical location of equipment and personnel in the chosen vehicle.

The target learners for the ECMO transport simulation will have different backgrounds and different roles, and thus different target objectives for the simulation (See Table 14.1). A brief didactic prior to simulation outlining these goals with some basic tutorials will likely be useful. The ultimate purpose of the simulation is not to have four equally interchangeable members and a physician lead. Rather, it is to introduce members to key concepts of the "other" provider's domain. For instance, safety is a primary focus of critical care transport teams; there are a number of checks and protocols in place to assure safety of both the patient and the team. Those concepts will need to be introduced to the ECMO team prior to participation in the simulation. Likewise, the non-ECMO focused members of the transport team need to become familiar with some of the broader concepts with regard to ECMO (such as the difference between veno venous and veno arterial cannulations) in order to care appropriately for the patient in an emergency situation.

Table 14.1 Potential learning objectives for transport simulation based upon provider role

	Transport Team	ECMO Specialist	Physician Lead
Basics of ECMO	X		
Transport team safety		X	X
Circuit mobilization safety	X	X	X

Principles of ECMO Transport to Incorporate into Practical Simulation

There are two main areas of ECMO transport that need to be incorporated into practical simulation sessions: ECMO considerations and transport medicine considerations. As in all simulations, to the degree that it is possible it is desirable to provide participants in ECMO simulation with a replication of the actual clinical environment. As such, it is important to have a manikin that is "cannulated" to allow the team to assess and manage the patient in addition to a functioning full ECMO circuit. In clinical practice, we recommend transitioning all patients, regardless of size, to a centrifugal pump prior to transport for ease of transport and safety of the circuit. Therefore, a centrifugal pump, as well as the equipment needed to transition over to the transport circuit, is necessary as well. Participants will need to have access to traditional resuscitation equipment (including devices for airway management, vascular access, and various medications) as well as emergency equipment for the circuit (such as clamps and syringes) to improve the realism of the scenario. As noted previously in Chap. 7, making adjustments to the circuit, the manikin, and the various monitoring devices can effectively replicate numerous patient and circuit emergencies that may be encountered during ECMO transport.

With regard to transport medicine considerations, several issues need to be incorporated for ECMO simulations such as weather, distance to referring institution, and patient stability. Given the complexity of transporting ECMO patients, it is our institutional policy to only proceed with transport once the patient is stably on ECMO for a minimum of 30 min. Any successful transport of a critically ill patient requires particular attention to communication/team behaviors. For optimal communication, the roles of each team member need to be explicitly delineated. One of the challenges of transport medicine is the potential for a high-stakes emergency situation to develop in a confined space such as the back of an ambulance or airplane. To optimize outcomes, these situations call for a previously defined understanding of responsibilities and clarification of roles. The traditional members of the transport team should continue to have primary responsibility for management of the patient. The ECMO-trained members of the team should have responsibility for the circuit. The physician lead should facilitate communication between all providers. In addition, communication between bedside providers at the referring institution and the transport team, as well as between the transport team and receiving team members at the accepting institution, is key. Ensuring a respectful and open dialogue between teams will help to establish a good working relationship despite providers potentially having just met.

Transport Simulation Design

Transport simulation design can be divided into three major areas for consideration: goals/learning objectives, location/setting, and equipment.

Goals and Objectives

The goals and learning objectives for each ECMO transport scenario will vary significantly depending on what topic is being addressed. Various topics may be considered depending on the level of experience and needs of the individual providers, as well as institutional preferences. A list of potential topics will be provided in the next section in this chapter. However, one of the primary goals of most ECMO transport simulation is to combine individual skill sets to create a functioning team for a rare high-risk scenario. Ideally, after participating in an ECMO simulation, team members will feel more comfortable performing their clinical roles despite the addition of the more unfamiliar elements (ECMO for transport team members, transport medicine for ECMO providers). In addition to being practically easier to schedule and execute a transport simulation at one's own institution, creating simulations in a local environment can also serve to unmask unforeseen difficulties (latent threats) in transporting patients, such as elevators that cannot hold the necessary equipment/personnel or turns in hallways that cannot be accommodated.

Setting

Simulation design for ECMO transport is dependent on the location or setting that is desired, though many elements (such as checklists and designated time outs) will overlap. Possible settings for ECMO simulation would be at the referring institution, or in the transport vehicle (ambulance, helicopter, or fixed wing). As noted previously, this chapter will focus on the transport of a patient on ECMO between institutions using ground transport, but concepts can be adapted for other modalities.

Equipment

ECMO transport simulations require significant amounts of equipment for both the care of the patient as well as the circuit. Having realistic equipment placed in typical locations will be most beneficial for participants in order to transfer learning to clinical practice. Another unique need for ECMO transport is the requirement for blood products. Patient transfusion needs should be assessed ahead of time and emergency blood products should be available during transport. To decrease the impact of potential bleeding exacerbated by movement/driving, we recommend blood priming the transport circuit on arrival to the patient's referring institution. Blood priming should be a standard part of the training required for at least one of the team members comprising the ECMO providers. It should be done in the standard fashion even at the outside institution and as such, does not need replication during the transport simulation itself.

Transport Simulation Scenarios

There are several elements of an uncomplicated transport that will be incorporated at baseline in every event (Table 14.2). Each stage involves a significant amount of communication amongst team members under the guidance of the physician lead. Full transport simulation scenarios should include all aspects of transporting a patient from start to finish, and therefore will need to include the following:

1. Predeparture checklist: Prior to leaving the home institution, the entire transport team should review a predeparture checklist to ensure that all necessary equipment is available. An example of this checklist is below (Fig. 14.1). During the circuit change, the patient is transitioned to the transport circuit. This will require a minimum of two people accustomed to local circuit change procedures. The circuit change should happen prior to transition to the transport gurney or isolette.
2. Transition of pumps/gurney: Once the patient has stabilized after the circuit change, the intravenous infusions need to transition to the transport pumps. The members of the regular transport team who have experience completing this task on a daily basis should guide the transition. Care must be given to plan how the patient will be situated in the back of the critical care ambulance. The schematic

Table 14.2 Recommended scenarios for hands-on ECMO simulation training

1. Conversion of patient to mobile ECMO circuit
Team handoff from referring providers
Review equipment checklist and repeat roles and responsibilities
Clamp and cut in new centrifugal circuit
Go back on ECMO flows
2. Patient transfer and mobilization of circuit
Practice move of patient to transport gurney
Roll gurney with mobile ECMO circuit on a short trip (consider an elevator trip)
Use bridge technique using a team member's arms to be holding on to both the circuit and the gurney
Move patient from gurney into bedspace
3. Roll patient and mobile ECMO circuit into transport vehicle
Low -technology simulation is adequate for these training simulations

Fig. 14.1 ECMO transport checklists

MOBILE ECMO

ECMO INTAKE:

Perfusionist:

Referring Hospital:

Patient Name:

Wt. kg:
Ht. cm:
BSA m2:

Reason for ECMO:

Cannulae brand, style, dimensions and connector size
Drainage 1:
Drainage 2:
Re-infusion 1:
Re-infusion 2:
LA vent:

Blood flow rate:
Sweep gas:
Pre/Post Oxy pressure:
Negative Ven pressure:
Anticoagulation:
Bleeding: Yes No
Open chest: Yes No
Target Temperature:
Other considerations:
RBC & Blood Products:

DEPARTURE CHECKLIST

- ☐ ECMO Mobile bag
- ☐ Cardiohelp
- ☐ Disposable setup
- ☐ Clamps (sterile and non-sterile)
- ☐ Extra oxygen tank
- ☐ Extra flowmeter
- ☐ Confirm Perfusion has spoken to outside facility regarding ECMO specifics and
- ☐ blood products requested
- ☐ Cooler for blood products
- ☐ Priming medication +(2) 250 ml 0.5% albumin
- ☐ Warm packs

PRE-RETURN CHECKLIST

Attending:

Perfusionist: ECMO RN:

Transport RN: Transport RT:

Time of Circuit Change: Time of Departure

- ☐ Oxygen tanks fully pressurized; re-check in 10 minutes
- ☐ Patient covered with several layers of blankets
- ☐ Mobile ECMO bag
- ☐ Volume available
- ☐ Lab values clinically acceptable
- ☐ Lines secured and immobilized
- ☐ Cooler with Blood Products

shown here (Fig. 14.2) provides an example of a relatively small rig with the necessary placement of individuals based on their clinical responsibilities. For instance, the critical care transport team member who will have the responsibility of administering medications will need to have access to the pumps and therefore the infusions should be set up on that side. Likewise, the team members responsible for the ECMO circuit will need to be able to access it for monitoring and interventions. Moreover, one person from the ECMO team is responsible for holding cannula position at the insertion site during all stages of patient movement and transfer. We recommend situating the pump at the foot of the bed. The ventilator will need to be situated toward the patient's head.

Movement of the patient to the transport gurney should involve all members of the ECMO transport team with each individual's role clearly laid out and reiterated by the physician lead during a huddle that will also review how the transition will occur (i.e., in one move or staged smaller moves to the gurney). Team members should be reminded that they are empowered to say "STOP" at any point in the transfer if they notice something wrong.

3. Moving the patient to the ambulance bay: Once the patient has been successfully moved onto the gurney and all supplies have been packed, the physician lead should go through the departure checklist to ensure all equipment/medications/products have been accounted for, the tanks supplying the circuit are fully pressurized and the battery of the pump is adequately charged for the transport. The route to the ambulance should be determined ahead of time and cleared of any equipment. Ideally, security should be holding elevators. One member of the two ECMO providers should be designated as the "bridge." As such, one hand should be on the patient's bed and the

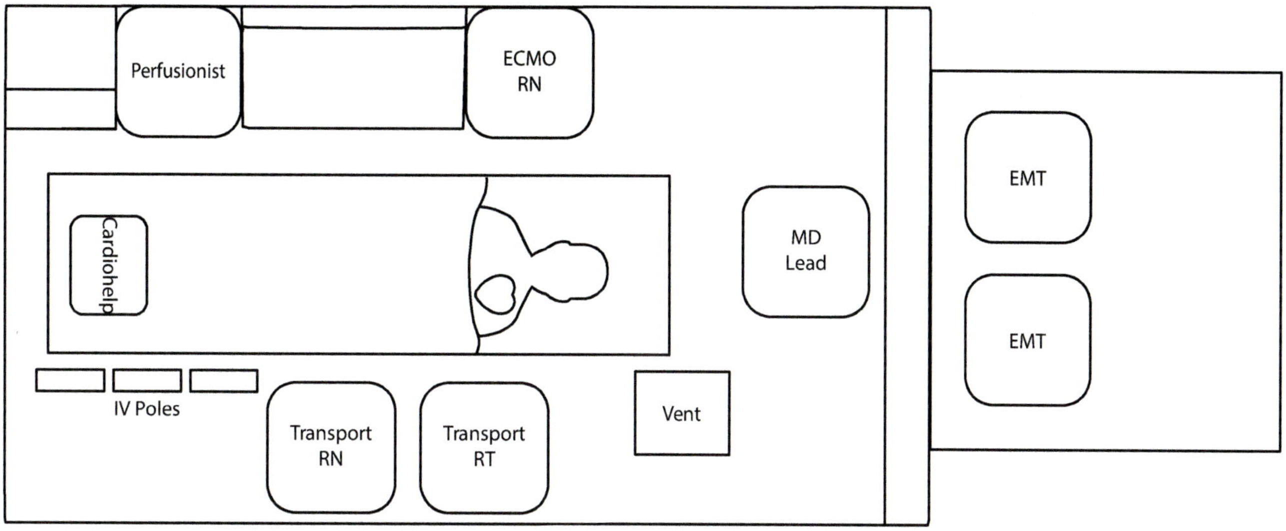

Fig. 14.2 ECMO transport ambulance configuration example

other on the ECMO circuit. This ensures that during the move, the circuit is not under tension if the bed and circuit are moving at different speeds. An initial move of only a short distance (e.g., 6 in.) will help to ensure that all equipment is unplugged and able to move freely.

4. Transporting the patient into the ambulance: The next stage of transport will involve getting the patient into the ambulance. As with all stages, good communication will be necessary to ensure lines are not disconnected and that undue tension is not placed on the circuit.
5. Transport back to home institution: The transport ambulance should physically leave the hospital to mimic what a true ECMO transport will feel like. This is especially key for members of the ECMO team who may not have experience working in the back of ambulance.
6. Getting out of the ambulance/transport back to ICU: The team should be physically responsible for moving the patient out of the rig and back to ICU.
7. Transition to inpatient bed: Similar to transition of patient onto the gurney, the simulation should involve moving the patient onto the inpatient bed. In this situation, we recommend the ECMO transport team remain the primary team caring for the patient. Transition of the care of the patient should not be completed until AFTER the patient has been moved to the inpatient bed. As such, only the team members who have been caring for the patient up until this point should be managing the patient. There will be a tendency for the team in the receiving inpatient unit to want to help, but in our experience, the safest, most efficient way of moving the patient involves keeping the team small and organized.

In addition to simulating the logistics of an uncomplicated transport, educators training ECMO teams will often-

Table 14.3 Example emergency scenarios for hands-on ECMO simulation training

1. Code event in transport vehicle
Learn the importance of predefined roles based on physical location in vehicle
Understand that a patient on VV ECMO is not hemodynamically supported
2. Circuit Air Emergency
Learn circuit clamping technique
Air evacuation procedure
Restart ECMO circuit
Recognize that CPR may be necessary during this time
3. Battery Shutdown
Know where handcrank equipment is located
Learn handcranking technique specific to your ECMO circuit
High-technology simulation may be needed to provide a high-fidelity experience in these scenarios

times include a patient or circuit emergency in their learning objectives (Tables 14.3 and 14.4). As patients requiring ECMO transport between institutions are dependent on the support provided by the ECMO circuit, circuit emergencies that involve an interruption to that support are life-threatening events. ECMO specialists and providers should undergo training on how to deal with various scenarios involving circuit disruption, but as noted above, on transport these instances are likely taking place in an unfamiliar environment with limited workspace and, potentially, with an unfamiliar team makeup. Undergoing these challenges in simulation will likely reveal unrecognized issues with the team and environment that could prevent optimal management of the patient in an actual emergency if not addressed proactively. There are a number of ECMO emergency scenarios that would be useful to conduct in simulation to familiarize the team with the adjustments needed to safely rescue the patient. Some of these include:

Table 14.4 ECMO transport bag

Safety straps (4)	500 ML NS (2)	
Chloroprep swabs	Alcohol pads	Stopcocks – High flow (8)
4 × 4 Gauze 2 × 2 Gauze	Blenderm tape (1) Elastaplast (1) White label Roll (1)	Clave IV access Connector Mini spike dispensing pin
Sterile clamps (4)	#10 Blades (2) Sterile scissors (2)	Bovie/cautery (2)
Sterile 3/8" Tubing (1)	Sterile 1/4" Tubing (1)	Sterile towels 2 Double pack
60 ml syringe (10)	10 ml syringe (10)	5 ml syringes (10)
3 ml syringe (10)	1 ml syringe (10)	Red Caps
NS flush 10 ml (10)	Sterile pack NS flush 10 ml (10)	Blunt needle
1/4" × 3/8" connect 1/4" × 1/4" connect	3/8" × 3/8" connect	1/4" × 3/8" × 3/8" Y connector
M/M connector (2)	Press.Tubing (4)	150 u blood filter/syringe adapter (3)
Dead enders pack (2)	Transducer kit (2)	CDI (2)
Tie band gun Tie bands (10)	Secondary set (2)	High-flow stopcocks (6)
Sterile gloves 7 (2)	Sterile gloves 7.5 (2)	Sterile gloves 8 (2)

1. Circuit air entrainment: Circuit air entrainment is a disastrous scenario that can and will occur if the circuit and all of the connectors are not properly checked prior to transport. Circuit air emergencies are an integral part of any standard ECMO training program and should be reinforced in team training for ECMO transport. The simulation should involve effective communication on management of the patient during air entrainment. During a massive air entrainment, the circuit should be clamped, source of air leak located and fixed, air removed and flushed out with saline, and circuit restarted. During this entire scenario, the patient will not be receiving circuit flow and therefore will need medical management and possibly CPR to stay alive. Again, the scenario should be performed in the back of the critical care transport rig to replicate the challenges of working in that environment.
2. Pump failure: Common causes of pump failure are transducer errors, severe hypovolemia, pump cone failure, or obstructed cannulae. It is uncommon for the actual electrical panel and pump to fail, but in this situation, changing the circuit over to a new pump may be a quick way to reset any issues. Any ECMO transport should carry a backup pump for this specific emergency. During pump failure, the patient will not be receiving mechanical circulatory support and will need to be entirely managed medically. As noted above, it is especially important to delineate provider roles. For instance, in the schematic demonstrated in Fig. 14.2, the physician lead managing the code situation is also the only person available to manually ventilate the patient, as the provider stationed to one side of the head of the bed will have to perform CPR given the size constraints of this small vehicle.
3. Hemodynamic instability is a surprisingly common event on ECMO. On transport, the most common time for hemodynamic instability is at the time of circuit change, especially if transitioning from roller head pump to a centrifugal pump. Both hypertension and hypotension have important consequences for the patient and the circuit individually. Centrifugal pumps are very afterload sensitive and the pump flow may be poor if the patient has been managed with high-dose SVR altering agents. Knowing this allows the team to prepare in advance for the potential swings occurring during the pump changeover. Transport team members may be accustomed to managing patient hypotension independently just as ECMO specialists may be accustomed to managing this clinical situation with circuit adjustments. Experiencing these events in simulation will help the team to develop a shared mental model regarding the potential derangements in blood pressure during pump changeover and transport, and to prepare for these in advance. To facilitate this, it is therefore vital that all clinical interventions are filtered through the physician lead to prevent overlap in treatment or worse, interventions that may be detrimental to the patient and circuit as a whole.

Conclusion

The goals of an ECMO transport simulation program center around creation of a team dynamic amongst providers to prepare for low-frequency, high-risk events. Simulation can help identify and address unforeseen systems issues (latent threats) that would otherwise have only been noted during a live transport. Simulation training should prepare the ECMO transport team for how to handle crisis situations in unfamiliar and potentially restrictive environments (i.e., the back of an ambulance for ECMO specialists) with unfamiliar physiology and equipment (i.e., for the core transport team, who may have limited familiarity with ECMO). Evaluating the competency of the ECMO transport team following simulation is difficult as the number of times a true transport comes up is likely to be infrequent and not all providers will have the chance to see their training borne out into real-world experience. For that reason, simulation experience should be a part of annual training with the theory consistent and repeated simulation experiences will achieve a shared mental model and comfort level between team members ultimately resulting in safe, successful transports.

References

1. Biscotti M, Agerstrand C, Abrams D, Ginsburg M, Sonett J, Mongero L, et al. One hundred transports on extracorporeal support to an extracorporeal membrane oxygenation center. Ann Thorac Surg. 2015;100:34–9; discussion 39-40.
2. Clement KC, Fiser RT, Fiser WP, et al. Single institution experience with inter-hospital extra- corporeal membrane oxygenation transport: a descriptive study. Pediatr Crit Care Med. 2010;11:533–5.
3. Sauer CM, Yuh DD, Bonde P. Extracorporeal membrane oxygenation use has increased by 433% in adults in the United States from 2006 to 2011. ASAIO J. 2015;61:31–6.
4. Extracorporeal Life Support Organization. Available at: https://www.elso.org/Resources/Guidelines.aspx. Accessed on 29 July 2019.

Debriefing ECMO Simulations: Special Considerations

15

Taylor Sawyer and Megan M. Gray

Learning Objectives

1. Define *post-event debriefing* and *within-event debriefing*.
2. Compare the *Reaction, Analysis, Summary* to the *Gather, Analyze, Summarize* debriefing conversational structure.
3. List conversational techniques, educational strategies, and debriefing adjuncts used in debriefing.
4. Explain special considerations for debriefing ECMO simulations.

Introduction

The most important components of healthcare simulation are feedback and debriefing [1–4]. The terms "feedback" and "debriefing" are often used interchangeably; however, there are important distinctions between the two. Feedback is the one-way conveyance of information from a facilitator to a learner on the gap between their performance and optimal performance standards, with suggestions on how the gap might be bridged [4, 5]. Debriefing is a bi-directional, interactive, and reflective discussion [4, 6–8]. Simulation debriefing involves varying levels of facilitation or guidance – either by a facilitator, or the learners – to assist in the reflective process that allows learners to develop suggestions for improving performance [4–11]. Debriefing is a form of "reflective practice," and provides a means of reflection-on-action in the process of continuous learning [12]. This reflection-on-action is a key tenet of Kolb's experiential learning theory, which describes how human experience provides a primary source of learning and development [13]. Central to the ideas of both reflective practice and experiential learning is the belief that experience alone does not lead to learning, but rather that deliberate reflection on the experience leads to learning [14].

In this chapter, we explore the particular nuances of debriefing ECMO simulations. The goal of this chapter is to provide a general overview of debriefing techniques and strategies that simulation educators can use when debriefing ECMO simulations. We begin by examining debriefing timing and facilitation methods. We then review different conversational structures used in debriefing. Next, we explore debriefing process elements including essential elements of debriefing, conversational techniques, educational strategies, and debriefing adjuncts. We have also provided an analysis of special considerations for debriefing ECMO simulations and conclude with a brief discussion of debriefing training and assessment for facilitators.

Debriefing Timing and Facilitation

Debriefing can occur either after a simulation scenario has ended or during the simulation scenario itself [4]. Debriefing conversations conducted after the simulation are referred to as "post-event debriefing" [4], while those occurring during the simulation are referred to as "within-event debriefing" [4]. Post-event debriefing is the most common debriefing method, as it provides a logical time to review individual and team performance, without interrupting the flow of the scenario. Multiple conversational frameworks for post-event debriefing have been described. A detailed review of the various frameworks is provided by Sawyer et al. [4]

T. Sawyer (✉)
Department of Pediatrics, Seattle Children's Hospital, Seattle, WA, USA
e-mail: tlsawyer@uw.edu

M. M. Gray
Department of Pediatrics, University of Washington, Seattle, WA, USA

L. C. Johnston, L. Su (eds.), *Comprehensive Healthcare Simulation: ECMO Simulation*, Comprehensive Healthcare Simulation,
https://doi.org/10.1007/978-3-030-53844-6_15

Table 15.1 Conversational frameworks for post-event debriefing

Debriefing with Good Judgment [18, 19]	G.A.S [20].
Reaction – Simulation participants express initial emotional reactions to the simulation.	*Gather* – Simulation participants review events during the simulation so no one is confused about what happened (establishes a shared mental model).
Analysis – Facilitator notes performance gaps related to the predetermined objectives, provides feedback on the gap by describing what they observed, investigates the basis for this gap and helps close the performance gap through discussion or teaching.	*Analyze* – Questions are used to stimulate conversation and examine performance around predefined learning objectives. Can follow "plus" (*what went well?*) and "delta" (*what could be improved?*) format.
Summary – Distill lessons learned into memorable rules-of-thumb or concepts to improve practice.	*Summarize* – Review lessons learned and take away points.

Table 15.1 provides an overview of two commonly used post-event debriefing frameworks: Debriefing with Good Judgment [18, 19], and Gather, Analyze, Summarize (G.A.S.) [20]. Each framework progresses through three "phases" and shares common elements of analysis and summary. The beginning phase, however, differs between the two. In the Debriefing with Good Judgment framework described by Rudolph et al. [18, 19], the initial phase of the conversation is aimed at allowing participants to express emotions and "blow off steam" prior to the debriefing conversation. In the G.A.S. framework described by Phrampus et al. [20], the debriefing conversation starts with a gathering of the facts around the simulation case in order to develop a shared mental model among the simulation participants. There are no data comparing the various post-event debriefing formats, and each may have strengths for different learners and situations [4]. Simulation educators generally use the framework with which they are most familiar and comfortable.

Within-event debriefing is less commonly used but can be a powerful educational strategy in the right situations. Within-event debriefing is typically conducted as part of mastery learning sessions or as part of "rapid cycle deliberate practice" (RCDP) [15, 16]. Within-event debriefing is shorter and more focused than post-event debriefings as the conversation usually covers only one or two learning objectives. Such "microdebriefings" are conducted during a short "pause and rewind" in the simulation scenario, allowing learners to consider their strategy and try again until they reach mastery of the skill in question [16]. The technique can be used for both technical and behavioral skill training. Figure 15.1 provides a schematic overview comparing post-event and within-event debriefing with three learning objectives. As noted in the figure, each within-event microdebriefing covers only one learning objective. This keeps the conversation short and concise. There are limited data comparing the educational efficacy of post-event debriefing versus within-event debriefing. One systematic review of RCDP found diverse and heterogeneous results from the 15 studies analyzed, which limited the ability to perform a quantitative synthesis [17].

Both post-event debriefing and within-event debriefing require some sort of conversational guidance or structure for facilitation. Following a predefined framework (Table 15.1) ensures that the debriefing conversation stays on track and that all relevant learning objectives are discussed. The debriefing facilitation can be "facilitator-guided" (e.g., done by a trained debriefing facilitator), or can be "self-guided" (e.g., done by the simulation participants themselves). In reports of self-guided debriefing methods, the participants typically utilize a cognitive aid or written guide to help standardized the conversational flow and to ensure that all important learning objectives are covered [9, 10]. Studies comparing facilitator-guided to self-guided debriefing are limited, however, evidence suggests that self-guided debriefing may be as effective as a facilitator-guided debriefing for behavioral skills training [9, 10]. Either method may be acceptable in certain situations. With junior learners, it may be advantageous to use facilitator-guided debriefing, where the facilitator can teach within the context of debriefing as a subject matter expert, providing input to the debriefing discussion and answering questions based on their experience and expertise [4]. Self-guided debriefing may be more feasible and appropriate for experienced teams [4], as the groups' cumulative experience and expertise are necessary to answer questions and teach each other within the context of the debriefing. This type of self-guided debriefing mirrors debriefings performed during clinical care, such as those performed after a code or difficult ECMO cannulation. By having simulation participants self-debrief, they can learn tactics and techniques that will improve their clinical debriefing skills [21]. Figure 15.2 compares facilitator-guided and self-guided debriefing.

Debriefing Process Elements

Debriefing process elements are the elements used to optimize learning and maximize the impact of the debriefing experience [4]. Some process elements are considered essential and should always be used. Others are conversational techniques, educational strategies, and debriefing adjuncts that can be added to the debriefing if desirable or appropriate to the situation. For example, novice learners may need more directive feedback whereas advanced learners may benefit from self-assessments. Table 15.2 provides an overview of the various process elements within their respective categories.

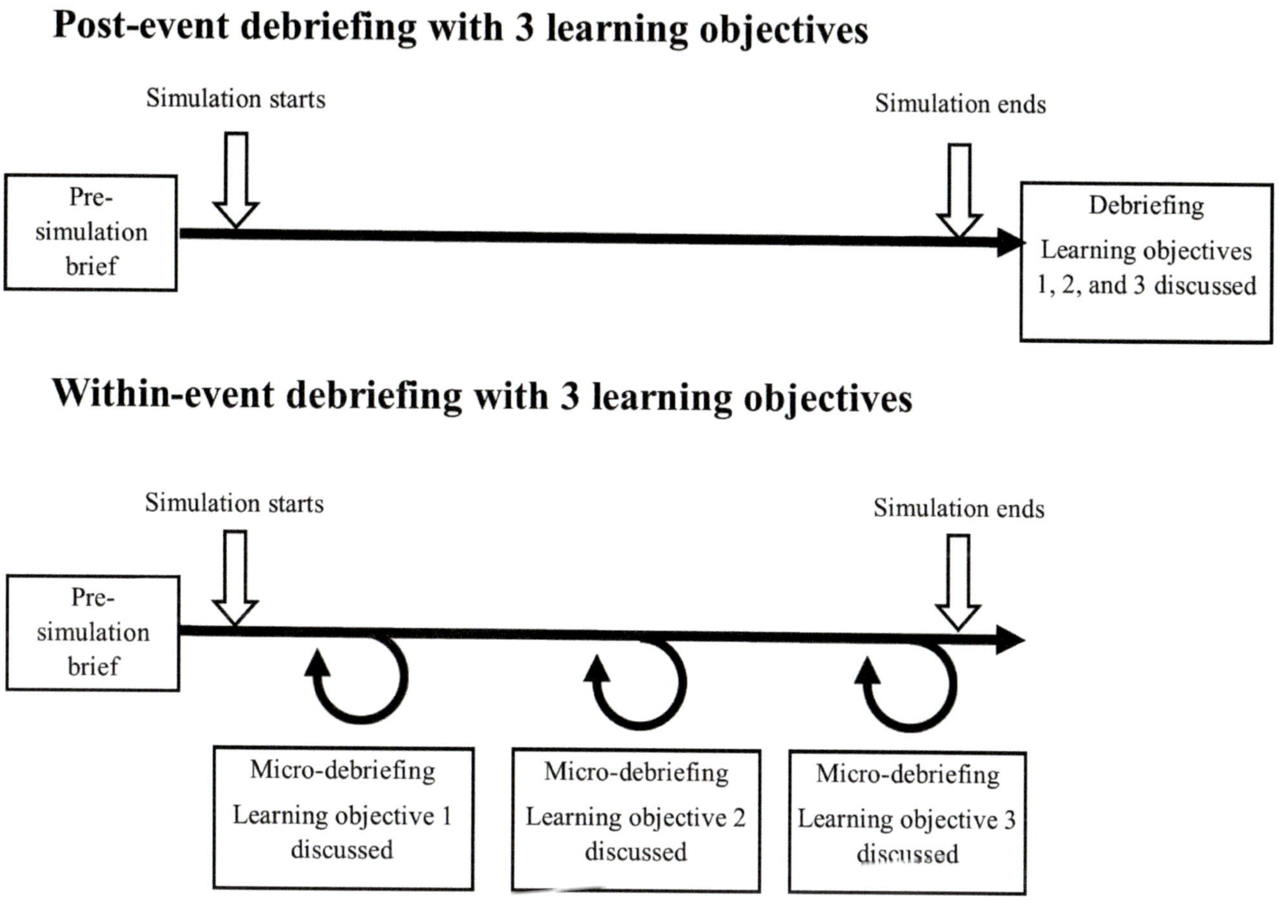

Fig. 15.1 Schematic overview comparing post-event and within-event debriefing with three learning objectives

Fig. 15.2 Comparison of facilitator-guided and self-guided debriefing

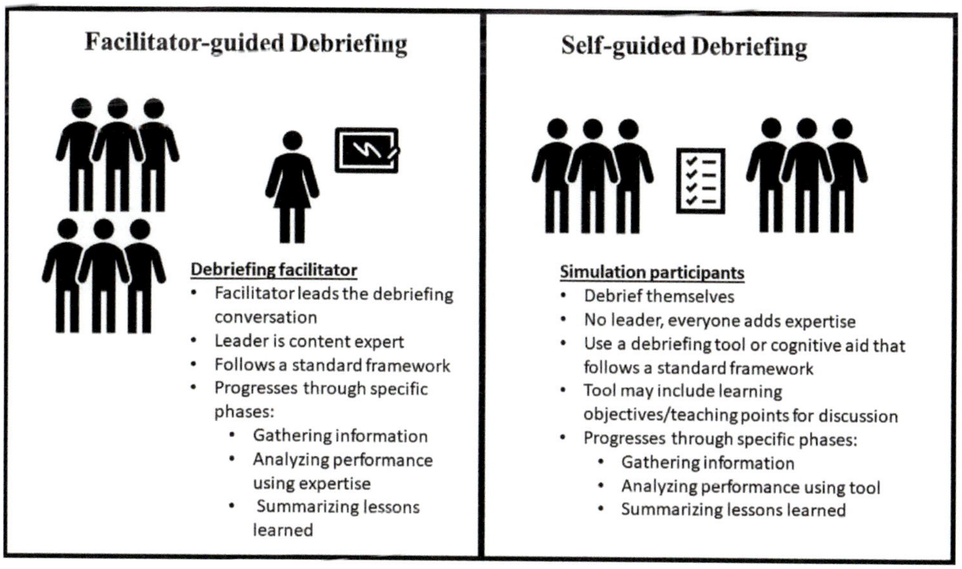

Table 15.2 Debriefing process elements

Categories of elements	Process elements in this category
Essential elements	Psychological safety Debriefing stance or "basic assumption" Establishing debriefing rules Addressing learning objectives Establishing a shared mental model Asking open-ended questions Using silence
Conversational techniques / educational strategies	Directive feedback Learner self-assessment Focused facilitation
Debriefing adjuncts	Video review Co-debriefer Debriefing script

Essential Elements of Debriefing

As noted above, some process elements are essential to effective debriefing and should be included in all simulation debriefings. These include ensuring psychological safety, having a debriefing stance or "basic assumption," establishing debriefing rules, establishing a shared mental model, addressing learning objectives, using open-ended questions, and effectively using silence [4]. The first three elements (psychological safety, debriefing stance or "basic assumption," and debriefing rules) should be made clear before the debriefing. The last four should all be done during the debriefing conversation itself.

Psychological safety Psychological safety is the ability to "behave or perform without fear of negative consequences to self-image, social standing, or career trajectory" [22], and its establishment within the learning environment during simulation and debriefing is essential [23]. Psychological safety is accomplished by conducting a pre-simulation brief by the simulation facilitator(s) [23], during which the participants are told that they can speak freely, without fear that their words will lead to personal harm or rejection [23]. One example of a way to create psychological safety is the use of the "Vegas rule," where all the comments and observations made in the simulation debriefing stay in the simulation debriefing and are not discussed outside that context.

Debriefing stance, or "basic assumption" An example of a basic assumption is: *we believe that everyone participating in this simulation is intelligent, capable, cares about doing their best, and wants to improve*. Sharing this basic assumption with simulation participants, and keeping it in mind encourages both the facilitator and learners to be curious – instead of accusatory – in instances where participants do not perform as expected [18]. This stance of *curiosity* drives the facilitator to examine the "mental frames" (e.g., frame of mind) that led to the observed actions [19]. Identifying these mental frames is an important way to facilitate learning in the process of formative assessment through simulation [19]. This also serves to frame participants' internal assessment of their own performance and reorient negative thoughts back to a growth mindset.

Establishing debriefing rules Some debriefing rules include the need for all members to be active participants in the discussion, assurance that the discussion is confidential, and the debriefing conversation will focus on performance improvement, rather than individual criticism. Informing simulation participants of the rules of debriefing can improve psychological safety and prevent potential problems [24].

Establishing a shared mental model Providing time in the debriefing conversation to establish a shared mental model of the events that transpired during the simulation allows a group of participants to have a shared understanding on which to build their learning [4]. A shared mental model is typically established by having a team member review the events of the scenario, with clarification from other team members or the facilitator, as needed.

Addressing key learning objectives In simulation, it is important to develop clear learning objectives for each simulation event [4, 25]. Addressing these learning objectives during the debriefing conversation is an important step in optimizing learning through simulation [19]. A discussion of the learning objectives is the primary purpose of the analysis phase of the debriefing conversation. Depending on the context of the simulation, these learning objectives can be revealed to the simulation participants prior to the simulation, or not. In simulations in which the team responds to an unexpected event, or diagnostic dilemma, withholding the objectives until the debriefing is best. While predefined learning objectives should ideally guide the debriefing discussion, participant's actions in a simulation can sometimes deviate far from the intended learning objectives. In such cases the facilitator needs to consider addressing the predefined learning objectives or addressing the learnings that emerged from the team's actions. In these situations it is usually better to address the emergent learnings objectives and not perseverate on the learning objectives that were initially planned.

Asking open-ended questions Open-ended questions foster reflection and self-assessment on the part of the simulation participants [4, 18]. Examples of open-ended questions include, "can you tell me what happened when the ECMO pump alarmed?" and "how was your teamwork during the cannulation?" A key skill of an effective facilitator is to avoiding close-ended, or "yes/no," questions, like "did you notice ECMO pump was alarming?" and "did you have good teamwork during the cannulation?". Open-ended questions encourage conversation, discussion, and learning; closed-ended questions do not.

Using silence After a facilitator asks an open-ended question, a period of silence follows. During this silence, the debriefing participants are reviewing their memories of the events, analyzing their mental frames, and formulating a response to the facilitator's inquiry. This period of silence is essential and required and may be as long as 20 s in some cases. Debriefing facilitators must be patient after posing open-ended questions and use silence as a tool, allowing it to take place as needed [4, 6]. A debriefing facilitator who is not patient – and jumps in with their own comments and observations to fill the silence – will stifle fruitful insight and discussion amongst the simulation participants.

Conversational Techniques/Educational Strategies

There are several conversational techniques and educational strategies that can be used during debriefing to skillfully facilitate the discussion [4]. These are classified by Eppich et al. into three broad categories: learner self-assessment, directive performance feedback, and focused facilitation [26].

Learner self-assessment Asking simulation participants to assess their own performance is called learner self-assessment [26]. A common method of facilitating learner self-assessment during debriefing is the "plus/delta method" [26–28]. Using the plus/delta method, the facilitator, or team member, asks open-ended questions regarding "what went well?" (*plus*) and "what could be changed or done differently next time?" (*delta*). After issues are identified through learner self-assessment, the facilitator can provide directive feedback and/or use focused facilitation to promote discussion on each topic [26]. Occasionally, the learner self-assessments do not agree with the facilitator's assessments. For example, a team member may state that they felt leadership went well during the simulation, but the facilitator may have noticed several opportunities for leadership improvement. In such situations, the technique of focused facilitation – using advocacy-inquiry (discussed below) – works well to investigate areas where the facilitator's observations do not match with the participant's experiences.

Directive feedback As noted in the introduction, *feedback* is a one-way conveyance of information to a learner on the gap between their performance and a standard, along with suggestions on how the gap might be bridged. When feedback is provided within a debriefing conversation it is directed at a specific area of performance, and is thus called "directive feedback." Directive feedback is most commonly used during the debriefing of junior participants with limited clinical experience, who might otherwise not be able to generate the insight needed to identify and bridge the knowledge gap [4, 26]. An example of directive feedback in a debriefing could be "in this simulation, I noticed you treated the patient with multiple saline boluses for hypovolemia. The problem, however, was a pneumothorax (*directive feedback*). Pneumothorax is sometimes hard to detect clinically in patients on ECMO. You should consider pneumothorax in the differential for a patient when the pump keeps cutting out after volume repletion (*filling gap between observed performance and expected performance*)." As seen in the example, the directive feedback is one-way, from the facilitator to the participant. These short, one-way, directive feedback events can be used during the longer, bi-directional, debriefing conversation as needed when knowledge gaps are identified.

Focused Facilitation Focused facilitation is a method to promote in-depth discussion with the goal of identifying and exploring the simulation participant's frame of mind, or mental frame [26]. The conversational technique known as "advocacy-inquiry" was first described in the business and organizational behavior literature [29], and is an effective way to gain insight into another person's frame of mind [18]. Using advocacy-inquiry, the debriefing facilitator first *advocates* their observation of an action or behavior and then *inquires* about the participant's frame of mind in relation to the action [18]. An example of an advocacy-inquiry exchange could be an instructor saying; "I saw that the team stopped the pump because there was air in the circuit. I wasn't sure, however, if the team leader knew the patient was off ECMO" (*facilitator advocates his/her observation).* "Let's talk about what you did to make the team aware that you were off ECMO" (*facilitator inquires about the underlying mental frames that led to the action*). Focused facilitation using advocacy-inquiry is an excellent way for the facilitator to spark conversation on a performance gap in a nonconfrontational way.

Debriefing Adjuncts

Educators can use debriefing adjuncts to maximize the impact of the debriefing experience. Three adjuncts that can be used during debriefing include co-debriefing, debriefing scripts, and video review [4].

Co-debriefing Using more than one person to facilitate a debriefing conversation is called co-debriefing. Co-debriefing for simulation-based education was evaluated extensively by Cheng et al. [30]. Advantages of co-debriefing include the potential to have two facilitators with complementary styles, the ability to provide a larger pool of expertise and viewpoints by having debriefing facilitators from various disciplines, and it allows for cross-monitoring and management of learner expectations and needs [30]. Possible challenges to co-debriefing include: a lack of knowledge of learning objectives by one of the debriefing facilitators; differing personal agendas amongst the facilitators; not using facilitator's expertise optimally during debriefing; one facilitator interrupting another facilitator's train of thought; one facilitator dominating the discussion; one facilitator speaking directly to only learners from one group of participants (e.g., only to physicians, or only to nurses); and open disagreement between facilitators [30]. Mitigation strategies for these challenges identified by Cheng et al. include facilitator pre-briefing; open negotiation; nonverbal communication; post-debriefing huddle; previewing; setting the stage for learners; pulse check; and a practice of listening, observing, and reflecting [30].

Debriefing scripts A debriefing script is a tool that a debriefing facilitator can use as a guide during the debriefing conversation. The use of a standardized debriefing script by novice debriefing facilitators has been associated with improvements in the acquisition of knowledge and team leader behavioral performance [31]. A debriefing script based on the G.A.S. framework has been used in the Pediatric Advanced Life Support Course offered by the American Heart Association [32]. The script does not need to be complex, and can simply provide a reference to the phases of the debriefing conversation (gather, analyze, summarize) and some example questions for the facilitator to use in each phase. Specific scripts can be developed for specific cases; that way the learning objectives of the case can be included as part of the script. This ensures that a discussion of each of the learning objectives takes place during the debriefing.

Video review Reviewing video during debriefing is common practice in many locations providing simulation-based healthcare education. The video provides objective evidence of what occurred during the simulation, thus avoiding memory bias. Despite its widespread use, however, several studies have failed to find educational benefits from the use of video-enhanced debriefing [33, 34]. A meta-analysis by Cheng et al. found that video-enhanced debriefing had similar learning outcomes to debriefing without video [35]. Important points to consider when using video during debriefing are to use video clips judiciously and focus on short segments that highlight learning objectives, or areas of excellent or suboptimal performance [4]. Excess time spent watching the video can limit the time available in the debriefing for meaningful conversation and exploration of learning objectives. Some simulation video software programs allow facilitators to bookmark specific times on a video to reduce time spent looking for the relevant segments.

Special Considerations for Debriefing ECMO Simulations

There are several special considerations for debriefing ECMO simulations. The timing of ECMO simulations debriefing can be either post-event or within-event (Fig. 15.1 and Table 15.2); debriefing ECMO simulations can follow different conversational structures (Table 15.1); and debriefing ECMO simulations can incorporate various conversational techniques, educational strategies, and debriefing adjuncts (Table 15.3). In this section, we explore some of these special considerations.

Most commonly, ECMO simulations debriefings are done post-event; however, within-event debriefing can also be used. The post-event debriefing method works well when debriefing simulations focusing on teamwork and communication. An example of this is a large interdisciplinary simulation in which the ECMO team responds to a pump emergency and must work together to stabilize the patient and reestablish ECMO flow. During the post-event debriefing, the facilitator guides the conversation to cover learning objectives geared toward improving teamwork and communication. The within-event debriefing method is better suited to simulations aimed at improving individual skills. An example

Table 15.3 Conversational techniques and educational strategies in ECMO debriefings

Conversational techniques/ educational strategies	ECMO simulations debriefing example
Learner self-assessment	As part of the "plus/delta" evaluation of team performance the debriefer asks the team: "What aspects of this case were managed well?" and "What aspects would you want to change?"
Focused facilitation	Using the technique of "advocacy-inquiry" the debriefing facilitator advocates his/her observation of performance, and then inquiries about the mental processes that underpinned the behavior: "I saw that the surgical team struggled with cannula placement. Can you tell me more about that?"
Directive feedback	Directive feedback is used by the debriefer, or a subject matter expert participating as a co-debriefer, to provide education on a specific knowledge gap: "I noticed in this case you gave platelets into the circuit. When giving platelets into the circuit we always give them post-oxygenator. This avoids thrombus formation in the oxygenator."

could be a simulation-based training session where each ECMO perfusionist is required to respond to an "air in circuit" alarm and quickly take the patient off ECMO, locate the air in the circuit, and safely complete the de-airing process. Using the within-event debriefing method, each perfusionist can participate in RCDP and can improve their skills toward mastery-level.

ECMO simulation post-event debriefings can follow several conversational structures. The two most commonly used structures are: the *Reaction, Analysis, Summary (RAS)* and the *Gather, Analyze, Summarize (GAS)*, discussed above. The primary difference between the two structures is the first phase. In the RAS structure, the debriefing starts with a consideration of the emotions and reactions of the simulation participants to the simulation experience. In the GAS structure, the debriefing starts with a review of the events of the simulation in order to establish a shared mental model amongst simulation participants. Neither structure is better than the other, and either can be used [4]. Some things to consider when deciding which structure to use include: the debriefing facilitator's preference, the context of the simulation experience (if it was emotionally charged, or not), and the experience level of the simulation participants. For emotionally charged simulation scenarios (like a patient death or a difficult conversation) and when working with inexperienced simulation participants, the RAS structure may be beneficial as it allows simulation participants some time to discuss the emotional impact of the experience prior to analyzing performance. For simulation sessions that are not emotionally charged and when working with experienced simulation participants, the GAS structure works well as it allows rapid movement of the conversation into the analysis phase where learning occurs.

Debriefing ECMO simulations can incorporate various conversational techniques, educational strategies, and debriefing adjuncts. Every debriefing should incorporate the seven essential elements of psychological safety, a debriefing stance or "basic assumption," debriefing rules, addressing learning objectives, establishing a shared mental model, asking open-ended questions, and effective use of silence. These seven essential elements provide the basic foundations for an effective debriefing no matter the experience level of the participants. Some examples of conversational techniques and educational strategies that can be used in ECMO debriefings are provided in Table 15.3. Debriefing adjuncts including co-debriefing, video review, and debriefing script may be useful in some ECMO debriefings. Because ECMO is an interprofessional undertaking, having debriefing facilitators from different backgrounds and disciplines – including intensivists, surgeons, perfusionists, and nurses – may be beneficial, as dictated by case and learner group. Video review provides objective evidence of team performance during debriefing. Debriefing scripts can be developed for ECMO simulations and may be beneficial for inexperienced debriefing facilitators.

Debriefing Training and Assessment

Debriefing is a skill, just like any other. Improving one's skill at debriefing takes training and practice. Training in debriefing can be obtained either at local simulation instructor courses, which are available at most academic medical centers or through national (fee-based) simulation instructor courses. Such courses offer an excellent opportunity to learn from experienced simulation educators and to practice debriefing in a constructive and supportive environment with feedback and coaching. Following participation in such a course, continued practice is essential. This can be obtained by participating in simulation-based training and taking an active role as a debriefing facilitator. If available, soliciting peer feedback on one's debriefing performance can be very helpful to improve debriefing quality [36].

Two tools are available to help evaluate debriefing skills, the Debriefing Assessment for Simulation in Healthcare (DASH), and the Objective Structured Assessment of Debriefing (OSAD). The tools can be used to provide either formative or summative assessment of debriefing skill. The DASH is a behaviorally anchored rating scale that evaluates performance and behaviors in six dimensions pertinent to debriefing including: establishing an engaging learning environment, maintaining an engaging learning environment, structuring the debriefing in an organized way, provoking engaging discussion, identifying and exploring performance gaps, and helping trainees achieve or sustain good performance [37]. Perceived performance in each area is rated on a 7-point scale from "extremely ineffective/detrimental" (1) to "extremely effective/outstanding" (7). The OSAD is a behaviorally anchored rating scale that evaluates performance in eight categories of debriefing identified from the literature and end-user opinion [38]. The categories include approach; establishes learning environment; engagement of the learners; reaction; descriptive reflection; analysis; diagnosis; and application. Each category is rated on a 5-point scale with descriptive anchors for scores of 1, 3, and 5. For example, Approach: 1 = "Confrontational, judgmental approach," 3 = "Attempts to establish rapport with the learner (s) but is either over-critical or too informal in their approach," and 5 = "Establishes and maintains rapport throughout; uses a non-threatening but honest approach, creating a psychologically safe environment." Both tools have shown good reliability and evidence of validity in specific contexts [37, 38].

Conclusion

The goal of this chapter was to provide a general overview of debriefing techniques and strategies that simulation educators can use when debriefing ECMO simulations. We began by examining debriefing timing and facilitation, including post-event debriefing and within-event debriefing. We then reviewed different debriefing conversational structures. Next, debriefing process elements including essential elements of debriefing, conversational techniques and educational strategies, and debriefing adjuncts were explored. We then provided an overview of special considerations for debriefing ECMO simulations. Finally, we concluded with a brief discussion of debriefing training and assessment. Understanding these debriefing techniques and using these strategies can improve the quality of ECMO simulation debriefings, and increase learning during ECMO simulations.

References

1. Issenberg SB, McGaghie WC, Petrusa ER, Lee Gordon D, Scalese RJ. Features and uses of high-fidelity medical simulations that lead to effective learning: a BEME systematic review. Med Teach. 2005;27(1):10–28.
2. Cheng A, Eppich W, Grant V, Sherbino J, Zendejas B, Cook DA. Debriefing for technology-enhanced simulation: a systematic review and meta-analysis. Med Educ. 2014;48:657–66.
3. Raemer D, Anderson M, Cheng A, Fanning R, Nadkarni V, Savoldelli G. Research regarding debriefing as part of the learning process. Simul Healthc. 2011;6(Suppl):52–7.
4. Sawyer T, Eppich W, Brett-Fleegler M, Grant V, Cheng A. More than one way to debrief: a critical review of healthcare simulation debriefing methods. Simul Healthc. 2016;11(3):209–17.
5. Voyer S, Hatala R. Debriefing and feedback: two sides of the same coin? Simul Healthc. 2015;10(2):67–8.
6. Fanning RM, Gaba DM. The role of debriefing in simulation-based learning. Simul Healthc. 2007;2(2):115–25.
7. Arafeh JM, Hansen SS, Nichols A. Debriefing in simulated-based learning: facilitating a reflective discussion. J Perinat Neonat Nurs. 2010;24:302–9.
8. Dismukes RK, Gaba DM, Howard SK. So many roads: facilitated debriefing in healthcare. Simul Healthc. 2006;1(1):23–5.
9. Boet S, Bould D, Bruppacher H, Desjardins F, Chandra D, Naik V. Looking in the mirror: self-debriefing versus instructor debriefing for simulated crises. Crit Care Med. 2011;39(6):1377–81.
10. Boet S, Bould D, Sharma B, Revees S, Naik V, Triby E, et al. Within-team debriefing versus instructor-led debriefing for simulation-based education: a randomized controlled trial. Ann Surg. 2013;258(1):53–8.
11. Jones I, Alinier G. Supporting students' learning experiences through a pocket-size cue card designed around a reflective simulation framework. Clin Simul Nurs. 2015;11(7):325–34.
12. Schön DA. The reflective practitioner: how professionals think in action. 1st ed. New York: Basic Books; 1984.
13. Kolb DA. Experiential learning: experience as the source of learning and development. Englewood Cliffs: Prentice Hall; 1984.
14. Kolb AY, Kolb DA. The learning way: meta-cognitive aspects of experiential learning. Simul Gaming. 2009;40(3):297–327.
15. Hunt EA, Duval-Arnould JM, Nelson-McMillan KL, Bradshaw JH, Diener-West M, Perretta JS, et al. Pediatric resident resuscitation skills improve after "rapid cycle deliberate practice" training. Resuscitation. 2014;85(7):945–51.
16. Eppich WJ, Hunt EA, Duval-Arnould JM, Siddall VJ, Cheng A. Structuring feedback and debriefing to achieve mastery learning goals. Acad Med. 2015;90(11):1501–8.
17. Taras J, Everett T. Rapid cycle deliberate practice in medical education - a systematic review. Cureus. 2017;9(4):e1180.
18. Rudolph J, Simon R, Dufresne R, Raemer D. There's no such thing as "nonjudgmental" debriefing: a theory and method for debriefing with good judgment. Simul Healthc. 2006;1(1):49–55.
19. Rudolph JW, Simon R, Raemer DB, Eppich WJ. Debriefing as formative assessment: closing performance gaps in medical education. Acad Emerg Med. 2008;15(11):1010–6.
20. Phrampus P, O'Donnell J. Debriefing using a structured and supported approach. In: Levine A, Demaria S, Schwartz A, Sim A, editors. The comprehensive textbook of healthcare simulation. 1st ed. New York: Springer; 2013. p. 73–85.
21. Sawyer T, Loren D, Halamek LP. Post-event debriefings during neonatal care: why are we not doing them, and how can we start? J Perinatol. 2016;36(6):415–9.
22. Ganley B, Linnard-Palmer L. Academic safety during nursing simulation: perceptions of nursing students and faculty. Clin Simul Nurs. 2012;8(2):e49–57.
23. Rudolph JW, Raemer DB, Simon R. Establishing a safe container for learning in simulation. Simul Healthc. 2014;9:339–49.
24. Der Sahakian G, Alinier G, Savoldelli G, Oriot D, Jaffrelot M, Lecomte F. Setting conditions for productive debriefing. Simul Gaming. 2015;46(2):197–208.
25. Lopreiato J, Sawyer T. Simulation-based medical education in pediatrics. Acad Pediatr. 2015;15(2):134–42.
26. Eppich W, Cheng A. Promoting excellence and reflective learning in simulation (pearls): development and rationale for a blended approach to healthcare simulation debriefing. Simul Healthc. 2015;10(2):106–15.
27. Sawyer T, Deering S. Adaptation of the U.S. Army's after-action review (AAR) to simulation debriefing in healthcare. Simul Healthc. 2013;8(6):388–97.
28. Ahmed M, Arora S, Russ S, Darzi A, Vincent C, Sevdalis N. Operation debrief: a SHARP improvement in performance feedback in the operating room. Ann Surg. 2013;258(6):958–63.
29. Senge P. The fifth discipline fieldbook. 1st ed: New York: Crown Business; 1994.
30. Cheng A, Palaganas J, Rudolph J, Eppich W, Robinson T, Grant V. Co-debriefing for simulation-based education – a primer for facilitators. Simul Healthc. 2015;10:69–75.
31. Cheng A, Hunt E, Donoghue A, Nelson-McMillan K, Nishisaki A, LeFlore J, et al. Examining pediatric resuscitation education using simulation and scripted debriefing: a multicenter randomized trial. JAMA Pediatr. 2013;167(6):528–36.
32. Cheng A, Rodgers D, Van Der Jagt E, Eppich W, O'Donnell J. Evolution of the pediatric advanced life support course: enhanced learning with a new debriefing tool and web-based module for pediatric advanced life support instructors. Ped Crit Care Med. 2012;13(5):589–95.
33. Savoldelli GL, Naik VN, Park J, Joo HS, Chow R, Hamstra SJ. Value of debriefing during simulated crisis management: oral versus video-assisted oral feedback. Anesthesiology. 2006;105(2):279–85.
34. Sawyer T, Sierocka-Casteneda A, Chan D, Berg B, Lustik M, Thompson M. The effectiveness of video-assisted debriefing versus oral debriefing alone at improving neonatal resuscitation performance: a randomized trial. Simul Healthc. 2012;7(4):213–21.

35. Cheng A, Eppich W, Grant V, Sherbino J, Zendejas B, Cook DA. Debriefing for technology-enhanced simulation: a systematic review and meta-analysis. Med Educ. 2014;48:657–66.
36. Cheng A, Grant V, Dieckmann P, Arora S, Robinson T, Eppich W. Faculty development for simulation programs: five issues for the future of debriefing training. Simul Healthc. 2015;10(4): 217–22.
37. Brett-Fleegler M, Rudolph J, Eppich W, et al. Debriefing assessment for simulation in healthcare: development and psychometric properties. Simul Healthc. 2012;7:288–94.
38. Runnacles J, Thomas L, Sevdalis N, Kneebone R, Arora S. Development of a tool to improve performance debriefing and learning: the paediatric Objective Structured Assessment of Debriefing (OSAD) tool. Postgrad Med J. 2014;90:613–21.

Controversies on Certification of ECMO Practitioners Using Simulation

16

Evan F. Gajkowski and Bishoy Zakhary

Abbreviations

ABMS	American Board of Medical Specialists
ACLS	Advanced cardiac life support)
CESAR	Conventional ventilatory support versus Extracorporeal membrane oxygenation for Severe Adult Respiratory failure
ECLS	Extracorporeal Life Support
ECMO	Extracorporeal Membrane Oxygenation
ELSO	Extracorporeal Life Support Organization
MOC	Maintenance of Certification
NRP	Neonatal Resuscitation Program
OSCE	Objective structured clinical examination
PALS	Pediatric advanced life support

Learning Objectives

1. Explain the need for standardized ECMO practitioner certification
2. Describe the role of simulation in medical education and certification
3. List three limitations of simulation-based ECMO certification

The Need for Standardized ECMO Practitioner Certification

The ECMO Practitioner

ECMO provision requires specialized healthcare professionals to care for patients from ECMO cannulation and initiation through ECMO weaning and decannulation. Utilized primarily in neonates during the 1980s and 1990s, bedside monitoring of the complex ECMO circuit was managed by perfusionists or biomedical engineers [1]. However, in the last decade, extracorporeal support devices have been simplified to allow for a variety of healthcare professionals, including nurses, respiratory therapists, perfusionists, and physicians to care for the ECMO circuit and patient. This has led hospitals and ECMO programs to develop and implement in-house training programs for ECMO practitioners. Without a standardized ECMO practitioner certification requirement, however, these programs have developed their own local standards for training leading to significant variability across programs [2].

Growth of ECMO Utilization

The Extracorporeal Life Support Organization (ELSO), established in 1989, maintains an international database of ECMO utilization and outcomes [3]. Among adult patients, ECMO utilization has grown with a 433% increase in ECMO utilization since 2009 [2]. Contributing to this growth is the 2009 influenza pandemic with respiratory failure refractory to mechanical ventilation as well as the publication of the CESAR trial, which demonstrated a benefit in disability-free survival for adult patients with the acute respiratory distress syndrome referred to an ECMO center versus conventional management. The number of ECMO programs and ECMO runs has continued to grow since [1].

E. F. Gajkowski
Department of Cardiology, Geisinger Medical Center, Danville, PA, USA
e-mail: efgajkowski@geisinger.edu

B. Zakhary (✉)
Division of Pulmonary and Critical Care Medicine, Oregon Health & Science University, Portland, OR, USA
e-mail: bzakhary@elso.org

L. C. Johnston, L. Su (eds.), *Comprehensive Healthcare Simulation: ECMO Simulation*, Comprehensive Healthcare Simulation,
https://doi.org/10.1007/978-3-030-53844-6_16

Risks Associated with ECMO

ECMO is a simplified form of cardiopulmonary support adapted for long-term use at the bedside. Despite significant advancements in the extracorporeal circuit, the management of the ECMO patient remains complex and risky. Each component of the ECMO circuit has a risk of failure and mechanical complication. Artificial pumps, for instance, risk air embolism and tubing rupture necessitating constant monitoring of blood flow and circuit pressures. While oxygenator membranes have improved efficiency compared to earlier models, the risk of oxygenator failure or membrane rupture remains [4]. In an effort to improve biocompatibility, tubing packs are now heparin-bonded and bio-coated. Nevertheless, clot formation remains a major concern requiring systemic anticoagulation, which carries its own risks [4]. A recent review of ECMO for respiratory failure reported rates of bleeding approaching 20% [5]. Vigilance in circuit setup and maintenance, meticulous cannulation technique, and adherence to management protocols are necessary to minimize adverse events [5].

High-Risk, Low-Frequency Events

As patients on ECMO are typically dependent on the circuit for full or partial life-support, complications can be catastrophic. At the same time, the occurrence rate for ECMO is less than ten cases per million population per year [1]. As such, ECMO complications are considered high-risk, low-frequency events, highlighting the need for proper education. Simulation has been promoted as the ideal modality for teaching management of high-risk, low-frequency events by offering repeated exposure in a safe and controlled setting. Recent evidence supports this with simulation-based education improving critical care fellow performance managing ECMO emergencies [6].

Variability in ECMO Center Training and Center Volume

ELSO has developed training courses to educate healthcare professionals on how to care for ECMO patients. To date, however, there is no standard process for ECMO practitioner certification. Despite being a complicated and risky technology, only about half of US ECMO centers have established local credentialing requirements [2]. Additionally, variability in center volume exists with studies demonstrating that higher volume ECMO centers have lower mortality [1]. This suggests that, in addition to appropriate education, ongoing ECMO patient exposure is an important determinant in outcome and should be an element of maintenance of ECMO practitioner credentialing.

Standardization

ECMO provision remains a highly technical but potentially life-saving technology. As the number of ECMO centers increase and the volume and indications of ECMO utilization expand, standardization of ECMO training and practitioner certification will be needed. Elements of standardization should delineate ECMO curricular requirements, didactic and simulation-based need and hours, mechanism for assessment of competency, minimum ECMO patient-hours exposure, and recertification requirements. Standardization of ECMO certification may increase training rates and reduce variability in certification practices across the United States [2].

The Role of Simulation in Certification

Miller's Model of Medical Competence

In competency-based educational methods, establishing a mechanism to evaluate the degree of competency attained is essential. This requires a simple, clear, and accurate description for each competency level [7]. Miller's model of medical competency outlines the relationship between knowledge and skill set (see Table 16.1) by classifying competence as "knows, knows how, shows how, or does" in a pyramid scheme. "Knows" and "Knows how" is classified by Miller as "I have the knowledge and know how to do it"; "Shows how" refers to one's performance during a simulation or objective structured clinical examination; "Does" correlates with one's clinical practice in the workplace.

One of the most broadly used and researched methods for assessing physician competency is the multisource assessment methodology. This assessment tool [7] is among those recommended by the ACGME/ABMS outcome project and

Table 16.1 Millers Model of Medical Competence [7] can assist educators in matching clinical competencies with expectations of what the learner should be able to do at various educational stages

Knows little	I know almost nothing
Knows and knows how	I have knowledge and know how to do it
Exercised does	I can do it, relying on rules
Selected does	I can do it, while recognizing situations and selecting and planning
Experienced does	I can do it based on similar experiences
Intuitive does	I can do it by intuition based on sufficient experience

relates to Miller's model concerning the "does" level. Using Miller's pyramid linking learning and performance, a multi-source feedback assessment can provide information on how to improve training opportunities. Those at the lower levels of Miller's Pyramid require knowledge; as such, didactic sessions rather than practical sessions are most helpful. Those at the higher levels of the pyramid need an opportunity to practice practical skills; as such, simulation and role-playing would be more beneficial. Those individuals who are at the "Show" level benefit from exploring the barriers to implementation.

Simulation in Medical OSCE

The objective structured clinical examination (OSCE) is an assessment tool used in various types of healthcare professions (medicine, physical and occupational therapy, physician assistant, nursing, and paramedicine). The OSCE uses a simulated environment to test a clinician's performance and hands-on skill with procedures, communication, manipulation techniques, troubleshooting, and interpretation of tests [8]. The OSCE style of clinical assessment allows for uniformity while offering versatility in clinical application by allowing for the evaluation of students at varying levels of training within a short period of time and over a broad range of skills. Specifically, the OSCE can assess problem-solving, communication skills, decision-making, and patient management abilities [14]. The primary limitations are the costs associated with its application, as well as the time for faculty to develop and implement these sessions.

Maintenance of Certification

Maintenance of Certification (MOC) is an active process of assessment and continuous professional development that allows participants to demonstrate ongoing competency with advances in the field of medicine throughout their careers. The MOC concept originated with the American Board of Medical Specialists (ABMS) in 1999 [9]. The **MOCA ®** (MOC in Anesthesiology, **MOCA ®**), in particular, has incorporated simulation-based assessment to ensure their specialists are up-to-date with quality outcomes and patient safety. The inclusion of simulation has allowed for an active hands-on approach and for structured clinical examination with real-time feedback on performance. Challenges regarding incorporation of simulation include an increased use of resources such as time spent preparing for simulation and recruitment of experts for administration.

Simulation in the Neonatal Resuscitation Program (NRP), Pediatric Advanced Life Support (PALS), and Advanced Cardiac Life Support (ACLS)

Cardiopulmonary resuscitation (CPR) has advanced life support certifications for registered nurses, certified nurse practitioners, physician assistants, and doctors. These advanced life support courses are divided into three categories: neonatal resuscitation (NRP) for professionals practicing in the neonatal population; pediatric advanced life support (PALS) for professionals caring for patients 1-day old to 18-years old; and advanced cardiovascular life support (ACLS) for professionals caring for patients greater than 18 years of age. Of note, simulation makes up approximately 50% of these educational courses and is also an integral part of the certification assessment. Instructors for these courses are certified through hospital or national organizations with a requirement to complete an instructor course, pass a discipline-specific test, and subsequent monitoring by a training center coordinator or mentor [11]. Training for the individuals who would like to obtain certification typically need to complete a 4–6 h course administered once every 2 years to maintain clinical competency. Instructors utilize hands-on simulation in addition to online educational videos and computerized simulations to teach and assess proper resuscitation efforts.

Controversies in Simulation-Based Certification of ECMO Practitioners

ECMO Certification

As discussed above, simulation has been used to train and credential medical professionals in all realms of medicine. In like manner, simulation-based training has recently been applied to ECMO practitioners [1], but several challenges limit its application in ECMO certification.

Defining Minimal Competency

Despite being used clinically for many years, minimal criteria for ECMO competency remain to be defined. In particular, there is no agreed-upon ECMO didactic or hands-on curriculum that outlines the knowledge and practical requirements an ECMO practitioner should master. One challenge is determining whether the criteria should be applicable across specialties and disciplines or whether different specialties require individual competency assessments. Another challenge relates to defining standards that are consistent across geographies accounting for different ECMO pumps and circuits as well as regional practice variations. Furthermore, once minimal competency is defined, validity assessment of the knowledge and hands-on assessment tools will be required before widespread implementation. While standardization of practice will allow for defining minimal competency, there are limitations to be noted. First, there may be a burden placed on both educators and learners who will be required to accept this new standard with potential remediation for certification. In addition, depending on the rollout and on the degree of uptake of the certification process, patients may not necessarily have access to certified providers. Whether this will affect local practice or credentialing, remains to be seen.

Differentiating Performance in Clinical Practice Versus in Simulation

In simulation-based medical education, the concept of deliberate practice refers to performing a task several times over with the goal of improving skill acquisition and procedural confidence through repetition with real-time formative feedback. A simulation-based mastery learning program increased residents' skills in simulated central venous catheter insertion and decreased complications during clinical care [12]. It is not clear, however, that competence in the simulated environment without this rigorous structure necessarily transfers to the bedside. Moreover, it has been described that learners behave differently in the simulated environment, where they are aware of being observed, versus the clinical setting. As such, it is argued that "the notion that theoretical training and simulation alone would be sufficient to produce competency in managing ECLS patients without adequate clinical exposure may have counterintuitive effects by creating pseudo-experts unaware of the potential risks and complications of ECLS as well as their limitations, resulting in deleterious consequences for patient outcomes" [10]. Whether simulation-based ECMO certification will correlate with clinical performance or outcomes remains to be determined, and further study in this area is needed. Of additional note, while simulation will appropriately assess hands-on objectives, additional assessment methodologies may be needed for a complete certification exam.

Lack of Evidence of the Efficacy of Simulation Training in Improving Patient Outcomes

Simulation-based education has been promoted as ideally suited for ECMO management training. Evidence supporting the beneficial role of simulation training on clinical outcome, however, is sparse, leading experts to comment that "relying solely on competency assessed in a simulation context cannot adequately replace real-life expertise" [10]. ECMO circuit emergencies, however, are low-frequency events that can be associated with significant patient morbidity and mortality. As such, while the clinical exposure is paramount, it seems prudent to incorporate simulation-based training as a critical adjunct. Standardizing the training experience amongst participants regardless of existing clinical experience will be an important challenge. Additionally, ensuring high-quality structured simulation debriefings with qualified instructors is paramount to ensuring a positive and effective educational experience.

Buy-in from ECMO Centers

As the primary consortium of healthcare institutions dedicated to improving the ECMO provision and research, ELSO has defined the standard for ECMO education through offering educational programs for ECMO centers worldwide. The development of a certification process will likely require a certain amount of ECMO training in line with the ELSO training guidelines. As such, ECMO centers will need to send ECMO team members to external ECMO training courses or to invest in the equipment and resources to run their own institutional simulation-based ECMO courses. Whether a hospital pursues external or internal training, a substantial cost will be necessary to achieve the educational and certification requirements. ECMO certification, therefore, must offer a significant perceived or proven value to ECMO centers to justify the time, effort, and resources associated with its widespread adoption. Potential benefits of standardization of policies and procedures include increasing patient safety by standardizing best practice as well as limiting legal issues associated with providing ECMO care.

Assessment of Multidisciplinary Team

ECMO is a team sport with a typical ECMO team composed of an intensivist, surgeon, bedside nurse, and ECMO practitioner whose background can be nursing, respiratory therapy, or perfusion. Management of the ECMO patient requires optimally coordinated teamwork with effective communication, planning, and decision-making. This is particularly true for troubleshooting circuit emergencies where practitioners have to be familiar with managing the patient, the ventilator, and a complex ECMO circuit simultaneously. Simulation-based assessment typically focuses on individual performance separate from team members. As such, practitioners participating in an individual simulation-based assessment may be required to troubleshoot ECMO emergencies without the assistance typically found in the clinical setting.

Unfortunately, complex team dynamics inherent in managing the ECMO patient is thus not well captured in this setting [2], though educators may consider introducing standardized participants into scenarios to allow for assessment of communication, leadership, and teamwork skills. Whether a simulation-based assessment of the team approach to ECMO management will be effective is unclear but can be considered.

Instructors/Assessor Training

An ECMO certification process will require a sufficient infrastructure to allow for comprehensive assessment. Paramount to this is the need for sufficiently trained ECMO instructors and assessors who have adequate knowledge and understanding of extracorporeal support as well as best educational/simulation practices. Moreover, formal simulation instructor training is necessary to run effective simulation scenarios and conduct effective debriefing sessions. The benefits of training a core group of instructors who assess practitioners in a central location(s) versus training a large number of instructors in varying locations will need to be determined. Rater training and calibration will be an important challenge that will likely depend on train-the-trainer courses.

Recertification Criteria

It is well documented that deterioration of skills can occur shortly after training with variability in rates of knowledge and skill decay [13]. As such, most existing medical certification programs are typically valid for a time-limited period and require recertification to ensure practitioners maintain competency over the long term. For ECMO certification, challenges regarding recertification include degree and mode of testing as well as defining duration for recertification to occur. Individual ECMO centers typically require annual competency assessments of ECMO practitioners via verbal testing, simulation, online questions, and minimal patient care hours. Whether these elements should factor into recertification remains to be defined.

Conclusion

ECMO practitioners are providers who have expertise in the management of the ECMO patient and circuit. As ECMO technology continues to improve and indications expand, it is likely that utilization will continue to increase. Simulation-based certification is a natural expectation though several challenges to its implementation exist. Nevertheless, overcoming such limitations to defining minimal competency and implementing ECMO certification is imperative to ensure best clinical practice is provided on a global level.

References

1. ACLS. ACLS Certification Institute. 2018. From: https://acls.com/.
2. American Heart Association. 2018. Retrieved from https://ahainstructornetwork.americanheart.org/AHAECC/CPRAndECC/Training/AHAInstructors/UCM_476669_AHA-Instructors.jsp.
3. Harden, et al. Assessment of clinical competence using objective structured examination. Br Med J. 1975;1(5955):447–51. http://www.bmj.com/cgi/content/abstract/1/5955/447.
4. Barsuk JH, McGaghie WC, Cohen ER, et al. Simulation-based mastery learning reduces complications during central venous catheter insertion in a medical intensive care unit. Crit Care Med. 2009;37:2697–701.
5. Brodie D, Bacchatta M. Extracorporeal membrane oxygenation for ARDS in adults. N Engl J Med. 2011;365:1905–14. https://doi.org/10.1056/NEJMct1103720.
6. Brum R, Rajani R, Gelandt E, Morgan L, Raguseelan N, Butt S, et al. Simulation training for extracorporeal membrane oxygenation. Ann Cardiac Anesth. 2015;18(2):185–90.
7. Combes A, Brodie D, Bartlett R, Brochard L, Brower R, Conrad S, et al. Position paper for the organization of extracorporeal membrane oxygenation programs for acute respiratory failure in adult patients. Am J Respir Crit Care Med. 2014;190(5):488–96.
8. David Brown MD. Guide to maintenance of certification in anesthesiology (MOCA); The American Board of Anesthesiology, Inc; 2011.
9. Guillaume A, Ibrahim F, Hassan AA, Mohammed AD, Ali Ait H, Ahmed L, Yahya A, Fayçal B, Abbes A, Abdulsalam Saif I. Addressing the challenges of ECMO simulation. Perfusion. https://doi.org/10.1177/0267659118777194.
10. Lequier L, Horton SB, McMullan DM, Bartlett RH. Extracorporeal membrane oxygenation circuitry. Pediatr Crit Care Med A Journal of the Society of Critical Care Medicine and the World Federation of Pediatric Intensive and Critical Care Societies. 2013;14(5 0 1):S7–12. https://doi.org/10.1097/PCC.0b013e318292dd10.
11. Muratore S, Beilman G, John R, Brunsvold M. Extracorporeal membrane oxygenation credentialing: where do we stand? Am J Surg. 2015;210(4):655–60. e2.
12. Stentz M, Kelly M, Jabaley C, O'eilly-Shah V, Groff R, Moll V, Blum J. Trends in extracorporeal membrane oxygenation growth in the United States, 2011–2014: American Society of Artificial Internal Organs; 2018. https://doi.org/10.1097/MAT.0000000000000872.
13. Weems MF, Friedlich PS, Nelson LP, Rake AJ, Klee L, Stein JE, et al. The role of extracorporeal membrane oxygenation simulation training at extracorporeal life support organization centers in the United States. Simul Healthc. 2017;12(4):233–9.
14. Zakhary B, Kam L, Kaufman B, Felner K. The utility of high-fidelity simulation for training critical care fellows in the management of ECMO emergencies. Crit Care Med. 2017;45(8):1367–73.

Research in ECMO Simulation: A Review of the Literature

17

Kristen M. Glass

Learning Objectives

By the end of this chapter readers will be able to:

1. Describe the current state of ECMO simulation science in the literature
2. Identify themes in ECMO simulation research
3. Recognize the importance of research in ECMO simulation

Introduction

As a high-stakes, low-frequency therapy, extracorporeal membrane oxygenation (ECMO) lends itself well to simulation for multiple purposes including: initial training, maintenance of competency, and ensuring quality and safety of care. While ECMO simulation in the form of water drills and animal labs has been practiced for decades, manikin-based ECMO simulation has emerged only recently. Early studies in ECMO simulation focused on the development of equipment and models for ECMO simulation as well as the feasibility and effectiveness of new ECMO simulation programs. Effectiveness was most often measured by learner confidence level and knowledge acquisition [1–3, 5, 6, 9]. Knowledge, behavior, and attitude are crucial in the ability of a provider to perform or deliver complex care. Research in ECMO simulation is expanding to include assessment of training methods for sources of validity and assessment of the impact of ECMO simulation on patient outcomes. Additional areas of study include quality improvement and systems-based research. The following sections will explore the available literature in those areas, as well as comment on the strength of the evidence and describe unanswered questions.

ECMO Simulation for Training Providers

Guidelines for initial training of ECMO specialists recommends hands-on practice with a water-filled circuit to reinforce technical skills and to learn to troubleshoot complications [13]. This training is typically referred to as "water drills"on a closed-loop circuit, or in an animal laboratory using a blood-filled circuit hooked up to a cannulated, anesthetized animal. More recently, ECMO centers have shifted away from the use of animal labs for training and instead, have adopted the use of manikin-based ECMO simulations [14]. While commercially available ECMO-ready manikins are not yet widely available [15], multiple ECMO-compatible modified manikins have been described in the literature [2, 5–8, 16]. Simulation based ECMO programs have existed since 2006 and have been rated highly by participants; however, research on the educational effectiveness of these programs is only beginning to emerge [3, 5, 16].

Initial training for ECMO specialists also includes a significant didactic component covering topics from the history of ECMO to physiology and pathophysiology, as well as daily management of ECMO patients [13]. Newer teaching methodologies such as the "flipped classroom," and computer-based simulations or serious games are gaining acceptance and have shown improved learner satisfaction, knowledge retention, and even improved patient outcomes [17–19]. However, these techniques have not yet been uniformly applied or rigorously studied in ECMO education. Computer-based programs have been developed for ECMO training and may be useful adjuncts to classroom teaching and ECMO simulation but still require validity assessment before their use is adopted universally [20].

K. M. Glass (✉)
Department of Pediatrics, Penn State Health Milton S. Hershey Medical Center/Penn State College of Medicine, Hershey, PA, USA
e-mail: kglass1@pennstatehealth.psu.edu

L. C. Johnston, L. Su (eds.), *Comprehensive Healthcare Simulation: ECMO Simulation*, Comprehensive Healthcare Simulation,
https://doi.org/10.1007/978-3-030-53844-6_17

While a comprehensive guideline is provided by ELSO for training of ECMO providers and simulation programs have increased in prevalence, ELSO does not currently require the use of simulation for ECMO training. One study by Weems et al. found that of ELSO centers, 72% reported the current or planned use of manikin-based ECMO training [14]. Most of these training programs have been in existence for fewer than 5 years and many are still in development. However, the characteristics of these programs are not standardized. Some programs report using simulation for individual training while other programs use simulation in team training. Other characteristics that may differ among programs include simulation models, scenarios, and use of simulation for assessment of trainees.

Common themes exist in scenarios used in ECMO training, including circuit emergencies (such as component failure and circuit rupture) as well as patient emergencies (such as bleeding complications and anticoagulation management). Patient management scenarios were found to be used less commonly than circuit emergency scenarios in the survey study of ELSO centers by Weems et al. This is likely due to multiple factors, not the least of which is complexity and need for a well-designed scenario targeting specific learning objectives. These scenarios are developed individually by programs so may differ in content and lack robust assessment for sources of validity evidence. While there is a multi-center collaborative effort underway to develop a bank of peer-reviewed scenarios for neonatal and pediatric ECMO simulation, the process of development and validity assessment of these scenarios will likely take several years [21].

The conduct of ECMO simulation may also differ between programs. While the use of simulation in ECMO training likely has benefits based on the hands-on nature of the teaching modality, debriefing is a key step of the process allowing learners to reflect on their experience and build a conceptual framework for newly acquired knowledge leading to better understanding [22]. Of the ELSO centers surveyed in the study by Weems et al., most reported the use of debriefing following scenarios but less than half of those programs utilized video debriefing [14]. Differences in the conduct or implementation of simulation may affect knowledge acquisition and retention. Scenarios must be developed with a great degree of specificity and should be peer reviewed and pilot tested to ensure efficacy. Standardization is also lacking in training and expectations of simulation instructors teaching these courses.

Evidence for the feasibility of implementation of simulation into training programs exists in the Neonatal Resuscitation Program (NRP) and Pediatric Advanced Life Support (PALS) [23, 24]. The cognitive, technical, and behavioral skills required for mastery by ECMO providers are similar; however, the current training environment lacks standardization. The current literature on the use of simulation in the training of ECMO providers has exposed a need for further research in numerous areas including: standardization and validity assessment of simulation practices, scenarios, and models used for ECMO simulation. The process of peer review will be necessary for curricular development and validity assessment of scenarios will be key in the creation of a standardized training platform. Future studies should focus on answering questions such as the effectiveness of high- versus low-technology manikins for ECMO simulation, and the use of interprofessional versus single disciplinary training and investigating which educational modality (didactic vs. self-study vs. sim, etc.) is most effective for each skill.

Development of ECMO Simulation Equipment

An active area of investigation in ECMO simulation is the development of realistic, high-technology simulators. Early simulators for neonatal ECMO simulation were low-technology manikins adapted with ECMO circuit tubing with or without a fluid reservoir placed in the body cavity or under the manikin [2]. The manikin was then attached to an ECMO circuit. Simulated participants or simulation instructors would intervene during the simulation to "cause" an emergency such as circuit rupture, or pinch tubing to induce changes in circuit pressures. Over time, more sophisticated models have been developed for both neonatal and adult ECMO with enhanced realism [6–8, 15]. More information on available simulators can be found in Chap. 7. These models are often developed in coordination with simulation centers and may be cost-prohibitive to smaller ECMO programs. The development of simulation equipment that is both affordable and promotes realism in ECMO simulation is continuing to emerge [25, 26]. It will be necessary to test this equipment on a large scale and compare simulators in the clinical and research settings to determine which is the most appropriate for the learning environment. While ECMO is a complex therapy, it may not prove necessary to have learners work with the most technologically advanced equipment to become effectively trained.

Evidence for Improvement in Knowledge and Skills

The use of ECMO simulation in educational curricula is multipurpose. Programs have been developed and described in the literature targeting technical and behavioral skills. Technical skills are extremely important to all ECMO providers but perhaps most important to ECMO specialists or perfusionists who are primarily responsible for managing the circuit. These individuals must have a firm understanding of the physiology and the technology that drives the therapy and, most importantly, they must be able to recognize and respond quickly to an emergency. The conduct of ECMO requires a team of individuals, so behavioral skills are equally important in handling emergencies. The required skills are diverse and include situational awareness, workload distribution, communication, role assignment, leadership, and professionalism.

The first ECMO simulation program described in the literature was developed by Anderson et al. in 2006 [2, 3]. This program was developed to give ECMO nurse specialists hands-on practice with technical and behavioral skills needed to handle ECMO emergencies. Participants were evaluated on technical skills such as: identifying an emergency and calling for help, isolating the patient from the circuit when an emergency was recognized, discontinuing the oxygen source from the circuit, and increasing ventilator support once off ECMO. Data collected on these variables was both discrete (yes/no) and continuous (time-based). Learners participated in two randomly chosen scenarios with facilitated video debriefing following each scenario. Timed technical skills did improve between the first and second scenarios; however, this difference was not statistically significant, possibly due to their small sample size (nine subjects.) Study participants were evaluated on behavioral skills, and performance was noted to improve significantly using a scoring tool that had previously been evaluated for validity evidence. This study marked the first of a series of studies looking at high-technology ECMO simulation as a tool to teach technical and behavioral skills to ECMO providers, and demonstrated positive effects on the skills of experienced providers. It is unknown whether those skills persist long term or if they translate into the clinical environment.

Since the 2006 study by Anderson et al., several studies have emerged lending support for ECMO simulation improving knowledge and skills in ECMO specialists [3]. A similar study evaluated the use of ECMO simulation training on technical skills, teamwork and safety attitudes in experienced ECMO specialists [4]. Quarterly simulation sessions were instituted wherein subjects participated in scenarios simulating cannulation and ECMO emergencies. Technical skill outcomes evaluated as part of this study were similar to prior work including time intervals for completion of certain tasks such as time to cannulation as well as adherence to institutional protocols and a cannulation checklist. While no statistically significant improvement was seen in time intervals or adherence to the protocol in the simulation setting, improvement was noted in provider attitudes toward safety and knowledge of safety protocols. Unlike prior studies, this research assessed technical and behavioral outcomes in the patient care setting as well. There was a statistically significant improvement in adherence to the cannulation checklist in the clinical setting, adding to the literature on clinical outcomes of ECMO simulation. Another strength of this study was the use of a validated scale to assess team performance, the Mayo High Performance Teamwork Scale (MHPTS) [27]. Qualitative data from similar studies shows that ECMO simulation training is well-received by learners, improving confidence and increasing awareness the importance of teamwork and communication [28].

There is evidence of improvement in knowledge and skill in other provider groups exposed to ECMO simulation training. A study by Fouilloux et al. described the impact of a 2-day ECMO training course using simulation for ICU nurses [10]. This program included didactic sessions as well as one full day of simulated scenarios. The effectiveness of the training program was then assessed using pre- and post-course written tests; however, the effect of the simulation component itself was not examined independently in this observational study. Burkhart et al. in 2013 investigated the effect of a post-cardiotomy ECMO crisis training course in thoracic surgery residents [9]. Unique to this study was the inclusion of a diverse population, consisting of 23 residents from different training programs. A pre-post course study design was used to assess confidence and knowledge in the components of the ECMO circuit and management of several crisis scenarios. The training successfully improved self-reported confidence, identification of circuit components, and crisis management.

Most of the training programs described previously target learners, primarily ECMO specialists, with at least some ECMO experience. This experience may bias results evaluating the effectiveness of the simulation program in teaching knowledge or skill. An interprofessional training course was developed by Chan et al. for novice learners, including fellows, nurses, respiratory therapists, and nurse practitioners [5]. The study demonstrated improved perceptions of knowledge, skills, and confidence. In addition, unlike similar assessments of ECMO simulation training programs performed previously, this study demonstrated retention of knowledge and skills in responding to ECMO emergencies upon 6–8 months' follow-up assessment. Skill degradation following training in resuscitation skills has been reported in other studies [29]. Future studies with longitudinal follow-up will be necessary to more formally evaluate the optimal interval for effectiveness of training programs.

Interprofessional training of ECMO providers is becoming more popular. ECMO requires a carefully orchestrated team effort, including effective communication and interactions between nursing staff, ECMO specialists and the physicians caring for the patient. It follows then that simulations for team training and practicing or refining responses to emergencies should involve all participants from the clinical environment. The training course developed by Chan et al. was interprofessional in nature but team behaviors and outcomes were not specifically assessed. Allan et al. developed an in situ interprofessional simulation training program for Crisis Resource Management (CRM) for the pediatric cardiac intensive care team caring for ECMO patients [1]. Participants were exposed to principles of CRM and had the opportunity for hands-on practice using high-technology simulation. The program was highly rated by participants and there was significant improvement in self-reported confidence and perceived ability to function as a team member in a code. This is one of the first studies to demonstrate the feasibility of an interprofessional in situ ECMO simulation program.

The literature contains several examples of incorporating interprofessional ECMO simulation training for specialized procedures involving ECMO, as well as the development of new ECMO programs. One such example describes the development of an interprofessional simulation for an ex utero intrapartum treatment (EXIT) to ECMO for an infant with complex congenital heart disease [30]. Simulating this complex procedure prior to the actual case allowed the team to prepare for and uncover potential problems. Another innovative program utilized in situ ECMO simulation to set up a regional ECMO program in Poland. Scenarios included both patient care simulations lasting 48 h and intra- and interhospital transport simulations [31]. These types of simulation programs are important for improving patient safety by identifying latent safety threats and improving team functioning; however, the level of evidence is relatively low given the small number of participants and the single-center nature of these investigations.

All of these studies lend support to the feasibility and effectiveness of ECMO simulation in imparting knowledge and skills on ECMO providers. However, significant variability in equipment utilized, scenario design, and skill and experience of instructors across centers have contributed to challenges with universal implementation of this instructional method. In addition, several features of existing research limit generalizability, including the fact that these studies are often conducted at a single center, have small sample sizes, lack control groups, and are not randomized. (Table 17.1). The assessment tools utilized in these studies have often not undergone formal evaluation for sources of validity evidence. More recent authors have utilized observational assessment tools that have been evaluated for validity and reliability evidence [4] and are using these tools in assessing the performance of ECMO providers [32].

Table 17.1 Level of evidence by study type

Type of Evidence	Level
Systematic review with homogeneity of RCTs	1a
Individual RCT	1b
All or none related outcome	1c
Systematic review with homogeneity of cohort studies	2a
Individual cohort study (or low-quality RCT)	2b
Outcomes research	2c
Systematic review with homogeneity of case-control studies	3a
Individual case-control study	3b
Case series (or poor-quality cohort and case-control studies)	4
Expert opinion without critical appraisal	5

Adapted from Oxford Centre for Evidence-Based Medicine. https://www.cebm.net/index.aspx?o=5653 [34]
RCT randomized control trial

Evidence of Improved Clinical Outcomes

Until very recently, much of the current research in ECMO simulation has focused on the impact of various ECMO simulation programs on learners, specifically with regard to their confidence and acquisition of clinical and teamwork skills. These investigations are primarily single-center studies evaluating a single discipline or clinical skill. While the importance of these investigations cannot be underscored, the ultimate question is whether this training translates to improved patient care and patient outcomes. ECMO simulation research is getting closer to answering those questions.

In a study by Allan et al. in 2013, an embedded surgical neck cannulation trainer and a curriculum were created to develop surgeons' skills at ECMO cannulation during cardiopulmonary resuscitation [7]. As part of the curriculum, surgical trainees participated in two cannulations using the task trainer with video-assisted feedback. The study showed improvement in time to cannulation between the first and second attempt from over 15 min to 12 min. A third cannulation performed on the simulator 3 months later revealed sustained improvement in the time to cannulation. This study is notable not only for the sustained improvement shown after the training but also for the sustained improvement shown in performance using a global rating scale that had been previously evaluated for validity evidence. Participants rated this training highly for realism and stated that participation in the training better prepared them to perform cannulation in a clinical setting. Unfortunately, clinical outcomes were not assessed in this study.

An improvement in a clinical outcome was demonstrated in one study investigating the development of a strategy for rapid deployment of extracorporeal cardiopulmonary resuscitation (ECPR) on time to initiation of ECMO flow [12]. ECPR is extracorporeal support that is used on patients with refractory cardiopulmonary collapse receiving CPR. In this scenario, shorter time to initiation of ECMO support is associated with improved patient outcomes [33]. Su et al. used systems-based analysis and process mapping of ECPR in their unit to create an "ideal rapid deployment" process complete with assigned roles and tasks [12]. Eight interprofessional simulations with structured debriefing and video review were used to further refine tasks and create a checklist. Time to deployment, defined as the time the call to the ECMO team was placed to the page operator until the start of

Table 17.2 Summary of ECMO simulation research studies

Author	Subjects (N)	Intervention	Outcome	Results[a]	Study design
Allan et al. [7]	CT surgery residents/ fellows (10)	ECMO cannulation skills training program with follow-up assessment 3 months after training	Time to cannulation; global rating scale (GRS) score; composite ECMO cannulation scale (CESC) score	Decrease in time to cannulation Higher scores on GRS and CESC	Observational
Anderson et al. [3]	Nurse ECMO specialists (9)	High-fidelity ECMO simulation training program for ECMO emergencies	Technical skill and behavioral skill performance	Improvement in technical and behavioral skills between first and second simulation session	Observational
Burton et al. [4]	ECMO providers (19)	Simulations of ECMO emergencies over 16 months (divided into quarters with 1 quarter initiation training, 3 quarters maintenance training)	Identification of latent safety threats (LSTs); time to circuit readiness and initiation checklist compliance	Identification of 99 LSTs; improvement in checklist compliance	Observational
Chan et al. [5]	Interprofessional provider group in pediatric CICU (26)	Interprofessional ECMO training curriculum incorporating in situ simulation	Knowledge, ability, and confidence as measured by pre-post course questionnaires	Improvement in participant perception of knowledge and confidence; maintenance of competency skills on 6 month follow up	Observational
Sanchez-Glanville et al. [11]	Interprofessional provider group (56)	Interprofessional simulation training for new ECMO center	Self-reported changes in knowledge and confidence in providing ECMO care	Improvement in knowledge and confidence	Observational
Su et al. [12]	Pediatric patients requiring ECPR (43)	"Ideal rapid deployment" strategy for ECPR; in situ interprofessional simulation sessions over 36-month period	Deployment time to ECPR initiation	Decrease in median deployment time (51 min to 41 min)	Observational; quality improvement

[a]All results in table were statistically significant ($p < 0.05$)

ECMO flow, was found to decrease significantly from the pre-intervention to post-intervention time period. While this was a retrospective study lacking a true control group, it highlights the critical role of simulation in ECMO systems improvement and interprofessional team training.

Educators are hopeful that increased interprofessional team training in ECMO will improve patient outcomes. A study by Sanchez-Glanville et al. investigated the effects of an interprofessional ECMO curriculum utilizing simulation on learners and patient outcomes in a center introducing a new pediatric ECMO program [11]. The curriculum consisted of a 2-day didactic course, as well as animal labs, interprofessional in situ simulations in the pediatric intensive care unit (PICU) and debriefings following clinical cases. Simulation sessions were conducted over a 6-month period following the introduction of the ECMO program and were eventually expanded to include in situ simulations in the emergency department and in the operating room. Survey data revealed that the simulation component of the curriculum was rated "important" to "very important" to future ECMO education by all respondents and was more favorably rated than animal labs and lectures. Self-reported learner confidence and knowledge were statistically higher following participation in the curriculum. This study also collected data on patient outcomes including time to cannulation, complications, and survival. Over the study period, the ECMO team was activated 44 times with 21 patients proceeding to cannulation. Successful cannulation was reported in 100% of patients with an overall survival rate to discharge of 76%, which compares favorably to ELSO registry survival data. Lack of a control group limited conclusions about the effects of the training program on patient outcomes; however, this data could serve as baseline data for future investigations.

The difficulty in linking clinical outcomes to simulation training is multifactorial and is not limited to ECMO simulation. Current studies on ECMO simulation are attempting to link a multifaceted training strategy with outcomes of a complex low-frequency clinical therapy. A summary of some of these studies and their impact on the state of the science can be found in Table 17.2. Future studies will benefit from multi-institutional collaboration both for standardization of simulation training curricula and to achieve sufficient outcome data to assess for statistical significance.

Conclusion

ECMO simulation research has emerged in the last 15 years and has advanced both ECMO training and simulation science, leading to the development of effective models and innovative educational programs. Future studies should focus on development and validation of simulation scenarios and curricula for initial training and maintenance of competency, identifying novel methods of improving the realism of

ECMO simulations, and evaluating the effect of ECMO simulation training on patient outcomes.

References

1. Allan CK, Thiagarajan RR, Beke D, Imprescia A, Kappus LJ, Garden A, et al. Simulation-based training delivered directly to the pediatric cardiac intensive care unit engenders preparedness, comfort, and decreased anxiety among multidisciplinary resuscitation teams. J Thorac Cardiovasc Surg. 2010;140(3):646–52.
2. Anderson JM, Boyle KB, Murphy AA, Yaeger KA, LeFlore J, Halamek LP. Simulating extracorporeal membrane oxygenation emergencies to improve human performance. Part I: methodologic and technologic innovations. Simul Healthc. 2006;1(4):220–7.
3. Anderson JM, Murphy AA, Boyle KB, Yaeger KA, Halamek LP. Simulating extracorporeal membrane oxygenation emergencies to improve human performance. Part II: assessment of technical and behavioral skills. Simul Healthc. 2006;1(4):228–32.
4. Burton KS, Pendergrass TL, Byczkowski TL, Taylor RG, Moyer MR, Falcone RA, et al. Impact of simulation-based extracorporeal membrane oxygenation training in the simulation laboratory and clinical environment. Simul Healthc. 2011;6(5):284–91.
5. Chan SY, Figueroa M, Spentzas T, Powell A, Holloway R, Shah S. Prospective assessment of novice learners in a simulation-based extracorporeal membrane oxygenation (ECMO) education program. Pediatr Cardiol. 2013;34(3):543–52.
6. Thompson JL, Grisham LM, Scott J, Mogan C, Prescher H, Biffar D, et al. Construction of a reusable, high-fidelity model to enhance extracorporeal membrane oxygenation training through simulation. Adv Neonatal Care. 2014;14(2):103–9.
7. Allan CK, Pigula F, Bacha EA, Emani S, Fynn-Thompson F, Thiagarajan RR, et al. An extracorporeal membrane oxygenation cannulation curriculum featuring a novel integrated skills trainer leads to improved performance among pediatric cardiac surgery trainees. Simul Healthc. 2013;8(4):221–8.
8. Atamanyuk I, Ghez O, Saeed I, Lane M, Hall J, Jackson T, et al. Impact of an open-chest extracorporeal membrane oxygenation model for in situ simulated team training: a pilot study. Interact Cardiovasc Thorac Surg. 2014;18(1):17–20; discussion.
9. Burkhart HM, Riley JB, Lynch JJ, Suri RM, Greason KL, Joyce LD, et al. Simulation-based postcardiotomy extracorporeal membrane oxygenation crisis training for thoracic surgery residents. Ann Thorac Surg. 2013;95(3):901–6.
10. Fouilloux V, Gran C, Guervilly C, Breaud J, El Louali F, Rostini P. Impact of education and training course for ECMO patients based on high-fidelity simulation: a pilot study dedicated to ICU nurses. Perfusion. 2018:267659118789824.
11. Sanchez-Glanville C, Brindle ME, Spence T, Blackwood J, Drews T, Menzies S, et al. Evaluating the introduction of extracorporeal life support technology to a tertiary-care pediatric institution: smoothing the learning curve through interprofessional simulation training. J Pediatr Surg. 2015;50(5):798–804.
12. Su L, Spaeder MC, Jones MB, Sinha P, Nath DS, Jain PN, et al. Implementation of an extracorporeal cardiopulmonary resuscitation simulation program reduces extracorporeal cardiopulmonary resuscitation times in real patients. Pediatr Crit Care Med. 2014;15(9):856–60.
13. Extracorporeal Life Support Organization. ELSO Guidelines for Training and Continuing Education of ECMO Specialists, version 1.5. 2010. Available from: https://www.elso.org/Portals/0/IGD/Archive/FileManager/97000963d6cusersshyerdocumentselsoguidelinesfortrainingandcontinuingeducationofecmospecialists.pdf.
14. Weems MF, Friedlich PS, Nelson LP, Rake AJ, Klee L, Stein JE, et al. The role of extracorporeal membrane oxygenation simulation training at Extracorporeal Life Support Organization Centers in the United States. Simul Healthc. 2017;12(4):233–9.
15. Lansdowne W, Machin D, Grant DJ. Development of the orpheus perfusion simulator for use in high-fidelity extracorporeal membrane oxygenation simulation. J Extra Corpor Technol. 2012;44(4):250–5.
16. Brazzi L, Lissoni A, Panigada M, Bottino N, Patroniti N, Pappalardo F, et al. Simulation-based training of extracorporeal membrane oxygenation during H1N1 influenza pandemic: the Italian experience. Simul Healthc. 2012;7(1):32–4.
17. Martinelli SM, Chen F, DiLorenzo AN, Mayer DC, Fairbanks S, Moran K, et al. Results of a flipped classroom teaching approach in anesthesiology residents. J Grad Med Educ. 2017;9(4):485–90.
18. McLaughlin JE, Roth MT, Glatt DM, Gharkholonarehe N, Davidson CA, Griffin LM, et al. The flipped classroom: a course redesign to foster learning and engagement in a health professions school. Acad Med. 2014;89(2):236–43.
19. Wang R, DeMaria S Jr, Goldberg A, Katz D. A systematic review of serious games in training health care professionals. Simul Healthc. 2016;11(1):41–51.
20. Antonius T, Hogeveen M, Peeters T, Hejst AV. Serious gaming in ECMO simulation. Int J Artif Organs. 2013;36(4):272.
21. Johnston L, Su L. Personal communication.
22. Anderson JM, Aylor ME, Leonard DT. Instructional design dogma: creating planned learning experiences in simulation. J Crit Care. 2008;23(4):595–602.
23. Neonatal Resuscitation Program. Available from: http://www.aap.org/nrp.
24. Pediatric Advanced Life Support. Available from: http://cpr.heart.org/AHAECC/CPRAndECC/Ttraining/HealthcareProfessional/Pediatric/UMC_476258_PALS.jsp.
25. Al Disi M, Alsalemi A, Alhomsi Y, Bensaali F, Amira A, Alinier G. Revolutionizing ECMO simulation with affordable yet high-Fidelity technology. Am J Emerg Med. 2017;36:1310.
26. Alinier G, Hassan IF, Alsalemi A, Al Disi M, Ait Hssain A, Labib A, et al. Addressing the challenges of ECMO simulation. Perfusion. 2018;33(7):568–76.
27. Malec JF, Torsher LC, Dunn WF, Wiegmann DA, Arnold JJ, Brown DA, et al. The mayo high performance teamwork scale: reliability and validity for evaluating key crew resource management skills. Simul Healthc. 2007;2(1):4–10.
28. Brum R, Rajani R, Gelandt E, Morgan L, Raguseelan N, Butt S, et al. Simulation training for extracorporeal membrane oxygenation. Ann Card Anaesth. 2015;18(2):185–90.
29. Chamberlain D, Smith A, Woollard M, Colquhoun M, Handley AJ, Leaves S, et al. Trials of teaching methods in basic life support (3): comparison of simulated CPR performance after first training and at 6 months, with a note on the value of re-training. Resuscitation. 2002;53(2):179–87.
30. Auguste TC, Boswick JA, Loyd MK, Battista A. The simulation of an ex utero intrapartum procedure to extracorporeal membrane oxygenation. J Pediatr Surg. 2011;46(2):395–8.
31. Puslecki M, Ligowski M, Dabrowski M, Stefaniak S, Ladzinska M, Ladzinski P, et al. BEST life-"bringing ECMO simulation to life"-how medical simulation improved a regional ECMO program. Artif Organs. 2018;42(11):1052–61.
32. Fehr JJ, Shepard M, McBride ME, Mehegan M, Reddy K, Murray DJ, et al. Simulation-based assessment of ECMO clinical specialists. Simul Healthc. 2016;11(3):194–9.
33. Topjian AA, Berg RA, Nadkarni VM. Pediatric cardiopulmonary resuscitation: advances in science, techniques, and outcomes. Pediatrics. 2008;122(5):1086–98.
34. Oxford Centre for Evidence-Based Medicine. May 1, 2016. https://www.cebm.net/index.aspx?o=5653.

Faculty Development for ECMO Simulation

18

Roberta L. Hales and David L. Rodgers

Learning Objectives

At the end of this chapter, you will be able to:

1. State the evolution of faculty development in higher education, particularly simulation-based education
2. Explain the theoretical frameworks that guide ECMO Simulation Faculty development
3. Compare and contrast the different approaches of ECMO Simulation Faculty Development
4. Describe the structure and components of a Simulation Faculty Development Program

ECMO Faculty Development for Simulation

Concepts of faculty development have changed significantly as the role of faculty has transitioned to meet modern needs. In the 1950s, the Age of the Scholar put emphasis on improvement and advancement in scholarship and competence. Today's fast-paced, twenty-first-century explosion of knowledge and information place faculty in the Age of the Network, requiring faculty to balance multiple, complex, and demanding roles and responsibilities in conjunction with the changing nature of teaching, learning, technology, and scholarship. In the past, it was assumed that clinical expertise equated to competence in teaching [2]. Similarly, there was a postulation that intellectual healthcare professionals, who have learned and trained for many years, needed little to no faculty development and/or support. In the present day and age, that thinking is no longer suitable. In some sense, the rapid increase in faculty development programs is related to the growth of public scrutiny and accountability. Some may perceive that faculty are ill-prepared for their various roles, given the changing nature of healthcare delivery and technology, the ongoing pursuit of excellence, and professionalization of teaching and healthcare education [3]. Furthermore, an emphasis on safety and quality assurance in healthcare, a desire to offer high-quality training programs for trainees and staff, along with the influence of regulatory and international accrediting bodies attests to the need for faculty development [3, 4]. For these reasons, there has been a significant increase in faculty development programs over the past 10 years to help support the healthcare professionals to fulfill these various roles.

This chapter will briefly discuss the evolution of faculty development in higher education and the fundamentals of faculty development in the context of ECMO simulation. The aim is to focus on the development of ECMO faculty, including the relevant theoretical frameworks, approaches to development, and design of a faculty development training program. In this chapter, "faculty" are assumed to be those individuals who are learning to become ECMO educators/instructors in simulation-based education.

Evolution of Faculty Development

The definition of faculty development in higher education has transformed from scholarly competence in the 1950s, to a broad range of activities that institutions use to renew or assist faculty [5]. These include all activities that health professionals pursue to improve their knowledge, skills, and

R. L. Hales (✉)
Center for Simulation, Advanced Education, and Innovation, The Children's Hospital of Philadelphia, Philadelphia, PA, USA

Drexel University, Graduate School of Biomedical Sciences and Professional Studies, Philadelphia, PA, USA
e-mail: hales@email.chop.edu

D. L. Rodgers
Clinical Simulation Center, Penn State Health Milton S. Hershey Medical Center, Hershey, PA, USA

L. C. Johnston, L. Su (eds.), *Comprehensive Healthcare Simulation: ECMO Simulation*, Comprehensive Healthcare Simulation,
https://doi.org/10.1007/978-3-030-53844-6_18

behaviors as teachers and educators, managers and leaders, and researchers and scholars, in both individual and group settings [3]. Faculty development is not a new phenomenon in higher education; however, it is viewed as a young profession that is still in development. In fact, it is referred to by numerous names (educational development, professional development, staff development) as a result of lack of consensus among the members of the profession [6]. Nonetheless, faculty development has transformed from the traditional classroom style of teaching into self-directed formal and informal approaches attributable to the accelerated dynamic and demanding nature of higher education, the healthcare environment and patient safety.

The oldest faculty development practice, sabbatical leave, originated at Harvard University in 1810 [7]. This was intended to promote and support the faculty's development as scholars within their field of study. Faculty development as it is defined today emerged and transformed from the United States' higher education system with initial work in the 1950s and 1960s. To appreciate the future of faculty development, it is important to briefly explore the evolution of the goals, practices, and structures that characterize this profession. Sorenelli et al. [8] categorized the evolution of faculty development into five stages: Age of the Scholar, Age of the Teacher, Age of the Developer, Age of the Learner, and Age of the Network (See Table 18.1) [4].

The fundamental goal of faculty developmental is to foster, promote, and reinforce the knowledge, skills, and attitudes in teaching, assessing, professionalism, and research to enhance professional education and competence in a myriad of healthcare and educational environments, both now and in the future. Emerging trends and innovations are creating numerous opportunities and challenges for faculty. This paradigm in teaching and learning requires faculty to transform and adopt innovative curricula and altered educational frameworks/strategies (simulation, competency-based education, interprofessional education) with little to no experience in educational theory and learning. Unfortunately, this lack of knowledge regarding theory and how to utilize these new/revised frameworks and strategies could translate into poor educational instruction and outcomes. By the same token, current-day learners possess a "heightened awareness of multiculturalism and diverse populations and have high expectations for the value and quality of their own education" [9]. Faculty development of healthcare professionals is an essential component of healthcare education at both the individual and organizational levels. Its primary focus has been teaching and instructional effectiveness. This mindset needs to shift to preparing faculty for various roles in their practice with the intention of sustaining productivity and vitality at all levels of the learning continuum as well as being aligned with societal needs and expectations [10].

Table 18.1 Five stages of the faculty development (FD) profession [4, 15]

Stages	Year	Key Aspects
Age of the Scholar	1950s–1960s	Primary focus: research and scholarly competence No formal faculty development (FD) programs Very few studies
Age of the Teacher	1960s–1970s	Primary focus: quality and instructional improvement Teacher-centric Beginning of formal FD programs Creation of two professional associations in United States
Age of the Developer	1980s	Rejuvenation of FD programs Robust curriculum design Increase in FD programs supported by internal and external funding Canada creates FD society
Age of the Learner	1990s	Change in faculty role to facilitator Learner-centric Variety of learning methods Technology evolution Advancement in assessment and performance measures
Age of the Network	2000–present day	FD programs continue to expand Explosion of technology Assessment and performance measure focus on outcomes High performance expectations at the individual, departmental, institutional, and state levels Expansion of FD leadership, research Less funding for FD programs

Permission obtained from Elsevier, Ref. [4]

Faculty Development for Simulation

Simulation is a methodology that replicates real-life experiences to facilitate learning in the cognitive, psychomotor, and affective domains. It is widely used to allow learners to engage in impactful scenarios and team exercises to facilitate the development of individuals and high-functioning teams. It creates meaningful learning experiences that promote skill acquisition, critical thinking, clinical decision-making, and problem-solving skills. The situation evokes reflection and construction of new or revised meanings of experiences and ideas as a guide to future action (transformative learning/reflective practice). Nonetheless, the metacognitive skills necessary for learners to examine and analyze their thought processes are challenging to acquire; therefore, substantial guidance and feedback from faculty may be necessary. In addition, learners might need direction on how to incorporate their new knowledge and experience into existing knowledge and apply it, a basic tenet of Constructivist learning theory [11]. And so, faculty may be the catalyst to creating and enhancing the learning experience resulting in positive behavior change in the learning and healthcare environments.

The role of simulation faculty is complex and requires a level of knowledge and expertise in numerous areas, including learning theory, curriculum design, learning strategies, facilitation, debriefing, and assessment. To be effective and efficient, it is necessary for faculty to be trained specifically in the simulation methodology they are employing. Within the broad band of healthcare simulation, debriefing has been identified as the most important element to the learning activity [1]. This facilitated self-reflection of the learner is a critical component for fostering deep learning and promoting transfer of skills and behaviors to clinical practice [12]. To this end, faculty must be competent in learner-centered teaching and be able to create and maintain a psychologically safe and supportive learning environment, manage the personalities and behaviors of the learners, and bring structure and direction to the conversation [1]. If immersive simulation is utilized for a specific content focus, such as Extracorporeal Membrane Oxygenation (ECMO), then faculty may need experience in the knowledge, skills, and behaviors to optimize the teaching effectiveness of this particular educational activity. If the faculty are not an expert in the content (ECMO), a subject matter expert (SME) can be utilized for the clinical knowledge and expertise in the simulation design, activity, and debriefing. Today's faculty development programs need to be tailored to the overall development of both new and seasoned faculty, and to assist them in their lifelong journey of change and growth that will help them and the learners to be successful.

Theoretical Frameworks to Guide ECMO Simulation Faculty Development

Simulation faculty and educators must be well versed in learning theories in order to select the best teaching methodologies in their practice. Defining the difference between *learning* theory and *teaching* theory requires making a distinction between theory and practice. Theories of learning deal with the ways a person learns, while theories of teaching address the ways a person influences the learner to learn. Therefore, the learning theory subscribed to by faculty will guide the application of teaching theory through the methods of instruction.

The five core learning theories (Experiential Learning Theory, Constructivism, Adult Learning Theory, Self-efficacy Theory, and Social Learning Theory) that are commonly referenced in healthcare simulation literature and that introduced a newer theory, Brain-Based Learning are provided in more detail in Chap. 5. This chapter will introduce the learning theories applicable to faculty development, which draw upon the core learning theories.

Situated Learning Theory

Situated Learning Theory emphasizes the need to engage learners in real activities found in everyday life including healthcare work. The learning environment itself becomes part of the learning experience. Many learning modalities, such as classroom or online learning, present information outside of the environment in which it will be applied. Simulation offers the opportunity to involve learners in activities where the subject matter is directly linked to its application. Situated Learning Theory overlaps with the previously discussed theories very well in healthcare simulation. As an example, consider this learning experience:

> A group of learners participate in a hands-on session to learn how the ECMO pump works and how to troubleshoot possible issues. The pump is connected to an ECMO circuit, which flows through a simulator. Physiological data is displayed in real time on monitors in the room. The room contains the relevant equipment that would be present in the clinical setting. The simulator is intubated and on a ventilator, and has numerous points of vascular access and pumps infusing medications and fluids. As complications occur, the simulator's status changes and the care team must decide what is happening and act.

Clearly, this is an example of situated learning as learners are actively engaged in a realistic simulation and not learning complication identification and management in the abstract form, as would occur in a traditional classroom. Examining this scenario more closely, the relationships with other learning theories become evident:

- Experiential Learning [13] – Learners are actively involved in the learning environment, experiencing the situation and deriving meaning from it (see Fig. 18.1 – Kolb [4, 13]).
- Adult Learning Theory [14] – This scenario is practical, complex, problem-based learning in a realistic environment that adds relevance (see Fig. 18.2 – Adult learning principles [4, 14]).
- Constructivism – Learners entered this scenario with a baseline level of ECMO knowledge. As the situation unfolds in the exercise and debriefing, the learners draw upon prior knowledge of ECMO complications, examine and filter the new information against their knowledge, beliefs, and practices, and push themselves to create new insights and meanings. The simulation faculty assists by building a framework in the debriefing by using dialogue or conversation to help the learners navigate and formulate these new experiences and meanings into their existing knowledge and practice.
- Social Learning Theory – Situated Learning Theory works best as a cooperative interaction with others. Learners and faculty share knowledge to advance all learners (and faculty, as well).

Other teaching practices associated with situated learning are cognitive apprenticeship, collaborative learning

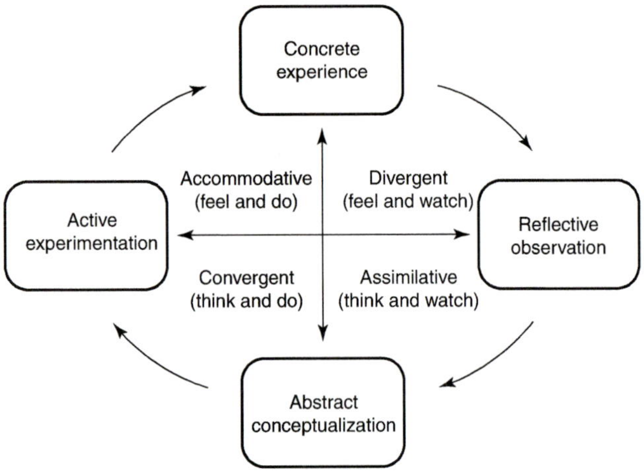

Fig. 18.1 Kolb's four-stage experiential learning cycle and styles [13]. (Permission granted from Elsevier, Ref. [4])

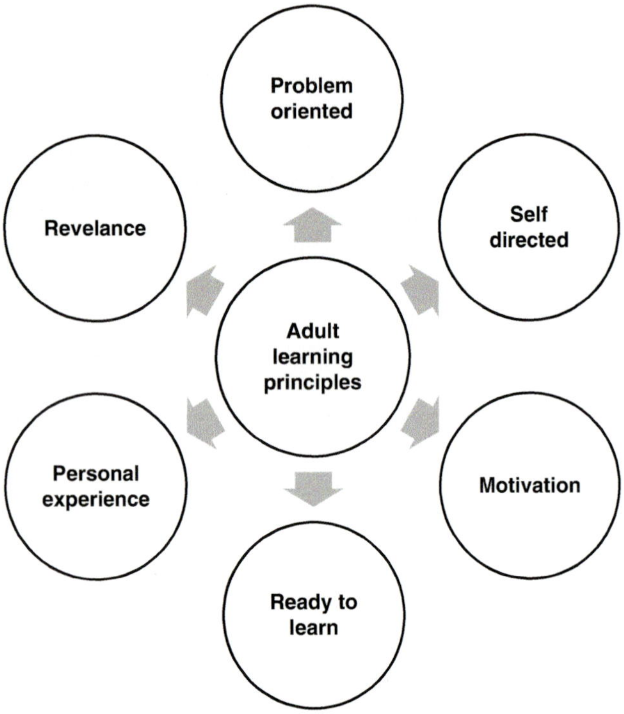

Fig. 18.2 Adult learning principles. (Permission granted from Elsevier, Ref [4])

reflection, deliberate practice, and articulation of learning skills [15].

Communities of Practice (CoP)

Closely linked with Situated Learning Theory is the concept of Communities of Practice [16]. There are four elements needed for a CoP:

- Domain – This is the topic of knowledge; the subject for which the community has interests in participating. For our purposes, this is ECMO.
- Community – These are the people that are working together to build knowledge and skill on the topic. For our ECMO example, this is the interprofessional healthcare team.
- Practice – This represents the activities and tools in which the community engages to learn more about the domain.
- Improvement – The goal of the CoP is continuous improvement in the domain, the community, and the practice.

Membership in a CoP is widely varied in terms of expertise. Lave and Wenger [16, 17] introduced "legitimate peripheral participation" as the way new members are introduced to the community. At the edge, or periphery, are the newcomers, those who would be considered novices. As individuals evolve in their knowledge and abilities, they migrate closer to the center of the CoP, eventually becoming experts (much as the progression from novice to expert of the Dreyfus model) [17]. Central to this model is the need for more knowledgeable and experienced expert members of the CoP to work with those at the periphery to help build competence and proficiency on their way to eventually becoming experts.

All professions, including ECMO educators/faculty, have Communities of Practice (CoP) [16]. Individuals may belong to more than one CoP, depending on their role within that profession. This is true for ECMO educators/faculty. One CoP for ECMO healthcare providers includes those in the role of clinician. For this CoP, the ECMO healthcare provider may be at the center of clinical practice. However, this role as clinical expert does not automatically transfer to other related CoPs such as an educator/faculty. The purpose of this book (especially this chapter) is to engage individuals who are expert in the clinical CoP to help them move toward expertise as simulation educators/faculty.

Transformative Learning Theory

Finally, we will discuss Transformative Learning Theory [18, 19]. Central to this theory is the concept of perspective transformation. Incremental learning is not the goal. What is needed is a shift in thinking, a new perspective about self-beliefs. This is accomplished through critical self-reflection. In simulation, this can occur through interprofessional education (IPE). In IPE, as learners learn with, from, and about each other, new perspectives are gained as the contributions of each team member are realized by others. This is also a part of the process found in a CoP. Part of the responsibility of the simulation faculty is to generate discussion that leads to new understandings about the role of the team members and how each person contributes to the patient care goals.

Methodology (Approaches) of ECMO Simulation Faculty Development

Educational theory, curriculum development, assessment, and research and system integration are all elements that contribute to healthcare simulation. The use of simulation has become widespread for many different healthcare professions and specialties in the undergraduate and postgraduate levels. As stated earlier, faculty should be well versed in each of these areas. The growth and popularity of simulation will require faculty to participate in formal and informal development programs to become proficient in the fundamentals, standards, and methods to ensure learner outcomes. This section will briefly review formal and informal approaches that can be used to educate ECMO simulation faculty.

Formal Approaches

Workshops/Seminars/Conferences/Short Courses

Workshops, seminars, conferences, and short courses are among the mainstays of faculty development programs in simulation-based education [20]. They can vary in duration, modality, and content, and include topics pertaining to educational theory, curriculum design, facilitation and debriefing, assessment and research. These formal approaches combine interactive lectures, small and large group discussions, and experiential learning to achieve the learning outcomes. The major emphasis is the acquisition of knowledge and skills, and changes in attitudes and behaviors with the intention of enhancing faculties' motivation, self-awareness, and enthusiasm [21]. There are two ways to attain further education in simulation-based education and faculty development in this realm: attend a wide range of simulation conferences and/or simulation instructor courses. Specialized instructor courses integrate the best practices in teaching and learning into simulation-based education. Currently, 13 simulation-based instructor courses are published in the literature and available nationally and internationally to the healthcare professional (Table 18.2) [22].

Faculty Simulation Fellowships/Longitudinal Programs (6 Months–2 Years)

An intense longitudinal fellowship program typically refers to a subspecialty training utilized by numerous disciplines. In definition, it is a cohort of faculty members selected to participate in a longitudinal set of faculty development activ-

Table 18.2 Sample multiday continuing education instructor courses

Name of course	Location	Collaborating simulation center	Approx. length
Institute for Medical Simulation (IMS): Comprehensive Instructor Course	Boston, MA	Center for Medical Simulation (CMS)	5 days
Improving Simulation Instructional Methods (ISIM)	Pittsburg, PA	Winter Institute for Simulation Education and Research (WISER)	3 days
Train the Trainer	Bristol, UK	Bristol Medical Simulation Center	2 days
International Workshop	Tel Hashomer, Israel	Israel Center for Medical Simulation (MSR)	5 days
Instructor Training Course	Sydney, Australia	Sydney Clinical Skills and Simulation Center	2 days
Center for Immersive and Simulation-Based Learning (CISL) Instructor Course	Stanford, CA	Center for Immersive and Simulation-based Learning (CISL) Stamford Medical School	2.5 days
Certificate in Simulation	Philadelphia, PA	Drexel College of Nursing and Health Professions	5 days
Australian Simulation Educators and Technician Trainers (AusSETT)	Rotating locations within Australia	Monash University (lead), The University of Melbourne, Edith Cowan University, Flinders University, The University of Queensland and Queensland Health	3 days
Coordinated Approach to Simulation Training (CAST)	East Bentleigh VIC, Australia	Southern Health Simulation Center, Monash Medical Center	5 days
Instructor Development: Simulation-Based Education Design and Debriefing	Rochester, MN	Mayo Clinic	3 days
Certificate in Simulation	Philadelphia	Center for Interdisciplinary Clinical Simulation and Practice, Drexel University College of Nursing and Health Professionals	5 days
The Basic EuSim Simulation Instructor Course and the Advanced EuSim Simulation Instructor Course	Copenhagen, Tuebingen, Bilthoven, London	Danish Institute for Medical Simulation (DIMS), Center for Patient Safety and Simulation (TuPASS), BARTS and The London NHS Trust	3 days
Keystones of Healthcare Simulation Certificate	Toronto, Canada	SIM-One, Ontario Simulation Network, University of Toronto and Waters Family Simulation Center	Three multiday courses and presentation at conference required
Master Debriefing Course	Calgary, AB, Canada	The Debriefing Academy	3 days

ities with the goals to improve the participant's teaching and coaching skills, and build a new cadre of healthcare educational leaders [23]. Within the simulation community there are two main types of fellowship programs. One type combines a clinical experience for which the fellow is compensated with the simulation learning experience. In the United States, the American College of Surgeons and the American College of Emergency Physicians offer hybrid programs of this nature. The other type of fellowship program is solely a learning experience and may be an uncompensated or a tuition-based educational program. The comprehensive and selective curriculum of simulation fellowship addresses a wide range of skills, behaviors, and attitudes to promote development of skills to become a well-rounded professional and academic leader in healthcare simulation. As of this publication, there were no formal standards for simulation fellowship programs. The lack of an accreditation process for fellowship has been recognized as an essential area of development by various national and international entities.

Advanced Education

Certificate and graduate degree programs are becoming more prevalent in advanced studies on simulation-based education. Some of the courses are completely asynchronous learning (on-line) while others may include an on-site requirement. The goal of these programs is to educate the healthcare professional in the essential knowledge and skills to be exemplary educators, leaders, and researchers who possess the qualifications and experiences to advance knowledge, research, and technology of healthcare simulation. Some of the master's degree programs are based on the education degree models so the curricula may include research methods in education, technology in education, leadership and organizational change, and scholarly writing [22].

At present, there are approximately five graduate certificate and five graduate degree programs specializing in simulation-based education in the United States and United Kingdom [22]. With the advancement of education methodologies and the desired shift toward learner-centric teaching approaches, healthcare professional faculty may need to seek higher education to be knowledgeable and effective simulation faculty.

Informal Approaches

Work-Based Learning

Work-based learning, often defined as learning for work, learning at work, and learning from work, is fundamental to faculty development [24, 25]. Actually, learning at work is related to experiential learning, whereby healthcare professionals acquire the knowledge, skills, and attitudes to become the role model and teacher in education. In reality, healthcare professionals influence their workplace and their own learning, which is often dependent on the conditions of the work environment. If it is a nurturing environment, they will be able to acquire the basic knowledge and skills of simulation education. By the same token, if the work environment is dysfunctional, this lessens their knowledge, skill transfer, and internal motivation toward learning and education. It is important to sanction these "on the job" encounters as learning experiences and encourage reflection to better understand the actions and outcomes [4].

In simulation, work-based learning is the first line of exposure and experience to learn and teach the fundamentals of simulation-based education. As such, it is an apprenticeship model. This model is founded upon behavioral, cognitive, and social learning concepts. One common and oft-cited apprenticeship model that focused on the cognitive domain is a six-stage process developed by Collins, Brown, and Newman [26] (See Table 18.3). Though developed for childhood learning, the model has been adapted to adult education, and specifically to healthcare [27]. Fundamental to this model, is the learner's ability to engage in practice to gain experience, reflect critically to identify opportunities for improvement, and apply in future activities. While it is important to hold fast to the apprenticeship model in simulation, it is equally as important to encourage faculty to pursue further education via other approaches.

Peer Coaching and Feedback

Peer coaching is a form of work-based learning and commonly involves observation of teaching and feedback [28].

- Peer coaching is a dynamic individualized faculty development approach that depends on collaborative and supportive relationships [28].
- Feedback is defined as constructive information provided back to the recipient that addresses specific areas of performance [29].

Table 18.3 Cognitive Apprenticeship Model [26]

Stages	Element
Modeling	Allow the learner to observe your practice in order to build up a conceptualization of that practice.
Coaching	Watch the learner practice, offering them guidance, critique, and feedback.
Scaffolding	Offer the learner more opportunities to practice, gradually and purposefully increasing complexity of the work undertaken while slowly fading out your input.
Articulation	Use questioning and supervision time to encourage learner to talk you through what they are doing, why and how, providing a rationale for approaches taken.
Reflection	Encourage learner to consider his/her performance analytically and to compare it with that of the expert to identify ways to further enhance his/her own performance.
Exploration	Provide opportunities for the learner to undertake new task and activities, prompting the learner to become more independent in his/her activity and his/her thinking.

The aforementioned involves coaching and feedback by a more experienced individual or by a peer with similar experience [28]. This learner-centric approach may be a suitable means to enhance the development and growth of faculty in simulation-based education. A recent publication by Cheng et al. holds that the integration of peer coaching into the flow of teaching offers everyday opportunities for educators to maintain and expand their skills [30]. To boot, it can provide the benefit of continuous reinforcement and improvement of skills in faculty's learning journey. This shared and collaborative practice enhances reflection, and encourages new strategies and approaches in a safe and supportive learning environment [28]. Cheng et al. identified debriefing as one component of simulation that could benefit from peer coaching. Debriefing is a conversation between two or more people to explore and analyze performance, as well as to gain insight to improve and sustain individual and group performance. Effective debriefings are the critical component in simulation-based learning because they provide the opportunity for learners to constructively self-reflect and become more aware of performance gaps [31]. However, the quality of the debriefing and eventual impact on learning outcomes is highly dependent upon the performance of the faculty facilitator(s) [30]. Through the use of peer coaching, ECMO faculty can tap into unique opportunities to create a sense of camaraderie as they teach together, learn together, and nurture each other to become knowledgeable and skillful simulation faculty.

Professional Community of Practice (See Theory Section for Further Details)

Wenger et al., [32] developed seven principles for cultivating communities of practice for faculty development including:

- Design of evolution: faculty communities should be built on preexisting development networks and allow for natural growth and development.
- Open dialogue between insider and outsider perspectives: faculty communities need an insider perspective for discovery and outsider perspective to think "outside the box."
- Invite different levels of participants: faculty communities offer individuals in all levels of faculty development to participate and engage for different reasons.
- Develop public and private community spaces: faculty communities have public events where faculty gather to exchange ideas, solve problems, and/or explore novel concepts; however the core is the one-on-one networking that occurs informally between them.
- Focus on value: faculty communities deliver value to organizations, to teams on which they serve and to the individual members themselves.
- Combine familiarity and excitement: successful faculty communities offer familiar workings and provide interesting perspectives on new concepts to keep new members cycling in.
- Create a rhythm for the community: the heart and livelihood of faculty communities revolve around the relationships among the members and their participation in familiar and new events. This creates the ebb and flow of members into active participation, which is the strongest indicator of the growth of an active community [32].

As evidenced by Wenger [32], building a simulation community of practice is essential for the success of the profession. It allows the simulationist to engage and network in conversation to discuss and share various facets of simulation practice. They explore the benefits and challenges, as well as share ideas, resources, and experiences. In addition, they share pointers, tips and tricks, best practices, insights, and innovations [33]. Informal activities may include regular or ad hoc meetings, journal clubs, literature reviews, a lecture series, webinars, or virtual media (Facebook, Twitter, Blogs, Wiki, Video-sharing sites, Podcasts). What will make the simulation community of practice robust is accretion of relevance and the network of local, national, and international people coming together to increase their expertise and skills for their profession.

Mentorship

"Mentor" or "mentorship" has been defined in many ways. The Institute of Medicine defines a mentor as a faculty advisor, career advisor, skills consultant, and role model [34]. It is a common strategy to promote development, socialization, and maturation of faculty by providing guidance, direction, support, and expertise [35]. Then again, it is an underutilized strategy for professional development and should be considered as an unequivocal approach to faculty development [36]. Mentorships are invaluable as they provide the support, challenge, and vision of the mentee's future through formal or informal processes [37]. Moreover, it assists mentees in understanding the organizational culture, and introduces them to the professional networks and CoP. The additional component of mentorship is reflective practice. Reflective practice is a deep-rooted self-analysis whereby the mentee thinks critically about former experiences with the intent to improve one's self; "however reflection on the experience of others, in this case the mentor, can be extremely valuable too,... particularly in making career decisions or work-life balances" [28].

Role Modeling

One part of mentoring is for the mentor to serve as a role model. Role modeling is a powerful approach for teaching and learning in simulation. It is a spontaneous learning process that happens naturally via passive observation and reflection, and is a complex mix of conscious and unconscious activities [38]. While we are aware of the conscious observation of behaviors, understanding the power of the unconscious component is essential to effective role modeling [38]. Through active reflection, the unconscious component can be transformed to a conscious component with meaning and actions. In fact, all healthcare professionals participate in this informal, unscripted role modeling; indeed, many of the corrosive effects of negative role modeling are experienced here [38]. Therefore, role models must be consciously aware of all their actions and reactions because they have a significant influence on the observing faculty's professional values, attitudes, and behaviors.

Standards of Practice
Simulation Faculty

The International Nursing Association for Clinical Simulation and Learning (INACSL) Standards for Best Practices: Simulation Facilitation (36).

Society for Simulation Council of Accreditation (37)
Teaching/Education Standards-Qualified Educators

The National Council of State Boards of Nursing (38)
Faculty checklists to assess faculty/staff development.

Fig. 18.3 Standards of practice: faculty development

Structure and Components of Simulation Faculty Development Program

As simulation-based learning has increased, the growing cadre of simulation faculty has challenged many simulation programs on how to educate and support their own team. Though there are many formal options, most healthcare professionals cannot afford the time and money to allow team members to attend workshops, conferences, and simulation instructor courses. Therefore, access to viable opportunities to achieve the same education, development, and learning outcomes is critically important in the local environment. In addition, the diverse nature of the recipient faculty may warrant the curriculum designer to develop different levels in the comprehensive program targeted audience members. As Peterson et al. states, a tiered method provides the recipient the needed confidence in conjunction with the "opportunity to gradually grow in simulation expertise" [31]. This tiered approach recognizes that faculty novice to simulation, regardless of their past and present clinical experience, skill, or knowledge, may also be novice to simulation methodology [31]. Similarly, not all faculty have the same skill sets so tailoring the faculty development program will help to provide them with a solid foundation for simulation practice.

For homegrown structured simulation faculty development programs, there are several sources that provide guidelines and standards for consideration. These programs should aim to integrate evidence-based practice and standards to ensure quality and structure in developing faculty to use simulation as an effective teaching tool [31, 39–41] (See Fig. 18.3).

ECMO Faculty Development

Establishing a faculty development program is particularly important to ECMO governance [42]. ECMO is arguably one of the most complex therapies in the ICU environment that "requires comprehensive knowledge, expertise in complex circuits, and skills to rapidly respond to potential life threatening complications" [42]. Presently, Extracorporeal Life Support Organization (ELSO) recommends education via didactic lectures with hands-on water drills, animal laboratory and/or bedside training, and a written exam [43]. Water drills are hands-on training with a closed-loop water-filled circuit to practice assembly and repair in a controlled environment [44]. Animal laboratories provide hands-on training with live animals that undergo real-time ECMO management in a controlled environment, while bedside training allows the trainee to assist the experienced ECMO specialist [44]. While these options are feasible, water drills offer limited opportunities for real-time troubleshooting, and the use of live animals is difficult, expensive [45] and not always equivalent to human pathophysiology [42]. Furthermore, trainees are not given the opportunity to incorporate real-time changes in the patient's clinical status into their plan of care and perhaps most importantly, these methods do not address the aspects of team behavior and effective communication amongst the interprofessional team [46]. Currently, approximately 41 ELSO sites are incorporating ECMO simulations in their training programs [44] to practice urgent and emergent management, in tandem with teamwork and communication in real-time simulated pressure environments. Nevertheless, these ECMO simulation programs are not standardized and utilize varying simulation methods, hence stressing the need and importance for standardization of training and faculty development. Faculty need to be trained on how to use "simulation as a teaching method to create the meaningful learning experiences that promote reflective practice and significant behavior change that results in measurable outcomes" [47].

Development of a Simulation ECMO Faculty Development Course

Designing a simulation ECMO faculty development course begins with understanding of the audience, culture, and leadership of the organization to ensure success of the program. Once established, it begins with using curriculum design principles. This chapter will use the Kern six-step curriculum model to build a simulation ECMO faculty development course [48]. Please see the Simulation ECMO Faculty Course example in the Appendix 18.1. For further detail on how to build an ECMO simulation curriculum, please refer to Chap. 6.

Faculty Assessment

Before we discuss faculty assessment methods, let us briefly review the reasons why it is so important to provide constructive feedback and reflection to simulation ECMO faculty. Debriefing is the crucial component of the simulation, which can promote positive or negative learning experiences. As discussed in a Chap. 15, debriefing is a facilitated discussion that requires skill and experience as a below-par debriefing could dismantle the learning and experience. Faculty are expected to evaluate and appraise a learner's performance [31]. Often faculty perceive performance differently on the basis of a combination of life experiences, academic training, and clinical experience [49]. This can lead to variance in debriefing, and how simulation is facilitated as a whole [31]. Moreover, if faculty do not have the right tools and skills, the environment may be unsafe for the learners to fully participate. For these reasons, faculty development is imperative for the success of the ECMO simulation program.

A broad array of assessment possibilities exist including simple dialogue to formal objective assessments with instruments that have been evaluated for sources of validity evidence. Assessment of faculty effectiveness involves exploring and gathering data about the processes and practices, such as educational strategies and debriefing, along with consequential data (experience and outcomes) from the learners. A valid assessment tool provides objective feedback on performance by providing an unbiased critique of competence. In her recent review of faculty development, Yvonne Stewart notes that intensive feedback was one of the most effective techniques in improving faculty performance [21]. In addition, Rebecca Minehart reported improvement in the quality of simulation faculty feedback to residents after just 1 hour of a structured educational intervention [50]. Therefore, appropriate training in debriefing methodologies and structure is imperative, as is the use of assessment tools for debriefing effectiveness, which have been evaluated for sources of validity evidence [31]. Faculty need ongoing training, mentoring, and coaching, along with multiple opportunities for practice and regular evaluations to ensure debriefing skills and techniques are maintained [31].

Several rating instruments have been designed to assist in developing and evaluating the effectiveness of debriefing by faculty. This chapter will briefly review these tools: the Debriefing Assessment for Simulation in Healthcare (DASH) © [51] and the Objective Structured Assessment of Debriefing (OSAD) [52].

DASH is a behaviorally anchored rating scale that evaluates the faculty's technique and strategy of the debriefing. There are three versions of DASH. One designed for trained raters, one designed for students to rate their instructors, and one designed for instructors to rate themselves. The rating scale ranges from 1(detrimental) to 7 (outstanding). The rating is a holistic view of each element. The tool contains six elements deemed pertinent to execute an effective debriefing [51]:

- Establishes an engaging learning environment
- Maintains an engaging learning environment
- Structures the debriefing in an organized way
- Provokes engaging discussions
- Identifies, explores, and closes performance gaps
- Help learners achieve and sustain good performance

The OSAD is a behaviorally anchored scoring rating tool across eight categories to provide feedback to faculty to improve the effectiveness and quality of the debriefing [52]. The rating scale ranges 1 (minimum) to 5 (maximum) regarding how well the element was conducted by the faculty. Descriptive anchors at the lowest point, mid-point, and high-point of the scale are used to guide the raters to construct the global score for OSAD [52]. The eight categories include:

- Approach – Constructive, supportive, and nonthreatening
- Learning environment – Clear expectation, safe, and supportive
- Learner engagement – Learner-centric discussion, active listening, silence
- Reaction – Exploration of the initial emotions/reactions
- Reflection – Self-reflect on one's actions
- Analysis – Examination of the reasons/consequences behind the actions
- Diagnosis – Positive and constructive feedback, close the gaps
- Application – Reinforcement of learning points, application to practice

These instruments of faculty assessment provide a guide to ECMO simulation programs to help maintain high-quality simulations and debriefings. Moreover, these tools provide guidelines for the novice/inexperienced faculty to rate themselves and reinforce the essentials of the effective debriefing. Lastly, faculty assessment tools provide the simulation program with objective data that can be used to make decisions about continued involvement as ECMO simulation faculty, and/or identify individuals who might benefit from further training, mentoring, and/or coaching.

Future Directions and Sustainment

This chapter has addressed the scope of ECMO simulation faculty development including informal and formal approaches, theoretical frameworks to guide learning, and the design and development of an ECMO faculty simulation training program. The healthcare environment is rapidly evolving due to changes in care delivery, advanced technology, and increased patient expectations. Accordingly, simulation faculty will need ongoing education to help maintain and update their skills as new evidence emerges on the best practice(s) to employ in simulation-based education in the healthcare environment. Thus, an infrastructure should be established to promote skill building and networking in conjunction with the establishment of a professional simulation CoP. The CoP will provide opportunities for meaningful exchange of information to build new knowledge and understanding, and develop approaches to problems faced in facilitating simulation-based education [53]. Equally important is the recognition that the needs of the ECMO simulation program will evolve and change, necessitating constant monitoring to identify when to adapt or replace the existing curriculum as new trends or needs emerge [54]. In many ways, it may be time to alter the thinking from formal faculty workshops to home-grown faculty workshops guided by the current and future simulation training standards, a standardized ECMO curriculum and ELSO guidelines for training and practice. In addition, faculty development requires organizational support as evidenced by financial support and/or protected faculty education time because it is a critical component to the sustainment and success of the ECMO simulation and faculty development programs. Highly motivated and trained faculty are a valuable resource. Promotion and facilitation of the faculties' career advancement and their development in simulation-based education will enhance, improve, and increase the ECMO simulation program's value, worth, and outcomes.

Appendix 18.1: Simulation Faculty Program Example

1. Problem identification and general NA:

   After the release of the 1999 Institute of Medicine report "To Err is Human… [48]" the Committee on Quality of Healthcare in America stated that healthcare system and policy must drastically change to ensure safe, quality healthcare. One of the recommendations was reformation of healthcare education by using simulation. Simulation education may possibly improve healthcare by improving the healthcare professionals' performance to enhance safety and quality of patient care.

   - Current approach: Simulation centers are using content experts as faculty to conduct ECMO simulation exercises. This teacher-centric approach is demonstrating deficiencies in the knowledge, skills and attitudes in simulation practice.
   - Ideal approach: Simulation ECMO faculty should be trained to the performance standards in the knowledge, skills, and behaviors of the learner-centric approach in simulation-based education to produce high-quality simulation learning experiences.

2. Targeted needs assessment (NA)
   - Targeted learners: all personnel functioning as simulation ECMO faculty
   - Needs assessment/Targeted learners:
     - Performance deficiencies

       Previous training in simulation facilitation or debriefing –none to moderate level of experience

       Faculty lecture material, no questioning, and no active reflection

       Don't allow learners to make mistakes

       Debriefing is biased and one-sided, and excessive negativism
     - Causes of deficiencies

       No formal facilitator training program

       Inefficient on the job training of facilitation and debriefing

       Knowledge and skills deficiency of facilitation and debriefing

       Knowledge deficiency in adult learning principles and theories

       Time constraints

       Content experts are assumed to be good facilitators

       Self-confidence of facilitator
   - Needs assessment/Learning environment:
     - No developed curricula for simulation faculty development.
     - There are no funds available to support this program.
     - There is not dedicated space to conduct this program
     - There is little demand/awareness by the organizational leaders.

3. Goals and Objectives

   (a) Goal:

   The simulation ECMO faculty workshop is a combination of didactic and experiential learning to increase your knowledge in concepts of adult learning and improve your skills as an effective simulation facilitator.

   (b) Objectives:

   (i) Describe the fundamentals and theories in simulation-based education.

   (ii) Create a comprehensive ECMO simulation exercise utilizing the step-by-step approach in simulation design.

  - (iii) Practice conversation strategies to promote critical thinking and clinical reasoning in debriefing exercises.
  - (iv) Demonstrate effective debriefing using reflective learning and integration of knowledge to close performance gaps.
  - (v) Evaluate effectiveness of your simulation design on meeting learning outcomes on multiple evaluation levels.

4. Educational Strategies (mixed mode approach)
   - (a) Describe the fundamentals and theories in simulation-based education.
     - (i) Content: Basic principles of simulation, terminology, theory
     - (ii) Lectures, readings, small group discussion, interactive games
   - (b) Create a comprehensive ECMO simulation exercise by using a systematic approach in simulation design.
     - (i) Content: Simulation design – Needs assessment to evaluation, matching modalities to learning outcomes, scenario development
     - (ii) Learning project, discussion, lecture, team-based learning
   - (c) Practice conversation strategies to promote critical thinking and clinical reasoning in debriefing exercises.
     - (i) Content: Debriefing, questioning techniques, disruptive behaviors, debriefing the debriefer
     - (ii) Role play, reflective learning, feedback on performance, video, discussion
   - (d) Demonstrate effective debriefing using reflective learning and integration of knowledge to close performance gaps
     - (i) Content: Develop, operate, and debrief a scenario
     - (ii) Reflective learning, discussion, feedback on performance, role plays, video
   - (e) Evaluate effectiveness of your simulation design on meeting learning outcomes on multiple levels.
     - (i) Content: Evaluation and assessment methods
     - (ii) Small group learning, discussion
5. Implementation
   - (a) Resources
     - (i) Personnel:
       1. A simulation interprofessional workgroup developed the workshop curriculum as per the needs assessment.
       2. Simulation Trained Faculty: 3:1 ratio for a 3-day workshop at 8.5 h/day.
       3. Support Staff:
       4. Administrative Assistant/secretary: assists with the copying and collating of the workshop materials, reservation of the facilities, data tabulation, and workshop certificates.
       5. Simulation Technician: assists with set up and break down for the various learning activities for the entire workshop.
     - (ii) Facilities, Equipment, Materials
       1. Facilities: Large conference room for lecture and several breakout/simulation rooms to execute simulation exercises. Debriefing rooms would be ideal but if not available, the large conference room will suffice.
       2. Equipment: Projector, computer with PPT, flip charts, AV equipment for videotaping, various simulators to utilize for simulation exercises and the availability of a Xerox machine for handouts.
     - (iii) Funding
       1. External funding: If applicable, what is the cost for external participants? Is there funding to pay the workshop faculty? Is there funding to assist with development of faculty?
       2. Internal funding: Is there funding from organization/department for snacks, drinks, and/or lunch? Is there funding for the workshop materials?
     - (iv) Internal and External Support
       1. Internal Support:
          - (a) Is the workshop supported by the Simulation Center Leaders (Medical Director, Administrative Director, Manager, Educators) and Administration of the organization?
          - (b) Is there support from the learners? Does the workshop help learners to achieve their personal goals?
       2. External Support:
          - (a) Is there funding from external agencies, governing bodies, and grants to support the workshop?
          - (b) Are there accreditation standards for the workshop?
     - (v) Administration
       1. There should be one designated person to serve as the Course Coordinator/Director. She/he coordinates the lectures, simulations, agenda-syllabus, updating of materials, and review of evaluation results. Additionally, this person is responsible for the recruitment and communication to faculty and learners regarding the curriculum.
     - (vi) Barriers
       - (i) Commitment-simulation workshop faculty to participate in the 3-day Simulation Facilitator Workshop on a volunteer basis
       - (ii) Faculty Turnover – change in interest or responsibilities to the organization. Need a

faculty development feeder program to mitigate this potential issue
- (iii) Time – Request for shorter, focused workshops from the learners and faculty because they cannot commit for the 3 days. Need to be adaptable
- (iv) Space – Adequate to conduct the workshop so there is ample space to do all activities. Should try to schedule workshop at minimum 1 year in advance
- (v) Motivation and Buy-in: faculty to participate in the workshop
- (vi) Resources: lack of institutional support and resources for the workshop

1. Introduction of curriculum
   - (a) There are several ways to introduce the curriculum of the faculty workshop.
     - (i) Pilot – test segments or the entire curriculum with designated audience.
     - (ii) Review of the curriculum evaluations, modifications should be implemented prior to full implementation.
   - (b) Phasing-in (also known as stratification and/or tiered approach) is a progressive build of content from simple to complex one segment at a time geared toward the level of learner – novice to expert. The tiered approach allows the faculty to develop a personalized plan of development on the basis of a structured level of progression [2]. It creates a learning experience with ongoing support, continuous feedback and redo from peers and mentors to develop a wide range of skills before progressing to the next level. The tiered approach enhances the faculties' confidence in their abilities which is beneficial for themselves and the learners [2]. Breaking down the skill sets can make the process more manageable for the novice faculty, plus lessen the resistance and increase acceptance especially if the stakeholders and/or healthcare organization is involved in the process.
   - (c) Full implementation – occurs after piloting or phasing-in unless there is a demand from the audience/healthcare organization to start immediately.

Step 6: Evaluation (see Appendices 18.2, 18.3, and 18.4)

- It determines if the goal and objectives have been met.
- It determines if the content is appropriate for the level of learners.
- It identifies the aspects of the curriculum activities that are working.

Appendix 18.2

THE CHILDREN'S HOSPITAL OF PHILADELPHIA
Overall Evaluation Facilitator Simulation Workshop (Reaction)

Date ______________________

Name (optional) ______________________

Instructors

We value your feedback, please take the time to complete this evaluation by answering the questions below.
Please check the most appropriate answer to each of the questions using the code given.

Poor	1
Fair	2
Good	3
Very Good	4
Excellent	5

Overall Rating of Workshop	1	2	3	4	5
Content					
Materials					
Trainer					
Presentations					
Methods of Instruction					
Environment					
Training Atmosphere	1	2	3	4	5
General atmosphere enhanced learning					
Course fostered teamwork					
Training Methods	1	2	3	4	5
Lectures with Questions and Anwers					
Whole Group Discussion					
Small Group Activities					
Simulation					
Video Review					
Debriefing Exercise					

THE CHILDREN'S HOSPITAL OF PHILADELPHIA
Overall Evaluation Facilitator Simulation Workshop (Reaction)

Strongly Agree	1
Agree	2
Neither agree or disagree	3
Disagree	4
Strongly Dusagree	5

Course Design and Content	1	2	3	4	5
Material presented was understandable					
Pace of course was appropriate					
Objectives were achieved					
Covered topics I needed to learn					
Difficulty level is appropriate					
Enough time devoted to each module					
Enough time given for feedback/questions					
Training met my expectatin					
Training is related to my job assignements					
Training covered will improve my performance					
Exercises contributed to learning					
Trainers Delivery	1	2	3	4	5
Sufficient knowledge of subject					
Communicate well					
Open, honest and fair to all					
Effectively presented material					
Organized					
Modules Covered adequately	1	2	3	4	5
Module 1: Simulation Medical Education					
Module 2: Adult Learning Principles					
Module 3: Role of Facilitator					
Module 4: Debriefing					
Module 5: Crisis Resource Management					

THE CHILDREN'S HOSPITAL OF PHILADELPHIA
Overall Evaluation Facilitator Simulation Workshop (Reaction)

Instructors performed well			1	2	3	4	5	N/A

What part of the course did you enjoy the most? Why?

What part of the course did you enjoy least? Why?

What is the most important thing that you have learned in the course?

Please write briefly any suggestions or recommendations for improvements or additions to the this course?

Thank You for completing the Evaluation!

Appendix 18.3

THE CHILDREN'S HOSPITAL OF PHILADELPHIA
Simulation Facilitator Course Session Evaluation

Date ________________ **Day 1: Modules 1, 2 & 3**

Name (optional) ________________________________

Instructors:
____

1. What part of the session was most useful? Why

2. What part of the session was least useful today? Why?

3. What is the most important thing you learned today?

4. If you found it difficult to participate today, please give your reasons and suggestions on how the situation could be improved.

5. Were the session objectives met?

6. Any feedback and/or suggestions regarding my facilitation please?

7. Additional Comments

Appendix 18.4

Date ________________ **Day 2: Module 4**

Name (optional) ________________________________

Instructors: ________________________________

1. What part of the session was most useful? Why

2. What part of the session was least useful today? Why?

3. What is the most important thing you learned today?

5. Were the session objectives met?

6. Any feedback and/or suggestions regarding my facilitation please?

7. Additional Comments

References

1. Issenberg BSMW, Petrusa ER, Lee GD, Scalese RJ. Features and uses of high-fidelity medical simulation that lead to effective learning: a BEME systematic review. Med Teach. 2005;27(1): 10–28.
2. Hendricson WDAE, Andrieu SC, Chadwick DG, Cole JR, George MC, et al. Does faculty development enhance teaching effectiveness? J Dent Educ. 2007;71(12):1513–33.
3. Steinert Y. Faculty development: core concepts and principles. In: Faculty development in the health professions. New York/London: Springer; 2014. p. 3–25.
4. French H, Hales RL. Neonatology faculty development using simulation. Semin Perinatol. 2016;40:455–65.
5. Centra JA. Types of faculty development programs. J High Educ. 1978;49(2):151–62.
6. Beach ALSM, Austin AE, Rivard JK. Introduction. In: Faculty development in the age of evidence. Sterling: Stylus Publishing Inc; 2016. p. 1–15.
7. Eells WC. The origin and early history of sabbatical leave. AAUP. 1962;48(3):253–6.
8. Sorenelli MD, Austin AE, Eddy PL, Beach AL. The evolution of faculty development creating the future of faculty development. Bolton: Anker Publishing Company, Inc; 2006. p. 1–28.
9. Sorcinelli M, Austin AE, Eddy PL, Beach AL. Current issues addressed by faculty development. In: Creating the future of faculty development: learning from the past, understanding the present. Bolton: Anker Publishing Company, Inc; 2006. p. 69–99.
10. Bland CJSC, Stritter F, Henry R, Aluise J. Successful faculty in academic medicine: essential skills and how to acquire them. New York: Springer Publishing; 1990.
11. Dewey J. Experience and education. New York: Macmillan; 1997.
12. Paige JTAS, Fernandez G, Seymour N. Debriefing 101: training faculty to promote learning in simulation based training. Am J Surg. 2015;209:126–31.
13. Kolb DA. Experiential learning: experience as the source of learning and development. Englewood Cliffs: Prentice Hall; 1984.
14. Knowles MS, Holton EF, Swanson RA. The theory of adult learning, andragogy. In: The adult learner. 7th ed. New York: Routledge; 2012. p. 34–71.
15. Brown JSCA, Duguid P. Situated cognition and the culture of learning. Educ Res. 1989;18(1):32–42.
16. Lave JWE. Situated learning; legitimate peripheral participation. New York: Cambridge University Press; 1991.
17. Dreyfus SDH. A five stage model of the mental activities involved in directed skill acquistion 1980 [cited California University Berkley Operations Research Center (monograph).
18. Perspective Transformation JM. Adult education quarterly. In: Mezirow J, Taylor EW, editors. Transformative learning in action: a handbook for practice, vol. 28. San Francisco: Jossey-Bass; 2009.
19. EW Taylor. Transformative learning theory. In: Jovita M. Ross-Gordon Joellen E. Coryell editor. New directions for adult and continuing education. Waco, Texas: Wiley. Periodicals Inc.; 2008.
20. de Grave WZA, Mansvelder-Longayroux DD, Molenaar WM. Workshops and seminars: enhancing effectiveness. Faculty development in the health professions: a focus on research and practice. New York: Springer; 2014. p. 181–95.
21. Steinert Y, Mann K, Centeno A, Dolmans D, Spencer J, Gelula M. A systematic review of faculty development initiatives designed to improve teaching effectiveness in medical education. Med Teach. 2006;28:497–26.
22. Navedo DSR. Specialized courses in simulation. In: Levine AL, Bryson EO, DeMaria S, Schwartz AD, editors. The comprehensive textbook of healthcare simulation. New York: Springer; 2013. p. 593–7.
23. Searle NSTB, Perkowski LC. Making it work: the evolution of the medical educational fellowship program. Acad Med. 2006;81(11):984–9.
24. Steinert Y. Developing medical educators: a journey not a destination. In: Understanding medical education, evidence, theory and practice Chichester. West Suussex: Wiley Blackwell; 2014. p. 455–71.
25. Swanwick T. See one, do one, then what? Faculty development in postgraduate medical education. Postgrad Med J. 2008;84:339–43.
26. Collins ABJ, Newman S. Cognitive apprenticeship: teaching the crafts of reading, writing and mathematics. In: Knowing, learning and instruction: essays in honour of Robert Glaser. Hillsdale: Lawrence Erlbaum Associates; 1989. p. 453–94.
27. Wooley NNJY. Situated cognition and cognitive apprenticeship: a model for teaching and learning clinical skills in a technologically rich and authetic learning environment. Nurs Educ Today. 2007;27(1):73–9.
28. Boillat MEM. Peer coaching and mentorship. In: Faculty development in the health professions. New York: Springer; 2014. p. 159–79.
29. Lopreiato JODD, Gammon W, Lioce L, Sittner B, Slot V, Spain A. Healthcare simulation dictionary. society of simulation in healthcare [Internet]. 2016. Available from: http://wwe.ssih.org/dictionary.
30. Cheng AGV, Huffman J, Burgess G, Szyid D, Robinson T, Eppich W. Coaching the debriefer: peer coaching to improve debriefing auality in simulation programs. Simul Healthc. 2017;12(5):319–25.
31. Peterson DTWP, Chapps CA, White ML. Simulation faculty development: a tiered approach. Simul Healthc. 2017;12(4):254–9.
32. Wenger EMR, Snyder W. Cultivating communities of practice. Boston: Harvard Business School Press; 2002.
33. Kaufman DMMK. Teaching and learning in medical education: how theory can inform practice. In: Understanding medical education: evidence, theory and practice. 2nd ed. Chichester/West Sussex: Wiley Blackwell; 2014. p. 7–29.
34. National Academy of Sciences NAoE, Institute of Medicine. Advisor, teacher, role model, friend: on being a mentor to students in science and engineering. Washington, DC: National Academy Press; 1997.
35. Steinert Y. Developing medical educators: a journey, not a destination. In: Understanding medical education-evidence, theory and practice. West Sussex: Wiley Blackwell; 2014. p. 455–73.
36. Steinert Y. Facutly development: from workshops to community practice. Med Teach. 2010;32(5):425–8.
37. Jackevicius CALJ, Nazer L, Hess K, Wang J, Law AV. Faculty development-A formal mentorship program for faculty development. Am J Pharm Educ. 2014;78(5):1–7.
38. Cruess SRCR, Steinert Y. Role modelling—making the most of a powerful teaching. BMJ. 2008;336:718–21.
39. Commitee I. INACSL standards of best practice: simulation-facilitation. Clin Simul Nurs. 2016;12:S16–20.
40. Simulation CfAoH. Teaching/education standards and measurements. Washington, DC: Society of Simulation in Healthcare; 2016.
41. Alexander M, Carol Alexander M, Durhan C, Hooper JI, Jeffries P, Goldman N, Kardong-Edgren S, et al. NCSBN simulation guidelines for prelicensure nursing programs. J Nurs Regul. 2015;6:39–42.
42. Banfi CBK, Giraud R. High-fidelity simulation for extracorporeal membrane oxygenation training, utile or futile? J Thorac Dis. 2017;9:4283–5.
43. ELSO. ELSO Guidelines for ECMO Centers. Ann Arbor: ELSO; 2014.
44. Weiss MFFP, Nelson LP, Rake AJ, Klee L, Stein JE, TA S. The role of extracorporeal membrane oxygenation simulation training at Extracorporeal Life Support Organization Centers in the United States. Simul Healthc. 2017;12(4):233–9.

45. Brazzi LLA, Panigada M, Bottino N, Patroniti N, Pappalardo F, et al. Simulation-based training of extracorporeal membrane oxygenation during H1N1 influenza pandemic: the Italian experience. Simul Healthc. 2012;7:32–4.
46. Johnston LSS. Development of ECMO simulation program: Experience at Yale New Haven Hospital. Medical Training Magazine [Internet]. 2012 July 2. Available from: https://medical-simulation.training/technology/development-of-an-ecmo-simulation-program-experience-at-yale-new-haven-hospital/.
47. Zigmong JON, Szyld D, Maestre J. Educator training and simulation methodology courses. In: Defining excellence in simulation programs. Philadelphia: Wolters Kluwer; 2015. p. 546–72.
48. Thomas PAKD, Hughes MT, Chen BY. Curriculum development for medical education: a six step approach. 3rd ed. Baltimore: The John Hopkins University Press; 2016.
49. ME C. Effect of faculty training on improving the consistency of student assessment and debriefing in clinical simulation. Clin Simul Nurs. 2015;11(1):64–71.
50. Minehart RDRJ, Pian-Smith MCM, Raemer DB. Improving faculty feedback to resident trainees during a simulated case: a randomized controlled of an educational intervention. Anesthesiology. 2014;120(1):160–71.
51. Simon RRD, Rudolph JW. Debriefing Assessment for Simulation in Healthcare (DASH)© Rater's handbook. Boston: Center for Medical Simulation; 2010.
52. Arora SAM, Page J, Nestel D, Runnacles J, Hull L, et al. Objective structured assessment of debriefing: bringing science to the art of debriefing in surgery. Ann Surg. 2012;256(6):982.
53. Steinert Y. Faculty development: Future directions. In: Steinert Y, editor. Faculty development in the health professions: a focus on research and practice. Philadelphia: Springer; 2014. p. 421–42.
54. Lieff SJ. Faculty development: yesterday, today and tomorrow: guide supplement 33.2 – viewpoint. Med Teach. 2010;32:429–31.

19 Quality Improvement

Kimberly W. Kyle, Lara P. Nelson, and Rachel L. Chapman

Learning Objectives

1. Define continuous quality improvement and describe importance in optimizing ECMO team performance and outcomes
2. Define the concepts of Safety I, Safety II, and the relevance to simulation in your own ECMO program
3. Describe the potential use of simulation to improve a specific process or outcome measure relative to ECMO

K. W. Kyle
ECMO Department, Children's Hospital Los Angeles, Los Angeles, CA, USA

Department of Pediatrics, Keck School of Medicine, University of Southern California, Los Angeles, CA, USA

L. P. Nelson
ECMO Department, Children's Hospital Los Angeles, Los Angeles, CA, USA

Department of Pediatrics, Keck School of Medicine, University of Southern California, Los Angeles, CA, USA

Division of Critical Care Medicine, Department of Anesthesiology Critical Care Medicine, Children's Hospital Los Angeles, Los Angeles, CA, USA

R. L. Chapman (✉)
Department of Pediatrics, Keck School of Medicine, University of Southern California, Los Angeles, CA, USA

Fetal and Neonatal Institute, Division of Neonatology, Children's Hospital Los Angeles, Los Angeles, CA, USA
e-mail: rachapman@chla.usc.edu

Introduction

A commitment to quality improvement is critical when performing a low-volume, but high-stakes, high-intensity therapy due to the high risk for complications, including significant morbidity and mortality. As it pertains to an ECMO program, simulation can be utilized for both Continuous Quality Improvement (CQI) and as a key component of Total Quality Management (TQM), including identification and mitigation of safety threats and development of resilient systems. In this chapter, we will review key concepts in quality improvement science and provide examples from the literature and our experiences of how simulation can be utilized to enhance the function of our ECMO teams, optimize patient safety, and improve patient outcomes.

Background and Terminology

Simulation

Simulation is a training and educational tool being used with increasing frequency in healthcare. The underlying principle of simulation is to create as realistic a clinical environment as possible to allow learners the opportunity to perform "as they would" in a real patient situation. Instructors are afforded the opportunity to observe learners' likely realistic responses while in a stressful environment, as opposed to theoretical verbal descriptions of what they would do while sitting in a classroom, and then to provide real-time feedback to improve performance.

Simulation may be implemented in low- to high-fidelity models and encompassing simple to complex clinical scenarios. Due to the unique nature of the simulation environment, factors beyond clinical knowledge or technical skills may also be evaluated. The potential for simulation as a method for testing changes to optimize performance of the

L. C. Johnston, L. Su (eds.), *Comprehensive Healthcare Simulation: ECMO Simulation*, Comprehensive Healthcare Simulation,
https://doi.org/10.1007/978-3-030-53844-6_19

team is enormous, and is being increasingly described in the literature, including in extracorporeal support, as a strategy to facilitate sustainable improvement in actual clinical performance and will be described in greater detail later in this chapter [1–3].

Continuous Quality Improvement (CQI)

CQI is a process defined by the US Department of Health and Human Services as "the systematic process of identifying, describing, and analyzing strengths and problems and then testing, implementing, learning from, and revising solutions [4]." It is a formalized way of:

- Examining and describing what we currently do
- Determining what does and does not work
- Identifying and implementing a change
- Learning from the results of the change
- Continuing to revise the process to optimize outcomes.

The opportunity to identify potential changes to improve patient outcomes and avoid adverse events demands systematic collection, review, and utilization of comprehensive institutional data, including review of adverse events and near misses.

Within a clinical ECMO program, this starts with a CQI Champion, who identifies a CQI team composed of multiple stakeholders in the program, which may include ECMO specialists, nurses, respiratory therapists, surgeons, critical care/neonatology physicians, perfusionists, and patient families. The CQI team is then charged with the identification of opportunities for improvement and determining the best means for implementing the change. One specific tool available for this process is simulation.

Total Quality Management (TQM)

In healthcare services, TQM is a management method utilized to optimize systems in order to improve outcomes for patients, reduce costs, and maintain a culture to enhance patient safety [5]. TQM requires a commitment to lead and champion culture change, and to develop a culture where employees continuously work to improve their ability to provide quality care. Employees need to feel or appreciate the reasons change is necessary. Therefore, in order to achieve effective organizational change, leadership needs to create this need or desire. "Lack of leadership support is the most frequently cited barrier to implementing and sustaining patient safety interventions" [6]. Here too, simulation allows a unique perspective by creating an environment to observe behaviors and interactions, unmasking previously unstated or unrecognized parts of the culture.

Systems Thinking

Systems thinking, at its core, is a theory aimed at evaluating how things are connected to each other [7]. Using simulation as a tool within systems thinking brings with it a wide application of possibilities. Simulation facilitates the bringing together of the multidisciplinary team, individual, or system with the ability to discover the broader "approaches," "perspectives," or "lenses" of an event [7]. This approach can focus on understanding and improving processes rather than focusing on the errors of individuals.

Utilizing these concepts, simulation can be used to facilitate program improvement through benchmarking performance and utilizing CQI and enhancing culture with TQM to improve outcomes. Simulation may also be used to enhance and optimize safety not only through mitigation of known risks, but additionally by identification of latent safety threats, as discussed further below.

Quality Indicators: Benchmarking Performance and Optimizing Safety

Benchmarking Performance

There are multiple opportunities for benchmarking performance within an ECMO program, including: (1) ECMO specific registries, such as the Extracorporeal Life Support Organization (ELSO); (2) patient population specific registries, such as the Congenital Diaphragmatic Hernia Study Group (CDHSG), Society for Thoracic Surgeons National Database (STS), the Children's Hospital Neonatal Consortium (CHNC); (3) complication/safety specific registries, such as Children's Hospitals' Solutions for Patient Safety (SPS) and the National Healthcare Safety Network (NHSN); and (4) program, unit, or hospital wide databases [8–13]. It is critical to identify key indicators for benchmarking within an ECMO program, and some or all of these databases can help to identify opportunities for improvement plus areas of strength, either locally or more broadly. Important qualities of benchmarking databases that relate to their capacity to define areas for improvement and allow for tracking of progress, include the granularity and clinical relevance of the data available, as well as the frequency of collection and reporting.

As pointed out in the most recent publication reporting outcomes from ELSO, variation in clinical outcomes, such as intracranial hemorrhage, frequency of mechanical complications, and duration of CPR prior to establishment of ECMO support in ECPR were correlated with survival and may be appropriate targets for quality improvement within and among ECMO Programs [14].

Performance Management for Optimizing Safety

When we think of safety, it is usually by reference to its opposite, the absence of safety. Historically, safety improvement was analyzed retrospectively, looking at events after they had transpired, the "what went wrong" approach that is now referred to as Safety-I. The traditional view of Safety-I has consequently been defined by the absence of accidents and incidents, or as the "freedom from unacceptable risk" [15]. As a result, the focus of safety research and safety management has usually been on *unsafe* system operation rather than on *safe* operation. This theory of safety improvement has been met with limited success due to its reactive nature. According to Woods, "a brittle system is the opposite of a resilient system" [16]. He further states that the value of disruptions in a system simultaneously shows how the system in question can stretch and adapt to given disruptions and the limits on the capacity to handle or buffer those challenges. The risk with only looking retrospectively is that there is the possibility of missing warning signs of possible increased safety risks that would be better addressed by looking proactively, allowing for organizations to identify when brittleness is increasing and evaluate effective sources of resilience [16, 17].

Resilience Engineering (RE) aims to move away from retrospectivity and evaluation of failures to learn from what goes right [17]. Ensuring things go right, proactive safety management, corresponds to a view of safety called Safety-II, which defines safety as the ability to succeed under varying conditions [15]. RE maintains that "things go wrong" and "things go right" for the same basic reasons. The understanding of everyday functioning is therefore a necessary prerequisite for the understanding of safety performance. This will change the definition of safety from "avoiding something going wrong" to "ensuring that everything goes right" – or increasing the ability to succeed under varying conditions so the number of intended and acceptable outcomes is as high as possible. The consequence of this is that the basis for safety and safety management now becomes an understanding of why things go right, which requires a thorough understanding of everyday activities [18]. RE focuses on the organizational level and stresses the importance of real-time flexibility in the work environment. A resilient system will adjust its functioning prior to, during, or following changes and disturbances, so it can sustain required operations and appropriately adjust for both expected and unexpected conditions.

RE perspectives, such as proposed by Anderson and Hollnagel, discuss the need to understand the work environment and the difference between "work as imagined" (WAI) in protocols, procedures and "work as done" (WAD) in practice [18, 19]. The gap between these two concepts can be viewed as a threat to safety. This use of WAI and WAD concepts can be useful when looking at innovation versus standardization and the ability of the system to adjust to the changing work environment.

The use of Safety-I/Safety-II and RE theories in combination with ECMO simulation can provide a platform to both proactively and retrospectively assess what works and what does not in the patient care environment. It can be used to fill the gap between WAI and WAD, allowing for the frontline provider working in the clinical environment to address the varying working conditions they encounter, including high census, high acuity, and lack of resources. Simulation creates an environment with the ability to respond, monitor, learn, and anticipate. Hollnagel et al. make a conditional case that training to respond to regular threats can make the system "more robust and less brittle," albeit if the temptation to standardize and reduce adaptive responses is avoided [20].

Improving and Sustaining Performance

The building blocks of quality improvement are centered on the improvement cycle, otherwise known as the Plan-Do-Study-Assess (PDSA) cycle (Fig. 19.1). The process entails

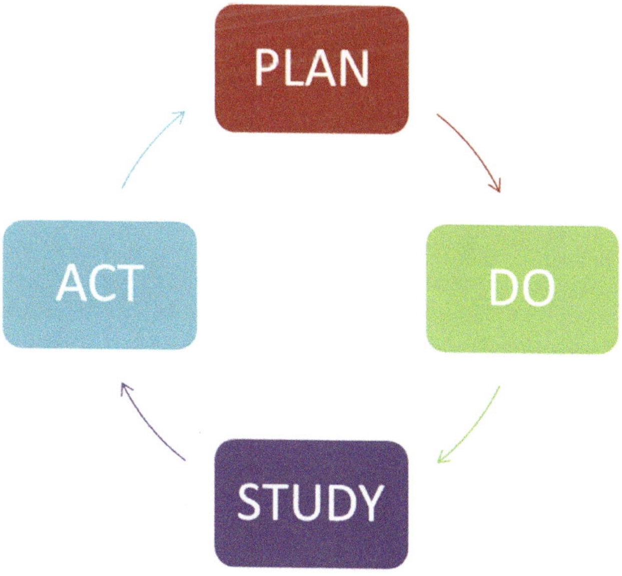

Fig. 19.1 PDSA cycle

planning a change (plan), testing the change (do), observing results (study), and acting upon what is learned (act), often leading to additional cycles or tests of change with a goal of achieving sustained improvement [21, 22]. Before initiating quality improvement work, however, it is important to define the following:

1. *What are we trying to accomplish?*

   Identification of a specific problem and what improvement is desired is crucial to beginning the process. It is often helpful to specify the patient population, in addition to the specific outcome desired. As an example, an ECMO team may wish to reduce the time from decision to proceed with ECMO to initiation of flow in neonates cannulated for respiratory failure over the next 2 years. The problem is prolonged time between decision and initiation (a complex system problem), it is measurable, and a timeline has been established. This particular outcome is a systems outcome, but one could also establish an additional clinical outcome, such as decreased time spent with preductal oxygenation saturation below 80% or time to normalization of serum lactate.
2. *How will we know that a change is an improvement*?

   Prior to initiating a QI initiative, it is critical to define metrics of success. This involves determining what will be measured (establishing measures), how often it will be measured, and what incremental change is desired. Returning to the example above, the team may start with assessing recent performance and benchmarking performance using a comparative database. Based on this information, the team would identify an initial goal for improvement. For example, if over the past 2 years, time from decision to initiation ranged from 90 to 130 min with an average time of 100 min, an initial improvement goal may be to decrease the average time to <90 min.

   It is critically important to be able to determine if improvement is actually happening and also to track sustainability of improvement efforts. This is often most effectively accomplished through the use of a run chart, which is a graph of outcome data (y axis) over time (x axis) [22]. A run chart is an effective way of displaying changes to your QI team, bedside staff, as well as program and hospital leadership. The Institute for Healthcare Quality offers run chart development tools that allow the team to graph data over time to help determine whether or not changes made are associated with improvement and whether improvement is sustained [23].

Examples

Two recent examples of the use of simulation for CQI to improve outcomes in the live clinical environment have been described in the literature. Su and colleagues described the use of a simulation program to improve performance of eCPR within a single institution. They used process mapping and identification of discrete teams, processes, and roles for the development of in situ simulations of deployment of eCPR in the setting of witnessed cardiac arrest occurring in the cardiac ICU or cardiac operating room during both day and night shifts over a 3-year period [2]. The primary outcome was time to initiation of ECMO support pre- and post-intervention and was significantly decreased from a median time of 51 min to 41 min in the post-intervention period, with a trend toward decreasing time in each of the 3 years post-intervention.

Di Nardo and colleagues retrospectively examined the association between the development of a simulation-based educational program and time to manage ECMO emergencies in a pediatric intensive care unit of a tertiary children's hospital [3]. The simulation-based educational program for the ECMO team started with 16 h of simulation-based instruction in the initial ECMO training and continued with quarterly simulation sessions, focusing on management of ECMO emergencies. Actual ECMO emergencies were evaluated as pre- and post-simulation based education eras, and were notable for a decrease in the median time to emergently change an oxygenator from 5.3 to 3.9 min and a decrease in the time to manage an air embolism from 22 to 15 min.

Similar to Di Nardo and colleagues, we have developed a simulation-based program for our ECMO team, which includes component change simulations (cone, bladder, tubing) and management of air embolism in an effort to reduce time off ECMO. The results of our center's simulations of actual ECMO emergencies were similar. For example, we decreased time off ECMO for a cone change from pre-simulation times of >5 min to post-simulation times of <2 min, which is graphically demonstrated in a run chart (Fig. 19.2, unpublished data.).

Sustaining Performance

According to the Institute for Healthcare Improvement (IHI), using the components of "Framework for Spread" is essential to any organizational initiative to help sustain the changes and guide the spread activities [24]. It is never too early to plan for spread, but they suggest having key stakeholders onboard first. The role of leadership cannot be emphasized enough when both initiating and actively supporting the spread once underway. Assessment of the readiness of the organization is crucial to the success or failure of the change, a key component of TQM. Making sure the reasons for the initiative are understood will provide a solid platform on which to sustain the initiative. The IHI suggest the initial

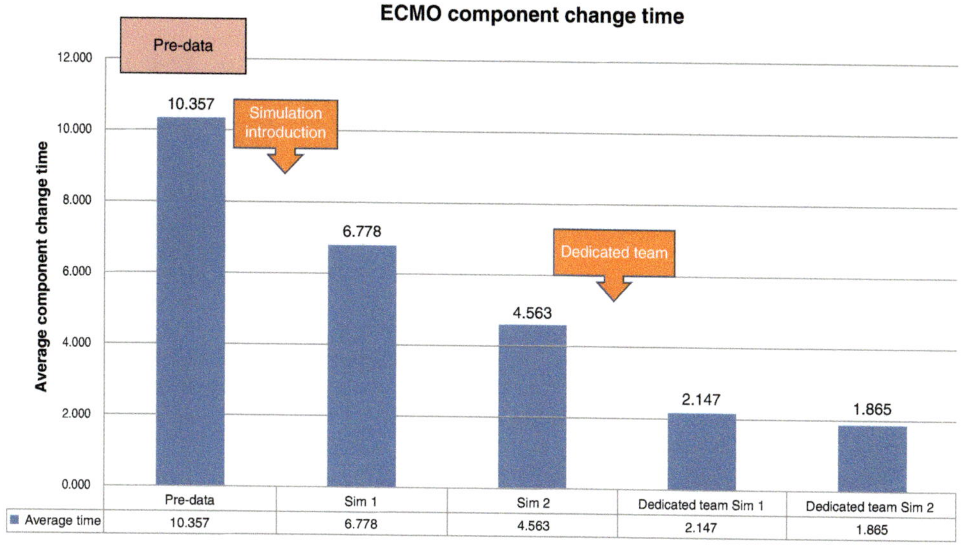

Fig. 19.2 Run chart: ECMO component change. Table represents time to change centrifugal pump-head (cone) before and after each PDSA cycle at a single institution (simulation-based training followed by transition to a dedicated specialist team); unpublished data

communication about the spread includes the "who, what, and where" and the following components:

1. *Establish an Aim for Spread*
   - The population (e.g., ECMO Department, surgeons, physicians, quality leaders, hospital administration)
   - The specific goals (e.g., improve time off ECMO while changing components, improve length of time to cannulation)
   - The specific improvements (e.g., decreasing the amount of time it takes to change a cone, reduce time from initiation of CPR to cannulation)
   - The time frame for the effort (e.g., 3 months, 6 months, 1 year)
2. *Develop an Initial Spread Plan*

   The spread plan addresses the "how" and includes communication and target population engagement, a measurement system to assess progress and the actions needed to make the changes in the organizations system [24]. Regular review of where the QI initiative is in the process (i.e., how many team members have completed simulation training) in the beginning, and then regular communication of the data, sharing run charts, clinical examples, and percentage of time an outcome goal has been made are all possible strategies. Regular reevaluations should be planned, including input from all team members and stakeholders, to allow ongoing reevaluation and assessment of sustainability of change or need for an additional PDSA cycle to achieve the desired goals.
3. *Disseminate Your Work*

   A local dissemination plan should include not only spreading to the clinical team, but should also consider spread of the components of change to other settings within your institution, as well as the spread to quality leaders and administrators within your institution. This will need to include the magnitude of change, how this has influenced outcomes and potential financial implications (e.g., fewer ECMO complications may mean less time on ECMO and is therefore likely both clinically and financially beneficial).

   It is also important to consider how to disseminate your work more broadly, including regional and national meetings. Target audiences could include attendees with particular interest in ECMO, as well as interest in quality improvement, simulation in healthcare, or specific neonatal, pediatric, or adult research meetings. While often daunting, it is also important to consider publishing your work since there remains a paucity of research into ECMO best clinical practices. The opportunities for dissemination are increasing because quality improvement science has become increasingly recognized as vital to patient outcomes and standard reporting guidelines have been developed to ensure rigorous standards. The SQUIRE (Standards for Quality Improvement Reporting Excellence) guidelines have been published by Ogrnic and colleagues, and were most recently revised in 2016 [25] and are also available through the SQUIRE website, which also includes multiple other resources for dissemination of quality improvement work [26].

Summary

Simulation as part of CQI can allow for optimization of performance of ECMO teams, and ultimately improve patient outcomes. A robust simulation program can provide the necessary tools to potentially mitigate the risks associated with ECMO (a low-volume, high-risk therapy), optimize team performance, and improve patient outcomes. Simulation can be incorporated into improvement efforts to optimize safety in the critical care environment. Planned assessment of change and development of a framework to sustain and spread change is critical in optimizing performance and outcomes.

References

1. Burton KS, et al. Impact of simulation-based extracorporeal membrane oxygenation training in the simulation laboratory and clinical environment. Simul Heathc. 2011;6:284–91.
2. Su L, et al. Implementation of an extracorporeal cardiopulmonary resuscitation simulation program reduces extracorporeal cardiopulmonary resuscitation times in real patients. Pediatr Crit Care Med. 2014;15:856–60.
3. Di Nardo M, et al. The introduction of a high-fidelity simulation program for training pedicatric critical care personnel reduces times to manage extracorporeal membrane oxygenation emergencies and improves teamwork. J Thorac Dis. 2018;10:1409–70.
4. Quality improvement. U. S. Department of Health and Human Services Health Resources and Services Administration, April 2011. [Internet] [cited 2019 October 13] https://www.hrsa.gov/sites/default/files/quality/toolbox/508pdfs/qualityimprovement.pdf.
5. Ovretveit J. Total quality management in European healthcare. Int J Health Care Qual Assur. 2000;13:74–80.
6. Deitsch ES, Dong Y, Halamek L, Rosen MA, Taekman JM, Rice J. Leveraging health care simulation technology for human factors: closing the gap between lab and bedside. Hum Factors. 2016;58:1082–95.
7. Peters DH. The application of systems thinking in health: why use systms thinking? Health Res Policy Syst. 2014;12:51.
8. Extracoporeal Life Support Organization [Internet] [cited 2019 October 13] Available from: https://www.elso.org.
9. Congenital Diaphragmatic Hernia Study Group [Internet] [cited 2019 October 13] Available from:https://med.uth.edu/pediatricsurgery/research/research-centers-and-programs/cdhsg/.
10. Society for Thoracic Surgeons National Database [Internet] [cited 2019 October 13] Available from: https://www.sts.org/registries-research-center/sts-national-database.
11. Children's Hospital Neonatal Consortium [Internet] [cited 2019 October 13] Available from: http://thechnc.org/.
12. Children's Hospitals' Solutions for Patient Safety [Internet] [cited 2019 October 13] Available from: https://www.solutionsforpatientsafety.org/.
13. National Healthcare Safety Network [Internet] [cited 2019 October 13] Available from: https://www.cdc.gov/nhsn/index.html.
14. Barbaro RP, et al. Pediatric extracorporeal life support organization registry international report 2016. ASAIO J. 2017;63:456–63.
15. Patterson M, Deutsch ES. Safety-I, safety-II and resilience engineering. Curr Probl Pediatr Adolesc Health Care. 2015;45:382–9.
16. Woods DD. Four concepts for resilience and the implications for the future of resilience engineering. Reliab Eng Syst Saf. 2015;141:5–9.
17. Woods DD, Branlat M, Herrera I, Woltjer R. Where is the organization looking in order to be proactive about safety? A framework for revealing whether it is mostly looking back, also looking forward or simply looking away. J Conting Crisis Manag. 2015;23:97–105.
18. Anderson JE, Ross AJ, Back J, Snell P, Walsh K, Jaye P. Implementing resilience engineering for healthcare quality improvement using the CARE mode: a feasibility study protocol. Pilot Feasibil Stud. 2016;2:61.
19. Hollnagel E. A tale of two safeties. Nucl Safety Simul. 2013;4:1–9.
20. Hollnagel E. How resilent is your organization? An introduction to the resilience analysis grid (RAG). In: Sustainable transformation: building a resilient organization. Toronto; 2010. Available at: https://hal-mines-paristech.archives-ouvertes.fr/hal-00613986.
21. AHRQ Innovations Exchange. U.S. Department of Health and Human Services Agencey for Health Related Quality [Internet] [cited 2019 October 13]. Quality tool: PDSA cycle. Last updated April 10 2013. Available at: http://innovations.ahrq.gov/qualitytools/plan-do-study-act-pdsa-cycle.
22. Managing data for performance improvement. U. S. Department of Health and Human Services Health Resources and Services Administration, April 2011. [Internet] [cited 2019 October 13] https://www.hrsa.gov/sites/default/files/quality/toolbox/508pdfs/managingdataperformanceimprovement.pdf.
23. Institute for Health Care Improvement [Internet] [cited 2019 October 13]. Run Chart Tool. Available at: http://www.ihi.org/resources/Pages/Tools/RunChart.aspx.
24. Massoud MR, Nielsen GA, Nolan K, Schall MW, Sevin C. A framework for spread: from local improvments to system-wide change. In: IHI innovation series white paper. Cambridge, MA: Institute for Healthcare Improvement; 2006. (Available on www.IHI.org).
25. Ogrinc G, Davies L, Goodman D, Batalden PB, Davidoff F, Stevens D. SQUIRE 2.0 (*Standards for QUality Improvement Reporting Excellence*): revised publication guidelines from a detailed consensus process. BMJ Qual Saf. 2016;25:986–92.
26. Standards for Quality Improvement Reporting Excellence [Internet] [cited2019 October 13] Revised Standards for Quality Improvement Reporting Excellence SQUIRE 2.0. http://www.squire-statement.org/index.cfm?fuseaction=Page.ViewPage&pageId=471.

Part VI

Special Considerations for Different ECMO Populations

Neonatology

20

Anne M. Ades, Danielle J. W. Reed, and Elizabeth A. Wetzel

Learning Objectives

- To identify specific neonatal disease processes for ECMO simulation scenarios
- To recognize considerations unique to neonates for ECMO simulation curriculum development
- To describe technical aspects of neonatal ECMO simulation

Introduction/Chapter Overview

Neonatal ECMO has been used for the care of acutely ill neonates for >30 years. As some studies suggest that neonatal noncardiac ECMO use is decreasing, the importance of developing rigorous ECMO curricula for acquisition and maintenance of ECMO skill by neonatal providers is paramount [1]. Given the uniqueness of neonatal ECMO indications, management, physiology, and circuit design, specific educational curricula are needed for neonatal ECMO providers. This chapter will discuss the distinctive characteristics of neonatal noncardiac ECMO with a brief overview including clinical indications, criteria, complications, and outcomes for neonates undergoing ECMO. Next, educational needs of different ECMO providers will be reviewed. Finally, unique technology needed for ECMO neonatal simulations will be outlined as well as delineation of neonatal-specific scenarios that should be considered for inclusion in a neonatal ECMO simulation curricula. Information relevant to neonatal cardiac ECMO will be addressed in Chap. 22.

Background

The first successful use of neonatal ECMO was reported in newborns with respiratory failure in 1975 [2]. Neonatal ECMO continued to gain momentum, supporting 40 newborns over the next 5 years with 50% survival. Increasing numbers of prospective trials performed at major children's hospitals over the next two decades showed increasing numbers of survivors. Thus, ECMO became a recognized standard of care for neonatal respiratory failure unresponsive to maximal medical management [3]. Interestingly, over the last three decades, neonatal noncardiac ECMO cases have steadily declined. The mean number of neonatal cases per ECMO center was 16.2 in 1990, decreasing by 50% by 2000, and averaging only 3.1 case per ECMO center by 2010 [1]. With changes in delivery room management recommendations from the American College of Obstetricians and Gynecologists, fewer infants are born post-dates, decreasing the incidence of meconium stained fluid and therefore meconium aspiration syndrome [4]. In addition, newer therapies for neonatal hypoxemic respiratory failure such as high-frequency oscillatory ventilation, surfactant administration, and inhaled nitric oxide have improved the medical management for infants who previously may have only been rescued by ECMO [1]. Therefore, infants requiring ECMO support may be more critically ill with more comorbidities, making the need for a highly -skilled, well-trained ECMO team all the more important.

A. M. Ades (✉)
Division of Neonatology, Children's Hospital of Philadelphia, Perelman School of Medicine at the University of Pennsylvania, Philadelphia, PA, USA
e-mail: ades@email.chop.edu

D. J. W. Reed
Division of Neonatology, Department of Pediatrics, Children's Mercy-Kansas City, University of Missouri-Kansas City School of Medicine, Kansas City, MO, USA

E. A. Wetzel
Division of Neonatal-Perinatal Medicine, Riley Hospital for Children at Indiana University Health, Indiana University School of Medicine, Indianapolis, IN, USA

L. C. Johnston, L. Su (eds.), *Comprehensive Healthcare Simulation: ECMO Simulation*, Comprehensive Healthcare Simulation,
https://doi.org/10.1007/978-3-030-53844-6_20

The Extracorporeal Life Support Organization, or ELSO, began a registry for ECMO data starting in 1990. Approximately 40,000 neonates have been treated with ECMO according to the ELSO registry by the end of 2018 [5]. Pulmonary disease is the most frequent reason neonates are placed on ECMO with congenital diaphragmatic hernia (CDH) now being the most common diagnosis [1]. Less common uses for ECMO in neonates include rescue therapy for failure of return of spontaneous circulation during cardiopulmonary resuscitation (E-CPR) and stabilization before or after airway/tracheal surgeries. In addition, there are unique neonatal cases where ECMO might be used, such as placement of a fetus on ECMO prior to full delivery. This strategy, *Ex Utero* Intrapartum Therapy (EXIT) to ECMO, may be a therapeutic option for those fetuses with suspected or known congenital anomalies that will cause extremis shortly after birth, for example severe CDH, thoracic masses, or left-sided cardiac lesions with restrictive flow. Other unique neonatal ECMO occurrences are the use of therapeutic hypothermia or surgical repair of CDH.

Per the ELSO registry, overall survival from decannulation is 87% for neonatal respiratory ECMO patients and survival to discharge is 73% [5]. Infants requiring ECMO for meconium aspiration have the best survival rate at 92% while infants cannulated for congenital diaphragmatic hernia complications have the lowest survival at 50% [5]. Infants cannulated via E-CPR also have a poor prognosis with 70% surviving to decannulation but only 41% surviving to discharge [5]. Long-term neonatal ECMO survivors are at increased risk of neurologic complications [1].

The decision to place an infant on ECMO is overall institution dependent. ELSO offers the general guideline that neonatal patients should be considered for ECMO if he/she has severe respiratory failure with a high likelihood of mortality with a potentially reversible etiology and at least one of the following: (1) inadequate tissue oxygen delivery despite maximal therapy (rising lactate, worsening metabolic acidosis); (2) severe hypoxic respiratory failure with acute decompensation ($PaO2 < 40$ mmHg); (3) oxygenation index with sustained elevation and no improvement; or (4) severe pulomnary hypertension with evidence of right ventricular dysfunction and/or left ventricular dysfunction [6].

Deciding who is not a candidate for ECMO is also generally institution dependent. Absolute contraindications per ELSO include a lethal chromosomal disorder or anomaly, severe brain damage, uncontrolled bleeding, significant intraventricular hemorrhage, and a vessel size that is too small for cannulation [6]. Relative contraindications include age and size of the patient (generally <34 weeks and <2 kg) and irreversible organ damage [6].

The neonatal ECMO circuit, like pediatric and adult circuits, varies by institution but has several consistent components. A cannula drains venous blood from the patient and moves it through a membrane lung or oxygenator, and with the aid of a pump, oxygenated blood is then returned to the patient. The main differences in neonatal circuits compared to pediatric and adult circuits are the size of the tubing, the membrane, and the cannulas. In addition, there is variability within neonatal ECMO centers on the use of roller or centrifugal pumps and the use of veno venous (VV) and veno arterial (VA) ECMO. Centers that provide ECMO across the neonatal–pediatric continuum might have different circuit configurations depending on the hospital unit or type of patient on ECMO. These differences can lead to unique considerations for management of the circuit and patient in routine and emergency situations. This highlights the need for an intense educational curriculum for neonatal ECMO caregivers to acquire mastery with each unique setup and frequent practice to ensure the ability to adapt easily to the potential differences. Please refer to Chap. 6 for further details on ECMO curriculum development. The use of VV versus VA ECMO as well as appropriate candidate selection for each modality is institution dependent and is beyond the scope of this chapter.

ECMO as a High-Risk Intervention

Types of ECMO complications are relatively universal even with the diverse neonatal disease processes; however, the incidence of complications varies across the age spectrum (Table 20.1) [5]. Complications may also be different based on whether a centrifugal or roller-pump is used and whether VA or VV is used. Thus, the response to prevent, diagnose, correct, or provide after-care may be different depending on the type of ECMO and circuit components in use as well as the patient physiology.

Acknowledging the uniqueness of ECMO use in neonates outlined above, the application of simulation as an

Table 20.1 Selected ECMO complication rates across age groups for respiratory ECMO, 2014–January 2019 [5]

Complications	Neonates	Pediatrics	Adults
Circuit component clots	36.8%	28.6%	13.1%
Hemolysis	15.3%	12.6%	4.1%
Cannula problems	12.8%	13%	4.8%
Cannulation site bleeding	11.8%	16.4%	7.8%
CNS hemorrhage	10.1%	5.1%	2.5%
Surgical site bleeding	6.4%	7.8%	6.8%
Pneumothorax requiring treatment	5.2%	7.7%	5.8%
Pulmonary hemorrhage	4.8%	6.6%	3.9%
Cardiac arrhythmia	4.5%	4.6%	7.9%
CPR required	2.7%	6.3%	4.1%
Hemorrhagic and non-hemorrhagic	2.4%	2.6%	1%
Myocardial stun by echo	1.3%	0.7%	0.6%

educational methodology to develop and maintain provider competence for routine and emergent procedures and care is critical.

Education Overview

While ELSO has specific recommendations for training of ECMO specialists and general recommendations for providers, there are no delineations for different populations of patients. ECMO specialists and bedside nurses may not have expertise in the general care of the acutely ill neonate. Since caring for ECMO patients is not a requirement to graduate from a neonatal–perinatal medicine fellowship training program, there are neonatal fellows that may not have any exposure to ECMO during their training. Even in institutions where neonatal ECMO is done in the neonatal intensive care unit, the relative rarity of neonatal noncardiac ECMO heightens the need for supplementation of ECMO experience with simulation. Thus, there is great need for rigorous development of simulation-based educational curricula for staff who are caring for neonates requiring ECMO.

ECMO Curriculum/Scenario Design

There are numerous neonatal cases that can be incorporated into ECMO simulation curricula as the clinical presentation and appropriate responses may vary from usual for the patient on ECMO. These include pneumothorax, cardiac tamponade, hypotension, hypovolemia, seizures, sepsis, and hemorrhage. In addition, scenarios that specifically involve risks to patients on ECMO such as accidental decannulation and mechanical or circuit emergencies could be incorporated into a neonatal ECMO simulation curriculum. Examples of these include component thrombosis, raceway rupture, membrane oxygenator failure, venous air embolism, and arterial air embolism. Equally essential inclusions for any neonatal ECMO simulation program include cannulation and decannulation scenarios where key management points can be embedded or complications specific to these procedures may occur, such as patient arrest during the event or excessive bleeding. In addition, other common procedures, such as component or full circuit changes, should be incorporated as the potential for error or patient decompensation during these events is not minimal. Transport scenarios with an arriving patient needing cannulation for E-CPR or coordinating the transport of a patient on ECMO would also be important in the development and maintenance of an ECMO program. All of these allow for the creation of simulation scenarios that involve the entire interprofessional care team incorporating technical skills, teamwork, and communication.

The mode of ECMO used, VA versus VV, also provides the opportunity for building scenarios around complications and situations unique to the method used. For example, recognizing the different ways oxygenation is monitored and managed in VA and VV ECMO and how blood gas interpretation is impacted can be incorporated into the objectives for simulation scenarios at centers that utilize both modalities. Specific scenarios could be created around recirculation on VV ECMO, cardiac stun, or pericardial tamponade. Given the potentially grave outcomes of these situations, the ability to recognize and intervene appropriately are critical to maximize patient outcomes. Additionally, optimal interventions may be different depending on whether the patient is on VA or VV support.

Neonatal physiology is unique and there are many neonatal procedures and diagnoses that lend themselves to ECMO simulation. Starting in the delivery room, organizations equipped with the personnel for EXIT to ECMO can use simulation in the setup and management of a program. Simulation in this instance is useful for physical logistics, such as floor plans and equipment location, as well as technologic logistics, like notification trees and team activations. Given the wide variety of fetal diagnoses that may be salvaged with EXIT, a variety of departments – maternal fetal medicine, obstetrics, otolaryngology, pediatric surgery, cardiology, cardiothoracic surgery, neonatology, perfusion – need to come together both in communication and hands-on procedures. Simulation can be used to rehearse for upcoming deliveries, with simulators that accommodate a pregnant uterus and fetus, to allow all the involved parties to gather together, test, refine, and practice the plan multiple times before implementation to ensure the best outcome for the patient.

Outside of the delivery room, ECMO simulation can be used for both daily management education and acute scenario training. Infants with meconium aspiration syndrome (MAS) accounted for 17–20% of neonatal ECMO patients in the last 5 years [1]. Early in their course, these infants are at risk for acute decompensation due to pneumothorax or pulmonary hypertensive crises with resulting severe hypoxia. A scenario can be developed for practice with urgent ECMO cannulation, including technical aspects using a cannulation trainer, troubleshooting the activation of the surgeons and perfusionists, as well as reinforcing the ongoing medical management of the bedside neonatal nursing and medical team as they await the gathering team. It can be taken a step further with a full arrest necessitating E-CPR, allowing the teams to work through cannulating during chest compressions. Simulation can also be used to facilitate discussion about the appropriate mode support for this patient population, VA versus VV. Once on ECMO, infants with MAS may still be at risk of air leaks depending on their lung dynamics and ventilation status. Recognition of hemodynamically significant pneumothorax or pneumomediastinum could be tested as well as the nuances of needle thoracostomy and chest tube placement while anticoagulated.

Congenital diaphragmatic hernia (CDH) is another common neonatal diagnosis necessitating ECMO support. These infants often struggle with varying degrees of pulmonary hypoplasia and pulmonary hypertension. Scenarios can be designed around cannulation, elective or emergent, in the delivery room or in the NICU. Infants with CDH often have their defect repaired on ECMO. Simulation can be used to facilitate discussions and work through logistics of such a surgery. As many specialties come together for repair, communication and teamwork would be a core objective of any scenario. Equipment placement, necessary personnel, anesthesia, and anticoagulation management could be addressed in the learning objectives. Following repair, infants are at risk for hemorrhage. Recognition and management of hemothorax and abdominal compartment syndrome could be simulated. Patient recovery with a focus on when to decannulate, the actual decannulation procedure, and post-ECMO management also lend themselves well to scenario development.

Infants who experience a severe perinatal event are at risk for hypoxic ischemic encephalopathy. Therapeutic hypothermia is the standard of care shown to improve neurodevelopmental outcomes [7]. Some of these patients develop critical hypotension and/or hypoxia secondary to their resulting multisystem organ dysfunction or to the cooling procedure itself. The support of this population on ECMO can have many complexities relating to the procedure for continuation of therapeutic hypothermia on ECMO as well as patient-specific issues. These patients can be exceptionally coagulopathic, facilitating discussion about ECMO parameters and management. A scenario involving insidious seizures in a heavily sedated patient could be designed. Head imaging for hemorrhage, stroke, or ischemia is commonly utilized in patients during or after completion of therapeutic hypothermia. ECMO simulation can be used to test the team's ability to safely transport a patient on ECMO to the radiology suite. In the case of a grave prognosis, an end-of-life scenario could also be designed to facilitate discussion on redirecting care within the team members and potentially incorporate standardized parent actors. Simulation could be used to help the teamwork through capping the cannulas and palliative care procedures.

Participants in ECMO Sim

ECMO can involve providers from many professions and disciplines. Different neonatal programs have differing professionals involved in the care of patients on ECMO and have different emergency response structures. Thus, participants in neonatal ECMO simulations should be decided by consideration of institutional requirements, team composition, and the learning objectives. The considerations for developing team-based simulations versus individual provider-based simulations are no different for neonatal ECMO simulation than it would be for other ECMO simulations. Certainly, any provider who will be caring for or interacting with neonates on ECMO should participate in simulation training.

While caring for neonates on ECMO is not mentioned in the Accreditation Council for Graduate Medical Education program requirements for graduate medical education in neonatal–perinatal medicine [8], ECMO is noted in the American Board of Pediatrics content outline for the examinations in neonatal–perinatal medicine [9]. The specific knowledge for ECMO in this outline is fairly general. Certainly, programs where neonates on ECMO are cared for by neonatal teams would be easily able to have this needed content covered and reinforced in simulations. For programs where neonates on ECMO are cared for elsewhere in the hospital, it would still be beneficial for neonatal fellows to be exposed at minimum through simulation to neonatal ECMO. Several residency and fellowship programs have developed ECMO electives to enhance the exposure of trainees to neonatal ECMO [10]. In addition, if fellows or faculty are joining programs where ECMO patients are cared for in the NICU, a simulation-based course would be useful to help them orient to different institutional ECMO management. This is particularly important if these providers have had minimal neonatal ECMO exposure.

Equipment Considerations for Neonatal ECMO Simulation

When running ECMO simulations in neonates you must consider the types of pumps that are being used, specifically a roller pump or a centrifugal pump. Roller pumps generate forward flow as a function of the tubing size and pump speed and utilize the addition of a bladder or transducer to deal with the suction that can be generated by the pump. The pump is stopped or slowed with excessive negative pressure and restarts when filling pressures exceed pump suction [11]. Tubing wear or raceway rupture is a unique emergency to roller pumps that can be incorporated into simulation scenarios at institutions that use these pumps. Centrifugal pumps have a spinning rotor that generates flow and pressure; perfusion pressure is limited by revolutions per minute (RPM). Thrombosis, cavitation, and hemolysis are key issues to consider with these pumps, as well as the potential for reversed flow with resulting hypovolemia. The disposable pump head can also fail in different ways. Centers that employ centrifugal pumps should consider simulation scenarios to address such occurrences [11].

One of the first decisions to make regarding manikins is if a low-technology or a high-technology manikin will be used. It is important to consider that the simulation environment can be made high-fidelity even with a low-technology manikin. Low-technology manikins might be preferred in scenarios where there is the potential for fluids that could come in contact with the manikin and potentially destroy electronics present in high-technology manikins. A popular method at many centers is to use a high-technology neonatal manikin that is modified for use with the ECMO circuit. This allows team members the ability to interpret feedback from the simulator without involvement by the facilitator. There are some simple modifications that can be made to a high-technology simulator to improve the realism of the scenario. One such method utilizes a silicone or similar type product to create a skin overlay that fits over the Laerdal Sim NewB manikin. The mold is made to include a longer neck portion to cover a neck pad that can be made instead of purchased (Fig. 20.1a, b). The neck pad is "cannulated" by a surgeon and the ECMO cannulas are fed through the skin overlay to give the appearance of direct neck cannulation. The tubing from the neck pad is draped across the abdomen of the manikin under the skin overlay but on top of the manikin skin to avoid any potential leakage of fluid into the manikin itself to ensure all electronics housed in the manikin are safe (courtesy of Riley Maternity and Newborn Health Simulation Team, Riley Children's Hospital).

Another adaptation using a high-fidelity manikin was done by Thompson et al., which used neck vessels constructed from latex rubber tubing attached to saline bags filled with simulated blood [12]. The inner components of the manikin are protected using DuoDERM reinforced with Tegaderm across seams. This is all covered by skin thus hiding components. This model allows for physical cannulation of the vessels (see Fig. 20.2a, b).

There are also low-technology modifications that can be made to neonatal manikins to help enhance the realism of the ECMO scenario. Anderson et al. utilized a manikin that could be intubated, receive positive pressure ventilation, and connect to a ventilator [13]. The manikin is cannulated, and the cannulas are connected within the cavities of the manikin exiting the back to remain hidden from view. The abdominal cavity contains a fluid reservoir for the umbilical lines permitting infusion of fluids. Tubing that connects to the modified ECMO circuit and then exits the manikin is routed to a control room and connected to a syringe that allowed facilitators to remotely remove or add air and alter fluid volume depending on the desired scenario [13].

High-technology systems also exist to help mimic the changes that can occur with the circuit during emergencies. The Orpheus perfusion system, initially intended for cardiopulmonary bypass training and educating of perfusionists, had been utilized as an ECMO simulation model. A hydraulic simulator, electronic interface unit, and computer worked together to recreate the circuit's response to normal and abnormal events on cardiopulmonary bypass in real time [14]. This system is no longer commercially available. Another commercial device is the EigenFlow. It is a wireless ECMO simulator that is incorporated directly into the existing neonatal ECMO circuit and allows for remote manipulation of various circuit emergencies such as air emboli, thrombi, and hypovolemia [15].

Other adaptations can enhance the fidelity of neonatal ECMO simulations even when low-technology manikins and modifications are used. For example, a low-technology manikin can be used in combination with a tablet and simple

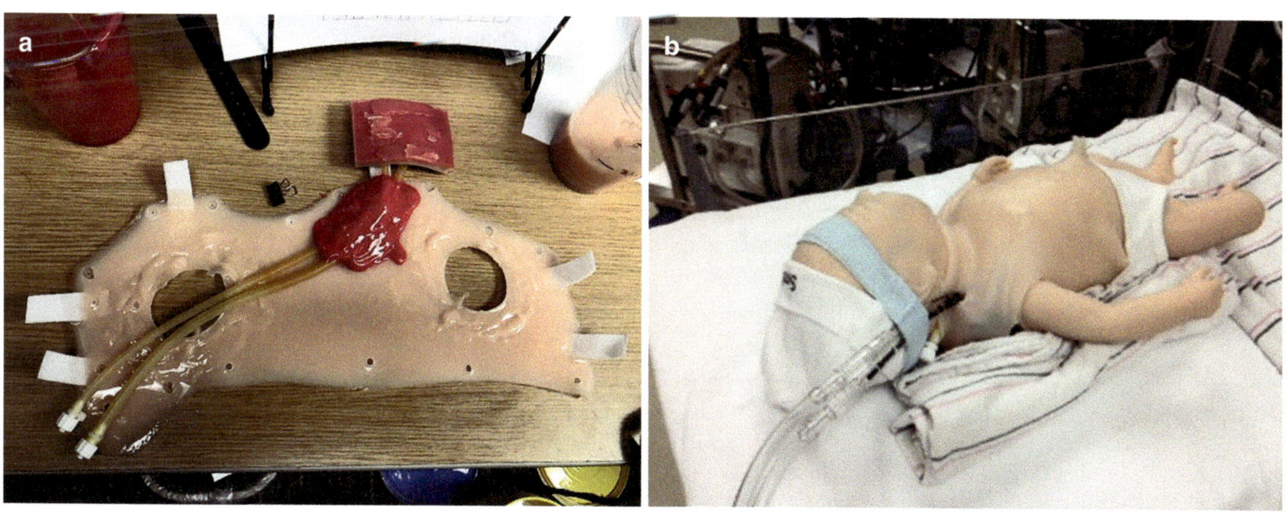

Fig. 20.1 (**a**) Neck pad created to allow for cannulation (underside visible below). (**b**) Neck pad in place on cannulated manikin connected to unprimed ECMO circuit. (Courtesy of Riley Maternity and Newborn Health Simulation Team, Riley Children's Hospital)

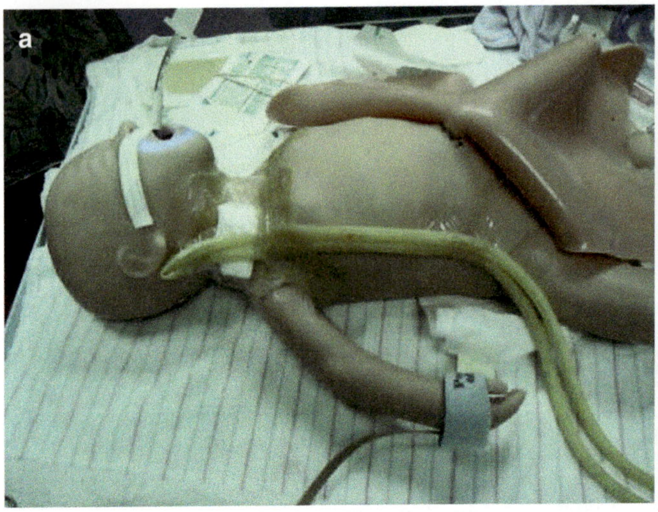

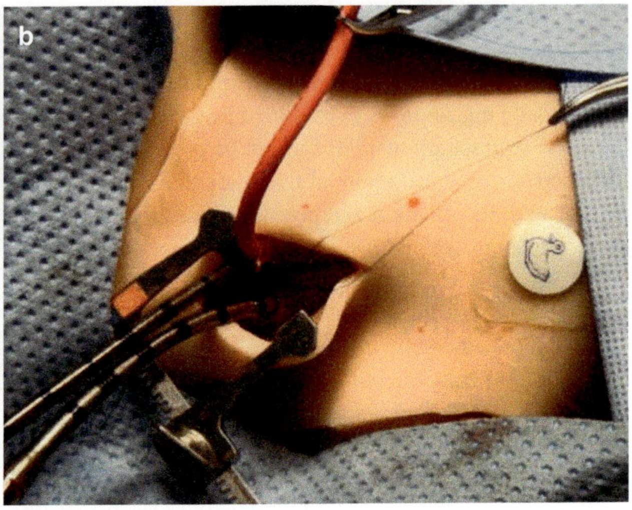

Fig. 20.2 (**a**) Preparation of the Neonatal SimNewB manikin. Tubing extends up to the neck, simulating the carotid and jugular vessels. It then travels down to connect to the reservoir. The skin is placed back in position prior to the simulation. (**b**). Cannulation of the simulated internal jugular vein and carotid artery using purse-string suturing method. (Reproduced with permission of Ref. [12])

monitor app that can be controlled by a simulation team member or by utilizing a computer monitor with input from simulator software [16]. When modifying simulators, considerations include where to have reservoir bags for blood, how to adapt the system to allow for altered hemodynamics (clamps, ports, etc.), and methods to simulate air in the circuit [13, 16, 17]. Both high- and low-technology manikins and various other technologies can be successful in creating ECMO simulation experiences as it is the overall interaction of physical, conceptual, and emotional fidelity that contributes to the overall realism and acceptance by learners [18].

Conclusions

The unique constellation of factors that need to be considered for neonates undergoing ECMO require the incorporation of neonatal-specific components into ECMO curricula. Simulation is an exceptionally critical educational methodology that should be used to ensure the acquisition and maintenance of the skills needed to optimize the management and outcomes of neonates on ECMO. Integrating neonatal-specific routine and emergent patient and circuit issues into a simulation-based ECMO educational program will help to ensure that safe care is provided for this high-risk therapy.

References

1. Mahmood B, Newton D, Pallotto EK. Current trends in neonatal ECMO. Semin Perinatol. 2018;42(2):80–8.
2. Bartlett RH, Gazzaniga AB, Jefferies MR, Huxtable RF, Haiduc NJ, Fong SW. Extracorporeal membrane oxygenation (EMCO) cardiopulmonary support in infancy. Trans Am Soc Artif Intern Organs. 1976;22:80–93.
3. Bartlett RH. Extracorporeal life support: history and new directions. Semin Perinatol. 2005;29(1):2–7.
4. Practice Bulletin no 146: management of late-term and post-term pregnancies. Obstet Gynecol. 2014;124(2 Pt 1):390–6.
5. ECMO Registry of the Extracorporeal Life Support Organization (ELSO). Ann Arbor, 2019, Jan.
6. Extracorporeal Life Support Organization (ELSO): Guidelines for Neonatal Respiratory Failure. ASAIO Journal. 2020, May.
7. Natarajan G, Pappas A, Shankaran S. Outcomes in childhood following therapeutic hypothermia for neonatal hypoxic-ischemic encephalopathy (HIE). Semin Perinatol. 2016;40(8):549–55.
8. ACGME Program requirements for graduate medical education in Neonatal-Perinatal Medicine. https://www.acgme.org/Portals/0/PFAssets/ProgramRequirements/329_NeonatalPerinatalMedicine_2019.pdf?ver=2019-02-19-132809-163. Accessed 23 Aug 2019.
9. American Board of Pediatrics. Content Outline: Neonatal-Perinatal Medicine. https://www.abp.org/sites/abp/files/pdf/neonatal_perinatal_content_outline.pdf. Accessed 23 Aug 2019.
10. Miller J, Piazza A, Keene S. Neonatal-perinatal medicine fellowship program focused ECMO training elective. Abstracts of the 35th annual symposium on ECMO and advanced therapies for respiratory failure. Children's National Medical Center, Keystone, CO. 24–28. February 2019.
11. Annich GM, Lynch WR, MacLaren G, Wilson JM, Bartlett RH. ECMO extracorporeal cardiopulmonary support in critical care. 4th ed. Ann Arbor: Extracorporeal Support Organization; 2012.
12. Thompson JL, Grisham LM, Scott J, Morgan C, Prescher H, Biffar D, et al. Construction of a reusable high-fidelity model to enhance extracorporeal membrane oxygenation training through simulation. Adv Neonatal Care. 2014;14(2):103–9.
13. Anderson JM, Boyle KB, Murphy AA, Yaeger KA, LeFlore J, Halamek LP. Simulating extracorporeal membrane oxygenation

emergencies to improve human performance. Part I: methodologic and technologic innovations. Simul Healthc. 2006;1(4):220–7.
14. Morris RW, Pybus DA. "Orpheus" cardiopulmonary bypass simulation system. J Extra Corpor Technol. 2007;39(4):228–33.
15. Eigen Flow ECMO simulator. http://curtisliferesearch.com/eigenflow-ecmo-simulator/.
16. Johnston L, Sudikoff S. Development of a ECMO simulation experience at Yale New Haven Hospital. Medical Training Magazine, 2012.
17. Raffaeli G, Ghirardello S, Vanzati M, Baracetti C, Canesi F, Conigliaro F, et al. Start a neonatal extracorporeal membrane oxygenation program: a multistep team training. Front Pediatr. 2018;6(151):1–9.
18. Choi W, Dyens O, Chan T, Schijven M, Lajoie S, Mancini M, et al. Engagement and learning in simulation: recommendations of the Simnovate Engaged Learning Domain Group. BMJ Stel. 2017;3:S23–32.

ECMO Simulation in Infants, Children, and Adolescents

21

Kelly D. Kadlec

Learning Objectives

After studying this chapter, the reader will be able to:

1. List the similarities and differences between pediatric, neonatal, and adult ECMO indications and complications
2. State the most common clinical indications for instituting VA or VV ECMO in the pediatric population
3. Describe how the following generally change throughout childhood: vital signs (particularly heart rate and blood pressure), cannula sizes, and age/weight-based flows.
4. Explain the potential clinical and physiological implications of younger pediatric ECMO patients requiring generally higher ECMO while typically requiring smaller cannula sizes.

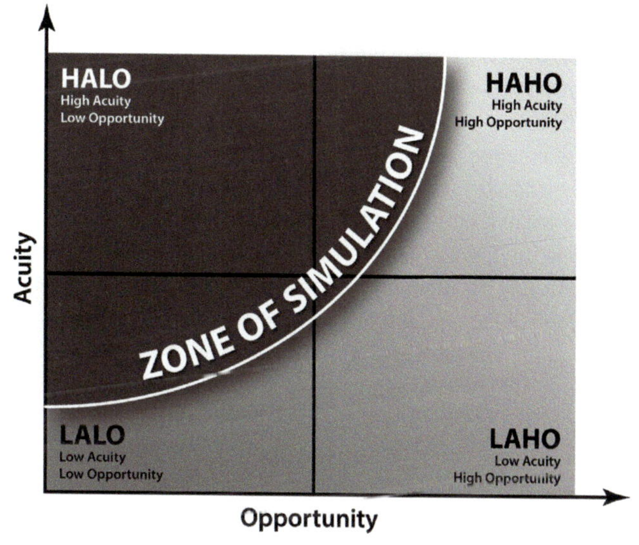

Fig. 21.1 Zone of Simulation Matrix [4]

Background

Internationally, in 2019, there were a total of 959 pediatric ECMO runs [1]. Of these runs, approximately 80% had at least one complication [2]. Given that there is an estimated 25% increase in the mortality rate associated with every complication [3], ECMO must be considered a low-frequency, high-risk process.

Chiniara [4] and colleagues, based on their publication, would likely agree that ECMO is an ideal clinical process for medical simulation. The authors developed a matrix to describe "zone of simulation" (Fig. 21.1) that takes into account the acuity and incidence of a particular clinical situation. Essentially, clinical situations that are encountered more frequently and are of lower acuity may be more appropriate for traditional educational modalities (e.g., classroom-based didactics, assigned readings). Conversely, clinical situations that are rare and have potentially severe implications (e.g., ECMO) may be circumstances where simulation may be preferred over other instructional methods; the authors refer to these as high-acuity, low-opportunity (HALO) situations.

Despite ECMO certainly being a HALO, as of 2017, only 46% of Extracorporeal Life Support Organizations (ELSO) sites reported incorporating simulation into their training programs, with an additional 26% stating they were in the process of developing institutional ECMO simulation training [5]. The authors attempted to describe the current state of ECMO simulation, at least in the United States. Of these

K. D. Kadlec (✉)
Department of Pediatric Critical Care, University of Nebraska College of Medicine, Children's Hospital and Medical Center, University of Nebraska Medical Center, Omaha, NE, USA
e-mail: kkadlec@childrensomaha.org

L. C. Johnston, L. Su (eds.), *Comprehensive Healthcare Simulation: ECMO Simulation*, Comprehensive Healthcare Simulation, https://doi.org/10.1007/978-3-030-53844-6_21

centers, 32% identified themselves as a combined adult and children's hospital, while another 28% were free-standing children's hospitals. Based on the survey's methodology, it is difficult to definitively state the percentage of pediatric ECMO programs that utilize simulation for pediatric ECMO training. A conservative estimate, based on the survey results, is that approximately 25–33% of pediatric ECMO programs incorporate some type of simulation into their training and educational curricula.

For programs that utilized simulation, the fidelity of the manikins was equally divided between low and high-fidelity, with 46 and 54% respectively. Access or affiliation of a clinical ECMO program with a simulation center correlated strongly with whether an ECMO program utilized simulation as a methodology for training, as programs with access to a simulation center were four times more likely to utilize simulation than those who did not have access to these resources.

Based on this data, over half of current ELSO ECMO centers *do not* currently utilize simulation, in any form, for ECMO-related education and/or training; the use of simulation for pediatric ECMO centers is likely even less. Simulation is an ideal educational modality to train ECMO providers and teams, but not many centers are incorporating it into their instructional design for ECMO training. This chapter is intended to serve as a practical resource for pediatric ECMO programs/educators as they seek to prioritize, design, and run pediatric ECMO simulations for a wide variety purposes and learners.

Scope

There are many topics related to pediatric ECMO simulation that may be considered interesting or worthy of discussion. However, not all of these topics are essential in meeting the objectives of this chapter. Accordingly, we will first outline which populations and topics the chapter *will* and *will not* cover.

First, this chapter will focus on patients between the ages of 28 days and 18 years, based upon the pediatric age categorizations utilized in the ELSO databases. We will review the following topics outlined in Table 21.1. We will also discuss perspectives on whether high(er)-fidelity manikins/environments are necessary for an ECMO simulation curriculum, enabling educators to more accurately simulate pediatric ECMO emergencies.

Subjects that will *not* be covered, because they are addressed elsewhere within this book include: neonatal ECMO simulation, simulation related to congenital heart disease, and adult ECMO simulations. Topics beyond the scope of this chapter include certain patient populations (children with genetic anomalies such as Trisomy 18, out-of-hospital cardiac arrests) and ethical considerations. Table 21.1 summarizes the scope of the chapter.

Table 21.1 Topics addressed/not addressed in this chapter

Pediatric ECMO-Related Topics	Covered	*Not* Covered
VA Versus VV ECMO? The Answer Lies in the Oxygen Delivery Equation	X	
Common Pediatric VA ECMO Indications	X	
Common Pediatric VV ECMO Indications	X	
Cannulation Considerations	X	
Pediatric ECMO Flows: Guidelines and Considerations	X	
Pediatric Anticoagulation/Hematologic Nuances	X	
Pediatric Vital Signs: One Size Does *Not* Fit All	X	
Systematic Approach to Develop, and Prioritize, the Most Appropriate Pediatric ECMO Simulations for Your Program	X	
ECMO Simulation: High(er) Fidelity Is Not, Necessarily, Better – Just More Complicated	X	
Neonatal ECMO		x
Pediatric Congenital Heart Disease		x
Adult ECMO		x
ECMO Weaning/Decannulation		x
Patient Populations		x
Ethical Considerations		x

VA Versus VV ECMO? The Answer Lies in the Oxygen Delivery Equation

In extracorporeal circulation, the ultimate goal is to provide adequate oxygenation to all end-organs and tissues. In all patient populations, if and when conventional modalities have failed, veno-arterial (VA) or veno-venous (VV) extracorporeal support can be considered. But which to use when? To answer this, it is helpful to review basic physiology as described in the oxygen delivery equation (Fig. 21.2).

Adequate systemic oxygen delivery is dependent on the ability to:

1. Maintain an adequate hemoglobin concentration
2. Adequately saturate hemoglobin with oxygen
3. Maintain adequate cardiac output

With rare exceptions (e.g., cyanotic congenital heart disease where higher hemoglobin levels can compensate for low baseline oxygen saturations), all three of these variables must be appropriate for oxygen delivery to be adequate. Depending on the clinical situation, if one or more of these variables is inadequate despite maximal medical therapy, extracorporeal circulation may be warranted.

VA ECMO is warranted when cardiac output, +/− adequate hemoglobin oxygen saturation, is insufficient to main-

Fig. 21.2 Oxygen Delivery Equation

Oxygen Delivery (DO_2) Equation

DO_2=CO X CaO_2

Cardiac Output (CO)

- Heart rate
- Stroke volume
  - Preload
  - Contractility
  - Afterload

Arterial O_2 Content (CaO_2)

- CaO_2(mL O_2/dL)=(1.34 X Hgb X SaO_2)+(0.003 X PaO_2)
  - Hgb: Hemoglobin concentration
  - SaO_2: Arterial hemoglobin saturation
  - PaO_2: Partial pressure of arterial oxygen
  - Normal CaO_2: ~ 20 ml O_2/dL

tain adequate oxygen delivery. In these situations, VA ECMO acts as a surrogate for both the lungs (e.g., oxygenation and ventilation) and the heart (e.g., cardiac output). Blood is removed from the venous side of the patient's body, oxygenated and ventilated by the extracorporeal circuit, and then returned to the arterial side of the body for delivery to the organs and tissues—thus the term VA ECMO.

VV ECMO is typically utilized in situations where cardiac output (to both the lungs and the body) and hemoglobin concentration are acceptable, but a primary pulmonary process interferes with oxygenation, such as in the case of acute respiratory distress syndrome (ARDS). This type of extracorporeal support removes blood from the venous side of the body, oxygenates it, removes carbon dioxide and then returns the blood back to the venous side – thus the term VV ECMO. This newly oxygenated and ventilated blood can return to heart and the patient's *own* systemic cardiac output delivers oxygenated blood to the body's tissues and organs. VV ECMO will be reviewed following this section.

As often is the case in clinical medicine, though, the appropriate initial extracorporeal strategy is not always simple to identify. For example, of 3128 ECMO runs primarily for respiratory support, 61.3% were VV while 36.5% were VA [1]. The higher than expected percentage of respiratory cases initially placed on VA support may be secondary to numerous possible reasons including center preference/familiarity for VA over VV ECMO, some degree of cardiac output compromise (although not the primary ECMO indication) and "preemptively" placing on VA ECMO to avoid a potential emergent conversion to VA. Indeed, about 5.5% of respiratory conditions for which VV ECMO was instituted initially needed to be converted to VA ECMO [1].

Common Pediatric VA ECMO Indications

According to the most recent ELSO data [1] (Table 21.2), VA ECMO for cardiac support is most frequently utilized in "other" conditions that do not fall neatly into other categories. The next most common indication for VA ECMO is

Table 21.2 Overview of Pediatric Cardiac Runs, 2014–2019—Includes Both VA (96.5%) and VV (1.6%) Modalities [1]

Cardiac Indication	Average Run Time (Hours)	% Survival
Other (43.5%)	191	59%
Congenital Heart Defect(s) (39.8%)	153	55%
Cardiogenic Shock (8.1%)	173	56%
Myocarditis (3.4%)	179	78%
Cardiomyopathy (2.8%)	264	60%
Cardiac Arrest (2.3%)	170	49%

congenital heart disease (CHD), which is a broad category for infants and children who are born with anatomically abnormal hearts. As previously noted, a full review of the various types of CHD is beyond the scope of this chapter; but, VA ECMO, when instituted for CHD, is typically done in the immediate postoperative period (either corrective or palliative) when patients are most vulnerable to developing cardiac insufficiency.

Cardiogenic shock, defined as inadequate systemic oxygen delivery primarily of cardiac origin, is another broad category for which VA ECMO is utilized, although at a substantially lower rate than the previous two categories. Cardiogenic shock can be due to septic shock or acute right heart failure due to a myriad of potential etiologies (e.g., pulmonary hypertension, pulmonary embolism, or arrhythmias). Although extremely uncommon in children, pulmonary embolism (PE) can occur in adolescents with certain risk factors, including thrombophilias, obesity, vascular trauma, sedentary status and oral contraceptive medications. A pediatric patient with a PE may require ECMO initiation in controlled manner if clinical status allows; alternatively, VA ECMO may emergently be required if the patient is unstable or if CPR is in process (e.g., ECPR, discussed shortly).

Initiating VA ECMO for pulmonary hypertension may be appropriate in certain clinical circumstances, particularly if the condition is expected to be transient or serves as a bridge to a definitive end-point (e.g., heart-lung transplant). VA ECMO may be considered for a wide variety of causes, including idiopathic pulmonary hypertension, chronic lung disease (e.g., severe bronchopulmonary dysplasia), systemic connective tissue disorders, obstructive left-sided heart lesions, and congenital heart defects with excessive, and/or long-standing, left to right shunts.

Children, like adults, can have arrhythmias, although these are exceedingly uncommon. Some arrhythmias can present acutely with complete loss of cardiac output (e.g., pulseless ventricular tachycardia (VT)), necessitating ECPR. Others may be more insidious in onset, with a more gradual decline in cardiac output and oxygen delivery (e.g., supraventricular tachycardia (SVT)), allowing clinicians more time to electively place a patient on ECMO. Arrhythmias in children can occur due to a variety of etiologies such as congenital channelopathies, postoperative myocardial irritation/injury, medications, myocarditis, and electrolyte abnormalities (e.g., hyperkalemia). VA ECMO is often appropriate for transient, acute dysrhythmias leading to shock, when refractory to other medical therapies.

VA ECMO can also be utilized in children who have decreased cardiac output due to decreased function of the myocardium itself, as occurs in myocarditis and cardiomyopathies. Progressive cardiomyopathies must be distinguished from acute myocarditis; the latter involves acute myocardial inflammation, often from a viral etiology. Patients with myocarditis can present in an acute or subacute manner and may require VA ECMO, urgently or emergently, if medical management fails. Typically, the outcomes for patients requiring ECMO due to myocarditis are excellent [1, 6].

Congestive heart failure is another condition for which VA ECMO support may be considered. It can occur in a variety of acute (e.g., ingestion of calcium channel blockers) or chronic circumstances (e.g., progressive worsening of cardiac function due to CHD). As with any clinical situation where ECMO is considered, clinicians need to proactively determine whether a particular patient is an appropriate candidate. ECMO is only a temporary solution; as such, patients without a reversible physiologic process (e.g., myocardial recovery after acute ingestion, transplant) and/or identifiable end-point are typically poor candidates for ECMO.

Finally, there are circumstances when VA ECMO is mobilized when CPR is in progress, or imminent; this is referred to extracorporeal cardiopulmonary resuscitation (ECPR). ECPR requires careful choreography and coordination of care provided by the multidisciplinary team. To an external observer, the scene can seem chaotic. At programs where ECPR is infrequently performed and/or there are few opportunities to practice this orchestration, chaos may in fact ensue. But, in programs where ECPR is utilized and/ or simulated frequently, the process is more choreographed, efficient, and timely. At minimum, ECPR requires highly detailed, and scripted, roles for each member of the team, excellent communications between individuals at bedside and services that are often remote (e.g., blood bank), equipment that is on standby and ready to be deployed at a moment's notice, optimization of space once CPR is in progress and the decision to go on ECMO has been made and, usually, designated positions for each member of the team in the room [7]. In many institutions, patients can be cannulated and on full ECMO support in less than 30 min from the time of CPR initiation [7].

The percentage of ECMO runs due to ECPR has doubled over the last 10 years, from ~12% to greater than 20% [7]. Historically reserved for patients with in-hospital cardiac arrest (IHCA), there are programs, nationally and internationally, utilizing ECPR for out-of-hospital cardiac arrests (OHCA). Survival rates for ECPR are variable, depending on the study, patient population, IHCA versus OHCA, and classification of the patient as cardiac versus noncardiac. However, survival outcomes for pediatric patients receiving ECPR have typically been better than adults (~35–50% vs. ~25–40%) [7].

Common Pediatric VV ECMO Indications

VV ECMO is primarily indicated when there is adequate pulmonary and systemic cardiac output, but there is difficulty achieving adequate systemic oxygenation despite optimizing medical therapies and mechanical ventilation settings. The most common indications, based on the most recent ELSO data [1], are outlined in Table 21.3.

Similar to the VA ECMO ELSO data, the most common respiratory indication for VV ECMO is "Other." It is difficult to specifically identify what conditions are included in this category but amongst them are likely pediatric patients with asthma exacerbations refractory to conventional medical and ventilatory therapies. Pediatric asthmatic patients requiring VV ECMO are an interesting subgroup of VV ECMO patients as the usual indication for them to extracorporeal support is not oxygenation but instead ventilation, which is a less common reason for ECMO support. The specific epide-

Table 21.3 Overview of pediatric respiratory runs, 2014–2019 – includes both VA (36%) and VV modalities (61%) [1]

Respiratory Indication	Average Run Time (Hours)	% Survival
Other (61.2%)	272	62%
Non-ARDS Respiratory Failure (11.2%)	315	64%
Viral Pneumonia (10%)	315	72%
ARDS, Not Due To Trauma/Post-Op (8.8%)	375	66%
Aspiration Pneumonia (1.6%)	247	66%
ARDS Due to Trauma/Post-Op (0.7%)	208	71%

miology of pediatric asthmatic patients requiring ECMO, both VV or VA, is not known.

Aside from the "Other" group, VV ECMO is used most frequently for non-ARDS respiratory failure, viral pneumonia/pneumonitis, and ARDS (not due to trauma or postoperative deterioration). In ARDS, there is severe bilateral injury to the lung parenchyma (typically with diffuse patchy alveolar infiltrates on chest radiographs) from various etiologies, which greatly impairs the patient's ability to effectively oxygenate and/or ventilate. In this population, the lungs can be further damaged by excessively high ventilator pressures or tidal volumes causing barotrauma and volutrauma, respectively. Thus, pediatric patients with ARDS, regardless of etiology, can be considered for VV ECMO to let their lungs heal and mitigate further potential lung damage from excessive ventilator pressures or tidal volumes.

Even if a child does not have ARDS, by definition, he/she can still have respiratory failure refractory to conventional medical and ventilator therapies. This pediatric patient population represents the second-most common indication for VV ECMO. Bacterial pneumonias, which do not meet ARDS criteria, often fall in this category. Other pneumonias resulting in profound pulmonary disease, such as those due to viruses or aspiration of gastric contents, can also result in the need for VV ECMO.

Cannulation Considerations

For VA ECMO, both venous and arterial cannulae need to be placed. The size of the cannulae is based primarily on weight, which generally correlates with a patient's age. However, as Appendix 21.1 shows, as the age increases, so does the degree of weight variation. For example, up until about 3 years of age, only two arterial and venous cannula sizes are typically utilized as children in this age group are of relatively consistent weight. As children get older, particularly by the early teenage years, there can be a considerable range of weights between the 5th and 95th percentiles, which precludes a "one size fits all" cannula selection. By 17 or 18 years of age, a significant difference still exists in weights between the 5th and 95th percentiles. However, there is less variability in cannula sizes as virtually all cannulae used in this population, whether a 23 or 29 French cannula, can achieve flows greater than 5.5 L/min, which is generally adequate for adults, regardless of size.

For all VA ECMO situations, including those involving pediatric patients, cannulation is categorized as *peripheral*, via the neck or femoral vessels, or *central*, directly into the heart/mediastinal great vessels. Each approach has particular advantages and disadvantages, which are outlined in Table 21.4. Nuances involved in VV ECMO cannulation will be discussed separately at the end of this section.

Table 21.4 Advantages and Disadvantages of Different Cannulation Approaches in Pediatric VA ECMO

Cannulation Route	Advantages	Disadvantages
Central	Quick/easy in children with recent sternotomy for cardiac surgery +/– open chest Higher ECMO flows attainable due to larger cannula size Brain and coronary arteries in closer proximity to oxygenated blood from arterial cannula	Increased infectious risk Increased bleeding risk Suboptimal CPR during cannula placement (e.g., ECPR) or with cannula already in position
Cervical	Relatively quick/easy Decreased infectious risk Decreased bleeding risk Ability to perform CPR during cannulation Brain and coronary arteries in closer proximity to oxygenated blood from arterial cannula	Increased risk of neurological injury due to emboli or decreased cerebral blood flow
Femoral	Relatively quick/easy Decreased infection risk Decreased bleeding risk Ability to perform CPR during cannulation	Inadequate distal limb blood flow, leading to ischemia (risk minimized with the addition of reperfusion cannula)

Benefits of central cannulation, typically into the right atrium and aorta, include relatively quick and easy access [8] in a child who has recently had a sternotomy for palliative or corrective heart surgery or has an "open" chest. In postoperative pediatric cardiac surgery patients, the chest is sometimes intentionally left "open," meaning the sternotomy remains, with variable distances between sternal edges, with an occlusive patch/dressing approximating the incisional edges. Reasons for the chest to remain "open" include: excessive bleeding and need to pack the mediastinum, inadequate cardiovascular or respiratory status after attempted sternal closure, and marginal cardiac output postoperatively where ECMO may be necessary. Another advantage for central cannulation includes the proximity of returned oxygenated blood, from the ECMO circuit, to the coronary arteries and the brain. A final advantage is that larger cannulas are able to be placed, allowing for higher flows [8] than what may be attainable through peripheral cannulation. Disadvantages of central cannulation include: increased risk of infection and bleeding [9], increased tissue fatigue [8] with risk for breakdown/bleeding, suboptimal cardiac compressions during

CPR that may have compromise outcomes [10], need for higher levels of analgesia and sedation, and consideration for the administration of neuromuscular blocking agents.

One form of peripheral cannulation is via the neck vessels. Cervical cannulation, utilizing the right common carotid artery (CCA) and the right internal jugular vein, is unique to neonatal and pediatric patients requiring VA ECMO. This is often the preferred choice of surgeons in children less than 2 years of age, although a specific age cutoff does not exist. In cervical cannulation, the right side of the neck is typically preferred over the left side due to technical aspects of venous cannulation. Cannulating the right internal jugular vein provides the most linear course (Fig. 21.3) for the venous cannula to reach the right atrium, where the confluence of all systemic venous return lies, via the superior vena cava (SVC) and the inferior vena cava (IVC). Cannulation of the left neck, using the left internal jugular vein, is a more circuitous route; therefore, appropriate placement of the distal portion of the catheter may be more challenging, particularly in an emergent situation.

The arterial cannula is typically placed into the right CCA (Fig. 21.4), not so much because it is preferred over the left CCA, but because of the preferential placement of the venous cannula is on that side. The distal end of the arterial cannula is placed between the insertion site and where the brachiocephalic artery branches off the aorta; the exact location is often based on surgical preference as long as the cannula is not in danger of becoming dislodged (e.g., too shallow) and or advanced into the descending aorta (e.g., too deep). With appropriate arterial cannula placement, the oxygenated blood from the ECMO circuit is in close proximity to the heart and brain to allow it to reach the coronary arteries and the head/neck vessels on the contralateral side. If the arterial cannula is too deep, in the proximal ascending aorta, there

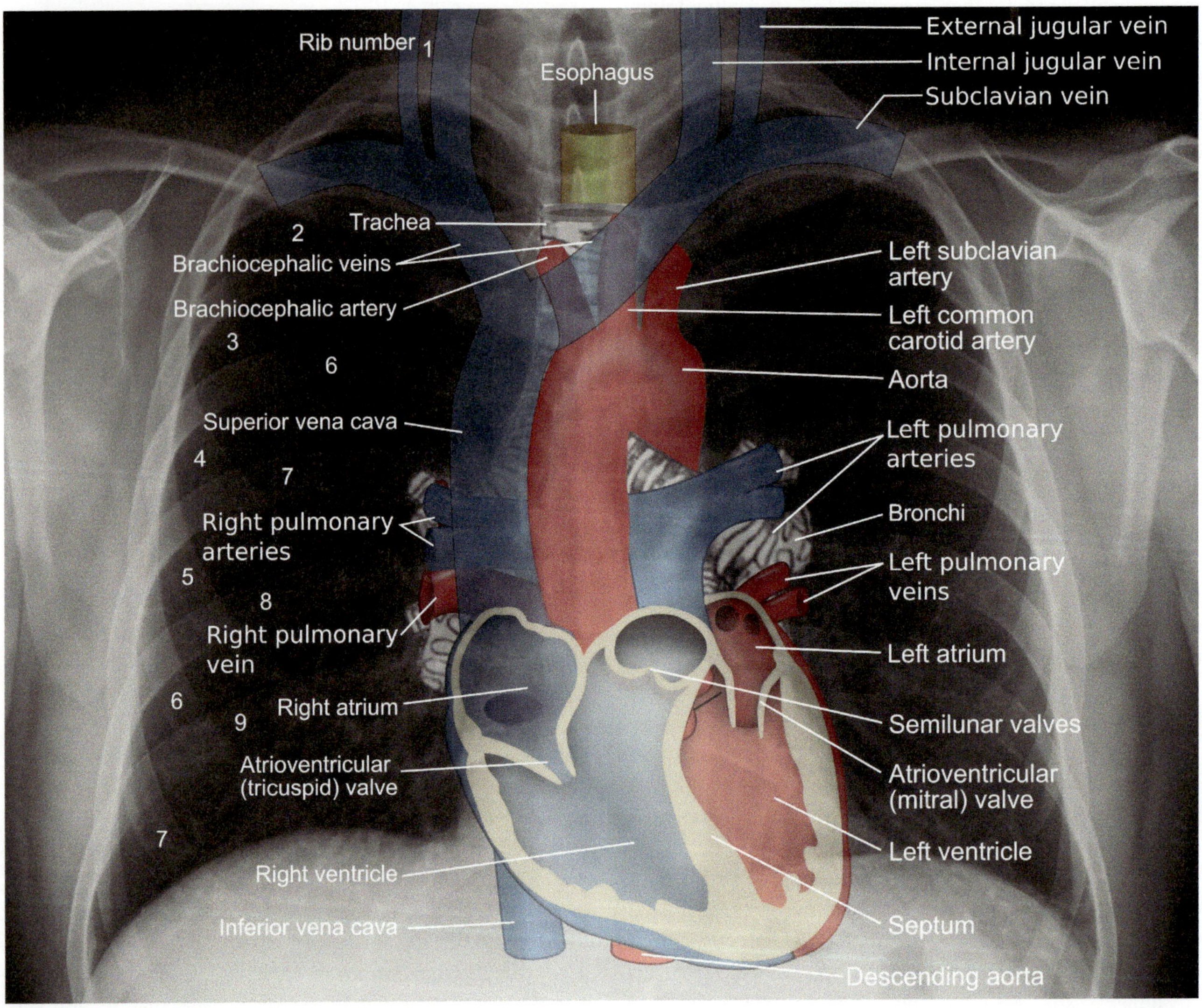

Fig. 21.3 Systemic Venous Drainage. (Obtained from: https://commons.wikimedia.org/wiki/File:Mediastinal_structures_on_chest_X-ray_annotated.jpg)

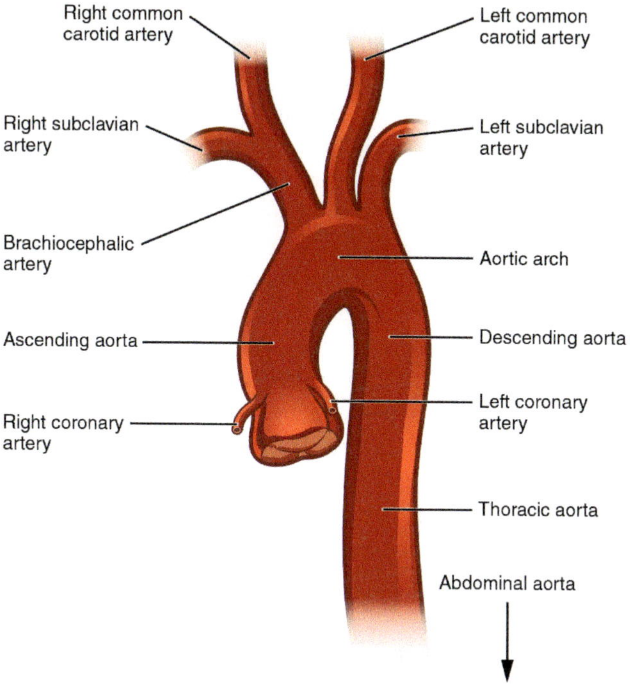

Fig. 21.4 Branches of the Aorta. (Obtained from: https://commons.wikimedia.org/wiki/File:2121_Aorta.jpg)

may be a lack of oxygenated blood delivered to the patient's brain and body. Additionally, retrograde blood flow into the left ventricle and left atrium can potentially cause left atrial dilation and pulmonary hemorrhage. Conversely, if the aortic cannula is placed too far into the aortic arch or descending aorta, the oxygen-rich blood from the ECMO circuit may fail to adequately oxygenate the coronary arteries or the left common carotid. A specific advantage of cervical cannulation includes proximity of returned oxygenated blood from the ECMO circuit to the coronary arteries and the brain (similar to the advantage of central cannulation).

However, a potential disadvantage of cervical cannulation is the risk of neurological injury due to emboli (clot or air) or inadequate cerebral blood flow [9]. Because one primary source of cerebral blood flow is eliminated due to cannulation, the remainder of the patient's cerebral blood flow is dependent upon cerebral blood flow via the left internal carotid artery, assuming the Circle of Willis is intact. The Circle of Willis (Fig. 21.5) allows for the rerouting of oxygenated blood throughout the brain in the event of compromised blood flow from the anterior (e.g., internal carotid arteries) or posterior (e.g., basilar artery) cerebral circulations. If the Circle of Willis is not intact, with right cervical cannulation, oxygenated blood entering the left carotid artery may not be able to reach the right side of the brain, potentially resulting in right hemispheric ischemia.

The second form of peripheral cannulation for VA ECMO is through cannulation of the femoral artery and femoral

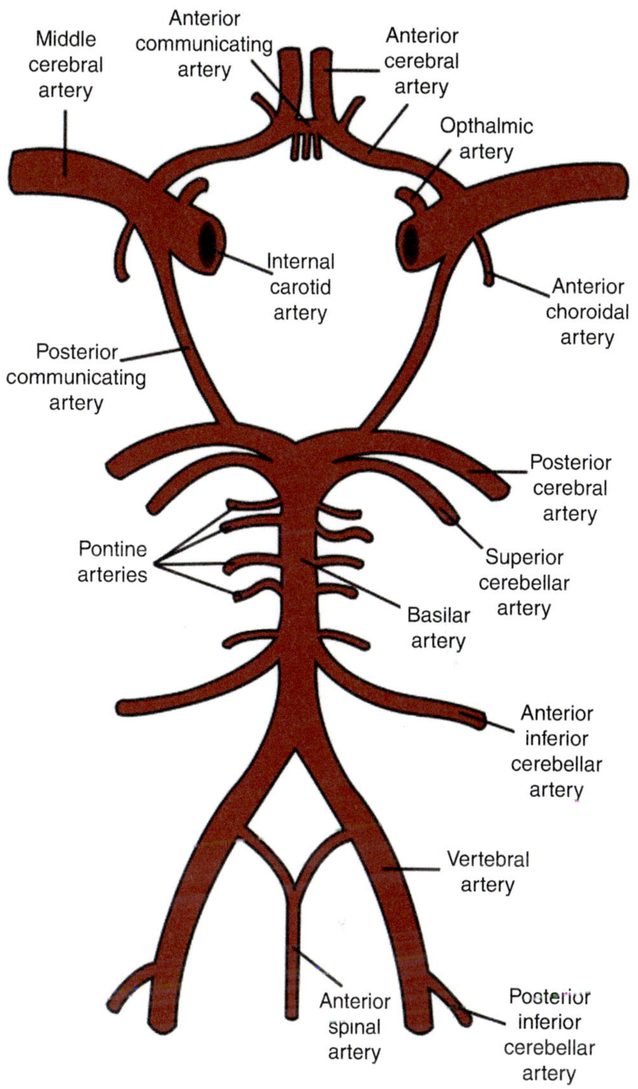

Fig. 21.5 Circle of Willis. (Obtained from: https://en.wikipedia.org/wiki/Partial_anterior_circulation_infarct)

vein. In this setting, an arterial catheter is placed into the common femoral artery with the tip terminating near the proximal internal iliac artery. Similarly, the venous cannula is inserted into the common femoral vein with the distal end of the cannula ideally being in or near the right atrium. This is the preferred peripheral cannulation method for all pediatric patients, including older adolescents, older than 2 years of age. Two primary disadvantages of femoral cannulation are related to the arterial cannula. First, because the distal end of the arterial cannula is in the lower abdominal area, it is less certain that the coronary arteries and brain will definitively receive oxygen-rich blood flow. Second, an arterial cannula in the common femoral artery can result in limb ischemia distal to the cannulation site. This risk can be mitigated by the addition of a reperfusion cannula, which comes off the arterial limb of the ECMO circuit and supplies oxygenated blood just distal to the main arterial cannula [11].

Although there are disadvantages to cervical and femoral cannulation, there are also general advantages that both peripheral techniques offer including decreased bleeding around cannulation sites, less analgesia/sedation requirements, and a lower risk of infection [8]. Finally, when the patient is decannulated from ECMO, the arteries and veins can be repaired, both in the cervical and femoral regions. In the past, after utilizing the neck vessels for ECMO, both the ICA and IJV were typically sacrificed, and subsequently ligated. Now, these vessels are commonly repaired at the time of ECMO decannulation [6].

Pediatric ECMO Flows: Guidelines and Considerations

Perhaps one of the most important concepts to understand in the clinical management of acutely ill pediatric patients is Pouiseille's equation (Fig. 21.6), which correlates the resistance to flow to both the length and radius of a tubular structure. This is relevant in clinical care of ECMO practice as it relates to cannula size. Compared to adults, children's anatomy (trachea, bronchi, veins, arteries, etc.) is smaller in diameter. Accordingly, in pediatric resuscitation, tubes or cannulae, therefore, have a relatively smaller radius; unfortunately, this has profound implications in all critically ill children, including those on ECMO.

Specifically, Pouiseille's equation states there is direct correlation between the length of a tube (e.g., endotracheal tube, intravenous catheter, or ECMO cannula) and the resistance to flow through that tube. Of even more significance, Pouiseille's equation states for every 50% decrease in the radius of a tube/cannula, flow resistance increases 16-fold (e.g., $(½)^4$ – where ½ represents the reduction of the radius by 50%.

Applying this concept, if child's airway radius decreases from 8 to 4 mm due to tracheal edema from a viral infection, the resistance goes up 16-fold. Because flow is inversely proportional to resistance, assuming unchanged pressures on either side of the tube, the flow within the airway drops 16-fold as well. The same changes in resistance and flow occurs if the radius of an IV or ECMO cannula is reduced; if the radius is reduced by 50%, the resistance increases 16-fold resulting in a 16-fold drop in flow.

Ideally, in pediatric patients, to minimize resistance and optimize flow, it is desirable to utilize the largest possible radius for any tube, catheter, or cannula inserted, which will not cause harm to the surrounding area/vessel(s). When it comes to pediatric ECMO, whether VV or VA, there exists an unfortunate paradox. Smaller and younger patients require proportionally smaller cannula, yet the ECMO flows need to be higher relative to the patient's weight to meet the body's typical aerobic oxygen demands (Table 21.5). This means the ECMO pump, in smaller patients, must generate higher pressures in order to: (1) counter the resistance of smaller cannulas and (2) achieve higher flows relative to those in older patients to meet the child's oxygen demands.

Most of the time, there are no issues achieving flows that the patient's physiologic status demands if age-appropriate cannulae are in place. Appendix 21.1 details the usual cannula sizes based on age and weight, as well as the typical maximum flows for the cannula. However, there are certain clinical situations, such as occurs in patients with sepsis or single-ventricle physiology, where the necessary higher flows are unable to be achieved due to limitations of the cannulae (due to excessive resistance) and/or pump (due to high pressures or revolutions per minute (RPM)). In these situations, larger cannulae, additional cannulae, and/or central cannulation all need to be considered.

Pediatric Anticoagulation/Hematologic Nuances

Considerations of anticoagulation, bleeding, and thromboses are important to review for simulation purposes as well. The younger a person is, the more likely they are to have an ECMO complication related to the hematologic system. Therefore, it is prudent for educators utilizing simulation for pediatric training to be aware of the increased incidence of these complications in pediatric and neonatal ECMO patients. Similarly, ECMO educators also need to be aware that neonatal and pediatric patients are physiologically more

$R=8nL/\pi r^4 \quad Q=1/R$

R	Resistance to Flow
n	Fluid Viscosity
L	Length of Tube/Cannula
r	Radius of Tube/Cannula
Q	Flow of Fluid/Air

Fig. 21.6 Pouiseille's Equation(s)

Table 21.5 Pediatric ECMO flow rates ranges, based on weight. (Reproduced with permission of Ref. [12])

Patient Weight (kg)	ECMO Flow Rate (mL/kg/minute)
1.8–3	100–200
3–10	100–150
10–15	80–125
15–30	50–100
30–50	50–75
>50	60–65

Table 21.6 Hematologic complications on ECMO [1] (ranges due to separate data for respiratory and cardiac ECMO indications)

	Adult	Pediatric	Neonate
Thromboses	9.3–12.8%	26.6–29.7%	31.2–40.5%
Bleeding	22.4–26.3%	36.4–39.2%	36.1–48.2%
Hemolysis	4.1–4.6%	11.7–17.9%	15.7–18.6%
DIC	1.5–1.7%	2.5–2.8%	3.3–4.1%

difficult to anticoagulate than adults when on ECMO. Both of these issues will be discussed in this section.

In reviewing the most recent ELSO Registry Report, for purposes of this chapter, complications were categorized as thrombotic, hemorrhagic, hemolytic, or related to disseminated intravascular coagulation (DIC); Table 21.6 summarizes these complications. Hemorrhagic complications included gastrointestinal (GI) hemorrhage, cannulation site bleeding (either peripheral or mediastinal), surgical site bleeding, central nervous system (CNS) hemorrhage, and pulmonary hemorrhage). Thombotic complications included hemofilter clots, thromboses within the oxygenator, and clots within the circuit.

Based on the data, neonates have the highest rate of thromboses, bleeding, hemolysis, and DIC, while adults have the lowest rates of these complications. The pediatric population has hematologic complication rates slightly lower those of neonates. On first consideration, one might think that as the thrombotic complication rate is increased, the rate of bleeding complications should be lower. In fact, that is most certainly not the case.

A full discussion regarding the reasons for the higher rate hematologic complications in neonates and pediatric patients is beyond the scope of the chapter; nonetheless, the multifactorial reasons are both intrinsic to the patient (e.g., native hematologic and coagulation systems, tissue friability) and extrinsic factors (e.g., smaller cannula in pediatric patients leading to increased resistance/decreased laminar flow, increased ECMO pump pressures in smaller children to meet their higher ECMO flow requirements). One of the intrinsic reasons neonates and children on ECMO are apt to develop thromboses relates to the relative difficulty achieving adequate anticoagulation as compared to adults.

Unfractionated heparin (UFH) is the most widely used anticoagulant across all ECMO patients, including children. Although other anticoagulants are available, such as bivalirudin (direct thrombin inhibitor) and argatroban (factor Xa inhibitor), no large-scale studies of these medications have been performed in the pediatric ECMO population [13]. Further discussion of these medications is beyond the scope of this chapter. UFH works by combining with the body's native antithrombin (AT), also known as antithrombin III (AT3), which has anticoagulation properties. When UFH combines with AT, the complex greatly potentiates the inhibitory coagulation effects of other proteins and factors. Neonates and younger children typically have lower levels of AT and, almost without exception, require higher doses of heparin relative to kilogram of body weight than adults, who have higher AT levels. It is not uncommon for neonates and younger children to require 30–40 units/kg/h of UFH to maintain adequate anticoagulation, whereas adults generally require 10–20 units/kg/hour. As with all UFH infusions, there can be significant variability; UFH should be titrated based on institutional standards. Because anticoagulation, particularly using UFH, is mandatory on ECMO in pediatric patients due to the high risk of thrombotic and bleeding complications, it is necessary for educators to have a basic understanding of these processes.

Pediatric Vital Signs: One Size Does *Not* Fit All

Perhaps the most important variable to consider when it comes to pediatric ECMO simulation is the patient's age. Unlike adults, whose normal vital signs are, typically, heart rate of 60–100, respiratory rate of 12–16, and blood pressure around 120/80, "normal" vital signs for children vary considerably by age. For example, a heart rate of 100 in an athletic, adolescent male may represent a relative tachycardia whereas a heart rate of 100 in a one-month female is more consistent with a relative bradycardia. It cannot be overemphasized that when performing pediatric ECMO simulations, those creating and executing the scenarios must have a thorough understanding of the normal range of vital signs for the patient in the scenario given their stated age. Not only should baseline vital signs for the scenario be realistic, but changes in the vital signs, based on the patient's changing condition or learner interventions, should be age appropriate as well. Appendix 21.1 shows the normal range of weight, heart rate, respiratory rate, systolic blood pressure, diastolic blood pressure, and mean arterial blood pressure for patients from 1 month of age through 18 years of age. Utilizing these normative values can assist educators in designing realistic, age-appropriate simulations for their learners.

However, there are several important caveats regarding vital signs for a pediatric patient on ECMO, specifically VA ECMO. To optimize ECMO flows and minimize bleeding risk, goal mean arterial blood pressures (MAP), while on ECMO, are often much lower than the normal MAPs listed in the chart. *In general, goal MAPs for pediatric patients on ECMO typically are much closer to the 50th percentile diastolic blood pressure for age*. This holds true for neonates, infants, children, and adolescents. For infants and young children, a goal MAP of 40–50 is generally sufficient. For older children on VA ECMO, a MAP goal of 50–60 is reasonable and for adolescents and adults, a MAP of >65 is typically considered a reasonable goal.

However, the aforementioned MAP goals are *exclusively* for VA ECMO patients; for patients on VV ECMO, the patient is going to retain his own native cardiac output and therefore, the blood pressure parameters should remain within the normal physiologic range for age, preferably closer to the 50th percentile than the 95th percentile to minimize bleeding risks, particularly intracranial.

The respiratory rate for patients on ECMO often differs substantially from typical physiologic vital signs presented in Appendix 21.1, due to the use of "rest" ventilator settings. Although resting ventilator settings, and modes, differ from center to center, a potential resting ventilator strategy for an infant or adolescent on VV ECMO is to place the patient in a pressure control mode with a mandatory respiratory rate of 10, positive end-expiratory pressure (PEEP) around 10, peak inspiratory pressure (PIP) around 20, and an inspiratory time (T_i) around 1.0 s. In adult patients, the mandatory respiratory rate on the ventilator may be decreased even further.

Systematic Approach to Develop, and Prioritize, the Most Appropriate Pediatric ECMO Simulations for Your Program

Similar to one range of vital signs not fitting all pediatric patients, learners participating in ECMO simulation may have unique backgrounds, considering both their discipline and expertise. To design the most appropriate ECMO simulation(s) for an institutional program, it is best to follow a systematic approach (Fig. 21.7):

1. Perform a comprehensive needs assessment of both the learners and the program; this is covered in detail in Chap. 6.
2. Consider all facets of the ECMO process to identify areas where knowledge gaps, inadequacies with teamwork/communication or issues with psychomotor skills exist, as well as where errors could possibly occur, and utilize this information to develop a preliminary list of scenarios.
3. Utilizing Fig. 21.9, develop a prioritized simulation scenario list.

Where Things Can Go Wrong: Common Pediatric ECMO Complications

First, we will review the common pediatric ECMO complications, based on the ELSO data [1], which will provide educators with an idea of high-yield areas on which to focus the efforts of the program. Tables 21.7 and 21.8 are provided to offer ECMO educators a quick resource regarding the complication types and frequencies for pediatric ECMO. Table 21.7 details many, not all, pediatric cardiac ECMO complications and includes both VA and VV ECMO data, although VV ECMO was only utilized in 1.6% of the cases. Similarly, Table 21.8 summarizes several pediatric respiratory ECMO complications. Of note, of these ECMO runs included in this

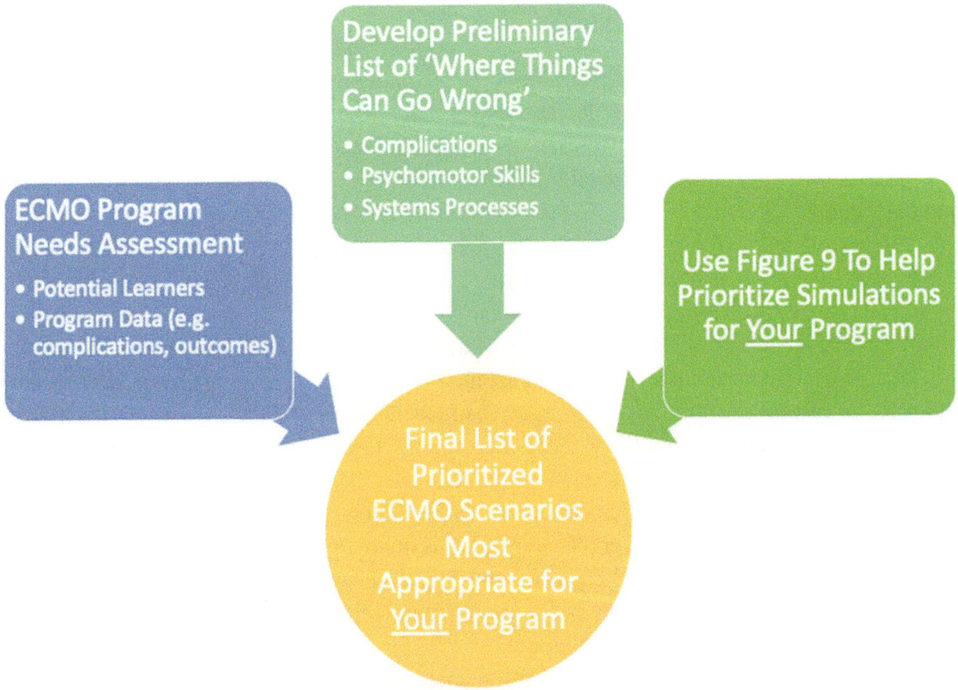

Fig. 21.7 Systematic Approach to Developing ECMO Scenarios

Table 21.7 Complications of pediatric cardiac runs, 2014–2019—includes both VA (96.5%) and VV (1.6%) modalities [1]

Mechanical	Hematologic	Neurologic	Cardiovascular	Pulmonary
Circuit Component Clots/ Air Emboli (21.3%)	Surgical Site Bleeding (19.2%)	Seizures (6.3%)	Inotrope Requirement (27.8%)	Pulmonary Hemorrhage (4.1%)
Cannula Problems (6.2%)	Cannulation Site Bleeding (12%)	CNS Infarction (5.7%)	Cardiac Arrhythmias (10.2%)	Pneumothorax Requiring Intervention (1.7%)
Circuit Change (3.8%)	Hemolysis (11.7%)	CNS Hemorrhage (5.4%)	Hypertension Requiring Vasodilators (9.9%)	
Hemofilter Clots (2.7%)	Mediastinal Cannulation Site Bleeding (4.3%)	Brain Death (1.9%)	Cardiac Tamponade Due to Blood (3.3%)	
Pump Failure (1.1%)	GI Hemorrhage (2.6%)	CNS Diffuse Ischemia (0.7%)	CPR Performed on ECMO (2.4%)	
Crack(s) in Pigtail Catheters (0.5%)	DIC (2.5%)	CNS Surgical Intervention Performed (0.1%)	Cardiac Tamponade Not Due to Blood (0.2%)	
Raceway/Tubing Rupture (0.3%)	Peripheral Cannulation Site Bleeding (1.1%)			
Heat Exchanger Malfunction (0.1%)				
Heat Exchanger Malfunction (0.1%)				

Table 21.8 Complications of pediatric respiratory runs, 2014–2019 – includes both VA (36%) and VV (61%) modalities [1]

Mechanical	Hematologic	Neurologic	Cardiovascular	Pulmonary
Circuit Component Clots/ Air Emboli (28.2%)	Hemolysis (17.9%)	CNS Hemorrhage (6.8%)	Inotrope Requirement (23.3%)	Pneumothorax Requiring Intervention (7.5%)
Cannula Problems (12.8%)	Cannulation Site Bleeding (14.7%)	CNS Infarction (4.6%)	Hypertension Requiring Vasodilators (11.4%)	Pulmonary Hemorrhage (6.3%)
Circuit Change (8.1%)	Surgical Site Bleeding (7.4%)	Seizures (3.9%)	CPR Performed on ECMO (6.3%)	
Hemofilter Clots (4.5%)	GI Hemorrhage (4.6%)	Brain Death (2%)	Cardiac Arrhythmias (4.4%)	
Pump Failure (1.1%)	DIC (2.8%)	CNS Diffuse Ischemia (0.6%)	Cardiac Tamponade Due to Blood (2.1%)	
Crack(s) in Pigtail Catheters (0.8%)	Peripheral Cannulation Site Bleeding (2%)	CNS Surgical Intervention Performed (0.2%)	Cardiac Tamponade Not Due to Blood (0.4%)	
Heat Exchanger Malfunction (0.4%)	Mediastinal Cannulation Site Bleeding (0.9%)			
Raceway/Tubing Rupture (0.3%)				

data, 61% were VV and 36% were VA. In both tables, complications are organized into the following categories: mechanical, hematologic, neurologic, cardiovascular, and pulmonary. Some complications are more amenable to replicating in a simulated environment (e.g., circuit component clot/air emboli) while others are more difficult, but not impossible (e.g., pulmonary hemorrhage). As noted in the previous section, hematologic complications are frequent. The next most common complication category is related to the cardiovascular system; most notably, almost half of cardiac and respiratory cases required inotropes or vasodilator administration or had arrhythmias develop.

Several other key points should be considered based upon the data. First, CPR while on ECMO was almost three times as likely to be required during respiratory cases, with the majority occurring with VV ECMO. Considering that these patients who primarily required ECMO for respiratory etiologies subsequently developed systemic (e.g., left ventricular) compromise requiring CPR, one can recognize the importance of *never* becoming complacent when *any* patient is on ECMO. This is especially relevant to patients on VV ECMO, as the ECMO circuit is merely oxygenating and ventilating the blood, but delivery of that blood is *completely* reliant on the patient's native systemic cardiac output, with or without vasoactive medications.

Pneumothoraces are almost twice as common in respiratory ECMO runs than in cardiac runs, likely secondary to the decreased compliance and need for higher ventilator setting prior to cannulation in respiratory runs. Cannula-related issues are also almost twice as common in respiratory ECMO compared to cardiac ECMO; this *may* be due to more frequent use of dual-lumen, single cannula that requires very precise intravascular/intra-atrial positioning for optimal function and avoidance of complications. Circuit changes are approximately twice as likely to occur on ECMO initiated for respiratory etiologies; the specific etiologies for this are likely multifactorial.

Recirculation in VV ECMO

There is one extremely important, well-known and frequent complication that has not been highlighted in these tables: recirculation during VV ECMO. Recirculation occurs when oxygenated blood returning from the ECMO pump immediately reenters the ECMO circuit instead of the patient's systemic circulation. Essentially, this is the same issue that occurs in certain physiologic left to right shunts (e.g., ventricular septal defects, patent ductus arteriosus) where oxygenated blood destined for systemic delivery reenters the pulmonary circulation instead. The end result of recirculation on VV ECMO is inadequate oxygen delivery to the patient's tissues and end-organs, similar to that which occurs in any type of shock state.

There are many different ways to provide VV ECMO (Fig. 21.8). These can be accomplished using one dual-lumen cannula (Fig. 21.8a, b) or two separate single-lumen cannulae (Fig. 21.8c–e). Dual-lumen single cannulae contain one lumen for systemic venous drainage and one lumen for oxygenated blood return. They offer the advantage of only one cannula having to be placed but often require more meticulous positioning than two single-lumen cannulae. VV ECMO using two cannula functions in the same way as the previous dual-lumen single cannulae; one cannula provides for systemic venous drainage from the body, toward the ECMO circuit, where it becomes oxygenated and ventilated. The newly oxygenated and ventilated blood is returned to the systemic venous vasculature via the second cannula.

Many factors contribute to the development of recirculation, including the rate of ECMO pump flow, cannula position, cannula design, native cardiac output and intravascular volume [14–18]. The hallmark of recirculation on VV ECMO is a decrease in the patient's systemic oxygen saturations with a simultaneous increase in the venous saturations. Since etiology can be multifactorial, the potential solutions vary depending on the underlying cause of recirculation. Sometimes the drainage and return catheters are too closely approximated. Dual-lumen single catheters may have malpositioning of the distal catheter resulting in altered flow patterns, increasing the risk of recirculation. Excessive flows and/or low intravascular volume are other common etiologies leading to recirculation. Higher flows can increase recirculation because it is more likely that newly oxygenated blood returned to the patient's body will be taken back up

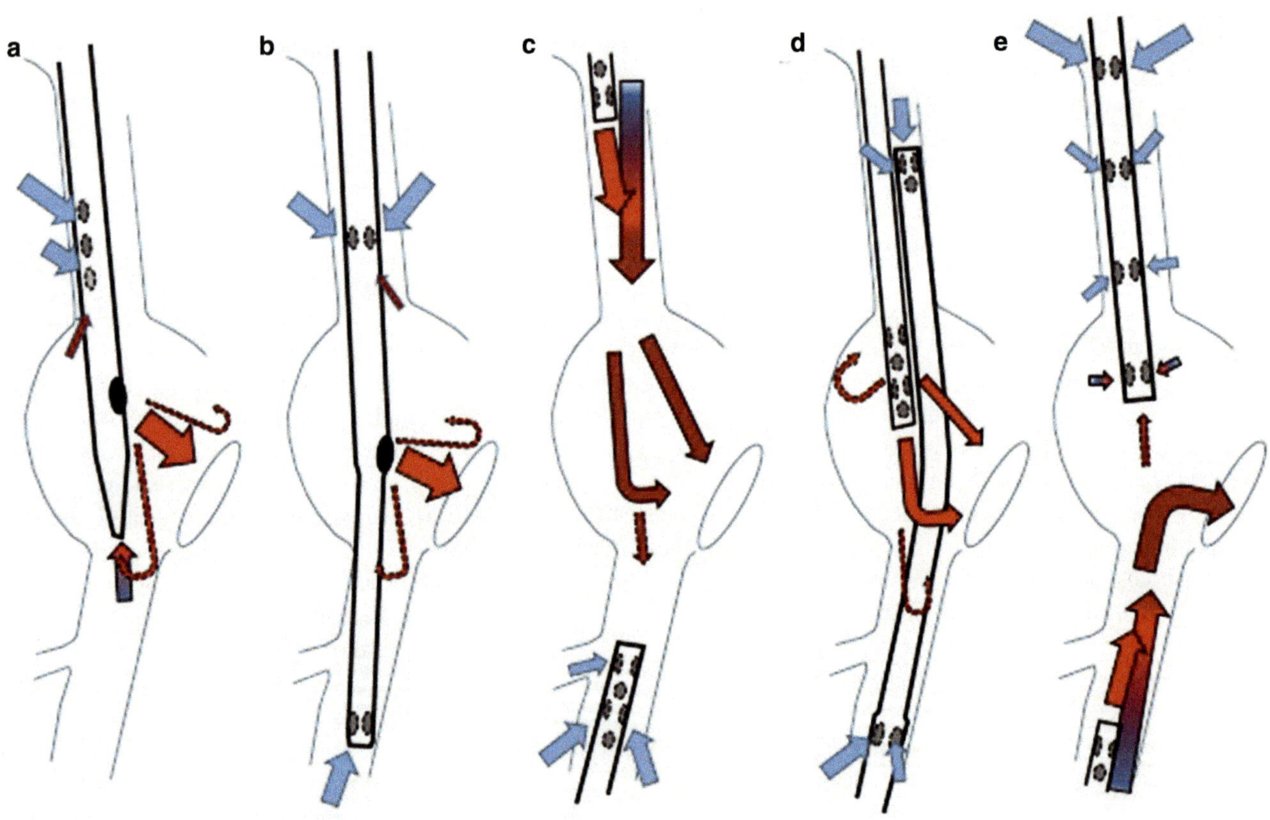

Fig. 21.8 Different VV ECMO Configurations. (Reproduced with permission of Ref. [19])

into the venous portion of the ECMO circuit, leading to further decline in the patient's systemic saturations. Oftentimes recirculation, if due to excessive flows, can be improved by decreasing the ECMO flows. Since this is a common issue on VV ECMO, ECMO educators should be very well versed in the physiology of VV recirculation to allow for incorporation of this topic into their simulation curriculum.

Where Things Can Go Wrong: Psychomotor Skills

Another area of potential focus for ECMO simulation concerns psychomotor skills, which are often related to cannulation or manipulation of the ECMO circuit. Perhaps the most common example of practicing or assessing psychomotor skills related to ECMO occurs during "water drills." These drills are ubiquitous in ECMO training conducted globally, as this format has been recommended as a learning modality by ELSO for many years. In water drills, ECMO specialists practice setting up, running, and trouble-shooting ECMO circuits filled with water instead of blood. These drills are designed to enhance the specialists' psychomotor skills in manipulating the circuit, which will ideally improve their confidence *and* performance in the clinical environment. Water drills can be performed with or without incorporation of a manikin. Additionally, the learner group participating in the water drill can vary depending on the objectives of the case, either incorporating specialists alone or utilized in an interdisciplinary training exercise.

Simulating ECMO cannulation, with realistic fidelity, is challenging. However, several options for cannulation models have been developed with very positive outcomes. Allan [20] et al. developed a task trainer specifically designed for ECMO cannula insertion. This trainer was utilized in combination with a curriculum for pediatric cardiothoracic surgical trainees to practice cannulation. In their study, the trainees found the experience to be highly useful and demonstrated sustained improvement in time to cannulation compared to their baseline performance [20]. Although incorporation of some types of cannulation trainers may be cost-prohibitive and time-consuming for many programs, Thompson [21] et al. described creation of a cannulation used as a part of a neonatal ECMO initiation simulation for ECMO specialists, costing only $25 USD to create and created in about 1 h.

Where Things Can Go Wrong: Systems Processes

Because ECMO is technologically complicated and requires the successful orchestration of providers across multiple disciplines *and* multiple professions, it is paramount that both communication and systems-related processes are optimized. Competency is not adequate; proficiency should be the goal so that children whose lives depend on this resource can have the best possible outcomes. Many studies have previously demonstrated benefits of ECMO simulations, including [22–29]:

- Improved individual and team preparedness
- Improved teamwork
- Enhanced communication
- Knowledge transfer/acquisition
- Increased self-confidence
- Improved performance (typically measured as less time to accomplish a task or fewer complications)
- Better recognition of safety concerns and latent safety threats (LSTs)
- Decreased times to critical actions (e.g., time from ECPR to initiation to cannulation)

Considering these findings, programs should incorporate assessment of systems processes into ECMO simulations. Indeed, in the seminal article, "To err is human" [30], the authors state:

"More commonly, errors are caused by faulty systems, processes, and conditions that lead people to make mistakes or fail to prevent them." This was true in 1999 and it remains true 20 years later; accordingly, any manner by which an ECMO program can practice to improve their local systems, processes, and communications can only result in improved performance and better patient outcomes. Pragmatically, however, designating time to practice in a simulated environment remains very difficult, if not impossible, given the many individuals, teams, and programs involved in the care of pediatric ECMO patients. As such, the types of simulations selected to be run in an interdisciplinary fashion need to be carefully considered and incredibly well-coordinated. This is where the program's needs assessment can be very useful. For example, if several different individuals across professions and disciplines endorse that getting a child onto ECMO during ECPR is chaotic, disorganized, and exhibits poor communication and lack of clarity around role definition, it follows that simulating this topic in an interdisciplinary fashion is likely high yield and likely to have positive clinical and programmatic impacts.

Prioritizing Simulations for Your Program

Once the needs assessment data has been analyzed and the program leadership has considered potential challenges in the ECMO process, the next step is to develop a prioritized list of pediatric ECMO simulation scenarios. This can be a rather daunting task, but by asking and answering three questions, this can be easily accomplished:

1. How likely is it that something will go wrong?
   (a) Refer to Tables 21.7 and 21.8 for known pediatric ECMO complications
   (b) Consider any psychomotor skills contributing to areas of known or suspected risk
   (c) Determine whether local systems-related issues contributed to the increased likelihood of adverse events
2. What is the likelihood of harm to the patient if a specific event occurs?
   (a) Not all complications have equal morbidity or mortality risks; a raceway rupture is far more likely to be catastrophic than a heat exchanger malfunction. A small clot within the venous portion of the VA ECMO circuit is not near as potentially harmful as a small clot located in the arterial limb of the tubing; the venous clot, if dislodged will likely just end up in the oxygenator whereas the arterial clot, if the circuit is not changed, could cause catastrophic neurological injury. These risks should be considered when determining which cases should be included in a program's simulation curriculum.
3. How easy will it be to accurately simulate the event locally, in a manner and fidelity that both the instructors and learners are comfortable with?
   (a) This consideration is a prelude to the next section, as not all simulation centers/programs offer the same technological fidelity. That is ok!
   (b) A program should realistically assess its capabilities in how to most effectively simulate a given clinical event. The key is NOT to try to make a simulation too complicated or technologically difficult if that is not what the educators, or the learners, are used to.

Figure 21.9 offers a schema that addresses the aforementioned questions for consideration. In this figure, numbers 1–4 represent areas of overlap and the author's recommendation for the order of prioritization for ECMO scenarios, with 1 being of the highest priority and 4 being of the lowest priority. A level 1 priority indicates a situation in which the likelihood of an event happening is high (e.g., clot in circuit), the potential for patient harm is high (e.g., clot is on the arterial side), and the educator feels it would be relatively easy to replicate in a simulation (e.g., put a dark dot near the arterial cannula). Taken together, this combination should render this case as a high-priority within an ECMO simulation curriculum.

For the other three regions (numbers 2–4), it is not as straightforward to prioritize; other experts in ECMO education and/or medical simulation, may have differing opinions. For purposes of this chapter, a *patient-centric approach* was taken, with the most important factor being "High Potential Harm to Patient if Event Occurs." The second-most important factor, again using a patient-centric framework, was

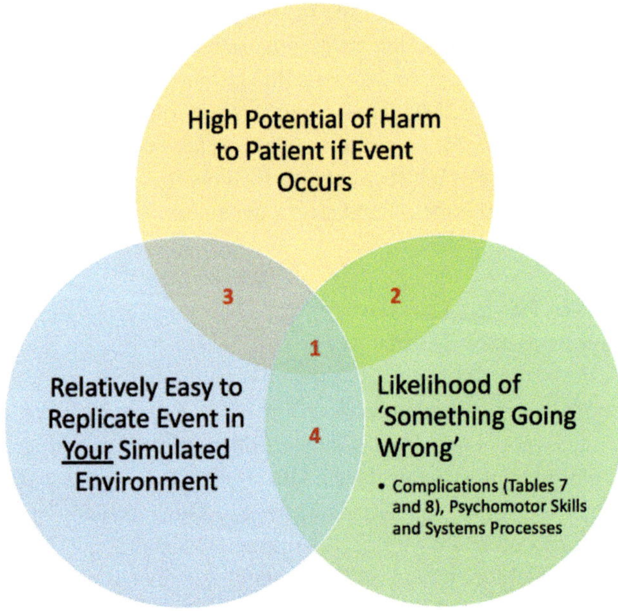

Fig. 21.9 Schema for Prioritizing Pediatric ECMO Simulation

"Likelihood of 'Something Going Wrong.'" The remaining factor, "Ease of Simulation Replication," was rated as the least important. Based on this stratification, one can then prioritize specific ECMO simulations for their institutional ECMO simulation program.

ECMO Simulation: High(er) Fidelity Is Not Necessarily Better – Just More Complicated

Considering that only approximately one-third of pediatric ECMO programs incorporate simulation training into their educational curriculum, it seems prudent to focus on highly complex ECMO simulations that are often conducted solely at large, quaternary academic institutions with high ECMO patient volume. Educators at each center must incorporate this information into the context of their local educational program in order to develop an educational product that best meets their needs and their abilities. One frequent misconception in simulation is that higher-fidelity simulation offers superior educational benefits and enhances transfer of knowledge; *however, the literature does not support this belief* [31]. Higher-fidelity manikins have a more realistic look and feel, but are more complicated to program and run. This additional level of complexity can lead to delays in enacting appropriate and timely changes to exam findings, vital signs, or circuit pressures. These challenges may detract from the ability of the learners to have the best possible simulation experience. In fact, higher-fidelity simulations may lead to overconfidence in self-perceived performance at the expense of actual performance, as measured by observer ratings [31]. In a randomized (low- versus high-fidelity) study of medical students participating an advanced life support session, both groups had similar theoretical knowledge acquisition with comparable observed overall performance. However, there were four areas where the higher-fidelity group statistically performed more poorly than the lower-fidelity group.

To further illustrate this point, consider an infant who requires treatment for septic shock. Using a low-technology manikin, after the learner verbally states that they have given an IV fluid bolus, they receive immediate feedback from the instructor that the tachycardia is improving. Alternatively, using a higher-technology manikin, after the IV fluid bolus is administered, there may be a delay in the heart rate coming down due to the need to alter the controls. This might also be missed altogether given the sheer number of things the simulation specialist is attending to at once. In many situations, the former situation would be preferable because the feedback is of higher physiologic fidelity, even though the manikin is of higher technical fidelity.

Far from recommending against the use of high-fidelity simulation, it is prudent to utilize a level of *technical* fidelity that both the educator and learners are comfortable with and which can be manipulated in a timely, appropriate manner to give learners an accurate representation of physiologic fidelity. Ultimately what matters most is providing opportunities for experiential learning to enable learners to provide the highest level of care for their future pediatric ECMO patients.

Conclusion

ECMO is a complex, high-risk, low-acuity treatment option for many patients, including those in the pediatric population – which makes it ideal for simulation-based training. What makes ECMO and ECMO simulation difficult in the pediatric population, compared to neonates and adults, is that there is no "one-size-fits-all" approach for the wide range of pediatric ages and sizes. In pediatric patients who require ECMO, there is considerable variation in patient age/size, ECMO equipment/flows and age-appropriate vital signs. By utilizing the information contained within this chapter, particularly the tables outlining age-based differences in flows, cannulae, and vital signs, educators designing and providing pediatric ECMO simulation should have all the tools necessary to ensure pediatric ECMO patients at their institution have the best possible outcomes via excellent simulation training of healthcare personnel who provide this life-saving measure.

Appendix 21.1: Pediatric Age-Based Vital Signs, Typical ECMO Flows and Cannula Sizes

	Male Wt in Kg (5%/50%/95%)	Female Wt in Kg (5%/50%/95%)	Heart Rate (5%/50%/95%)	Resp. Rate	SBP (5%/50%/95%)	DBP (50%/95%)	(50%/95%)	Typical Flow Ranges (mL/kg/min) ELSO Pg 118	Venous Cannula	Max Flow(s) (mL/min)	Arterial Cannula	Max Flow(s) (mL/min)
1 Month	3.4/4.4/5.4	3.2/4.2/5.1	121/149/179	30–50	65/80/95	46/55	57/68	100–200	8 10	600 800	8 10	600 800
2 Months	4.1/5.3/6.4	3.8/4.8/5.9	121/149/179	30–40	65/80/95	40/50	57/68	100–200	8 10	600 800	8 10	600 800
6 Months	6.5/7.9/9.6	5.9/7.2/8.7	109/134/169	25–35	65/80/95	40/50	53/65	100–150	12 14	1000 1500	12 14	1000 1500
1 Year	8.6/10.3/12	8.0/9.5/11.4	89/119/151	20–30	67/85/103	37/56	53/72	100–150	14 15	1500 2000	14	1500
2 Years	10.6/12/6/15	10.2/12/14/5	89/119/151	20–30	70/88/106	42/61	57/76	80–125	14 15 Art	1500 2000	14	1500
3 Years	11.7/14.3/17	11.6/13.8/17	73/108/137	20–25	72/91/109	46/65	61/80	80–125	15 Art 17 Art	2000 2500	14 15	1500 2500
4 Years	13.5/16.2/20	13/15.8/20.2	73/018/137	20–25	75/93/111	50/69	64/83	50–125	15 15 Art 17 Art	2000 2000 2500	14 15	1500 2500
5 Years	15/18.4/23.3	14.6/18/23.9	65/100/133	20–25	78/95/112	53/72	67/85	50–100	15 15 Art 17	2000 2000 2500	14 15	1500 2500
6 Years	16.8/20.6/27	16.3/20.2/27	65/100/133	20–25	78/96/114	55/74	69/87	50–100	15 17 Art 19 Art	2000 2500 3500	15 17	2500 3500
7 Years	18.6/23/30.8	18/22.7/31.3	65/100/133	20–25	79/97/115	57/76	70/89	50–100	15 17 17 Art 19 Art 21 Art	2000 2800 2500 3500 4500	15 17	2500 3500
8 Years	20.5/25.6/35	20/25.6/36	62/91/130	20–25	82/99/116	59/78	72/91	50–100	15 17 17 Art 19 19 Art 21 Art	2000 2800 2500 3500 3500 4500	15 17 19	2500 3500 4500

9 Years	22.6/28.5/40	22.2/29/41.5	62/91/130	20–25	82/100/118	60/79	73/92	50–100	15	2000	15	2500
									17	2800	17	3500
									17 Art	2500	19	4500
									19	3500		
									19 Art	3500		
									21	4800		
									21 Art	4500		
									23 Art	5500		
10 Years	24.8/32/45.8	24.7/32.9/48	62/91/130	16–20	85/102/119	61/80	75/93	50–100	15	2000	15	2500
									17	2800	17	3500
									17 Art	2500	19	4500
									19	3500		
									19 Art	3500		
									21	4800		
									21 Art	4500		
									23	5500		
									23 Art	5500		
11 Years	27.4/36/52.3	27.7/37/54.7	62/91/130	16–20	87/104/121	61/80	75/94	50–100	15	2000	17	3500
									17	2800	19	4500
									19	3500	21	5500
									19 Art	3500		
									21	4800		
									21 Art	4500		
									23	5500		
									23 Art	5500		
									25	6000		
12 Years	30.4/40.5/59	31/41.6/61.3	60/85/119	16–20	89/106/123	62/81	77/95	50–75	17	2800	17	3500
									19	3500	19	4500
									19 Art	3500	21	5500
									21	4800	23	6000
									21 Art	4500		
									23	5500		
									23 Art	5500		
									25	6000		
									27	6000		
									29	6000		
13 Years	34/45.5/65.8	34.5/46/67.3	60/85/119	16–20	90/108/126	62/81	77/96	50–75	17	2800	17	3500
									19	3500	19	4500
									21	4800	21	5500
									21 Art	4500	23	6000
									23	5500		
									23 Art	5500		
									25	6000		
									27	6000		
									29	6000		

(continued)

Appendix (continued)

	Male Wt in Kg (5%/50%/95%)	Female Wt in Kg (5%/50%/95%)	Heart Rate (5%/50%/95%)	Resp. Rate	SBP (5%/50%/95%)	DBP (50%/95%)	(50%/95%)	Typical Flow Ranges (mL/kg/min) ELSO Pg 118	Venous Cannula	Max Flow(s) (mL/min)	Arterial Cannula	Max Flow(s) (mL/min)
14 Years	38.3/51/72.4	37.8/49.3/72	60/85/119	16–20	94/111/128	63/82	79/97	50–75	19	3500	19	4500
									21	4800	21	5500
									23	5500	23	6000
									23 Art	5500		
									25	6000		
									27	6000		
									29	6000		
15 Years	43/56.3/78.5	40.6/52/75.7	60/85/119	16–20	95/113/131	64/83	80/99	50–75	21	4800	19	4500
									23	5500	21	5500
									23 Art	5500	23	6000
									25	6000		
									27	6000		
									29	6000		
16 Years	47/61/84	42.9/53.9/78	60/85/119	16–20	98/116/134	65/84	82/101	50–75	21	4800	19	4500
									23	5500	21	5500
									23 Art	5500	23	6000
									25	6000		
									27	6000		
									29	6000		
17 Years	51/64.5/88.6	44.4/55/79.5	60/85/119	16–20	100/118/136	67/87	84/103	60–65	21	4800	19	4500
									23	5500	21	5500
									23 Art	5500	23	6000
									25	6000		
									27	6000		
									29	6000		
18 Years	53.1/67.2/92	45.3/56/80.7	60/85/119	16–20	102/120/138	69/90	86/106	60–65	23	5500	19	4500
									23 Art	5500	21	5500
									25	6000	23	6000
									27	6000		
									29	6000		

References

1. ELSO ECLS Registry Report. International Summary. July 2019. Accessed 2019 Aug.
2. Van Meurs K, Lally K, Peek G, Zwischenberger J. ECMO extracorporeal cardiopulmonary support in critical care, vol. 134. Ann Arbor: Extracorporeal Life Support Organisation; 2005.
3. Anderson JM, Boyle KB, Murphy AA, Yaeger KA, LeFlore J, Halamek LP. Simulating extracorporeal membrane oxygenation emergencies to improve human performance. Part I: methodologic and technologic innovations. Simul Healthc. 2006;1(4):220–7.
4. Chiniara G, Cole G, Brisbin K, Huffman D, Cragg B, Lamacchia M, Norman D. Simulation in healthcare: a taxonomy and a conceptual framework for instructional design and medial selection. Med Teach. 2013;13:e1380–95.
5. Weems MF, Friedlich PS, Nelson LP, Rake AJ, Klee L, Stein JE, Stavroudis TA. The role of extracorporeal membrane oxygenation at extracorporeal life support organization centers in the United States. Simul Healthc. 2017;12(4):233–9.
6. Cicek S, Chan T, Dearani J. Neonatal, pediatric and adult cardiac extracorporeal life support. In: Brogan TV, Annich G, Ellis WC, Haney B, Heard M, Lorusso R, editors. ECMO specialist training manual. 4th ed. Ann Arbor: ELSO; 2018. p. 75–81.
7. Guerguerian AM, Gunnerson K, Thiagarajan RR. Extracorporeal membrane oxygenation for cardiopulmonary arrest and resuscitation. In: Brogan TV, Annich G, Ellis WC, Haney B, Heard M, Lorusso R, editors. ECMO specialist training manual. 4th ed. Ann Arbor: ELSO. 2018. p. 85–93.
8. Edwards L, Todd M. Patient management: neonatal and pediatric cardiac ECLS. In: Brogan TV, Annich G, Ellis WC, Haney B, Heard M, Lorusso R, editors. ECMO specialist training manual. 4th ed. Ann Arbor: ELSO; 2018. p. 187–94.
9. Butt W, Heard M, Peek G. Clinical management of the extracorporeal membrane oxygenation circuit. Pediatr Crit Care Med. 2013;14(5 Supplement 1):S13–9.
10. Chan T, Thiagarajan RR, Frank D, et al. Survival after extracorporeal cardiopulmonary resuscitation in infants and children with heart disease. J Thorac Cardiovasc Surg. 2008;136(4):984–92.
11. Peek GJ, Hammond I. Neonatal/pediatric cardiac cannulation. In: Brogan TV, editor. Extracorporeal life support: the ELSO red book. 5th. ed. Ann Arbor: ELSO; 2017. p. 347–55.
12. Lorusso R, Dinardo M, Wang I, Makdisi G. Patient management: neonatal and pediatric cardiac ECLS. In: Brogan TV, Annich G, Ellis WC, Haney B, Heard M, Lorusso R, editors. ECMO specialist training manual. 4th ed. Ann Arbor: ELSO; 2018. p. 113–9.
13. Cho HJ, Kim DW, Kim GS, Jeong S. Anticoagulation therapy during extracorporeal oxygenator support in pediatric patients. Chonnam Med J. 2017;53:110–7.
14. Heard M, Davis J, Fortenberry j. Principles and practice of venovenous and venoarterial ECMO. In: ECMO specialist training manual. 3rd ed. Ann Arbor: Extracorporeal Life Support Organization; 2010. p. 59–75.
15. van Heijst AF, van der Staak FH, de Haan AF, et al. Recirculation in double lumen veno-venous extracorporeal membrane oxygenation measured by an ultrasound dilution technique. ASAIO J. 2001;47(4):372–6.
16. Korver EP, Ganushchak YM, Simons AP, Donker DW, Maessen JG, Weerwind PW. Quantification of recirculation as an adjuvant to transthoracic echocardiography for optimization of dual-lumen extracorporeal life support. J Intensive Care Med. 2012;38(5):906–9.
17. Browman LM, Hultman J. Double lumen catheter placement during VV ECMO in an infant with persistent left superior vena cava-important considerations. ASAIO J. 2014;60(5):602–5.
18. Palmer O, Palmer K, Hultman J, Broman LM. The influence of cannula design on recirculation during venovenous extracorporeal membrane oxygenation. ASAIO J. 2016;62(6):7370742.
19. Browman LM, Wagoner S. Venovenous extracorporeal membrane oxygenation. In: Brogan TV, Annich G, Ellis WC, Haney B, Heard M, Lorusso R, editors. ECMO specialist training manual. 4th ed. Ann Arbor: ELSO; 2018. p. 123–7.
20. Allan CK, Pigula F, Bacha EA, Emani S, Fynn-Thompson F, Thiagarajan RR, Imprescia A, Hayes G, Weinstock P. An extracorporeal membrane oxygenation cannulation curriculum featuring a novel integrated skills trainer leads to improved performance among pediatric cardiac surgery trainees. Simul Healthc. 2013;8(4):221–8.
21. Thompson JL, Grisham LM, Scott J, Mogan C, Prescher H, Biffar D, Jarred J, Meyer RJ, Hamilton AJ. Construction of a reusable, high-fidelity model to enhance extracorporeal membrane oxygenation training through simulation. Adv Neonatal Care. 2014;14(2):103–9.
22. Chan SY, Figueroa M, Spentzas T, Powell A, Holloway R, Shah S. Prospective assessment of novice learners in a simulation-based extracorporeal membrane oxygenation (ECMO) education program. Pediatr Cardiol. 2013;34:543–52.
23. Su L, Spaeder MC, Jones MB, Sinha P, Nath DS, Jain PN, Berger JT, Williams L, Shankar V. Implementation of an extracorporeal cardiopulmonary resuscitation simulation program reduces extracorporeal cardiopulmonary resuscitation times in real patients. Pediatr Crit Care Med. 2014;15(10):856–60.
24. Burton KS, Pendergrass TL, Byczkowski TL, Taylor RG, Moyer MR, Falcone RA, Geis GL. Impact of simulation-based extracorporeal membrane oxygenation training in the simulation laboratory and clinical environment. Simul Healthc. 2011;6(5):281–91.
25. Sanchez-Glanville C, Brindle ME, Spence T, Blackwood J, Drews T, Menzies S, Lopushinsky SR. Evaluating the introduction of extracorporeal life support technology to a tertiary-care institution: smoothing the learning curve through interprofessional simulation training. J Pediatr Surg. 2015;50:798–804.
26. Atamanyuk I, Ghez O, Saeed I, Lane M, Hall J, Jackson T, Desai A, Burmester M. Impact of an open-chest extracorporeal membrane oxygenation model for in situ simulated team training: a pilot study. Interact Cardiovasc Thorac Surg. 2014;18:17–20.
27. Nardo MD, David P, Stoppa F, Lorusso R, Raponi M, Amodeo A, Cecchetti C, Guner Y, Taccone FS. The introduction of a high fidelity simulation program for training pediatric critical care personnel reduces the time to manage extracorporeal membrane oxygenation emergencies and improves teamwork. J Thorac Dis. 2018;10(6):3409–17.
28. Burkhart HM, Riley JB, Lynch JJ, Suri RM, Greason KL, Joyce LD, Nuttall GA, Stulak J, Schaff HV, Dearani JA. Simulation-based postcardiotomy extracorporeal membrane oxygenation crisis training for thoracic surgery residents. Ann Thorac Surg. 2013;95:901–6.
29. Zakhary BM, Kam LM, Kaufman BS, Felner KJ. The utility of high-fidelity simulation for training critical care fellows in the management of extracorporeal membrane oxygenation emergencies: a randomized controlled trial. Crit Care Med. 2017;45(8):1367–73.
30. Kohn LT, Corrigan J, Donaldson MS. To err is human: building a safer health system. Washington, D.C: National Academy Press; 2000.
31. Massoth C, Roder H, Ohlenburg H, Hessler M, Zarbock A, Popping DM, Wenk M. High-fidelity is not superior to low-fidelity simulation but leads to overconfidence in medical students. BMC Med Educ. 2019;19:29. https://doi.org/10.1186/s12909-019-1464-7.

ECMO Simulation in Patients with Cardiac Disease

22

Peta M. A. Alexander, Katie M. Moynihan, Susanna Price, and Catherine K. Allan

Learning Objectives

1. To understand the complexity of clinical microsystems characterized by ad hoc team formation and complex environments which are inherent in cardiac critical care and impact the delivery of ECMO to these patients.
2. To describe the simulation technology complexities in establishing high-fidelity adult education, particularly for those learners managing patients with complex congenital heart disease and varying cannulation strategies.
3. To highlight extracorporeal cardiopulmonary resuscitation as an example of a particularly complex cardiac management strategy. Team-based training can prepare clinical environments for these cognitively and technically challenging rare events.

Introduction

Extracorporeal membrane oxygenation (ECMO) is increasingly utilized in the management of critically ill patients with cardiovascular collapse who fail to respond to conventional therapies [1, 2]. High-fidelity simulation strategies are established methods for individual and team training in a structured environment remote from patient harm. These facilitate technical skill proficiency and identify systems hazards while reducing the risk of error due to human and interpersonal factors [3–6]. Multi-professional teams initiate ECMO, frequently in response to rapid changes in clinical condition, across a spectrum of ages, sizes, anatomical vascular configurations, and pathophysiologies [2]. Care is delivered within various clinical microsystems (prehospital, emergency room, operating room, catheterization laboratory, intensive care unit), often characterized by ad hoc team formation, complex environments, high technical and cognitive demands, and need for frequent handover (Fig. 22.1 and Table 22.1) [7–11]. These aspects must be addressed during simulation training with a degree of fidelity that facilitates experiential adult learning. ECMO simulation models have proven particularly useful for intensivists, with retention of knowledge and skills demonstrated in trouble-shooting complications [5, 6]. Specific cardiac simulation-based training programs need to be developed for these complex situations to improve team function and ultimately positively impact patient outcomes [4, 12].

Veno-arterial (VA) ECMO is a form of invasive mechanical support instituted for refractory cardiac, respiratory or cardiorespiratory failure. Specific goals of VA-ECMO in the cardiac population include addressing the etiology of cardiorespiratory compromise including identification and treatment of residual lesions while providing hemodynamic support to maintain tissue oxygen delivery and support end-organ function while facilitating myocardial recovery [2, 13]. The majority of mechanical circulatory support required for patients with underlying cardiac disease in the emergency

P. M. A. Alexander (✉) · K. M. Moynihan
Department of Cardiology, Boston Children's Hospital and Department of Pediatrics, Harvard Medical School, Boston, MA, USA
e-mail: peta.alexander@cardio.chboston.org; katie.moynihan@cardio.chboston.org

S. Price
Department of Cardiology and Intensive Care, Royal Brompton Hospital and Departments of Cardiology and Intensive Care, Imperial College London, London, UK
e-mail: S.Price@rbht.nhs.uk

C. K. Allan
Department of Cardiology, Boston Children's Hospital and Department of Pediatrics, Harvard Medical School, Boston, MA, USA

SIMPeds, Boston Children's Hospital Simulator Program, Boston Children's Hospital and Harvard Medical School, Boston, MA, USA
e-mail: catherine.allan@cardio.chboston.org

L. C. Johnston, L. Su (eds.), *Comprehensive Healthcare Simulation: ECMO Simulation*, Comprehensive Healthcare Simulation,
https://doi.org/10.1007/978-3-030-53844-6_22

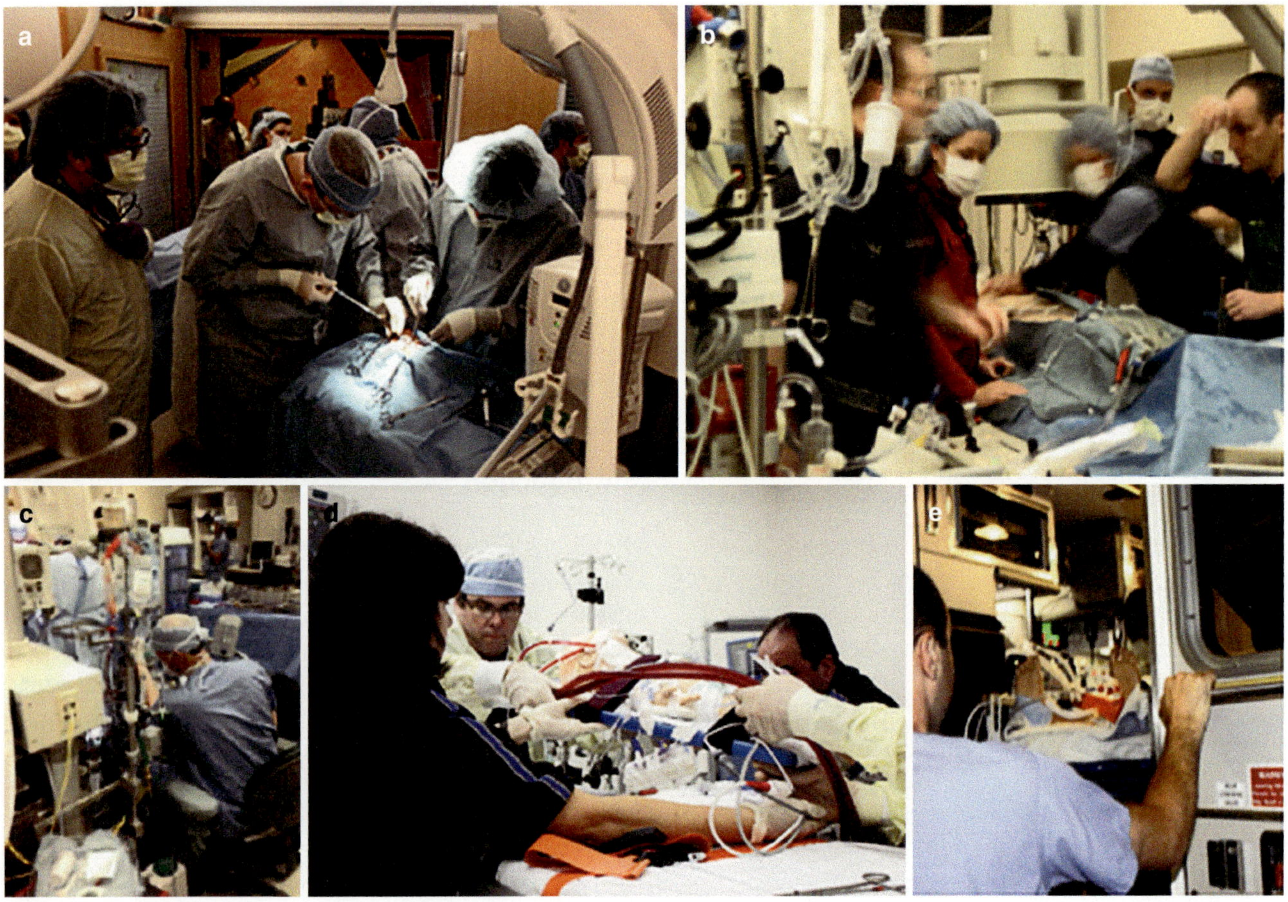

Fig. 22.1 Team training simulation across microsystems delivering care to patients with cardiac disease. (**a**) Cardiac intensive care unit, (**b**) cardiac catheterization laboratory, (**c**) cardiac operating room, and (**d**, **e**) ECMO transport

setting comprises veno-arterial (VA) ECMO [1, 14]. Veno-veno (VV) ECMO for isolated pulmonary support is addressed in Chap. 21. Decision-making around candidacy for ECMO is influenced by social, cultural, and institutional norms as well as patient factors and is outside the scope of this chapter. Technical advances in circuit componentry and increased familiarity with ECMO have resulted in broadening of the indications for ECMO support in the cardiac population. For example, institution of VA ECMO while undergoing cardiopulmonary resuscitation (ECPR) has expanded with evidence of acceptable survival and neurological outcomes [1, 14, 15]. Similarly, use of VA-ECMO to support patients with single-ventricle circulation is now common, when it was once considered a contraindication to ECMO support [16–18].

Both the growing use of ECMO in the cardiac population (Fig. 22.2) and the complexity of ECMO care in terms of technical and team requirements make it an ideal target for simulation-based training. ECMO is frequently deployed in the cardiac intensive care unit (CICU) and other environments during times of rapid clinical deterioration. Multiple care providers may need to come together emergently to form an ad hoc team, make cognitively demanding decisions, and perform technically challenging procedures. Variable patient ages, sizes, specific anatomical vascular configurations, and pathophysiologies impact the mode of support, choice of pump, cannulation strategy, and monitoring requirements. To address this complexity, simulation-based training programs need to be developed and delivered using rigorous, structured processes based on the principles of adult learning theory. Ideally this process includes a needs assessment, scenarios constructed to target defined learning objectives, and safe, supportive debriefing to facilitate learner self-reflection [3, 6, 12, 19].

Simulation for ECMO training has higher complexity than traditional manikin-based simulation. The need to integrate the ECMO circuit with the manikin, replicate ECMO emergencies, and provide complex physiologic data via both standard patient monitors and ECMO monitors with high levels of fidelity has required significant innovation. Recent technical and system developments have enabled educators to create simulation scenarios that accurately replicate the

Table 22.1 Clinical microsystems in cardiovascular care: complexity of personnel, equipment, and teams

Location	Personnel	Equipment	Clinical systems
Intensive care unit	Intensivist Cannulating interventionist or surgeon ICU nurses Respiratory therapist ECMO specialist or perfusionist Operating room nurses Trainees	ECMO circuit Resuscitation carts Defibrillator Surgical instrument table Surgical equipment (cautery, headlamp, etc.) Specialist equipment (flexible bronchoscopes, difficult airway, etc.) Ultrasound and echocardiography	Multiple patients Capacity constraints/bed availability Blended teams Hierarchy of personnel
Emergency room	Emergency physician(s) ER nurses Anesthesiologist/intensivist Respiratory therapist ECMO specialist/perfusionist Interventionist/surgeon Operating room nurses Trainees	Resuscitation rooms/equipment Portable radiography Surgical instrument table Surgical equipment (cautery, headlamp, etc.) ECMO circuit Ultrasound and echocardiography	Limited familiarity with ECMO Undifferentiated pathophysiology Limited patient background Multiple patients Capacity constraints/bed availability Blended teams Hierarchy of personnel Remote equipment
Cardiac catheterization laboratory	Interventional cardiologist Catheter technologist Anesthesiologist Nurses +/− surgeon +/− OR nurses Trainees	Fluoroscopy equipment Fixed catheterization table Cath instrument table Surgical instrument table Ultrasound and Echocardiography	Rapidly changing physiology Radiation exposure Multiple equipment changes Communication between control room and lab High level of technical skills Possible simultaneous interventions – catheter-based therapy and surgical cannulation Hierarchy of personnel
Cardiac operating room	Surgeon Assistant surgeon Anesthesiologist Scrub nurse Circulating nurse ECMO specialist Perfusionist Echocardiographer Trainees	CPB circuit ECMO circuit Anesthesia machine Minimally invasive equipment Echocardiography	Time pressure on cardiopulmonary bypass High level of technical skills Transition from CPB to ECMO Possible blended teams (CPB and ECMO) Hierarchy of personnel

complex physiology of ECMO-patient interactions by manipulating a mock ECMO circuit integrated with a manikin. For instance, infant, pediatric, and adult cannulation part-task trainers have been designed in collaboration with expert surgeons for training on technical skills, with a goal of shortened time to ECMO initiation [5, 20]. Accurate display of "monitored" physiologic data is now possible, including intra-cardiac pressures and ECMO parameters, which promotes suspense of disbelief of learners and increases the fidelity of these exercises. Lastly, simulations can be modified and adapted, with the goal of being able to conduct them in the various environments relevant to cardiac patients. These methods of increasing fidelity, which enable scenarios to closely mirror clinical reality, allow teams to practice integrating patient and circuit physiology under appropriate time pressure to diagnose and treat circuit emergencies and achieve management proficiency [6].

In this chapter, we describe simulation strategies to facilitate specific learning objectives for the interdisciplinary team managing cardiac patients requiring ECMO support, focusing on relevant anatomical and physiological considerations as well as ECPR. We then describe pertinent elements for various location-specific microsystems and unique interdisciplinary team dynamics relating to cardiac patients.

Simulation Design and Setup

The importance of technical, conceptual, and emotional realism in design and delivery of simulations to enhance learner engagement has been well described [21, 22]. Technical realism reflects how closely manikins, patient monitors, and equipment replicate "real life." For ECMO simulation, technical realism includes the integration of the ECMO circuit into the simulation. Conceptual realism refers to the accuracy and relevance of the clinical narrative portrayed by a simulation scenario. Emotional realism includes the learners' overall response to the delivery environment and can be

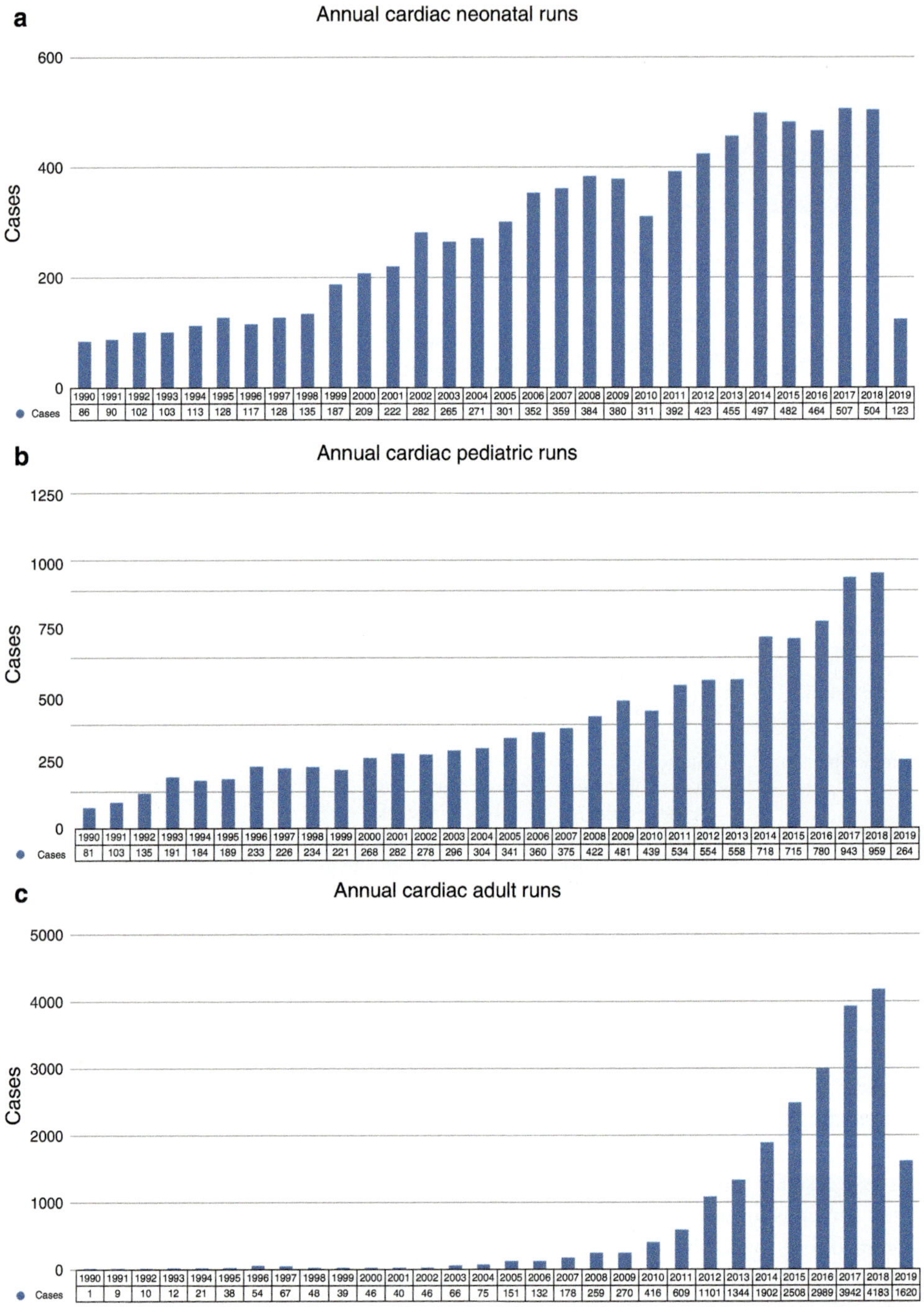

Fig. 22.2 Cardiac ECMO runs reported to the Extracorporeal Life Support Organization over time. (**a**) Neonates, (**b**) children, (**c**) adults. (With permission from the Extracorporeal Life Support Organization (ELSO), ECLS Registry Report International Summary, July 2019. ELSO 2800 Plymouth Road, Building 300, Room 303, Ann Arbor, MI 48109). Note: 2019 represents partial year ascertainment only

enhanced through simulation in the native environment with complete clinical teams. In order to increase fidelity of cardiac ECMO scenarios and encourage the learners to fully engage in simulations, elements of clinical care specific to the cardiac population must be faithfully replicated during scenario design and setup. Of note, because the physiology displayed is often non-standard (e.g., non-pulsatile flow, multiple intra-cardiac lines, multiple pulse oximeters, atypical cardiac rhythms), it is essential that simulationists understand the limitations of the simulation software or display of physiologic parameters used. Successful replication of cardiac ECMO physiology requires advanced planning and, often, work-arounds applied to typical simulation-software displays. In this chapter, we will review methods to enhance technical, conceptual, and emotional realism for simulation of cardiac ECMO, address issues related to use of specific ECMO circuits during simulation, and discuss training specific for ECMO cannulation, physiologic displays for ECMO

Box 22.1 Zone/Level 1 Simulation – Instruction of ECMO Cannulation

Target Audience: Cardiac surgical attending/instructor and cardiac surgical residents and fellows with scrub nurse or capable assistant
Learning Objectives:
At the end of this simulation scenario, the participants will be able to:
1. Identify and demonstrate the vascular anatomy of the neck/groin.
2. Under aseptic technique, dissect, identify, and isolate arterial and venous access for cannulation.
3. Insert venous cannula into identified vein and arterial cannula into identified artery.
4. Connect arterial cannula to arterial limb of the ECMO circuit and venous cannula to venous limb of the ECMO circuit.

Equipment:
High-fidelity vascular cannulating trainer manikin (neck and groin)
ECMO circuit and cannula
Surgical procedure cart

Evaluation:
Medicine –The following technical aspects were adequately demonstrated:
Aseptic setup
Initial surgical time-out
Dissection and identification of vascular structures
Insertion of appropriate cannula into vessels
Circuit connection with appropriate time-out
ECMO flows

simulation, management of circuit emergencies and complex cardiac ECMO physiology, and ECMO during cardiopulmonary resuscitation (ECPR). Example scenarios are included (Boxes 22.1, 22.2, and 22.3). In sum, creating an effective simulation-based experience related to cardiac ECMO requires the curriculum designer to meld real-to-life clinical narratives, accurate representations of patient physiology, and integration of circuit and circuit monitors using, at times, complex simulation technical methodology for optimal engagement of the learner.

ECMO Pump Type

There are two major types of ECMO pumps available, and either can be utilized during simulation. Roller pumps deliver a fixed output utilizing sequential compression of the circuit tubing, while centrifugal pumps deliver output in an afterload-dependent manner utilizing centrifugal force generated by a rotating impeller [23]. Institutional device preference for centrifugal versus roller pumps should define circuit component choice for local simulation education scenarios.

In a patient without native ejection, attention to nuances of arterial waveforms is required for the optimal simulation experience. As a centrifugal pump flow is continuous, in the setting of no ejection, no pulse pressure is discernible on invasive arterial monitoring. Alternatively, the mechanism of flow in roller pumps results in an apparent narrow pulse pressure of 4–8 mmHg, which is evident on invasive arterial monitoring and can be simulated on the monitor display. The limitation of available simulation software is such that a mean arterial pressure alone cannot be displayed, so blood pressure for either type of pump must be portrayed as a systolic and diastolic with a very narrow pulse pressure.

Cannulation Strategy – Anatomical Location and Implications

Simulation approach to cannulation strategy, including the anatomical location of cannulae and technical fidelity of cannulation mechanism, is driven by the scenario narrative and learning objectives. A primary peripheral (versus central) cannulation strategy is driven by operative status and timing of cardiopulmonary failure in most centers. Central cannulation is generally reserved for scenarios in the early post-operative period. Choice of neck or groin for peripheral cannulation is determined by patient and vessel size, body habitus, vessel patency, and potential access for percutaneous coronary interventions or adjunctive support strategies such as intra-aortic balloon pump. High-fidelity groin, neck, and intra-thoracic cannulation trainers have been developed for scenario narratives that encompass surgical cannulation as key learning objectives [5, 24]. Commercially available trainers can be costly, and "home-made" versions require significant preparation time (Fig. 22.3). Thus, these higher-fidelity trainers are generally reserved for use either for dedicated cannulation skills training or when required

Box 22.2 Zone/Level 2 Simulation – Management of an ECMO Complication by a Native Team

Target Audience: CICU attending/CICU fellow/nurse practitioner /ECMO specialist or perfusionist +/– cardiac surgeon/bedside nursing staff

Learning Objectives:

At the end of this simulation scenario, the participants will be able to:

Clinical:

1. Recognize and manage pump failure.
2. Demonstrate patient management during pump failure including CPR and hand cranking to temporarily maintain circuit flow.
3. Mobilize the personnel and resources required to change the pump/circuit.

Teamwork:

1. Verbalize a clinical summary at critical points during the event to ensure a shared understanding among team members.
2. Demonstrate effective closed-loop communication during the resuscitation.

Environment:

Manikin: Infant manikin with R internal jugular and common carotid neck cannulae in place

Lines/tubes: Full VA ECMO circuit with a centrifugal pump with visible clots in the venous inflow, chest tubes × 3, femoral line, arterial line

Respiratory: ETT, ventilator, settings SIMV PIP 27/Peep 10 × 20, FiO2 0.4

Monitor: CVP, HR, RR, SpO2, arterial blood pressure, temperature, ETCO2

Medications: Milrinone 0.5mcg/kg/min, morphine 0.05 mg/kg/min, dexmedetomidine 1mcg/kg/hr

Actors: May have a confederate ECMO specialist, allows for transmission of information from stem to case progression

Case Narrative:

Patient Name: Jessica Staples

Age/gender: 12-month-old male

Weight: 10 kg

All: NKDA

Patient history: 12-month-old male with double outlet right ventricle and pulmonary stenosis who failed to separate from cardiopulmonary bypass with no native ejection following Rastelli procedure with RV-PA conduit. Patient returned from the OR bleeding requiring blood product resuscitation, tranexamic acid, and a single dose of activated factor 7. You respond to a staff assist call for an ECMO circuit alarm and arrive to find no pulse pressure on invasive arterial monitoring and a MAP of 18 with no saturation trace. HR 70, NIRS- 32.

Scenario Progression: Fellow/ANP responds to a staff assist call for a patient on ECMO with no flow, no pulse pressure on invasive arterial monitoring, and a MAP of 18.

State	*Suggested vital signs*	*Learner's expected intervention*
PEA	HR 70 beats/min BP 18 mmHg, no waveform O2 sats not detected RR 20 breaths/min (SIMV) CVP (fem) 8 mmHg ETCO2 4	Recognize pump failure Commence CPR and/or trial hand crank to maintain cardiac output Maintain effective CPR/hand cranking, monitoring ETCO2 and arterial waveform as markers of cardiac output quality
Patient condition with successful hand cranking or high-quality CPR	HR 100 beats/min BP 72/40 mmHg during compressions or MAP 46 with cranking O2 sat 92% RR 20 breaths/min CVP 16 mmHg	Mobilize resources to replace pump/circuit Continue ALS including epinephrine boluses, blood requested immediately and volume prepared

Debriefing Plan:

Medicine: Patient returns from the operating room after failure to wean from bypass with no native ejection complicated by bleeding, blood product replacement, and circuit thrombosis resulting in pump failure. A trial of hand cranking may be effective in maintaining circuit flow but alternatively CPR should be initiated while preparations are made to replace pump/circuit.

Clinical aspects of scenario and teamwork: Exploration of team training and systems issues identified during the particular scenario may include recognition and management of ECMO circuit complications and mobilization of a team and resources to replace the ECMO circuit, and cardiopulmonary arrest management and crisis resource management principles are accomplished through open-ended questioning to encourage critical thinking.

Box 22.3 Zone/Level 3 Simulation – Resuscitation or E-CPR event with Full Native Team

Target Audience: CICU attending/CICU fellow/nurse practitioner/cardiac surgeon/ECMO specialist or perfusionist/bedside nursing staff

Learning Objectives:

Clinical:

1. To rapidly deploy ECMO during CPR in a patient with refractory cardiac arrest
2. To manage advanced life support including CPR during cardiac arrest and ECMO cannulation

Teamwork:

1. To mobilize the resources (equipment and personnel) necessary for ECMO cannulation during CPR
2. To maintain effective communication across the "Bermuda triangle" between the event manager, ECMO specialist, and cardiac surgeon during ECMO cannulation and initiation

Environment:

Location: Local CICU bedspace (in situ) or critical care-equipped simulation lab
Manikin: Adolescent manikin
Lines/tubes: Right internal jugular CVL, right radial arterial line, peripheral IV, ECMO cannulae (arterial and venous)
Respiratory: ETT, ventilator, baseline settings SIMV PC 25/5 × 12, FiO2 0.6
Monitor: CVP, HR, RR, SpO2, ABP, NIBP, ETCO2.
Medications: Dopamine 5 mcg/kg/min, morphine 2 mg/hr, midazolam 2 mg/hr
Equipment: Code cart, defibrillator

Case Narrative:

Patient Name: AJ Jones
Age/gender: 14-year-old male
Weight: 48 kg
All: NKDA

Patient history: AJ is a previously healthy adolescent, with recent viral illness and progressive exercise intolerance. He presented to the ER when he developed shortness of breath with minimal exertion. In the ER he was noted to be tachypneic with HR 136 with weak peripheral pulses and manual BP 76/39. A PIV was placed and patient given 20 ml/kg NS. Saturations were subsequently noted to be 87%, with minimal rise on supplemental oxygen and worsening respiratory distress. He was started on 5 mcg/kg/min dopamine and intubated and central venous and arterial lines placed. An echocardiogram showed an EF of 14% with a mildly dilated LV. He was transferred to the CICU with a presumed diagnosis of acute fulminant myocarditis.

Scenario Progression: Fellow/nurse practitioner called to room by bedside RN for hypotension frequent ventricular ectopics and non-sustained ventricular tachycardia

State	*Suggested vital signs*	*Learner's expected intervention*
Hypotension and non-sustained VT	HR 150; frequent PVCs/VT at 200 BP 78/40 O2 sat 94% RR 12 (on vent) CVP 12 ETCO2 32	Check laboratory results; lactate, MVSaO2, and electrolytes Consider additional inotrope Call in ECMO team (equipment, personnel, circuit, blood products)
Pulseless VT	HR 200, VT Asystole on arterial trace unless compressions RR 14 (or hand vent) CVP 20 ETCO2 6 *Does not convert to NSR with defibrillation	Recognize VT Initiate CPR and place defib pads and defibrillate Maintain effective CPR during cannulation, monitoring ETCO2 and arterial waveform as markers of CPR quality with minimal interruptions Surgical preparation for groin cannulation Beware excessive vasopressors if going on centrifugal pump
On ECMO	HR 220, VT BP 55/50 (gradual increase as flows approach 75 ml/kg/min) O2 sat 99% RR 14 (or as set by team) CVP 14 ETCO2	Consider cardioversion once on full flows

Debriefing Plan:

Medicine: Patient presents with acute fulminant myocarditis with decompensated heart failure and rapidly deteriorates with progressive ventricular arrhythmia to cardiac arrest. Optimizing CPR according to invasive arterial blood pressure, ETCO2, and minimization of CPR interruptions during cannulation to ECMO is associated with improved outcomes.

Clinical aspects of scenario and teamwork: Exploration of team training and systems issues identified during the particular scenario may include timing of ECMO activation and recognition, and cardiopulmonary arrest management and crisis resource management principles are accomplished through open-ended questioning to encourage critical thinking.

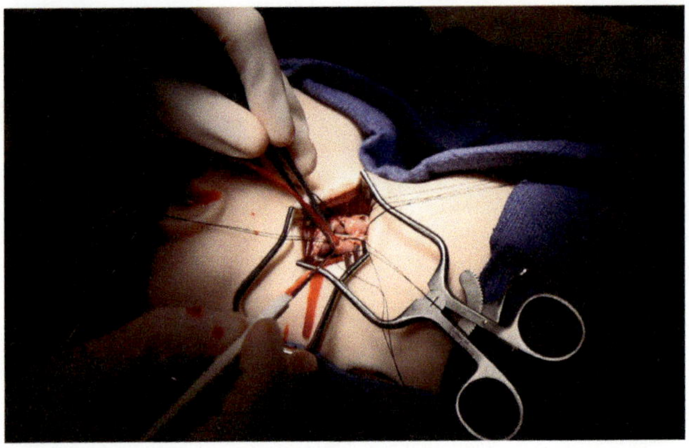

Fig. 22.3 Boston Children's Hospital SIMPeds™ Neonatal ECMO Trainer, manufactured by FracturedFX Inc., Monrovia, CA. (Designed in collaboration with Jill Zalieckas, MD, MPH)

for full participant engagement during multidisciplinary team training.

A lower technology alternative can be used in scenarios focused on troubleshooting ECMO complications on a 'previously cannulated patient.' ECMO cannulae can be inserted into a bag of intravenous fluids or a priming bag, which serves as a capacitance reservoir [25, 26]. *The bag can be concealed either adjacent to or inside the body cavity of a low fidelity manikin with cannulas emerging from the neck or groin line, and with manikin 'skin' reaffixed over the cannula insertion site. The reservoir bag, cannulae, tubing, and ECMO circuit then form a closed circuit that can be manipulated to simulate ECMO emergencies.*

The scenario narrative should drive participants to appreciate clinical consequences of a specific cannulation strategy. For example, a learning objective targeting the physiology of patients partially supported with peripheral VA-ECMO via the groin may include differential hypoxemia. Here, blood ejected across the aortic valve during myocardial recovery may not be fully saturated, leading to lower saturations measured by a pulse oximeter placed on the ear or hand, versus the foot. This may be further exacerbated with the use of an intra-aortic balloon pump [13, 27].

In this setting, a scenario of myocardial recovery could be simulated by demonstrating an increase in pulse pressure, with progressive upper body oxygen desaturation, and ST segment changes on ECG monitoring representing the development of myocardial ischemia. A chest radiograph with persistent evidence of lung disease should be available to show participants. However, of note, some simulation software packages do not allow for display of 2 simultaneous saturation waveforms. As differential saturations are key elements of this scenario, workarounds must be developed to ensure the conceptual fidelity of the scenario. For instance, a second pulse oximeter tracing can be superimposed on the monitor using open source software packages such as Rainmeter (https://www.rainmeter.net/); however this requires substantial technical know-how and is not amenable to rapidly changing saturation values in real time. For a lower technology alternative, participants can be verbally provided with information about differential saturations.

Cannulation Strategy – Number and Dimensions

Myocardial recovery on ECMO is reliant on adequate decompression of the systemic ventricle to reduce wall stress and myocardial oxygen consumption. Further, effective systemic venous drainage is essential for maintenance of ECMO flows and minimization of end-organ injury related to high central venous pressures. Thus, the adequacy of arterial and venous cannula size is essential to enable delivery of the required ECMO flows. Evaluating cannulation strategy as a mechanism of inadequate ECMO support is therefore an important cognitive task for cardiac ECMO teams and a relevant topic for simulation training. Here insufficient venous drainage, or arterial flow restriction, may lead participants to specific clinical interventions or to consider modifying the cannulation approach. For example, when ECMO flows are inadequate, interventions may include volume resuscitation, placement of additional venous drainage cannula, upsizing the arterial cannula, or introduction of vasoactive medications to reduce systemic vascular resistance depending on the specific physiology presented to learners.

Learning objectives related to the adequacy of cannulation strategy can be divided into venous versus arterial side problems, the physiology of both of which can be simulated by making simple manipulations to the ECMO simulation circuit (see Chap. 27).

To simulate flow limitation secondary to arterial cannula issues (e.g. small arterial cannula, arterial cannula malposition, or arterial cannula obstruction (such as from clot), a Hoffman tubing clamp placed on the arterial limb of the ECMO circuit can be discretely tightened, causing increased resistance to flow. This will manifest as increased pre-membrane and post-membrane pressures on integrated ECMO circuit pressure monitors. In a centrifugal pump system this will result in a decrease in ECMO flows. Alternative explanations of arterial side resistance secondary should be explored by the learner, with expected interventions including vasodilator infusions, increasing intravascular volume, sedation and neuromuscular blockade or cannula manipulation or exchange. In this setting resources describing standard arterial cannula dimensions per flow rate and patient size should be available for participant reference and/or during debriefing.

In a similar manner, obstruction to venous inflow to the ECMO circuit can be simulated by applying a Hoffman tubing clamp to the venous limb of the circuit and discretely tightening until the desirable effects are seen. Venous cannula issues as a mechanism for inadequate ECMO support will then manifest on the ECMO circuit monitor display as negative circuit venous pressures, escalating to turbulent flow or 'chatter' of the circuit, potentially leading to a reduction of ECMO flow on a centrifugal pump. Simultaneously, the expected accompanying changes in patient physiologic parameters, such as decreased arterial blood pressure and increased central venous pressure, are displayed. Additional clinical details provided to participants will enhance the conceptual fidelity of scenarios. For example, hemolysis seen in the case of high arterial resistance can be simulated by pink urine discoloration (hemoglobinuria), and participants can be provided with

Table 22.2 Simulation of inadequate cannulation strategies and circuit manipulations

	Simulator changes		Patient variables			ECMO circuit variables			
	venous limb clamp	Arterial limb clamp	HR	BP	CVP	Venous pressure	Pre-membrane pressure	Post-membrane pressure	Flow
Small venous cannula/venous cannula malposition	Tighten	No change	High	Low	High	More negative	No change	No change	Low*
Small arterial cannula/arterial cannula obstruction	No change	Tighten	High	Low	High	No change	High	High	Low*

laboratory evidence such as elevated plasma-free hemoglobin if they inquire, thereby completing the clinical picture. Table 22.2 *summarizes required circuit manipulations, expected changes in circuit monitor parameters, and active changes made to patient physiologic monitoring variables for simulation of inadequate ECMO support including cannulation issues and other ECMO complications.*

Additional Cardiac and ECMO Circuit Monitoring

Teams managing patients on ECMO must integrate data from the patient monitor and the ECMO circuit to understand and act on physiologic changes. Simulation provides an excellent opportunity for individual clinicians and teams to practice the critical thinking skills this requires. However, to be an effective educational tool to meet this objective, data must be displayed and changes fed back within a timeframe that closely replicates clinical practice. Post-operative cardiac patients often have invasive hemodynamic monitoring, including central venous pressure (CVP), arterial pressure, left atrial pressure (LAP), right atrial pressure (RAP), common atrial pressures (in patients with single-ventricle physiology), and pulmonary artery or Glenn pressure (superior cavopulmonary). In neonates with ductus arteriosus-dependent congenital heart disease, pre-ductal and post-ductal arterial saturation probes (usually measured on the right hand (pre-ductal) and a lower limb (post-ductal)) are routinely measured. Intra-aortic balloon pump integration and monitoring may also be incorporated into simulation.

Display of many of these parameters, such as LAP or RAP, is not supported by most commercially available simulation software packages; therefore, work-arounds must be found to ensure adequate technical and conceptual realism. If there is a limitation to the number of displayed parameters, then ventilation and hemodynamic monitoring including numbers and waveforms must be modified to best represent the scenario narrative.

Solutions may involve complex processes such as the use of software such as Rainmeter (https://www.rainmeter.net/), to create 'overlays' on the monitor. A simpler work-around would be to substitute an alternative waveform available in simulation software, such as intracranial pressure (ICP), and affix a label on the monitor next to the waveform, covering ICP and indicating what pressure measurement is actually represented. When the display arrangement deviates from what clinicians might expect to see, clinicians should be thoroughly oriented to those differences prior to the start of simulations so that they know where to readily find the anticipated monitoring data. In addition, a facilitator should be available and attentive to remind the participants of variations in the monitor display during the simulation. At times the total number of pressure monitoring lines used in clinical practice will exceed the capabilities of simulation software. In this situation, the most relevant hemodynamic parameters must be chosen for display while recognizing that this will by necessity limit fidelity.

Rhythm disturbances in the cardiac population should be similarly approached with rigor to maintain high fidelity of the scenario. Most simulation software packages provide a wide variety of options to simulate arrhythmias. It should be noted that these rhythm disturbances more typically simulate arrhythmias expected in the adult rather than pediatric population. In addition, in the situation where invasive hemodynamic monitoring is in use, attention should be paid not only to the arrhythmia but also to how hemodynamic waveforms might change.

For example, in the case of atrioventricular dyssynchrony seen in a post-operative junctional ectopic tachycardia, efforts can be made to demonstrate 'cannon waves' on a CVP or intra-cardiac pressure tracing by substituting an arterial waveform.

Left Heart Decompression on ECMO

Myocardial decompression and avoidance of vasoactive medications that increase oxygen consumption are key learning objectives for teams providing ECMO support [2]. Patients with severe myocardial dysfunction on peripheral VA-ECMO warrant specific consideration for the potential need for left-sided decompression [13, 28]. Institutional policies should inform locally relevant learning objectives and expected interventions.

Given the clinical importance of early evaluation of the adequacy of left-sided decompression, incorporation of this element of management into a cardiac ECMO training curriculum is highly relevant. This scenario logically follows an initial cannulation scenario. Effective simulation requires provision of an appropriate patient history, display of ancillary data, accurate representation of patient monitoring data, and manipulation of the manikin to represent the physiologic changes consistent with left atrial hypertension. Patient history includes severe left ventricular dysfunction prior to cannulation. As the scenario progresses, elevated LA pressure should be obvious (if appropriate monitoring is in place, such as in a post-operative patient) and a minimally pulsatile arterial waveform should be visible. Poor lung compliance can be simulated by increasing airway resistance on the manikin. Ancillary data to be provided includes a chest radiograph with evidence of pulmonary venous hypertension and verbal information regarding the presence of hemoptysis or blood-tinged secretions on suctioning of the endotracheal tube. Examples of possible early learner responses include increasing ECMO flows or institution of inotropes, and the pros and cons of these two approaches (increased myocardial oxygen consumption with inotropes and increased systemic afterload with increased flows) become important elements of the debriefing. Facilitators should always be prepared to provide reasonable ancillary data requested by the learner, including an echocardiogram with severe ventricular dysfunction, left ventricular and left atrial dilation, absence of aortic valve opening, left to right bulging of the inter-atrial septum, or a high trans-septal gradient when an atrial communication is present. In this setting a number of expected proposed interventions exist, including cardiac catheterization for atrial septostomy or stent and/or insertion of intra-aortic balloon pump, Impella device, or LA vent. These decisions by the participants become natural end points for the scenario.

Investigation for Cardiac Lesions Implicated in Cardiopulmonary Failure

Coronary artery lesions and anatomic lesions are common causes for cardiopulmonary failure requiring ECMO support and require urgent investigation [1, 2, 8, 14, 29]. Manifestations of low cardiac output, arrhythmia, or unbalanced pulmonary and systemic circulations in children with palliated single-ventricle circulation require investigation and intervention for unrecognized anatomical abnormalities or residual lesions in the post-operative patient. These important concepts can all be replicated through simulation, allowing the learner to work through the important cognitive tasks related to differential diagnosis of cardiopulmonary failure by integrating the relevant physiologic data.

For example, a case narrative of unexplained cardiac arrest related to coronary ischemia, a rare but catastrophic event in the post-operative congenital heart disease population, should prompt consideration of cardiac catheterization for urgent coronary intervention. Typical simulation software allows the display of ST segment changes of varying severities (e.g., scale of 0–10) allowing simulationists to modify how obviously the ischemia is presented. Alternatively, new bundle branch block or complete heart block shown can be simulated on cardiac monitoring to prompt participants to further investigate. Changes in physiologic monitoring, such as increase in left atrial pressure and tachycardia, all provide corroborating data.

Simulation of Complex Cardiac Anatomy and Physiology

Clinical narratives, high-fidelity equipment, and accurate representation of physiologic monitoring can be applied to address the diversity of patient size, ages, and cardiac anatomy and physiology seen in both the complex congenital heart disease and adult heart disease populations. Table 22.3 describes some of the related congenital surgical anatomy

Table 22.3 Basic congenital heart disease surgical anatomy and considerations for ECMO cannulation

Physiology	Circulation description	Circulation of blood flow	ECMO cannulation considerations
Structurally normal heart	Two ventricles in series without structural congenital anomalies	Systemic venous blood returns via the right heart, through lungs to left heart, to systemic circulation	Standard
Single-ventricle circulation: stage 1 palliation or systemic-to-pulmonary artery shunt	Single-ventricle parallel circulation with pulmonary blood flow dependent on patency of shunt or ductus arteriosus	Systemic venous blood to single ventricle, to systemic and pulmonary circulations	Small babies – neck cannulation if peripheral. Concern for excess pulmonary blood flow and potential for systemic hypoperfusion
Single-ventricle circulation: bidirectional Glenn and hemi-Fontan	Single-ventricle parallel circulation with pulmonary blood flow via superior vena cava	Inferior vena cava blood to single ventricle to systemic circulation, superior vena cava blood through lungs passively, to single ventricle to systemic circulation	May require multiple venous drainage cannulae to completely decompress (see Fig. 22.2). If cannula in IVC or atria alone – Glenn circulation must be maintained through lungs in order for upper-body (SVC) blood flow to return to atria
Single-ventricle circulation: Fontan	Single-ventricle series circulation	Systemic venous return through lungs passively to single ventricle to systemic circulation	Either standard or may require multiple venous drainage cannula to completely decompress – depending on surgical anatomy

and cannulation strategies referenced below, and a few examples of representative complex physiology and simulation approaches follow.

Biventricular Circulation

Aortic (or neo-aortic) valvular regurgitation: Severe aortic or neo-aortic regurgitation may be present immediately at cannulation or evolve while supported on VA-ECMO due to underlying anatomic defects or cannula positioning. Aortic regurgitation results in left ventricular distension and compromises myocardial decompression, coronary artery blood supply, and systemic blood flow. This can be simulated to prompt the need for intervention as a learning objective. Important elements of the simulation portrayal include left atrial hypertension when a monitoring line is available and evidence of progressive worsening lung compliance simulated through increased airway resistance, progressing to ST segment changes due to coronary run-off, low diastolic blood pressure, hypotension, and perhaps a diastolic murmur on auscultation (pediatric population). Ancillary data provided to participants would include rising lactate, a chest radiograph with evidence of pulmonary venous hypertension, and an echocardiogram with aortic regurgitation and left ventricular distension.

Acute Coronary Syndromes, Myocardial Infarction, and Pulmonary Embolism

Current guidelines relating to the assessment and management of cardiogenic shock in adults emphasize the importance of initiation of early mechanical circulatory support (ECMO) and exclusion and treatment of the underlying cause [30]. The commonest cause for cardiogenic shock in adults remains coronary ischemia, although pulmonary embolism is an important, potentially treatable time-critical diagnosis to exclude.

The case narrative may be of unheralded/unexplained cardiac arrest, or of a clinical context suggesting the underlying diagnosis/differential diagnosis. Where confounding factors (co-morbidities and/or the mixed-shock scenario frequently seen in older patient populations) are presented, these should not be presented in a way intended to deceive the learners. In complex scenarios, patient history and ancillary data are best taken from real case scenarios in order to maintain credibility.

Acute Coronary Syndromes and Myocardial Infarction

Cardiac arrest/cardiogenic shock in an adult should prompt urgent referral for coronary angiography with a view to revascularization if indicated, according to current guidelines [9, 31–33].

In a simulation scenario where ECMO has been successfully initiated, simulation of intermittent/ongoing ischemia may be achieved by demonstrating any one of the following features: continuous/intermittent/progressive elevation of pulmonary capillary wedge pressure, loss of pulsatility on arterial line, ventricular arrhythmias, heart block changing axis, or changing ST segments of varying severity, and evidence of progressive worsening lung compliance simulated through increased airway resistance. Intermittent ventricular arrhythmias are particularly suggestive of the diagnosis. Of note, once established on ECMO, changes in ST segments, rhythm and hemodynamics may be subtle.

In all ischemia scenarios, learners would be expected to request a 12-lead ECG, and where the diagnosis is uncertain, and/or ongoing features suggesting instability are present, earlier recorded ECGs and rhythm strips are utilized for comparison. Ancillary information provided may include a chest radiograph demonstrating pulmonary venous hypertension (or frank pulmonary edema) and elevation of relevant biomarkers (including high-sensitivity troponin). The request for BNP should promote later discussion regarding its sensitivity/specificity in the hyper-acute setting, depending upon the narrative presented (acute cardiogenic shock versus acute decompensated heart failure). Echocardiography will demonstrate significant left ventricular dysfunction, with/without evidence of complications of myocardial infarction (ruptured papillary muscle, ventricular septal defect, pericardial collection). Discussion should include the challenges of identifying regional wall motion abnormality in the context of a partially bypassed heart (false positive and negative). In the case of simulation of mechanical complications, the narrative might suggest a late/missed presentation of myocardial infarction.

Ruptured papillary muscle on ECMO can be simulated by disproportionately high pulmonary capillary wedge pressure and pulmonary oedema, lack of ejection, with/without hypotension, but in the context of an echocardiogram showing a well-decompressed left heart.

Discussion for all patients with suspected acute coronary syndrome/myocardial infarction should include timing and initiation of dual antiplatelet therapies, the potential options to confirm/exclude the diagnosis (institution-dependent), cautions (and alternative diagnostic strategies) considering coronary artery instrumentation where spontaneous coronary artery dissection (SCAD) is considered, and options for definitive exclusion of important differential diagnoses (aortic dissection, pulmonary embolism).

Aortic Balloon Pumps/Impella

Intra-aortic balloon pumps (IABP) are no longer recommended for routine use to support the circulation in cardiogenic shock complicating myocardial infarction, except in the presence of mechanical complications [2, 34, 35]. In some centers IABP are still used for offloading the left ventricle in patients on ECMO, although data regarding its benefit are lacking [36, 37]. Part-task training for insertion of IABP is well-established (arterial puncture, wire skills, cannulation, computer-generated pressure interpretation); however, inclusion of IABP insertion into high-fidelity ECMO simulation training is not routine [38]. Immersive high-fidelity simulation for IABP insertion is beyond the remit of this chapter; however, simulation of ECMO+IABP hemodynamic data may be useful, in particular to remind learners of the importance of understanding the relevance of the hemodynamics presented. In a simulation scenario of ECMO+IABP, interpretation of a pulsatile arterial waveform (either simulated or printed paper recording) should prompt the learner to ask for the IABP to be paused/simultaneous echocardiography in order to demonstrate ejection and aortic valve opening.

Combination of ECMO with left-sided Impella (ECPELLA) has been increasingly explored as an option to improve LV decompression on peripheral ECMO, although high-quality data confirming its benefit remain lacking, and complications, particularly related to limb ischemia, remain high, and alternative insertion routes (including axillary) are being proposed, each of which provides its own challenges when considering development of high-fidelity simulation training [39–41]. Thus, as with all catheter-based procedures, in addition to part-task trainers, simulation using silicone vascular models, commercially developed ultrasound and fluoroscopy-based simulation, and comprehensive, augmented reality simulation are available, but have not yet been widely/formally integrated into ECMO high-fidelity simulation training. As with ECMO+IABP, the concept of Impella usage may be introduced into ECMO simulation relating to (a) recognition of requirement for LV decompression and the device as a potential option, (b) interpretation of physiological monitoring in the context of initiation of Impella (worsening of Harlequin syndrome – described above – in case of initiation in the context of severe respiratory failure), and (c) in very advanced simulation, introduction of both Impella and ECMO simulation to the team for staged decision-making. Here, with predominantly left ventricular failure, initiation of Impella support may lead to worsening right-sided hemodynamics (rising right atrial pressure, progressive falling in systemic pressures and Impella flows, simulated using a commercially available Impella simulator) and should lead the learner to request for an echocardiogram. Here, demonstration of right ventricular dilatation and failure should lead to discussion around options including addition of peripheral ECMO, upgrade to ECMO, or addition of a right-sided device, each of which can be simulated using the appropriate proprietary software, within the high-fidelity simulation.

Single-Ventricle Circulation

Mechanical support in patients with single-ventricle physiology is increasingly utilized, representing a unique population with specific challenges [42]. Simulation offers teams caring for these patients a means of safely practicing the rapid integration of complex data from patient and ECMO circuit required to provide successful ECMO support to this population. To improve these skills, teams must be able to react based on the monitoring feedback with a high degree of realism for single-ventricle physiology. Several specific physiologic concepts unique to the single-ventricle population and appropriate simulation approaches are described. Of note, simulation facilitators should be aware of programmed characteristics of many simulation software packages that provide unique challenges in the congenital heart disease population. For instance, some packages have lower saturation limits below which plethysmography tracings manifest as flat line or unable to obtain. Pre-programmed parameters can be reset to reflect lower limits, but this must be done prior to the start of the scenario. Similarly, lower blood pressure limits may need to be reset to avoid display of a "flat line" below a certain threshold. Simulation facilitators and technicians should familiarize themselves with the limitations of the specific software packages they use in order to anticipate these problems.

Pre-operative patients (with patent ductus arteriosus [PDA] maintaining systemic circulation) or those palliated with a *systemic to pulmonary artery shunt.*

A key challenge for ECMO support in this setting is excessive pulmonary blood flow with systemic hypoperfusion. Recognizing and managing this complication represents important specific learning objectives. Creation of a realistic and relevant clinical scenario comes primarily through appropriate manipulation of vital signs and provision of ancillary data: The simulated patient will manifest high saturations, progressive systemic hypotension with low diastolic blood pressure unresponsive to increased ECMO flows, and tachycardia. Facilitators should be prepared to provide corroborating ancillary data when requested, including high lactate concentration and low mixed venous saturations if relevant monitoring lines are present. Expected interventions may include temporizing strategies such as further increasing ECMO flows to improve systemic perfusion, ventilation management to limit pulmonary blood flow, or surgical intervention with bilateral PA bands if medical interventions are unsuccessful. Simulation facilitators should be prepared to react to the spectrum of possible interventions through changes in patient vital signs and other physiologic monitoring data. Manipulation of the simulated ECMO circuit is not usually required in these scenarios.

Bidirectional Glenn Circulation

ECMO support in patients with a bidirectional Glenn (BDG) presents numerous challenges for clinicians that are amenable to experiential learning through simulation. Cannulation strategy is of particular importance, because of the separate superior vena cava (SVC) anastomosis to the pulmonary arteries, while the inferior vena cava (IVC) continues to drain into the common atrium. Evaluating the adequacy of support and venous drainage (central versus neck) denotes fundamental learning objectives for mechanical support in a BDG circulation. Promoting realism with specific simulation methods is essential to enhance experiential learning.

Central cannulation in the common atrium alone requires passive pulmonary drainage through the pulmonary vasculature (Fig. 22.4), with attendant risk of inadequate decompression of the Glenn circulation.

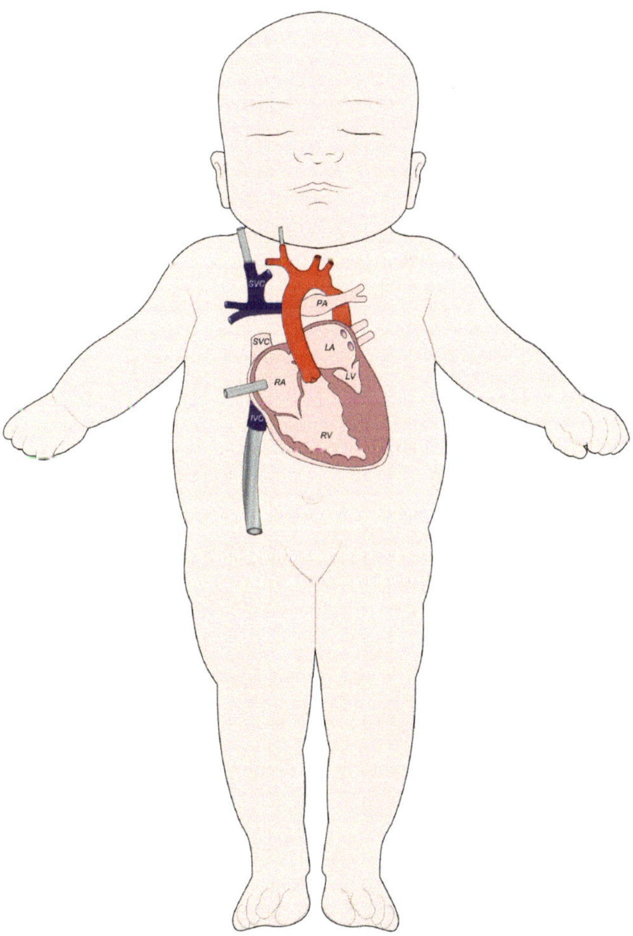

Fig. 22.4 Single-ventricle cannulation strategies. Superior cavopulmonary anastomosis (Glenn connection or shunt) results in upper-body blood moving passively through the lungs before returning to the single ventricle. Single venous ECMO cannulation strategy (inferior vena cava or common atrium) results in only partial support, and blood flow from the upper body must return to the common atrium via the lungs. Alternatively, a venous cannula inserted in the superior vena cava can facilitate additional support

Inadequate Glenn decompression can be simulated through a combination of presentation of typical hemodynamics (high central venous, or 'Glenn,' pressures and low common atrial pressures) along with ECMO circuit changes including highly negative circuit venous pressures. Highly negative circuit venous pressures can be simulated by applying a Hoffman tubing clamp to the venous limb of the circuit and discretely tightening until the desirable effects are seen. These measures should prompt learners to initiate ventilation strategies to promote pulmonary blood flow, start inhaled nitric oxide or consider addition of a second venous drainage cannula in the Glenn pathway.

Similarly, cannulation with an isolated neck (Glenn pathway) cannula in patients with this circulation can be simulated. In this scenario, IVC flow still returns to the common atrium. In patients with no/minimal native ejection, this leads to inadequate myocardial decompression. In contrast to the scenario with a single common atrial cannula, single Glenn cannula results in high common atrial pressures and a narrow transpulmonary gradient. The relationship between measured end tidal CO2 (ETCO2) and PaCO2 reflects the obligatory shunt at IVC to common atrial level, i.e., ETCO2 below PaCO2 indicative of reduced pulmonary blood flow (QP:S < 1). In addition, hepatomegaly, renal dysfunction/oliguria, and abdominal distension can be described in the scenario progression as additional indicators of inadequate atrial decompression. No specific manipulation of the ECMO circuit is required to simulate this scenario.

ECPR

Extracorporeal life support during active cardiopulmonary resuscitation (ECPR) is recommended for consideration by the American Heart Association (AHA) and the International Liaison Committee on Resuscitation (ILCOR) for children and adults in cardiopulmonary arrest when available for rapid deployment. ECPR is a low-frequency, high-complexity, time-critical, team-dependent event and represents the ultimate ECMO challenge [43–45]. Effective leadership has been shown to positively impact both simulated and actual clinical resuscitation events [20, 46–49]. The ability of an "event manager" to organize a team, avoid task fixation, and articulate a global assessment of patient status and a management plan has been associated with superior performance measures, including hands-on chest compressions and time to appropriate defibrillation. These important clinical metrics have been associated with improved survival after cardiac arrest [50–52]. The practical setting of ECPR requires simultaneous maintenance of effective patient resuscitation and preparation of the technology (ECMO circuit and cannula) during technical identification and manipulation of vessels to be cannulated. The individuals performing these three central roles – event manager, ECMO specialist, and cannulating interventionist or surgeon – are all at risk for task fixation.

Task fixation and associated lack of effective communication between these three key individuals during the resuscitation event result in poorly coordinated efforts, loss of critical information, and ultimately delays in cannulation or ineffective resuscitation (Fig. 22.5). For example, where technical difficulties during cannulation that will delay establishment of flows exist, the event manager is better able to anticipate resuscitation needs or recruit additional help, provided this information is clearly communicated to them. Effective communication across intensive care, surgical, and ECMO teams are similarly critical during management of ECMO circuit emergencies after ECMO cannulation. For example, if the ECMO specialist encounters a circuit complication that requires circuit clamping, such as large-volume air entrainment, communication of the intention to clamp to the event manager allows the resuscitation team to prepare for CPR and other resuscitative measures. Simulation provides important opportunities to practice these communication skills both among and between the micro-teams involved in ECPR (or management of ECMO circuit emergencies) – the intensive care unit team, ECMO specialists, and the surgical team. Targeted to address these issues, the principles of crisis resource management (CRM) can be effectively practiced in EECPR simulation for learning objectives related to event leadership, followership, communication, and team coordination [49, 53–55]. These principles include:

1. *Role clarity* – Team members are assigned specific tasks and responsibilities, as they would be in actual resuscitation event.
2. *Communication* – Effective communication strategies emphasizing explicit statements directed to specific individuals with "closed-loop" communication. Team members offer information and suggestions to the event manager across authority gradients.
3. *Global assessment* – Maintaining situational awareness of the entire event and environment is required to avoid fixation errors. A shared mental model is established through frequent updates by the event manager and team-based review of clinical status.
4. *Personnel support* – Identifying and mobilizing additional resources, including expert consultants.
5. *Resource utilization* – Leveraging systematic and institutional resources for critical event management. This includes understanding human and technical resource availability and operations, supported by a working knowledge of institutional policies and procedures.

For ECPR simulations in particular, involvement of the full native team is an important priority for enhancing emotional realism. Conduct of the ECPR simulations in the native clinical care environment allows teams to not only enhance emotional realism but also allows teams to troubleshoot systems issues that may arise in real-time cannulations. Technical realism is enhanced through attention to availability of all equipment and resources normally used in an ECPR event. For instance, surgical instruments, headlamps, ECMO circuit, and resuscitation equipment should, as much as possible, be those that are used in live cannulations. The simulation team will need to work closely with clinical leadership to ensure that these resources are available for simulation and that processes are put in place to avoid mixing of simulation supplies and clinical supplies. An example ECPR Zone 3 simulation is included below (Box 22.3).

Cardiovascular Care Microsystems

Cardiovascular care is delivered within the clinical microsystems of pre-hospital care, emergency rooms, operating rooms, catheterization laboratories, and intensive care units (Fig. 22.1)

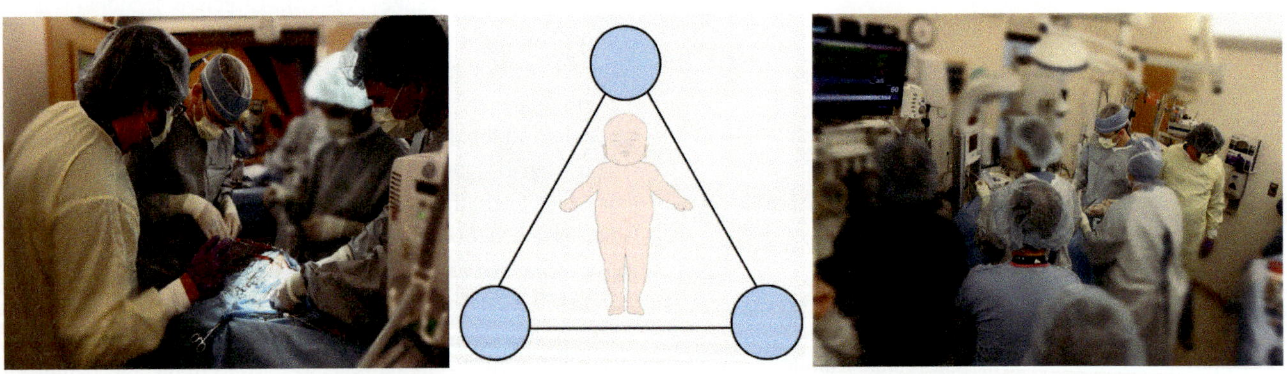

Fig. 22.5 Communication within and between clinical microteams during ECPR events. (**a**) The event manager, cannulating surgeon, and ECMO specialist are all focused on the same aspect of care. While this may facilitate communication related to one aspect of care, other tasks may be neglected. (**b**) Schematic of the clinical microteams during ECPR. Intensivist, ECMO specialist, and surgeon must all complete their individual task while communicating effectively across microteams to optimize coordination of care. (**c**) Task fixation in microteams. The event manager, cannulating surgeon, and ECMO specialist are physically separated and focusing on different aspects of management. This can be unavoidable during portions of resuscitation and ECMO initiation but risks task fixation and communication failure

[7–11]. Each of these is characterized by complex teams and environments with high technical and cognitive demands (Table 22.2). Formation of ad hoc teams within different settings has implications for team member psychological safety and communication across authority gradients [11]. Optimal team-member engagement depends on psychological safety as the team coexists, interacts, and potentially misaligns – with important implications for team learning, performance, and development. Programs incorporating simulation have been associated with improved trainee satisfaction, enhanced provider knowledge, and superior team performance [5, 56, 57]. To address the identified learning objectives, simulation of cardiac ECMO processes can be facilitated across any of the identified microsystems, including patient hand-off between different locations and teams (Fig. 22.1).

Conclusions

ECMO represents a high-risk low-frequency therapy and may involve management of complex physiology. Simulation-based education provides a valuable opportunity for exposure to these physiologic patterns, to test interventions, and to practice concepts related to team-based care. To create optimal educational experiences, educators must work to create simulations that faithfully replicate these complex patterns of physiology through attention to (1) creation of an accurate clinical narrative, inclusive of laboratory, imaging, and other ancillary data; (2) faithful replication of nuanced physiologic data on patient monitors, recognizing and adapting to limitations to commercially available simulation software; and (3) integration of an ECMO circuit with the manikin and physical manipulation of the circuit to replicate the varied pathophysiologies of ECMO.

References

1. Thiagarajan RR, Barbaro RP, Rycus PT, McMullan DM, Conrad SA, Fortenberry JD, et al. Extracorporeal life support organization registry international report 2016. ASAIO J. 2017;63(1):60–7.
2. Abrams D, Garan AR, Abdelbary A, Bacchetta M, Bartlett RH, Beck J, et al. Position paper for the organization of ECMO programs for cardiac failure in adults. Intensive Care Med. 2018;44(6):717–29.
3. Matteo Di Nardo PD, Stoppa F, Lorusso R, Raponi M, Amodea A, Cecchetti C, Guner Y, Taccone F. The introduction of a high-fidelity simulation program for training pediatric critical care personnel reduces the times to manage extracorporeal membrane oxygenation emergencies and improves teamwork. J Thorac Dis. 2018;10(6):3409–17.
4. Montero S, Combes A, Schmidt M. The extracorporeal membrane oxygenation (ECMO) high-fidelity simulator: the best complementary tool to learn the technique. J Thorac Dis. 2017;9(11):4273–6.
5. Allan CK, Pigula F, Bacha EA, Emani S, Fynn-Thompson F, Thiagarajan RR, et al. An extracorporeal membrane oxygenation cannulation curriculum featuring a novel integrated skills trainer leads to improved performance among pediatric cardiac surgery trainees. Simul Healthc. 2013;8(4):221–8.
6. Zakhary BM, Kam LM, Kaufman BS, Felner KJ. The utility of high-fidelity simulation for training critical care fellows in the management of extracorporeal membrane oxygenation emergencies: a randomized controlled trial. Crit Care Med. 2017;45(8):1367–73.
7. Morrow DA, Fang JC, Fintel DJ, Granger CB, Katz JN, Kushner FG, et al. Evolution of critical care cardiology: transformation of the cardiovascular intensive care unit and the emerging need for new medical staffing and training models: a scientific statement from the American Heart Association. Circulation. 2012;126(11):1408–28.
8. Neumann FJ, Sousa-Uva M, Ahlsson A, Alfonso F, Banning AP, Benedetto U, et al. 2018 ESC/EACTS Guidelines on myocardial revascularization. Eur Heart J. 2019;40(2):87–165. https://doi.org/10.1093/eurheartj/ehy394. PMID:30165437.
9. Sousa-Uva M, Neumann FJ, Ahlsson A, Alfonso F, Banning AP, Benedetto U, et al. 2018 ESC/EACTS Guidelines on myocardial revascularization. Eur J Cardiothorac Surg. 2019;55(1):4–90. https://doi.org/10.1093/ejcts/ezy289. PMID: 30165632.
10. Bacha EA. Patient safety and human factors in pediatric cardiac surgery. Pediatr Cardiol. 2007;28(2):116–21.
11. Christopher J Roussin TLM, Rudolph JW. The safety in unsafe teams: amultilevel approach to team psychological safety. J Manag. 2016;42(6):1409–33.
12. McBride ME, Su L, Allan CK. Education and training in pediatric cardiac critical care. Pediatr Crit Care Med. 2018;19(6):585–6.
13. Donker DW, Brodie D, Henriques JPS, Broome M. Left ventricular unloading during veno-arterial ECMO: a review of percutaneous and surgical unloading interventions. Perfusion. 2018;267659118794112
14. Barbaro RP, Paden ML, Guner YS, Raman L, Ryerson LM, Alexander P, et al. Pediatric extracorporeal life support organization registry international report 2016. ASAIO J. 2017;63(4):456–63.
15. Michels G, Wengenmayer T, Hagl C, Dohmen C, Bottiger BW, Bauersachs J, et al. Recommendations for extracorporeal cardiopulmonary resuscitation (eCPR): consensus statement of DGIIN, DGK, DGTHG, DGfK, DGNI, DGAI, DIVI and GRC. Clin Res Cardiol. 2018;108:455.
16. Ford MA, Gauvreau K, McMullan DM, Almodovar MC, Cooper DS, Rycus PT, et al. Factors associated with mortality in neonates requiring extracorporeal membrane oxygenation for cardiac indications: analysis of the extracorporeal life support organization registry data. Pediatr Crit Care Med. 2016;17(9):860–70.
17. McMullan DM. Is there a concerning trend in extracorporeal life support utilization for single-ventricle patients? Pediatr Crit Care Med. 2016;17(3):259–60.
18. Misfeldt AM, Kirsch RE, Goldberg DJ, Mascio CE, Naim MY, Zhang X, et al. Outcomes of single-ventricle patients supported with extracorporeal membrane oxygenation. Pediatr Crit Care Med. 2016;17(3):194–202.
19. Schmidt A, Cappucciati M, Radua J, Rutigliano G, Rocchetti M, Dell'Osso L, et al. Improving prognostic accuracy in subjects at clinical high risk for psychosis: systematic review of predictive models and meta-analytical sequential testing simulation. Schizophr Bull. 2017;43(2):375–88.
20. Su L, Spaeder MC, Jones MB, Sinha P, Nath DS, Jain PN, et al. Implementation of an extracorporeal cardiopulmonary resuscitation simulation program reduces extracorporeal cardiopulmonary resuscitation times in real patients. Pediatr Crit Care Med. 2014;15(9):856–60.
21. Rudolph JW, Simon R, Raemer DB. Which reality matters? Questions on the path to high engagement in healthcare simulation. Simul Healthc. 2007;2(3):161–3.
22. Dieckmann P, Gaba D, Rall M. Deepening the theoretical foundations of patient simulation as social practice. Simul Healthc. 2007;2(3):183–93.
23. Barrett CS, Jaggers JJ, Cook EF, Graham DA, Yarlagadda VV, Teele SA, et al. Pediatric ECMO outcomes: comparison of cen-

trifugal versus roller blood pumps using propensity score matching. ASAIO J. 2013;59(2):145–51.
24. Thompson JL, Grisham LM, Scott J, Mogan C, Prescher H, Biffar D, et al. Construction of a reusable, high-fidelity model to enhance extracorporeal membrane oxygenation training through simulation. Adv Neonatal Care. 2014;14(2):103–9.
25. Ninomiya S, Tokumine A, Yasuda T, Tomizawa Y. Development of an educational simulator system, ECCSIM-Lite, for the acquisition of basic perfusion techniques and evaluation. J Artif Organs. 2007;10(4):201–5.
26. Atamanyuk I, Ghez O, Saeed I, Lane M, Hall J, Jackson T, et al. Impact of an open-chest extracorporeal membrane oxygenation model for in situ simulated team training: a pilot study. Interact Cardiovasc Thorac Surg. 2014;18(1):17–20; discussion.
27. Thuys C, MacLaren G, d'Udekem Y, Eastaugh L. Vascular access for pediatric coronary angiography on extracorporeal membrane oxygenation. World J Pediatr Congenit Heart Surg. 2015;6(1):126–9.
28. Eastaugh LJ, Thiagarajan RR, Darst JR, McElhinney DB, Lock JE, Marshall AC. Percutaneous left atrial decompression in patients supported with extracorporeal membrane oxygenation for cardiac disease. Pediatr Crit Care Med. 2015;16(1):59–65.
29. Howard TS, Kalish BT, Wigmore D, Nathan M, Kulik TJ, Kaza AK, et al. Association of extracorporeal membrane oxygenation support adequacy and residual lesions with outcomes in neonates supported after cardiac surgery. Pediatr Crit Care Med. 2016;17(11): 1045–54.
30. Ponikowski P, Voors AA, Anker SD, Bueno H, Cleland JG, Coats AJ, et al. 2016 ESC guidelines for the diagnosis and treatment of acute and chronic heart failure: the Task Force for the diagnosis and treatment of acute and chronic heart failure of the European Society of Cardiology (ESC). Developed with the special contribution of the Heart Failure Association (HFA) of the ESC. Eur J Heart Fail. 2016;18(8):891–975.
31. Kirchhof P, Benussi S, Kotecha D, Ahlsson A, Atar D, Casadei B, et al. 2016 ESC guidelines for the management of atrial fibrillation developed in collaboration with EACTS. Europace. 2016;18(11):1609–78.
32. Neumann FJ, Sousa-Uva M, Ahlsson A, Alfonso F, Banning AP, Benedetto U, et al. 2018 ESC/EACTS Guidelines on myocardial revascularization. Eur Heart J. 2019;40(2):87–165.
33. Patel MR, Calhoon JH, Dehmer GJ, Grantham JA, Maddox TM, Maron DJ, et al. ACC/AATS/AHA/ASE/ASNC/SCAI/SCCT/STS 2017 appropriate use criteria for coronary revascularization in patients with stable ischemic heart disease: areport of the American College of Cardiology Appropriate use Criteria Task Force, American Association for Thoracic Surgery, American Heart Association, American Society of Echocardiography, American Society of Nuclear Cardiology, Society for Cardiovascular Angiography and Interventions, Society of Cardiovascular Computed Tomography, and Society of Thoracic Surgeons. J Am Coll Cardiol. 2017;69(17):2212–41.
34. Gerhard-Herman MD, Gornik HL, Barrett C, Barshes NR, Corriere MA, Drachman DE, et al. 2016 AHA/ACC guideline on the management of patients with lower extremity peripheral artery disease: areport of the American College of Cardiology/American Heart Association Task Force on Clinical Practice Guidelines. Circulation. 2017;135(12):e726–e79.
35. Ponikowski P, Voors AA, Anker SD, Bueno H, Cleland JGF, Coats AJS, et al. 2016 ESC guidelines for the diagnosis and treatment of acute and chronic heart failure: the Task Force for the diagnosis and treatment of acute and chronic heart failure of the European Society of Cardiology (ESC)Developed with the special contribution of the Heart Failure Association (HFA) of the ESC. Eur Heart J. 2016;37(27):2129–200.
36. Wang L, Xing Z. Short-term outcomes of intra-aortic balloon pump combined with venoarterial extracorporeal membrane oxygenation: a systematic review and meta-analysis. Artif Organs. 2019;43(6):561–8.
37. Li Y, Yan S, Gao S, Liu M, Lou S, Liu G, et al. Effect of an intra-aortic balloon pump with venoarterial extracorporeal membrane oxygenation on mortality of patients with cardiogenic shock: a systematic review and meta-analysisdagger. Eur J Cardiothorac Surg. 2019;55(3):395–404.
38. Young MN, Markley R, Leo T, Coffin S, Davidson MA, Salloum J, et al. Effects of advanced cardiac procedure simulator training on learning and performance in cardiovascular medicine fellows. J Med Educ Curric Dev. 2018;5:2382120518803118.
39. Patel SM, Lipinski J, Al-Kindi SG, Patel T, Saric P, Li J, et al. Simultaneous Venoarterial extracorporeal membrane oxygenation and percutaneous left ventricular decompression therapy with Impella is associated with improved outcomes in refractory cardiogenic shock. ASAIO J. 2019;65(1):21–8.
40. Abaunza M, Kabbani LS, Nypaver T, Greenbaum A, Balraj P, Qureshi S, et al. Incidence and prognosis of vascular complications after percutaneous placement of left ventricular assist device. J Vasc Surg. 2015;62(2):417–23.
41. Mastroianni C, Bouabdallaoui N, Leprince P, Lebreton G. Short-term mechanical circulatory support with the Impella 5.0 device for cardiogenic shock at La Pitie-Salpetriere. Eur Heart J Acute Cardiovasc Care. 2017;6(1):87–92.
42. Misfeldt AMKR, Goldberg DJ, et al. Outcomes of single-ventricle patients supported with extracorporeal membrane oxygenation. Pediatr Crit Care Med. 2016;17(3):194–202.
43. Marino BS, Tabbutt S, MacLaren G, Hazinski MF, Adatia I, Atkins DL, et al. Cardiopulmonary resuscitation in infants and children with cardiac disease: ascientific statement from the American Heart Association. Circulation. 2018;137(22):e691–782.
44. Link MS, Berkow LC, Kudenchuk PJ, Halperin HR, Hess EP, Moitra VK, et al. Part 7: adult advanced cardiovascular lifesupport: 2015 American Heart Association guidelines update for cardiopulmonary resuscitation and emergency cardiovascular care. Circulation. 2015;132(18 Suppl 2):S444–64.
45. de Caen AR, Berg MD, Chameides L, Gooden CK, Hickey RW, Scott HF, et al. Part 12: pediatric advanced life support: 2015 American Heart Association guidelines update for cardiopulmonary resuscitation and emergency cardiovascular care. Circulation. 2015;132(18 Suppl 2):S526–42.
46. Cooper S, Wakelam A. Leadership of resuscitation teams: "lighthouse leadership.". Resuscitation. 1999;42(1):27–45.
47. Hunziker S, Tschan F, Semmer NK, Zobrist R, Spychiger M, Breuer M, et al. Hands-on time during cardiopulmonary resuscitation is affected by the process of teambuilding: a prospective randomised simulator-based trial. BMC Emerg Med. 2009;9:3.
48. Marsch SC, Muller C, Marquardt K, Conrad G, Tschan F, Hunziker PR. Human factors affect the quality of cardiopulmonary resuscitation in simulated cardiac arrests. Resuscitation. 2004;60(1):51–6.
49. Fernandez Castelao E, Boos M, Ringer C, Eich C, Russo SG. Effect of CRM team leader training on team performance and leadership behavior in simulated cardiac arrest scenarios: a prospective, randomized, controlled study. BMC Med Educ. 2015;15:116.
50. Ali B, Zafari AM. Narrative review: cardiopulmonary resuscitation and emergency cardiovascular care: review of the current guidelines. Ann Intern Med. 2007;147(3):171–9.
51. Christenson J, Andrusiek D, Everson-Stewart S, Kudenchuk P, Hostler D, Powell J, et al. Chest compression fraction determines survival in patients with out-of-hospital ventricular fibrillation. Circulation. 2009;120(13):1241–7.
52. Chan PS, Krumholz HM, Nichol G, Nallamothu BK. American Heart Association National Registry of cardiopulmonary resuscitation I. Delayed time to defibrillation after in-hospital cardiac arrest. N Engl J Med. 2008;358(1):9–17.

53. Gaba DM, DeAnda A. A comprehensive anesthesia simulation environment: re-creating the operating room for research and training. Anesthesiology. 1988;69(3):387–94.
54. Howard SK, Gaba DM, Fish KJ, Yang G, Sarnquist FH. Anesthesia crisis resource management training: teaching anesthesiologists to handle critical incidents. Aviat Space Environ Med. 1992;63(9):763–70.
55. Reznek M, Smith-Coggins R, Howard S, Kiran K, Harter P, Sowb Y, et al. Emergency medicine crisis resource management (EMCRM): pilot study of a simulation-based crisis management course for emergency medicine. Acad Emerg Med. 2003;10(4):386–9.
56. Burkhart HM, Riley JB, Lynch JJ, Suri RM, Greason KL, Joyce LD, et al. Simulation-based postcardiotomy extracorporeal membrane oxygenation crisis training for thoracic surgery residents. Ann Thorac Surg. 2013;95(3):901–6.
57. Sanchez-Glanville C, Brindle ME, Spence T, Blackwood J, Drews T, Menzies S, et al. Evaluating the introduction of extracorporeal life support technology to a tertiary-care pediatric institution: smoothing the learning curve through interprofessional simulation training. J Pediatr Surg. 2015;50(5):798–804.

Surgical Considerations

23

ECLS Simulation in Surgery

Justyna Swol

Abbreviations

ACT	Activated clotting time
CPB	Cardiopulmonary bypass
ECLS	Extracorporeal life support
ECMO	Extracorporeal membrane oxygenation
ECPR	Extracorporeal cardiopulmonary resuscitation
ED	Emergency department
FAST	Focused assessment with sonography in trauma
GCS	Glasgow Coma Scale
HFES	High-fidelity extracorporeal simulation
ICU	Intensive care unit
NIRS	Near-infrared spectroscopy
OR	Operating room
OS	Operating system
POC	Point of care
SIRS	Systemic inflammatory response syndrome
TBI	Traumatic brain injury

Learning Objectives

1. Identify elements of various simulation techniques ranging from discussion of clinical scenarios to high-fidelity extracorporeal simulation.
2. Determine the most appropriate scenario and simulation technique prior to the team experience.
3. Describe trauma scenario in high-fidelity simulation.

J. Swol (✉)
Department of Respiratory Medicine, Allergology and Sleep Medicine, Intensive Care, General Hospital Nuremberg, University Hospital of Paracelsus Medical University, Nuremberg, Germany

Introduction

The use of extracorporeal heart and lung support systems has undergone fascinating technical improvements over the last 10–15 years [1]. Circuits have decreased in size and become more streamlined, and advances in percutaneous vascular cannula insertion, centrifugal pump technologies, and miniaturization of extracorporeal devices have simplified ECLS for deployment in a variety of settings, including the surgical environment. Extracorporeal membrane oxygenation (ECMO), also referred to as extracorporeal life support (ECLS), is a high-risk and complex life-saving procedure designed to support cardiac and/or pulmonary functions in cases of organ failure. ECLS simulation-based education plays an important role in preparing ECLS teams to handle routine procedures as well as emergency situations, ensuring patient safety. Various simulation techniques have been developed, ranging from discussion of clinical scenarios to high-fidelity extracorporeal simulation (HFES).

Simulation Techniques

The ECLS system consists of a pump, an oxygenator, and a console, where, inter alia, both the blood flow and pressure conditions on the oxygenator can be monitored. This system is connected to the patient via large-lumen cannulas (e.g., 15–21 French cannula in adults) that are percutaneously introduced with the Seldinger technique, usually under ultrasound guidance.

ECLS simulators are composed of several modules serving different functions required to simulate ECLS emergencies. The simulation of an ex vivo ECLS system can be built with increasing complexity [2]. Although the system of organization for simulation-based learning was largely discussed in terms of Boston's zones [2], this is another way to organize and understand complexity in simulation.

L. C. Johnston, L. Su (eds.), *Comprehensive Healthcare Simulation: ECMO Simulation*, Comprehensive Healthcare Simulation,
https://doi.org/10.1007/978-3-030-53844-6_23

Level 1 simulation is a simple simulation of the system by connecting the cannulas to a tubing system, provides a convenient visualization of the system, and is suitable for a basic beginner course (Fig. 23.1, 23.2, and 23.3).

A *Level 2* simulation system allows cannulation on a manikin, preferred in Seldinger technique for percutaneous cannulation. Ultrasound simulation can be implemented, especially for wire guidance and vessel approval [3]. Higher demands on the tubing system and an additional pump system for circuit simulation are required (Fig. 23.4).

Level 3, high-fidelity extracorporeal simulation (HFES), allows both the detection of pathophysiological relationships by changing the device function and the simulation of vital parameters of the patient (Figs. 23.5 and 23.6). As soon as a patient simulator is added to the simulator-based learning experience, additional scenarios can be recreated. Thermochromic fluid can be used to simulate oxygenated blood [4]. The jugular and femoral sites are fitted with ultrasound-compatible models to enable proper dilatation of venous and arterial cannulation [3]. To verify the positioning of the ECLS cannulas, the heart anatomy could also be reproduced with a software application with required scanner combinations and mounted readily into simulated training scenarios [3]. A variety of phantoms exists for training in ultrasound-guided vessel access [5–7]. Silicone tubing or balloon phantom visualizing vessels may be used. Commercially available and self-made models (meat and nonmeat based) can be created with materials such as agar, gelatin, tofu, chicken, or porcine meat [7]. However, they suffer from a short shelf life. Meat-based phantoms provide more realistic tissue feedback and have a background echogenicity [7].

The final solutions are various models of ECLS circuit simulators and ECLS patient simulators to reproduce realistic, typical patient and device emergencies.

The above-described simulation levels are primarily intended for educational purposes, providing a near-authentic experience and enhanced learning of the basic ECLS run. As discussed in other chapters, several commercial products have been released to the market [8, 9]. Passionate ECMOlogists have also developed self-engineered simulators consisting of a combination of reanimation manikins and closed-loop systems [8, 10–12]. In addition, an ex-vivo ECLS model can be used to scientifi-

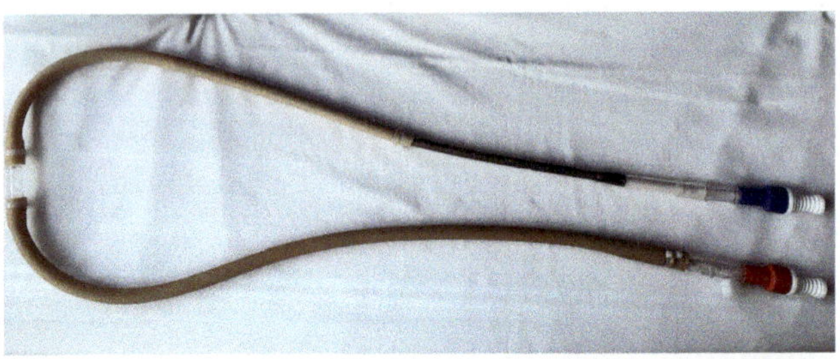

Fig. 23.1 Loop systems connecting the cannulas as a basic simulation tool

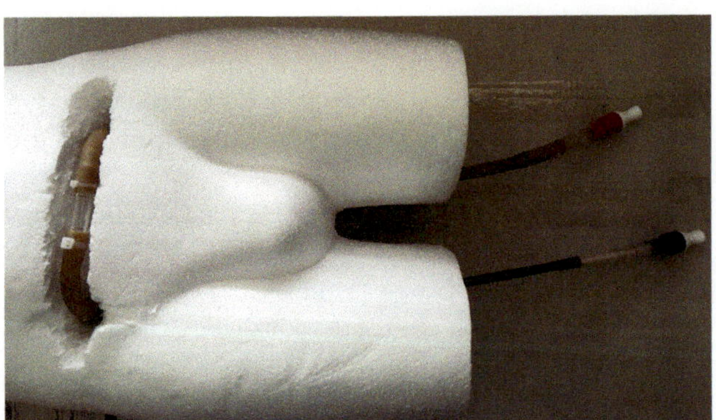

Fig. 23.2 Loop system connected to the cannulas, which is built into the manikin

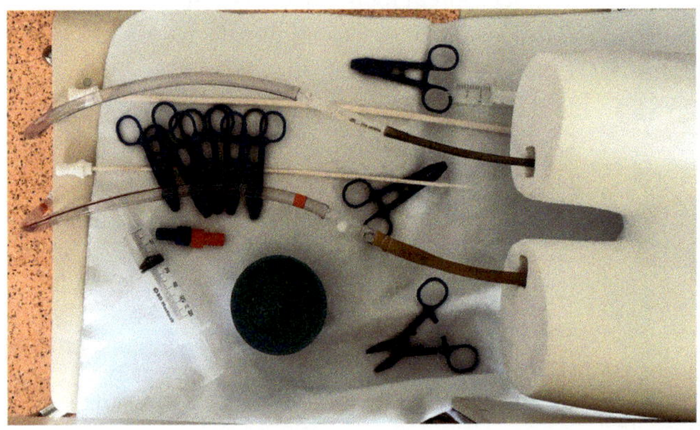

Fig. 23.3 The water-filled ECLS circuit connected to the loop system

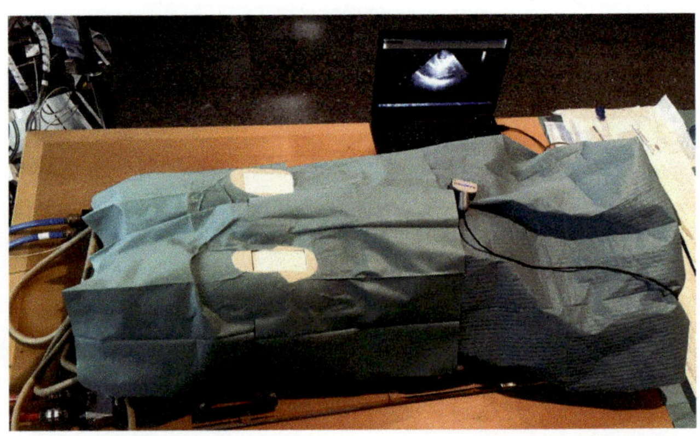

Fig. 23.4 Cannulation simulator[1]. Phantom prepared with silicon tubes and replaceable groins for vessel access. Fluid, e.g., water, circulation is ensured by a pump. Ultrasound simulation of wire placement for ECLS cannulation of femoral vessels[2]. [1]With courtesy of Emmanuel Bossavy, Global Therapy Development Manager Cardiopulmonary, Getinge, France. [2]Department of Cardiovascular Surgery, University Heart Center Freiburg, Faculty of Medicine, University of Freiburg, Germany

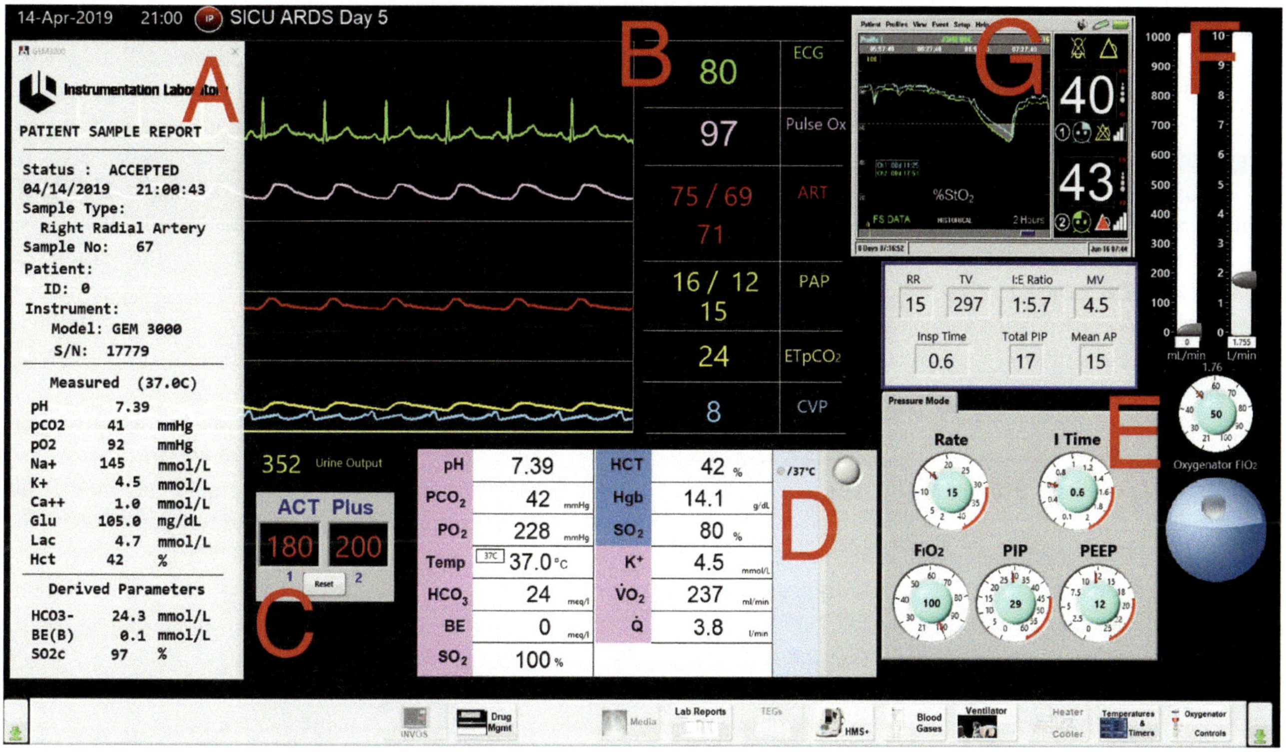

Fig. 23.5 Fig. Screenshot of Califia Simulator Version 3. Item A – Arterial blood analysis right radial artery. B – Monitor of patient's vital signs. C – Urine output and activated clotting time (ACT) measurement. D – Post-oxygenator blood gas analysis. E – Ventilator support settings. F – Sweep gas flow for ECLS. G – Near-infrared spectroscopy. (With courtesy of Richard Tallman, Biomed Simulation Inc., San Diego, CA 92126, USA)

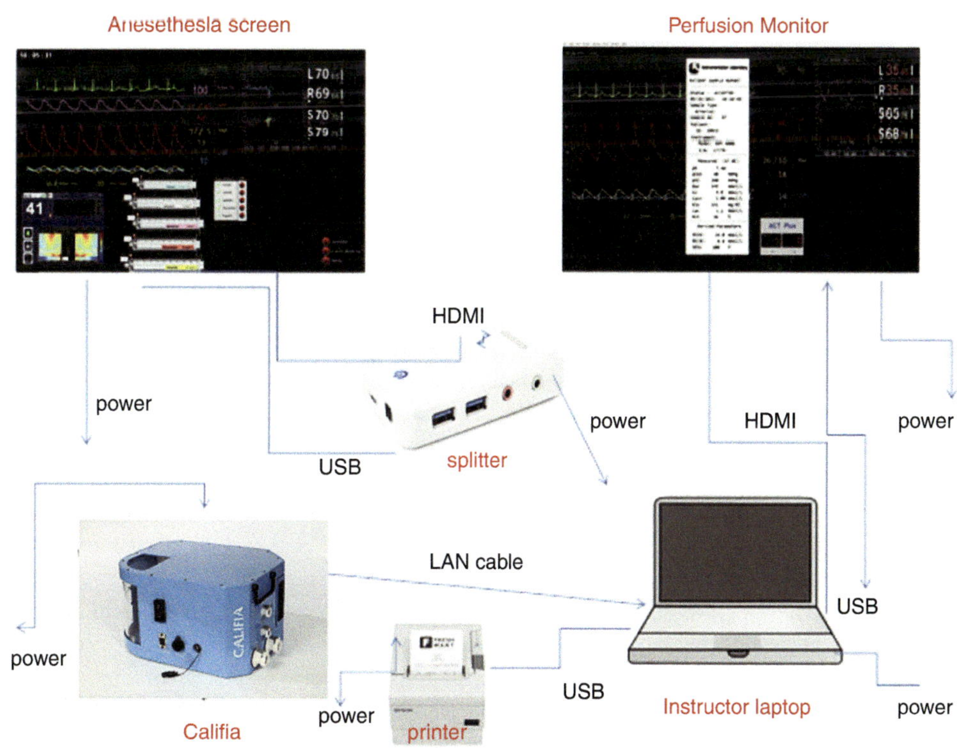

Fig. 23.6 Schematic of the simulation environment of the Califia Simulator Version 3. (With courtesy of Hans Seiler, Biomed Simulation Inc., San Diego, CA 92126, USA)

cally investigate clinical issues related to oxygenator membrane properties [13], optimal blood flow velocities [14, 15], or other research questions [16–19]. Most models consist of a reservoir bag and two connected circuits (pump, oxygenator, and heat exchanger), one simulating the patient and the other the ECMO, using a blood- or saline-primed circuit. Furthermore, diverse numerical models facilitate the understanding of oxygenation or hemodynamic physiology on ECMO and can be used to teach these principles [16–23] (Figs. 23.5 and 23.6). The establishment of ex vivo models allows identification of key factors likely to influence patient outcomes [13, 15, 24–26].

ECLS Scenarios in a Surgical Context

Any kind of ECLS simulator relies on scenarios similar to those in clinical practice in a controlled environment without negative consequences due to errors (e.g., tubing connections to the cannulas, troubleshooting, oxygenator changing, or clotting). The ECLS procedure involves cannulation and a risk of potential physiologic and mechanical complications. Simulator learning objectives for team or individual training include an identification of the problem, the intervention, a reassessment, and a debriefing. As soon as a patient simulator is added to the simulator-based learning experience, participants can be exposed to more scenarios (Table 23.1) and a wider spectrum of learning objectives compared with those achievable during water drills or animal models [27].

The origins of extracorporeal heart and lung support begin in adult and pediatric cardiac surgery. That is, when ECLS originated, many pediatric and adult cardiac programs already provided simulation-based education, including perfusion and cardiac surgery specific scenarios [28–37]. The perfusion simulator system (Califia Simulator, Biomed Simulation Inc., San Diego, CA 92126, USA) simulates a patient before, during, and after cardiopulmonary bypass (CPB) for open-heart surgery and is designed as a patient simulator to attach to any heart-lung or ECLS device circuit. Full CPB simulation program included the simulator system and an additional program on the controller display for blood, cardioplegia flow, and reservoir levels instead of using the sensor feedback from the patient module. This simulator allows for expanded teaching and testing opportunities without the use of a heart-lung or ECMO machine. The patient's side module has a reservoir system with several inducted transducers and valves attached and should be operated by a desktop computer, laptop, or tablet, defined as an operating system (OS). The OS also serves as the operating room's anesthesia monitor and displays a wide variety of patient data, e.g., cardiovascular parameters and several different ECG patterns, including sequentially stepping through to the asystole ECG rhythm upon sensing an adequate delivery of cardioplegia. Bypass blood flow rate, cardioplegia flow, circulating blood volume, and temperature should be integrated into the monitoring module. The activated clotting time (ACT), outputs from various point-of-care devices such as blood gas analyzers or anticoagulation management system printouts, radiological images, and videos can also be displayed. Output from ancillary monitors displaying physiological parameters related to the patient during the course of the clinical scenario is customizable using the controller display on the OS. A flexible teaching practice allows changes, comments, and sequentially stepping through a case or proceeding at predetermined intervals once a clinical scenario is loaded.

However, the scenario creator can also be used to input previous or current patient records as a retrospective review of patient courses and therapies. These data may include all parameters that occurred during therapy, such as labs, perfusion protocols, blood gas analyses, ACT values, NIRS values, and ventilation parameters. Observational assessment tools can be used for evaluating the performance of an operator in the conduct of simulated cardiopulmonary bypass or ECLS and are helpful for debriefing and providing feedback [28, 38]. Such tools are capable to train teamwork and non-technical skills and psychometrically sound to assess team behaviors during cardiac arrest resuscitation attempts, providing trainees with more specific feedback with regard to performance quality and areas requiring improvement [39]. Thus, existing findings and experiences can be repeatedly played for review or training purposes and adapted to other surgical subspecialty-related scenarios [40].

Moreover, the number of publications on ECLS use in surgical patients of all subspecialties, such as abdominal, thoracic, vascular, orthopedics, and trauma surgery, and surgery-associated complications, such as postoperative bleeding or sepsis, is increasing [41, 42]. Although these conditions, especially trauma and bleeding, were considered contraindications in the past, these scenarios should be included in current contemporary training and simulation-based education programs (Tables 23.1, 23.2, and 23.3).

Surgical patients may be in critical condition. Major trauma patients undergo systemic inflammatory response syndrome (SIRS) in the early posttraumatic phase and are hemodynamically unstable with a high risk of multiorgan failure. The risk of bleeding and the need for further interventions and operations during ECLS make extracorporeal therapy of trauma patients challenging. ECLS therapy requires a difficult balance between the need for anticoagulation and the persistent risk of bleeding [41, 42]. Second-hit complications and organ failure later in the course can also make extracorporeal support necessary. ECLS improves oxygenation and restores circulation in patients with parenchymal organ disruption and/or bleeding. The extracorporeal devices correct hypercarbia and help improve metabolic acidosis. Furthermore, they help to restore hemodynamics and rewarm patients in cases of hypothermia [41].

Table 23.1 Scenarios in ECLS simulation-based education

Scenarios prior to ECLS system	Technical requirements
Circuit-related complications Pump or oxygenator failure Inadequate drainage	ECLS device, clamps, demonstration of appropriate circuit pressures (pre- and post-oxygenator), membrane pressure, and drainage (venous) and return (arterial) pressures
Circuit- and cannula-related complications Recirculation	Closed-loop real-time simulation model, circuit filled with artificial blood and thermochromic ink, and visible fluctuations in the mixed venous oxygen saturation
Cannulation-related complications: Cannulation failure because of vessel perforation or dissection (also with retroperitoneal hemorrhage and cannula site bleeding) Cannulation of the wrong vessel Cannula malposition or migration Accidental decannulation	ECLS device, tubes suitable for cannula placement, pump-driven manikin circulation, plastic bag to drain the manikin circuit to demonstrate a bleeding condition/blood loss, upgrade for pulsatile circulation and ultrasound fitted materials
Cannula-related complications Kinking or clotting	ECLS device, clamps
Surgical context scenarios	
Veno-venous and pulmonary support for severe hypoxemia Pre-, intra-, and postoperative support and complications management in thoracic surgery, e.g., tracheal reconstruction Acute severe respiratory failure and/or injury of the trachea-bronchial tree, resulting in an inadequate gas exchange Near-drowning, inhalation trauma, burns, and a complete tracheal or bronchial obstruction Pulmonary contusion after blunt trauma or blast injury Fat or amniotic fluid embolism, air embolism, airway injury or obstruction	Customized circuit connected to the patient simulator to demonstrate ventilator settings Simulated blood gas analysis available Trauma manikin visualizing potential injuries Plastic bag to drain the manikin circuit to demonstrate a bleeding condition/blood loss
Venous-arterial (circulatory shock) support Postoperative cardiac arrest Cardiogenic shock (traumatic or ischemic) Massive pulmonary embolism with cardiogenic shock or cardiac arrest Acute traumatic cardiac failure (myocardial contusions and ruptures) resulting in inadequate circulation (cardiogenic shock or cardiac arrest) or hemorrhagic shock	Cannulation simulator for extracorporeal cardiopulmonary resuscitation (ECPR) Manikin ultrasound fitted Circuit connected to the patient simulator to demonstrate ventilator settings Simulated blood gas analysis Vital sign monitoring Trauma manikin visualizing potential injuries Plastic bag to drain the manikin circuit to demonstrate a bleeding condition/blood loss
Other conditions Sepsis Organ hypoperfusion Hypothermia Metabolic acidosis	Closed-loop real-time simulation model Circuit filled with artificial blood and thermochromic ink Visible fluctuations in the mixed venous oxygen saturation Simulated blood gas analysis

The scenarios for simulation-based ECLS education can be divided into device-/circuit-related education, education related to the cannulation procedure, and clinical scenarios (Table 23.1). The description in Tables 23.2 and 23.3 provides more examples of how existing simulation tools can be adapted for training purposes in trauma-related scenarios including ultrasound simulation (Tables 23.2 and 23.3).

Human Factors in ECLS Team Training

Medical educational services are usually based on lectures, multiple-choice questions, water drills, and animal labs. Several studies have demonstrated that simulation-based ECLS training improves team performance, safety culture, and patient-related outcomes [27–29, 32, 37, 38, 43–45]. In 2015, only 57% of the 173 US ECMO centers reported an established institutional ECMO credentialing program with recertification (16%), training elements, and barriers [46]. Lack of standardization for credentialing (36%) was the major barrier for program establishment [46]. Most high-risk industries, such as aviation, include simulation training as a mandatory requirement for their professionals and facilities. According to their statistical frequency, most aviation errors are based on psychological factors, overconfidence, and equipment malfunction. Recommendations made by the aviation industry regarding technical and team-based training care can be transferred to ECLS centers and ECLS team training [9]. Everyone involved is responsible for patient safety. Skills are achieved through a permanent change in behavior through practice and experience. Simulation has been accepted to complement or replace a predetermined

Table 23.2 Trauma scenario in high-fidelity extracorporeal simulation. Existing simulation tools and human factor aspects can be adapted for training purposes in trauma-related scenarios including ultrasound simulation

Parts of scenario trauma	Implemented simulation tools	Human factor aspects
Prepared case vignette	1. Model of ECLS circuit simulators (Figs. 23.1, 23.2, and 23.3) eventually including cannulation phantom (Fig. 23.4) 2. ECLS patient simulator, available with vital signs, monitoring, visualized mathematical model of physiology on extracorporeal support (Figs. 23.4 and 23.5) 3. Ultrasound simulator (Fig. 23.6)	1. Defined team of supervisors 2. Survey performed before the simulation to explore the experience of participants 3. Defined course of the simulation, roles, responsibilities, feedback, and debriefing modalities
Case vignette: A 16-year-old cyclist hit by a car on the roadway subsequently presented with blunt chest trauma, a pelvic fracture, and a penetrating injury to the left upper extremity. His Glasgow Coma Scale score was 6 at the scene. He was incubated in the ED and mechanically ventilated in instable condition.	1. Heart rate is 150 beats/min, blood pressure 60/40 mmHg, respiratory rate 12 breaths/min, and his oxygen saturation 83%. On vasopressors 2. Ventilatory settings: Tidal volume 200 mL, PEEP 16, inspiratory pressure 35 mm H_2O, FiO_2 of 1.0 3. Vital signs and monitoring visualized on patient's simulator 4. Ultrasound simulation for focused assessment with sonography in trauma (FAST) (Table 23.3)	1. Recognition of involved specialists 2. Interprofessional discussion and decision 3. Alert of ECLS team
1. Thoracic drainage placement after bilateral tension pneumothoraces are identified 2. The patient required increasing doses of vasopressors and increasing invasiveness of mechanical ventilation 3. Bleeding coagulopathy following vascular injury of the brachial artery and pelvic fracture	1. Arterial blood gas analysis: Arterial pO_2 of 68 mmHg, pCO_2 of 110 mmHg, and pH of 7.12 2. Ventilatory settings: Tidal volume less than 150 mL, "delta" $P > 20$, PEEP increased to 18, and increased inspiratory pressure at 38 mm H_2O with an FiO_2 of 1.0	Challenge to teamwork and communication related to: 1. Bridging to radiological vascular intervention and surgery for vessel reconstruction and pelvic fixation 2. Controversial indication to ECLS cannulation regarding TBI and bleeding
The patient experienced traumatic brain injury, blunt and penetrating trauma, bleeding coagulopathy, severe hypoxemia, hypercapnia, respiratory acidosis secondary to decreased lung compliance, and acute, severe lung failure. ECLS is indicated for respiratory support. TBI has been concerned as a relative contraindication and an option to run ECLS without anticoagulation for limited time have been discussed. Regarding bleeding, veno-arterial cannulation to restore the circulation has been performed	1. Visualization of pts vital signs deterioration and monitoring 2. Mass transfusion protocol 3. Ultrasound-guided cannulation 4. Adjusted ventilator setting after cannulation 5. Eventually, in cases of reduced lung compliance, additional venous return cannulas (V-A-V) to facilitate adequate gas exchange and ultra-protective ventilation 6. Interhospital transfer to OR	Team time-out and check lists Interpretation of the results: 1. Veno-venous ECLS is a lung support option in case of reduced lung compliance and can be used to prevent ventilator-induced lung injury 2. Veno-arterial ECLS is feasible to restore circulation and rewarming Hand over to anesthesia or ICU team Debriefing, survey, feedback

Table 23.3 Trauma-related ultrasound scenarios to simulate the whole process and decision-making during high-fidelity extracorporeal simulation

Clinical context	Ultrasound technique
Primary and secondary survey in emergency department (ED)	Focused assessment with sonography in trauma (FAST)
Intraabdominal bleeding, e.g., due to organ or vessels injury	Abdominal sonography
Traumatic cardiac tamponade (e.g., due to penetrating injury) Aortic dissection or rupture Traumatic cardiogenic shock (e.g., due to coronary vessel rupture)	Cardiac echography
Pneumothorax Atelectatic consolidation	Lung and pleural sonography
ECLS cannulation (veno-venous or veno-arterial)	Ultrasound-guided vessel identification Ultrasound-guided vessel puncture Wire location approval
ECLS cannulation during cardiopulmonary resuscitation (ECPR)	Cardiac echography Ultrasound-guided vessel identification Ultrasound-guided vessel puncture Wire location approval arterial and venous regarding intraabdominal view and echocardiography
Distal (retrograde) cannulation in case of arterial femoral cannulation	Ultrasound-guided vessel identification Ultrasound-guided vessel puncture Wire location approval

number of direct patient contact hours; thus, participants can transfer their learning to real clinical settings [43, 47] (Table 23.2). Implementation of an extracorporeal cardiopulmonary resuscitation simulation program reduces extracorporeal cardiopulmonary resuscitation times in real patients [32]. It proves the benefit of HFES regarding team behaviors and communication. Placing an emphasis on high-quality educational learning opportunities for participants, for both initial training and continuing professional development, provides opportunities to develop teamwork skills and expertise to decrease device- and patient-related risks. Team time-out procedure and checklists increase safety because operations can be systematically processed. Routine team meetings and regular safety briefings also promote safety culture in a unit. Even less critical mistakes or errors can be used as an important error avoidance experience if they are consciously perceived, analyzed, and handled appropriately.

Decision-making, especially in the treatment of surgical patients, requires an interdisciplinary consensus between an ECLS-specialized intensivist, surgeons, anesthetists, and all other physicians and medical and nursing team members involved. Successful resolution of a medical emergency also depends on the key parties' behavioral skills, leadership, communication, and teamwork [38]. Good communication with all persons involved in planned interventions can help to prevent errors and misunderstandings. Active listening and argumentation are the strategies that are the most likely to contribute to constructive solutions to interpersonal conflict.

The simulated scenarios should be followed by a debriefing session during which the decision-making process and actions of the participants can be analyzed to develop a better understanding of the issues addressed [28, 29, 48]. Additionally, pre- and post-participation questionnaires can be used to determine the effect of a proficient transfer of knowledge, technical and behavioral skills, and confidence levels of the participants to the live medical routine [48, 49].

The current literature indicates a large variation in in-hospital costs estimated for ECLS [50]. The financial costs of the simulation equipment limit the number of simulators and the availability for ECMO training purposes. The financial impact of simulator-based ECLS education is currently unknown and is difficult to predict. It is difficult to balance the cost of education against potential additional costs related to medical errors, which might be due to a lack of experience, qualifications and confidence, insurance costs, and estimated life loss.

Summary

Simulation-based learning is frequently used in medical education and skills training and is particularly suitable for complex technologies such as extracorporeal systems. The simulation tools serve as an alternative to real patients. They promote experimental and reflexive learning and help teach crisis management skills. Thus, medical simulation offers numerous strategies for comprehensive and practical training as well as safer patient care in the application of extracorporeal procedures. Repetitive training leads to skill improvement with clearly defined goals. Lessons learned can lead to effective improvements in the workplace and beneficial changes in how to cannulate and manage surgical patients on ECLS.

Acknowledgments Special acknowledgment goes to Prof. Dr. Richard Tallman, Founder and CEO of Biomed Simulation Inc., San Diego, CA 92126, USA, for providing helpful feedback from his experience about high-fidelity extracorporeal simulation and physiology.

References

1. Betit P. Technical advances in the field of ECMO. Respir Care. 2018;63(9):1162–73.
2. Roussin CJ, SimZones WP. An organizational innovation for simulation programs and centers. Acad Med. 2017;92(8):1114–20.
3. Damjanovic D, Goebel U, Fischer B, Huth M, Breger H, Buerkle H, et al. An easy-to-build, low-budget point-of-care ultrasound simulator: from Linux to a web-based solution. Crit Ultrasound J. 2017;9(1):4.
4. Al Disi M, Alsalemi A, Alhomsi Y, Bensaali F, Amira A, Alinier G. Using thermochromism to simulate blood oxygenation in extracorporeal membrane oxygenation. Perfusion. 2019;34(2):106–15.
5. Farjad Sultan S, Shorten G, Iohom G. Simulators for training in ultrasound guided procedures. Med Ultrason. 2013;15(2):125–31.
6. Hocking G, Hebard S, Mitchell CH. A review of the benefits and pitfalls of phantoms in ultrasound-guided regional anesthesia. Reg Anesth Pain Med. 2011;36(2):162–70.
7. Rippey JC, Blanco P, Carr PJ. An affordable and easily constructed model for training in ultrasound-guided vascular access. J Vasc Access. 2015;16(5):422–7.
8. Al Disi M, Alsalemi A, Alhomsi Y, Bensaali F, Amira A, Alinier G. Revolutionizing ECMO simulation with affordable yet high Fidelity technology. Am J Emerg Med. 2018;36(7):1310–2.
9. Lansdowne W, Machin D, Grant DJ. Development of the orpheus perfusion simulator for use in high-fidelity extracorporeal membrane oxygenation simulation. J Extra Corpor Technol. 2012;44(4):250–5.
10. Puslecki M, Ligowski M, Dabrowski M, Sip M, Stefaniak S, Klosiewicz T, et al. The role of simulation to support donation after circulatory death with extracorporeal membrane oxygenation (DCD-ECMO). Perfusion. 2017;32(8):624–30.
11. Puslecki M, Ligowski M, Kiel M, Dabrowski M, Stefaniak S, Maciejewski A, et al. ECMO therapy simulator for extracorporeal life support. Am J Emerg Med. 2018;36(3):506–8.
12. Puslecki M, Ligowski M, Kiel M, Dabrowski M, Stefaniak S, Sip M, et al. Prototype of extracorporeal membrane oxygenation (ECMO) therapy simulator used in regional ECMO program. J Thorac Dis. 2018;10(8):5073–9.
13. Rais-Bahrami K, Mikesell G, Seale WR, Rivera O, Hearty JP, Short BL. In vitro evaluation of the MeraSilox-S 0.5 and 0.8 m 2 silicone hollow-fibre membrane oxygenator for use in neonatal ECMO. Perfusion. 1992;7(4):315–20.
14. Sea P. Hemodynamic evaluation of novel i-cor pulsatile ECLS system during various cardiac arrhythmias: in vitro study. Artif Organs. 2014;38(5):A16–7.

15. Spurlock DJ, Ranney DN, Fracz EM, Mazur DE, Bartlet RH, Haft JW. In vitro testing of a novel blood pump designed for temporary extracorporeal support. ASAIO J. 2012;58(2):109–14.
16. Broman M, Frenckner B, Bjallmark A, Broome M. Recirculation during veno-venous extra-corporeal membrane oxygenation--a simulation study. Int J Artif Organs. 2015;38(1):23–30.
17. Sakamoto K, Saku K, Kishi T, Kakino T, Tanaka A, Sakamoto T, et al. Prediction of the impact of venoarterial extracorporeal membrane oxygenation on hemodynamics. Am J Physiol Heart Circ Physiol. 2015;308(8):H921–30.
18. Broome M, Donker DW. Individualized real-time clinical decision support to monitor cardiac loading during venoarterial ECMO. J Transl Med. 2016;14:4.
19. Messai E, Bouguerra A, Harmelin G, Di Lascio G, Bonizzoli M, Bonacchi M. A numerical model of blood oxygenation during veno-venous ECMO: analysis of the interplay between blood oxygenation and its delivery parameters. J Clin Monit Comput. 2016;30(3):327–32.
20. Stevens MC, Callaghan FM, Forrest P, Bannon PG, Grieve SM. Flow mixing during peripheral veno-arterial extra corporeal membrane oxygenation – a simulation study. J Biomech. 2017;55:64–70.
21. Hsu PL, Wang D, Ballard-Croft C, Xiao D, Zwischenberger JB. A numerical simulation comparing a cavopulmonary assist device and VA ECMO for failing Fontan support. ASAIO J. 2017;63(5):604–12.
22. Chicotka S, Burkhoff D, Dickstein ML, Bacchetta M. Extracorporeal membrane oxygenation for end-stage interstitial lung disease with secondary pulmonary hypertension at rest and exercise: insights from simulation modeling. ASAIO J. 2018;64(2):203–10.
23. Donker DW, Brodie D, Henriques JPS, Broome M. Left ventricular unloading during veno-arterial ECMO: a simulation study. ASAIO J. 2019;65(1):11–20.
24. Shekar K, Roberts JA, McDonald CI, Fisquet S, Barnett AG, Mullany DV, et al. Sequestration of drugs in the circuit may lead to therapeutic failure during extracorporeal membrane oxygenation. Crit Care. 2012;16(5):R194.
25. Shekar K, Roberts JA, McDonald CI, Ghassabian S, Anstey C, Wallis SC, et al. Protein-bound drugs are prone to sequestration in the extracorporeal membrane oxygenation circuit: results from an ex vivo study. Crit Care. 2015;19:164.
26. Wagner D, Pasko D, Phillips K, Waldvogel J, Annich G. In vitro clearance of dexmedetomidine in extracorporeal membrane oxygenation. Perfusion. 2013;28(1):40–6.
27. Brazzi L, Lissoni A, Panigada M, Bottino N, Patroniti N, Pappalardo F, et al. Simulation-based training of extracorporeal membrane oxygenation during H1N1 influenza pandemic: the Italian experience. Simul Healthc. 2012;7(1):32–4.
28. Anderson JM, Boyle KB, Murphy AA, Yaeger KA, LeFlore J, Halamek LP. Simulating extracorporeal membrane oxygenation emergencies to improve human performance. Part I: methodologic and technologic innovations. Simul Healthc. 2006;1(4):220–7.
29. Burton KS, Pendergrass TL, Byczkowski TL, Taylor RG, Moyer MR, Falcone RA, et al. Impact of simulation-based extracorporeal membrane oxygenation training in the simulation laboratory and clinical environment. Simul Healthc. 2011;6(5):284–91.
30. Pantalos GM, Sahetya S, Merkley TL, Horrell T, Austin EH 3rd, Mascio CE. Mock circulation simulation of extracorporeal membrane oxygenation support for systemic ventricular failure in an infant: the effect of atrial septostomy. ASAIO J. 2012;58(4):415–9.
31. Burkhart HM, Riley JB, Lynch JJ, Suri RM, Greason KL, Joyce LD, et al. Simulation-based postcardiotomy extracorporeal membrane oxygenation crisis training for thoracic surgery residents. Ann Thorac Surg. 2013;95(3):901–6.
32. Su L, Spaeder MC, Jones MB, Sinha P, Nath DS, Jain PN, et al. Implementation of an extracorporeal cardiopulmonary resuscitation simulation program reduces extracorporeal cardiopulmonary resuscitation times in real patients. Pediatr Crit Care Med. 2014;15(9):856–60.
33. Allan CK, Kleinman ME. Enhancing the power of simulation for complex clinical care. Pediatr Crit Care Med. 2014;15. United States:904–6.
34. Sanchez-Glanville C, Brindle ME, Spence T, Blackwood J, Drews T, Menzies S, et al. Evaluating the introduction of extracorporeal life support technology to a tertiary-care pediatric institution: smoothing the learning curve through interprofessional simulation training. J Pediatr Surg. 2015;50(5):798–804.
35. Weems MF, Friedlich PS, Nelson LP, Rake AJ, Klee L, Stein JE, et al. The role of extracorporeal membrane oxygenation simulation training at extracorporeal life support organization centers in the United States. Simul Healthc. 2017;12(4):233–9.
36. Raffaeli G, Ghirardello S, Vanzati M, Baracetti C, Canesi F, Conigliaro F, et al. Start a neonatal extracorporeal membrane oxygenation program: a multistep team training. Front Pediatr. 2018;6:151.
37. Di Nardo M, David P, Stoppa F, Lorusso R, Raponi M, Amodeo A, et al. The introduction of a high-fidelity simulation program for training pediatric critical care personnel reduces the times to manage extracorporeal membrane oxygenation emergencies and improves teamwork. J Thorac Dis. 2018;10(6):3409–17.
38. Anderson JM, Murphy AA, Boyle KB, Yaeger KA, Halamek LP. Simulating extracorporeal membrane oxygenation emergencies to improve human performance. Part II: assessment of technical and behavioral skills. Simul Healthc. 2006;1(4):228–32.
39. Walker S, Brett S, McKay A, Lambden S, Vincent C, Sevdalis N. Observational Skill-based Clinical Assessment tool for Resuscitation (OSCAR): development and validation. Resuscitation. 2011;82(7):835–44.
40. Whitmore SP, Gunnerson KJ, Haft JW, Lynch WR, VanDyck T, Hebert C, et al. Simulation training enables emergency medicine providers to rapidly and safely initiate extracorporeal cardiopulmonary resuscitation (ECPR) in a simulated cardiac arrest scenario. Resuscitation. 2019;138:68–73.
41. Swol J, Brodie D, Napolitano L, Park PK, Thiagarajan R, Barbaro RP, et al. Indications and outcomes of extracorporeal life support in trauma patients. J Trauma Acute Care Surg. 2018;84(6):831–7.
42. Ull C, Schildhauer TA, Strauch JT, Swol J. Outcome measures of extracorporeal life support (ECLS) in trauma patients versus patients without trauma: a 7-year single-center retrospective cohort study. J Artif Organs. 2017;20(2):117–24.
43. Chan SY, Figueroa M, Spentzas T, Powell A, Holloway R, Shah S. Prospective assessment of novice learners in a simulation-based extracorporeal membrane oxygenation (ECMO) education program. Pediatr Cardiol. 2013;34(3):543–52.
44. Fehr JJ, Shepard M, McBride ME, Mehegan M, Reddy K, Murray DJ, et al. Simulation-based assessment of ECMO clinical specialists. Simul Healthc. 2016;11(3):194–9.
45. Fouilloux V, Gran C, Guervilly C, Breaud J, El Louali F, Rostini P. Impact of education and training course for ECMO patients based on high-fidelity simulation: a pilot study dedicated to ICU nurses. Perfusion. 2018;267659118789824
46. Muratore S, Beilman G, John R, Brunsvold M. Extracorporeal membrane oxygenation credentialing: where do we stand? Am J Surg. 2015;210(4):655–60.e2.
47. Zakhary BM, Kam LM, Kaufman BS, Felner KJ. The utility of high-fidelity simulation for training critical care fellows in the management of extracorporeal membrane oxygenation emergencies: a randomized controlled trial. Crit Care Med. 2017;45(8):1367–73.
48. Brum R, Rajani R, Gelandt E, Morgan L, Raguseelan N, Butt S, et al. Simulation training for extracorporeal membrane oxygenation. Ann Card Anaesth. 2015;18(2):185–90.
49. Endo T, Kagaya Y, Arata Y, Imai H. Long-term efficacy of an extracorporeal membrane oxygenation simulation with a novel, low-cost vascular model "Endo-circuit.". Acute Med Surg. 2017;4(1):79–88.
50. Harvey MJ, Gaies MG, Prosser LA. U.S.and international in-hospital costs of extracorporeal membrane oxygenation: asystematic review. Appl Health Econ Health Policy. 2015;13(4):341–57.

24 Nursing Aspects of ECPR and ECMO Training

Dorothy M. Beke and Annette Imprescia

Learning Objectives

The objectives of this chapter are for the readers to:

1. Identify key aspects of developing a simulation-based ECMO program for critical care nurses.
2. Describe foundational nursing skills that are required and can be practiced through simulation in order to care for patients on ECMO support.
3. List crucial nursing roles for ECPR and ECMO-related emergencies that can be explored through simulation.
4. Outline critical elements of crisis resource management team-based skills including role clarity, communication, global assessment, resources, and personnel support.

Introduction

Nurses who care for patients on extracorporeal membrane oxygenation (ECMO) require specific knowledge and baseline competence for the provision of optimal care. Specialized skills development begins early during nursing orientation with learning and performing foundational practices inherent of critical care nursing. Orientation and continuing education and skills training may incorporate a variety of approaches to enhance both knowledge and technical proficiency. These varied approaches may appeal to individuals with different learning styles and preferences. Kolb describes several learning styles, which result from various combinations of individual preferences, such as feeling and watching, watching and thinking, doing and thinking, and doing and feeling [1]. By utilizing a combination of learning methods, including self-guided activities, didactic lectures, hands-on practice, team-structured activities, and simulation with interactive participation, instructors can meet the needs of all types of learners and contribute to knowledge acquisition and skills development [2]. Simulation training provides a realistic environment for nurses to practice and master skills that are necessary for ECMO deployment, management of ECMO-related emergencies, and provision of routine ECMO care as part of the team in a controlled setting before they are expected to perform these tasks with actual patients. By utilizing "SimZones" training, nurses develop their specialized skills and knowledge with a structured approach that initially begins with individual, distraction-free learning [3]. During progression through the various SimZones, practices are further developed over time by adding more complexity, distractions, and interdisciplinary team participation as providers progress to the acquisition of mastery-level skills. Expert instructors and facilitators are required to create psychological safety and provide an optimal educational and training environment [4].

The Extracorporeal Life Support Organization (ELSO) does not currently recommend one specific staffing model for providing care to patients requiring ECMO support; however, ELSO does support institution-specific models of staffing that maximize safe patient practices [5]. This chapter specifically focuses on aspects of training for nurses to care for patients on ECMO as the bedside clinician and not as an ECMO specialist. Please refer to Chap. 12 for details on dedicated training for ECMO specialist providers.

Description of SimZones

Roussin and Weinstock describe a unique organizational approach to simulation training with the use of SimZones, which helps to address challenges associated with simulation

D. M. Beke · A. Imprescia (✉)
Cardiac Intensive Care Unit, Boston Children's Hospital, Boston, MA, USA
e-mail: dorothy.beke@childrens.harvard.edu; annette.imprescia@childrens.harvard.edu

L. C. Johnston, L. Su (eds.), *Comprehensive Healthcare Simulation: ECMO Simulation*, Comprehensive Healthcare Simulation,
https://doi.org/10.1007/978-3-030-53844-6_24

training programs [3]. These challenges include balancing skills acquisition versus team-focused educational experiences, managing the training of faculty, augmenting the mix of participants to enhance the learning experience, balancing the delivery of simulation from a range of locations (in situ, in a designated hospital setting, or in the simulation center), and coordinating pertinent research related to simulation [3]. The SimZones model provides a longitudinal structured approach to ECMO skills training for new nurses. Initially, nurses learn and practice foundational skills that are necessary to care for patients in the critical care environment who require mechanical circulatory support. Training progresses from one zone to the next, from Zone 0 through Zone 4. As the level increases, there is an increase in the associated complexity of the cases with incorporation of distractions. Using this structure permits the development of individual mastery of skill sets within the interdisciplinary team.

The SimZones format is discussed in detail in Chap. 4. However, we will briefly describe the format here in the setting of nursing training and education. The emphasis of Zone 0 training is for the individual participant to focus on a specific skills training with no distractions and without the presence of an instructor. This type of training may include virtual reality tools with auto feedback technology [3].

Zone 1 simulations are instructor-led educational experiences that routinely involve several participants or groups of providers from specific disciplines. Instructors provide information on topics such as what to do in a particular circumstance, or how to perform specific skills within outlined standards of practice. A "pause and correct" methodology is usually utilized to allow individuals to perform activities with minor distractions. In this format, the instructor allows time for pauses during the simulation to teach or to correct any deviations to acceptable standards of practice. Typically, this provides an opportunity to discuss both the positive aspects of the activity and specific areas for improvement [3].

During Zone 2 training, partial or full interdisciplinary teams of individuals with varying levels of experience are formed to build on existing skill sets. The activities often proceed uninterrupted, are more complex in nature, and may involve skilled actors to enhance the realism and learning experience. The simulation activity is followed by a debriefing with an expert facilitator [3].

Zone 3 simulation typically involves the full complement of native, interdisciplinary team members for the purpose of strengthening team dynamics and for systems development. The training experience may involve more than one scenario and might incorporate different aspects such as equipment failures, human factors, and other distractions that often pose challenges to optimal team function [3]. A structured debriefing following each simulation activity encourages individuals to reflect on experiences and express feelings during specific phases. The facilitator guides discussions that include strategies for positive change.

Zone 4 does not include simulation. Zone 4 allows providers to utilize skills learned from prior simulation experiences (from Zones 0 to 3) and apply them in real-life clinical situations involving patients. Similar to Zone 3 training, skilled facilitators lead structured debriefings after a clinical event. Zone 4 provides a means for clinicians to bridge simulation practice into clinical experience [3].

Zone 0 Foundational Training with Simulation

Initiation of learning in Zone 0 provides novice nurses with the opportunity to review specific content and explanations of skills in a distraction-free learning environment [3].This allows for clear focus on clinical content to enhance further knowledge acquisition. Zone 0 learning may be accessed through on-line courses and virtual reality training tools. Educators are able to identify specific foundational modules for independent review by participants. Content and practice simulators may be accessed through educational platforms, such as OPENPediatrics [6]. Table 24.1 highlights educational sections that should be completed by novice critical care nurses prior to progressing to Zone 1 simulation training.

Modules contain pre- and post-tests that provide self-directed learners with instant feedback during educational experiences [6]. A major benefit at this level is that content may be reviewed multiple times until trainees have achieved a certain level of understanding and proficiency. A curriculum that is supplemented with on-line modules provides nurses the opportunity to review information asynchronously and practice on simulators. This allows for mastery of content by novice clinicians prior to application of Zone 1 simulation training. As a result of preparatory work in Zone 0, learners are competent to perform introductory skills that

Table 24.1 Foundational learning modules from OPENPediatrics

Cardiac anatomy and physiology	Interpreting central venous pressure waveforms
Cardiac output	Cardiac rhythms and arrhythmias
Cardiac assessment and monitoring	Electrophysiology and introduction to defibrillation
Congenital heart lesions	Postoperative assessment and monitoring
Non-invasive cardiac monitoring	Postoperative cardiac emergencies
Invasive cardiac monitoring	Event management in emergency situations
Interpreting arterial waveforms	Pain management

OPENPediatrics [6]

will be utilized and built upon as they progress through a prescribed simulation curriculum.

Creating Psychological Safety

One essential element to support the success of any simulation experience is ensuring that time is spent to introduce the "ground rules" of the simulation environment and provide clear expectations of educational goals and objectives for participants prior beginning any learning activities [4]. Creating a safe environment in which to practice and master skills promotes a more engaging learning experience, allows for free-flowing questions, and fosters an atmosphere that is critical for the optimal educational impact of the debriefings. Establishing a safe atmosphere for learning is instrumental to fostering knowledge and skills development throughout the learning continuum [4].

Zone 1 Foundational Instruction

Care of patients on ECMO requires competence with typical nursing critical care skills prior to managing emergency cannulation and circuit-related events. Through the application of simple clinical scenarios, Zone 1 simulation provides a learning experience in which basic skills training and introductory procedures (including safety checks, utilizing chain of commands, and effective communication) may be practiced. Instructors provide immediate feedback and/or correction on technical skill performance during simulations [3]. As trainees demonstrate improved abilities, instructors allow for longer periods of uninterrupted time and provide positive feedback for participants as they master each technique or skill. Examples of skills include physical assessment, ventilation with a resuscitation bag, endotracheal tube suctioning, cardiac rhythm assessment, and defibrillation, among others.

Establishing safe nursing practice is essential when caring for complex patients requiring mechanical circulatory support. Basic, uncomplicated scenarios provide clinical circumstances where nurses are able to deliberately review and discuss key elements of safe patient care, such as a beginning of a shift safety assessment. By exploring daily routines in a methodical fashion, learners are encouraged to discuss aspects of their safety checks, identify why components are necessary, and share real-life experiences. These experiences will ideally affirm the importance of these aspects of clinical practice.

The scenarios utilized can also highlight the importance of structure in providing critical care, as this organized approach allows crisis events to be identified and addressed in a rapid manner. Scenarios provide opportunities for thoughtful reflection and discussion on numerous aspects, including accessing the appropriate chain of command and use of communication frameworks. Structured critical language is utilized to deliver important information in a clear, organized, and concise manner, such as with situation-background-assessment-recommendation (SBAR) format, which is used to convey relevant information about a patient's status in an organized and logical fashion [7]. Other techniques, such as the use of closed-loop communication, improve time to task completion [8]. Initially these communication strategies may be challenging to perform; however, with practice in the simulation laboratory, nurses begin to develop these skills that will be used in clinical practice.

As learning and comprehension progress, the simulation curriculum is designed to incorporate scenarios that include content to stimulate the development of critical thinking skills. Scenarios with added complexity allow for the reinforcement and continued development of the basic skills that were initially highlighted. Each scenario is designed to expand clinical knowledge, reinforce utilization of structured communication tools, and encourage use of appropriate chains of command. Simulation allows for multiple opportunities for practicing communication and helps to ensure clear and concise transmission of information [9].

In addition to foundational knowledge, Zone 1 simulation scenarios progress in complexity to include resuscitation events. Advanced scenarios provide an opportunity for nurses to explore all aspects of managing emergency events while practicing in each role associated with resuscitation as supported by Pediatric Advanced Life Support (PALS) training (Table 24.2) [10]. By utilizing clinical pauses, both faculty and participants may intentionally halt the progression of scenarios to ask questions and elicit further clarification of technical aspects of the crisis, critical language, and nursing roles.

Beyond exploring the roles in a code, simulation allows for discussion related to specific pathophysiology that may precipitate emergency situations, along with common conditions that may occur while patients are on ECMO or are actively weaning from mechanical circulatory support. Scenario development focuses on specific conditions, which may include (1) hypovolemia, (2) coagulopathy, (3) cardiac arrhythmias, and (4) issues related to systemic and pulmonary vascular resistance. Understanding the physiology of these various states promotes early recognition of clinical changes or impending deterioration, as well as identification of ECMO-related emergencies requiring prompt treatment.

Zone 2 Acute Situational Instruction

Participation in Zone 2 simulation is enhanced by prior, multiple exposures to Zone 1 training. Transition into Zone 2 high-fidelity simulation occurs once learners have demon-

Table 24.2 Pediatric Advanced Life Support (PALS) recommended roles in a code

Team leader	Required for every resuscitation Assigns roles of team members Makes treatment decisions Provides feedback to the rest of the team as indicated
Compressor	Assesses patient Performs five rounds of compressions Alternates with clinician in charge of defibrillator every five cycles or 2 minutes (and earlier with signs of compressor fatigue)
Monitor/ defibrillator	Ensures availability and operation of defibrillator Alternates with compressor Ensures visibility of monitor for the team leader and team
Airway	Opens airway Provides bag-mask ventilation Inserts airway adjuncts as indicated
IV/IO medication	Initiates intravenous (IV)/intraosseous (IO) access Administers medications
Recorder	Records time of interventions and medications and announces when next emergency medications are due as indicated Records frequency and duration of interruptions in compressions Communicates issues to team leader (and the rest of the team)

Adapted from PALS [10]

strated comfort and confidence with the prerequisite material. Zone 2 training includes the introduction of staff from other disciplines to participate in mock codes with groups of nurses. Nurse practitioners, physicians, and respiratory therapists, in addition to other clinicians, all complement team training. Zone 2 scenarios continue to have increased complexity beyond Zone 1. They are allowed to proceed uninterrupted from inception to completion and incorporate formal debriefings to aid in reflection and acquisition of knowledge and skills. Crisis resource management (CRM) team concepts, including role clarity, personnel support, communication, global assessment, and resource utilization, are explored further in this zone [11]. Communication skills that were acquired in previous zones are practiced further with interdisciplinary team members, allowing nurses to develop strategies to manage the authority gradient.

A Zone 2 scenario might include a patient who decompensates quickly, requiring nurses to rapidly perform an assessment and notify the other members of the team. During these events, more distractions, such as inclusion of audible alarms and rapid changes in vital signs, add to the complexity and urgency of the scenario. Bedside nurses are required to activate an emergency response and provide succinct summaries to providers from other disciplines utilizing structured communication tools, as practiced in Zone 1 training. Scenarios may rapidly progress to include cardiac arrest; these events require delineation of nursing roles and completion of specified tasks while communicating with an event manager. Examples of specific nursing responsibilities are outlined in Table 24.3 under "nursing roles." During Zone 2 simulation, trainees are required to perform basic skills learned in previous zones, though during a more complex and potentially stressful situation, such as a patient who requires activation of ECMO deployment in the setting of a clinical deterioration. Events may conclude with clinical hand-off of pertinent information by nurses to medical and surgical team members called to perform cannulation. Structured debriefings follow each scenario and progress through phases: (1) exploration of reactions; (2) review of pertinent medical data and differential diagnosis; (3) understanding phase, which includes discussion of positive aspects of team function along with strategies for improvement; and (4) summary [12].

Educational curricula for nurses that include high-technology simulation may significantly augment learning experiences by enhancing the realism of the training environment [13]. Novice nurses benefit from being able to practice skills in a safe environment before performing them on actual patients. Studies have shown a positive correlation between participation in high- technology simulation and improvements in knowledge development and confidence of new nurses [9, 12, 14, 15].

ECMO-Specific Prerequisite Training

A focused curriculum to manage ECMO cannulation during cardio-pulmonary resuscitation (ECPR) events, ECMO-related emergencies, and general care of patients on mechanical circulatory support occurs once a structured orientation with SimZones training is complete. Nurses who have demonstrated competence with general cardiac intensive care knowledge and skills acquisition are required to participate in more advanced training. Orientation to ECMO is typically provided away from the clinical area and includes multiple aspects, including an overview of the circuit and its components, indications for both veno-venous (VV) and veno-arterial (VA) support, and institution-specific equipment. Didactic lectures often address the care and management of ECMO patients, including a review of potential complications and strategies to optimize outcomes, including adherence to anticoagulation protocols and other specific policies and guidelines. Interdisciplinary faculty members, including a seasoned ECMO specialist and an experienced nurse, provide pertinent information for care and management and promote various aspects of team communication that are essential in caring for patients on mechanical circulatory support [16].

Next, the nurses will complete several precepted shifts at the bedside of an ECMO patient along with an experienced ECMO-trained nurse. During this time, nursing preceptees must complete various items on a competency-based check

Table 24.3 Nursing roles for ECPR

Charge nurse	Nursing roles	Operating room nurses

Assists event manager
Assigns parent facilitator prn
Delegates calls/pages for:
  Attending surgeon and other surgical personnel
  Blood bank
  Operating room personnel
  Support staff
Organizes nursing team roles:
  Bedside nurse
  Emergency cart
  Documentation
  Defibrillator management
  Compressions
  Equipment/resource management/ mobilization
Crowd and environment control
Family notification
	Bedside nurse
	  Calls for help early/call code prn
	  Initiates CPR
	  Identifies open access and administers medications
	  Assists with patient preparation for cannulation
	  Attaches pacing wires to pacemaker and ensures pacemaker is accessible as applicable
	Emergency cart nurse(s)
	  Prepares medications
	  Prepares medication tubing for access under sterile drapes prn
	Compressor(s) as indicated
	Defibrillator management
	Documentation
	  Medications
	  Interventions
	  Interruptions to CPR
	  Time-outs
	Mobilizing and assisting other equipment and resources
	  Blood products
	  Mediastinal cart
	  Cannula cart
	  Bovie and equipment
	  Surgical loops
	  Antibiotic/chest irrigation solutions
	Parent facilitator
		Scrub and circulating nurses as indicated
		Preparation of patient for cannulation
		  Position patient and ensure surgical field lighting
		  Surgical preparation
		  Bovie pads/defibrillator pads prn
		  Sterile drapes
		  Facilitate appropriate team surgical attire
		Mediastinal cart management
		  Sterile field and equipment
		  Monitor sterile solutions
		  Ensure correct counts (needles, sponges, etc.)
		  Maintain perioperative safety (cautery, fire risk, sterility)
		  Monitor temperature of solutions on field

Table 24.4 Nursing ECMO competency outline

ECMO nursing competency check list
Locates resources
Identifies differences between VA versus VV ECMO
Describes major differences between centrifugal and roller pumps (as appropriate)
Identifies components of ECMO circuit and describes function
Describes pre-cannulation management
Describes nursing roles during cannulation
Identifies sites for cannulation
Identifies need for post-cannulation chest x-ray and specific laboratory studies
Identifies key aspects of care for patients on ECMO utilizing a systems approach
Neurologic
Cardiac
Respiratory
Hemostasis and coagulation
Fluid and nutrition management
Infection
Analgesia and sedation
Integument and mobility
Identifies key aspects of psychosocial care
Family
Interdisciplinary team involvement
Identifies key aspects of decannulation
Patient readiness
Anticipates need for:
Increased vasoactive support
Increased mechanical ventilation
Analgesia, sedation, and pharmacological paralysis
Anticoagulation management plan
Specific tests and laboratory assessments
Describes ECMO-related emergencies and management strategies

list, including identification of safety issues, indications for support, as well as basic ECMO care and management strategies (Table 24.4).After the completion of these competencies during precepted shifts, nurses progress to Zone 3 ECMO training.

Zone 3 Team and Systems Development Training

Zone 3 simulations involve additional clinicians from the clinical environment, including bedside nurses, charge nurses, operating room personnel, intensive care unit physicians, cardiac surgeons, and ECMO therapists, in specialized team training. For example, the native team might be asked to manage an ECPR event or another ECMO-related emergency during these simulation sessions. Team simulation training allows for practice and assessment of cognitive, technical, and behavioral skills required for optimal care delivery to patients on ECMO [16]. High-technology simulation enhances team training by engaging participants in realistic situations, utilizing functional equipment in familiar settings. This method has been shown to increase participant knowledge and confidence in managing ECMO-related events [17]. In situ training in the cardiac intensive care unit further promotes realism and assists with exposing latent safety threats in the clinical environment [12]. While didactic lectures, bedside orientation, and simulation are critical constituents of ECMO training [16], individual ECMO centers may have institution-specific practices for enhancing the effectiveness of team training during simulation sessions. One strategy may include beginning the simulation with introductions and an "ice breaker" activity, followed by a game that encourages participants to identify critical principles of crisis resource management (CRM) training [12]. Participants may be asked to share details about a situation that involved an ECMO-related event or crisis as a means of discussing and further exploring aspects of CRM principles. Expert instructors may provide a brief, formal didactic review of critical aspects of ECMO care and how these may relate to team function. An overview specifically addresses expectations of nursing roles, and roles of other disciplines, during cannulation and for ECMO-related emergencies. Please see Chap. 10 for further details on interprofessional education and training.

Studies have shown a positive correlation between ECMO simulation training and efficiency of team response [18, 19]. DiNardo and colleagues associated high-technology ECMO simulation training with improved teamwork and behavioral skills, along with decreased time to effective implementation of interventions [19]. ECMO team simulation training exercises were noted to significantly reduce time to cannulation in the clinical setting with actual patients [18]. ECMO training with the interdisciplinary team integrates cognitive, behavioral, and technical aspects of care. In this setting, effective communication and role clarity for all participants are highlighted.

Unique aspects of communication for ECMO care include calling for help early. Bedside nurses may be among the first clinicians to recognize a problem and are required to alert the appropriate disciplines of a crisis or an evolving problem as practiced in prior SimZones training. Rapidly calling for help and activating a "code" if required are key components of the communication process. Managing an ECPR event or ECMO-related crisis may present unique challenges, since many resources and additional personnel are often required for timely initiation of interventions. Depending upon the clinical environment and team composition, several roles are often specifically delegated to nursing staff. Nurses are crucial to ensure that systems and processes are in place so that an event manager may focus on clinical decision-making and resuscitation management. A designated member of the team, often the charge nurse, may assist the event manager by delegating certain activities, including communicating the need for additional assistance (e.g., notification of the blood bank for rapid product set-up, requesting presence of the attending cardiac surgeon and operating room personnel as indicated for an urgent surgical procedure) via phone/pager, and assigning specific nursing roles and activities of support staff. A clinical nurse specialist or experienced nurse may also fill the role of assisting the event manager in place of a charge nurse (see Table 24.3).

Optimal management of any crisis event, including rapid deployment of ECMO, requires the appropriate trained staff and resources. Nurses are key members of the team; their experience and expertise are critical for successful patient outcomes [20]. The Extracorporeal Life Support Organization (ELSO) describes several distinct nursing roles for rapid deployment. These include (1) the bedside nurse, (2) nurses at the emergency cart, (3) preparation of the patient for cannulation, (4) performance of chest compressions with other members of the team, (5) documentation of the event with monitoring of compressions, and (6) defibrillator management [21]. There is minimal evidence-based data defining specific nursing roles during ECPR and ECMO-related emergencies. Table 24.3 describes proposed responsibilities specific to charge, bedside, crisis assistance, surgical scrub, and circulating nursing roles. In the absence of operating room personnel, or during "off hours", nurses in the critical care environment may need to take on tasks and responsibilities of traditional surgical nurses. Ideally as many as six to eight nurses may be needed to fill essential nursing roles during rapid deployment of ECMO.

As in Zone 2, a structured debriefing in distinct phases (reactions, medicine, understanding with strategies for improvement, and summary) follows the initial ECPR simulation scenario. Experienced faculty often explores any existing barriers to effective communication, such as vocalizing concerns and managing the authority gradient, as well as issues related to role clarity for all team members.

In addition to an emergent cannulation scenario, team members are required to manage ECMO-related emergencies, such as pump or oxygenator failure, air entrainment, or cannula dislodgement, during simulation. These scenarios allow participants to practice rapid assessment of specific problems and intervene promptly in a safe learning environment prior to caring for actual patients. ECMO training activities incorporating interprofessional simulation have been shown to improve both knowledge and confidence in intervening with ECMO-related events [17].

Zone 4 Real-Life Debriefing and Development

After completion of nursing orientation with SimZones and advanced ECMO training, nurses may care for actual patients on mechanical circulatory support. They are expected to utilize the appropriate resources in the critical care environment with adherence to ECMO-related protocols and guidelines and to contact experienced clinicians, including nurses, ECMO therapists, and other team members, for questions or concerns. Following their training, nurses are prepared to anticipate problems and participate effectively as a part of the team during ECMO-related crisis events.

During Zone 4, structured team debriefings are performed after actual crisis events in the clinical environment involving patients who require ECPR or develop ECMO-related emergencies [3]. Debriefings emphasize aspects of events that went well and explore individual performance, interdisciplinary team processes, and systems issues that may require strategies for improvement [22]. "Hot" debriefings occur immediately following a crisis or resuscitation, involve all members of the team who were present, and are facilitated by one of the team members, which may include the event manager or charge nurse [23]. Nurse documenters, who have received training in debriefing methodology or utilization of debriefing tools, may be well-positioned to lead or co-facilitate debriefings, since they are able share specific information on timing and actions [21]. "Cold" debriefings occur within days or weeks of the event and may include both team members who participated in events and others who were not present at the time [23]. Structured debriefings after resuscitation or emergent events have been found to provide unique educational experiences for interdisciplinary team members and to be useful in improving care processes [22, 23].

Please refer to Table 24.5 for typical timeline for progression through SimZones.

Ongoing Education

Continuing education is an important aspect of ensuring safe ECMO care practices over the long-term [16]. Ongoing ECMO training is a necessary component of any ECMO program, regardless of center volume [16]. Educational activities for nurses, including team training with simulation, should be provided on a continuing basis and may include annual competency review. Procedures and guidelines should be refined as necessary [24], and training guidelines established by ELSO should serve as a reference tool for all centers providing ECMO support [16].

Table 24.5 Timeline and topics for nursing simulation curriculum utilizing SimZones

Simulation session topic and SimZone	Learning objectives for session	Scenario	Timeline in orientation	Timeline post-orientation

#1
Airway skills
SimZone1
	Shift change safety check
	Chain of command
	Structured communication
	Airway assessment
	Skills practice station
	Bag-mask ventilation
	Hand ventilation
	Suctioning endotracheal tube (ETT)
	  In-line
	  Open suction
	  High risk suction guidelines
	Discussion of extubation check list
	Discussion of intubation check list
		Extubation and intubation scenario
		Postoperative right ventricular outflow obstruction resection who is ready for extubation; if extubation fails, reintubation is required
			Week 1–2	N/A

#2 Ventilation strategies SimZone1	Shift change safety check Chain of command Structured communication Identification and treatment of pulmonary artery hypertension (PAH)	Advanced ventilation scenario Postoperative complete atrio-ventricular canal repair with episode of PAH	Week 3–4	N/A
#3 Admitting a postoperative cardiac case SimZone1	Admission safety check Chain of command Structured communication Preparation to receive postoperative cardiac admission Participation in structured sign-out Admission of patient	Receiving a postoperative admission Postoperative aortic coarctation repair with hypertension requiring initiation of antihypertensive infusion	Week 5–6	N/A

#4
Arrhythmias
SimZone1
	Shift change safety check
	Chain of command
	Structured communication
	Skills practice station
	  Rhythm identification
	  Hands-on synchronized cardioversion and defibrillation
	Identification and diagnosis of arrhythmias
	Demonstration of atrial-wire tracing
	Administration of adenosine
		Arrhythmia: supraventricular tachycardia (SVT)
		Postoperative ventricular septal defect (VSD) repair
		awaiting transfer to ward with acute onset of SVT
			Week 6–7	N/A

(continued)

Table 24.5 (continued)

Simulation session topic and SimZone	Learning objectives for session	Scenario	Timeline in orientation	Timeline post-orientation
#5 Roles in a code SimZone1	Shift change safety check Chain of command Structured communication Identification of impending cardiac arrest Review of policy and procedure for intracardiac line removal Recognition of cardiac tamponade and preparation for treatment	Left atrial (LA) line removal: Cardiac tamponade Postoperative arterial switch operation (ASO) de- intensifying requiring LA line removal with subsequent cardiac tamponade	Week 7–8	N/A
#6 Synthesis SimZone2	Shift change safety check Chain of command Structured communication Demonstration of crisis resource management (CRM) principles Identification of postoperative stage I Norwood physiology and potential complications Calculation and administration of appropriate code medications	Postoperative stage I Norwood with acute shunt thrombosis Postoperative stage I Norwood with acute shunt thrombosis requiring CPR and chest procedure	Week 10–12	N/A
CRM training SimZone3	Utilizing CRM principles with interdisciplinary team training Role clarity Communication Resources Personnel support Global assessment	ECMO CRM Two scenarios #1 Neonate admitted with suspected viral myocarditis anticipating emergent ECMO cannulation (ECPR event) #2 Same patient with an ECMO-related emergency (pump or oxygenator failure, air entrainment, or cannula dislodgement)	N/A	≥ 12 months
Real-life event SimZone4	Utilization of CRM principles during interdisciplinary team debriefing after an ECMO-related emergency Role clarity Communication Resources Personnel support Global assessment Debrief What went well Areas for improvement Solutions	N/A	N/A	N/A

Conclusion

Nurses who care for patients on ECMO must be knowledgeable and proficient in foundational critical care practices prior to caring for this critically ill subset of patients. An orientation that incorporates simulation opportunities throughout the training process in a deliberate manner adheres to adult educational principles, promotes retention of knowledge, improves team function, and fosters clinician confidence. SimZones training provides a longitudinal approach using a structured format for nurses to develop knowledge and competence in order to care for patients requiring mechanical circulatory support as part of the interdisciplinary team [3]. Ongoing educational activities with simulation are an integral part of the ECMO educational curriculum for critical care nurses and all members of the team.

References

1. McLeodS. Kolb-learning styles: learning styles. Available from: //www.simplypsychology.org/learning-kolb.html.
2. Johnston L, Williams SB, Ades A. Education for ECMO providers: using education science to bridge the gap between clinical and educational expertise. SeminPerinatol. 2018;42:138–46.
3. RoussinCJ, Weinstock P. SimZones: an organizational innovation for simulation programs and centers. Acad Med. 2017;92(8):1114–20.
4. RudolfJW, Simon R, Rivard P, Dufresne RL, Raemer DB. Debriefing with good judgement: combining rigorous feedback with genuine inquiry. AnesthesiolClin. 2007;25:361–76.
5. Morrison T, Heard ML. Staffing for the ECMO patient. In: Brogan TV, Annich G, Ellis WC, Haney B, Heard ML, Larusso R, editors. ECMO specialist training manual. 4th ed. Michigan: ELSO; 2018. p. 259.
6. OPENPediatrics [internet]. Boston: Pediatric cardiac intensive care nursing curriculum; 2015. Available from:https://www.openpediatrics.org.

7. Müller M, Jürgens J, Redaèlli M, Clingberg K, Hautz WE, Stock S. Impact of the communication in patient hand-off tool SBAR on patient safety: a systematic review. BMJ. 2018;8:1–10.
8. El-Shafy IA, Delgado J, Akerman M, Bullaro F, Christopherson NAM, Prince JM. Closed-loop communication improves task completion in pediatric trauma resuscitation. J SurgEduc. 2018;75(1):58–64.
9. Campbell JM. Education and simulation training of pediatric intensive care unit nurses to care for open heart surgery patients. CCN. 2015;35(3):76–81.
10. American Heart Association, Academy of Pediatrics. Effective resuscitation team dynamics. USA: Pediatric advanced life support; 2016. 110 p.
11. Allan CK, Weinstock P. Simulation-based training to enhance patient safety in pediatric cardiovascular care. In: Barach PR, Jacobs JP, Laussen PC, Lipshultz SE, editors. Pediatric and congenital cardiac disease: outcomes analysis, quality improvement, and patient safety. 2nd ed. London: Springer-Verlag; 2015. p. 425–39.
12. Allan CK, Thiagarajan RR, Beke D, Imprescia A, Kappus LJ, Garden A, Hayes G, Laussen PC, Bacha E, Weinstock PH. Simulation-based training delivered directly to the pediatric intensive care unit engenders preparedness, comfort, and decreased anxiety among multidisciplinary resuscitation teams. J Thorac CardiacSurg. 2010;140(3):646–52.
13. Raffaeli G, Ghirardello S, Vanzati M, Baracetti C, Canesi F, Conigliaro F, et al. Start a neonatal extracorporeal membrane oxygenation program: a multistep training. Pediatrics. 2018;6(151):1–9.
14. Boling B, Hardin-Pierce M, Jensen L, Hassan Z. Evaluation of a high-fidelity simulation training program for new cardiothoracic intensive care unit nurses. SeminThorac Card Surg. 2016;28(4):770–5.
15. Banfi C, Bendjelid K, Giraud R. High-fidelity simulation for extra corporeal oxygenation training, utile or futile? J Thorac Dis. 2017;9(11):4282–5.
16. Ogino MT, Froehlich CD, Moore EA. Education and training. In: Brogan TV, Lequier L, Lorusso R, MacLaren G, Peek G, editors. Extracorporeal life support: the ELSO redbook. 5th ed. Michigan: ELSO; 2017. p. 747–61.
17. Brum R, Rajani R, Gelandt E, Morgan L, Raguseelan N, Butt S, Nelmes D, Auzinger G, Broughton S. Simulation training for extracorporeal membrane oxygenation. Ann Card Anaesth. 2015;18(2):185–90.
18. Su L, Spaeder MC, Jones MB, Sinha P, Nath DS, Jain PN, Berger JT, Williams L, Shankar V. Implementation of an extracorporeal cardiopulmonary resuscitation simulation program reduces extracorporeal cardiopulmonary resuscitation times in realpatients. PCCM. 2014;15(9):856–60.
19. DiNardo M, David P, Stoppa F, Lorusso R, Raponi M, Amodeo A, Cecchetti C, Gunner Y, Taccone FS. The introduction of a high-fidelity program for training pediatric critical care personnel reduces the time to manage extracorporeal oxygenation emergencies and improves teamwork. J Thorac Dis. 2018;10(6): 3409–17.
20. Gaies MG, Clarke NS, Donohue JE, Gurney JG, Charpie JR, Hirsch JC. Personnel and unit factors impacting outcomes after cardiac arrest in a dedicated pediatric cardiac intensive care unit. PediatrCrit Care Med. 2012;13(5):583–8.
21. Jones MB, Heichel J, Beke DM. Nursing management of neonates and children with cardiovascular disease on ECLS. In: Brogan TV, Lequier L, Lorusso R, MacLaren G, Peek G, editors. Extracorporeal life support: the ELSO redbook. 5th ed. Michigan: ELSO; 2017. p. 379–84.
22. Kessler DO, Cheng A, Mullan PC. Debriefing in the emergency department after clinical events: a practical guide. Ann Emerg Med. 2015;65(6):690–7.
23. Couper K, Perkins GD. Debriefing after resuscitation. Crit Care. 2013;19(3):188–94.
24. Blum JM, Beca J, Ochiai R. Centralization and regionalization of ECLS resources. In: Brogan TV, Lequier L, Lorusso R, MacLaren G, Peek G, editors. Extracorporeal life support: the ELSO redbook. 5th ed. Michigan: ELSO; 2017. p. 741–5.

ECMO Simulation in the Adult Population – Proning, Awakening and Breathing Trials, and Mobilization

25

Bhavesh M. Patel, Rys Chapple, Simmie Kalan, Amelia A. Lowell, Amanda Key, Hannelisa E. Callisen, Cory M. Alwardt, Hussein D. Kanji, and Ayan Sen

Abbreviations

ECLS	Extracorporeal life support
ECMO	Extracorporeal membrane oxygenation

Learning Objectives

- The reader will understand basic physiology of adult prone positioning and mobilization while on ECMO.
- The reader will understand a method for simulation of prone positioning on ECMO.
- The reader will understand a method for simulation of emerging from sedation and mobilization on ECMO.
- The reader can list the potential simulation crisis events occurring during proning and mobilization.

Electronic Supplementary Material The online version of this chapter (https://doi.org/10.1007/978-3-030-53844-6_25) contains supplementary material, which is available to authorized users.

B. M. Patel (✉) · A. A. Lowell · H. E. Callisen · A. Sen
Department of Critical Care Medicine, Mayo Clinic College of Medicine, Mayo Clinic, Phoenix, AZ, USA
e-mail: Patel.bhavesh@mayo.edu

R. Chapple · S. Kalan
Vancouver General Hospital, Intensive Care Unit, Vancouver, BC, Canada

A. Key
Department of Nursing, Intensive Care Unit, Mayo Clinic, Phoenix, AZ, USA

C. M. Alwardt
Department of Critical Care Medicine, Mayo Clinic College of Medicine, Mayo Clinic, Phoenix, AZ, USA

Department of Surgery, Clinical Perfusion, Mayo Clinic, Phoenix, AZ, USA

H. D. Kanji
Department of Critical Care Medicine, Vancouver General Hospital, Vancouver, BC, Canada

Introduction

Compared to other extracorporeal life support (ECLS) populations, adult patients present unique challenges to the care team when considering proning and mobilization due to their size and weight. Despite possible risks, emerging literature supports the therapeutic benefit of proning and mobilization in adult ECLS [1–3]. Simulation-based interprofessional team training is well suited to practice the complex multiprofessional tasks required for routine proning, emergence from sedation, and mobilization of patients in addition to crisis event management during these interventions. Training with various simulation modalities provides opportunities for discovery of latent patient safety threats while allowing sequential skill development through real-time feedback and engagement in coordinated deliberate practice. Facilitation of these simulation events requires a clear understanding of relevant physiologic interactions, choreography of equipment and personnel, and knowledge of management strategies for rare but potentially catastrophic crisis events that are time-sensitive. In addition, simulation educators need to be prepared to facilitate the interactions of the interprofessional team in order to promote collaboration and leadership during crisis event rehearsal to ultimately help mitigate adverse events and optimize outcomes in this ECLS population [4, 5].

Overview of Prone Positioning (PP) and Mobilization on ECLS

Patients on ECLS are frequently totally dependent upon circuit function for critical oxygen delivery. The increased oxygen consumption created by proning, emerging from sedation, or mobilization may result in physiologic stress leading to inadequate global and/or regional oxygen delivery resulting in end-organ injury. This is a dynamic process dependent upon five major factors: metabolic demands, native cardiac

L. C. Johnston, L. Su (eds.), *Comprehensive Healthcare Simulation: ECMO Simulation*, Comprehensive Healthcare Simulation,
https://doi.org/10.1007/978-3-030-53844-6_25

function, native pulmonary function, blood oxygen carrying capacity (hemoglobin), and ECLS function.

Prone Positioning (PP) for Adult Respiratory Distress Syndrome (ARDS)

Prone positioning (PP), when a patient lays on their sternum and abdomen [6] (Fig. 25.1), has been used to improve oxygenation in severe ARDS since the 1970s and, in recent years, has been proven to improve mortality in randomized controlled trials [7–9]. PP decreases posterior lung compression caused by the heart and diaphragm and increases posterior pulmonary recruitment while homogenizing ventilation and ventilation/perfusion ratio thus improving oxygenation and potentially decreasing ventilation pressures. It has also been shown to improve cardiac output, likely because venous return improves as the right atrium moves ventrally and pulmonary vascular resistance decreases from the relief of hypoxic vasoconstriction [10]. Combined with ECLS, PP has the potential to permit ultraprotective lung ventilation and possibly improve outcomes [11, 12]. This is not without risks and complications which include cannula, invasive tube, or line obstruction, malposition, or dislodgement, bleeding from cannulae or invasive line sites, cutaneous pressure ulcers, facial edema, corneal abrasions, and hemodynamic instability [13]. The three most concerning complications are bleeding from cannulation sites, endotracheal or thoracostomy tube obstruction and dislodgment, and hemodynamic instability during positioning [13].

Emerging from Sedation and Mobilization on ECLS

Preparing for and awakening the mechanically ventilated patient on ECMO for mobilization can present some challenges. The ABCDEF protocol, of which the letter "B" stands for "Both Spontaneous Awakening Trials (SAT) and Spontaneous Breathing Trials (SBT)," defines a process for evaluating patients to undergo a daily sedation interruption and spontaneous breathing trial [14] which are necessary preliminary steps prior to mobilization [15]. Only half of ECLS patients undergo sedation interruption; midazolam, propofol, and fentanyl are the most commonly utilized drugs [15]. Incorporating this "sedation-vacation" step into a pre-mobilization simulation scenario would help to highlight the interaction between spontaneous breathing, patient-ventilator dyssynchrony (PVD), and the ECMO circuit prior to engaging in the more complex interprofessional task of mobilization. In addition, it may identify perceived barriers to early mobilization and SAT [15].

Most often when patients are awakened, they experience some type of PVD. Patients on V-V ECMO for ARDS should be treated with low tidal volumes and low respiratory rates for lung protection which initially may require heavy sedation to be tolerated [16]. However, emerging from sedation often results in ventilator flow mismatch and unmet patient demand, seen as double triggering or "bucking the vent" when awake on an assisted mode with a set respiratory rate, flow rate, or inspiratory time [17, 18]. The potential for elevation in intrathoracic pressure to occur during PVD is high and can result in decreased venous return, increased ECMO inflow negative pressures, and decreased ECMO flow rates [19]. Additionally, if the patient's diaphragm has become weakened, they will be dyspneic and tachypneic when the work of breathing is transitioned back to them. The same issues often arise during more vigorous activity as the work of breathing increases. PVD can be simulated in the various phases of patient mobilization.

Engaging in mobilization of the critically ill confers many benefits including lower rates of delirium, more ventilator-free days, and improved functional status [20]. Early data on mobilization of patients on ECLS suggest that it occurs in 22% of patients and it is relatively safe; however, the data comes from centers with specialized and experienced teams

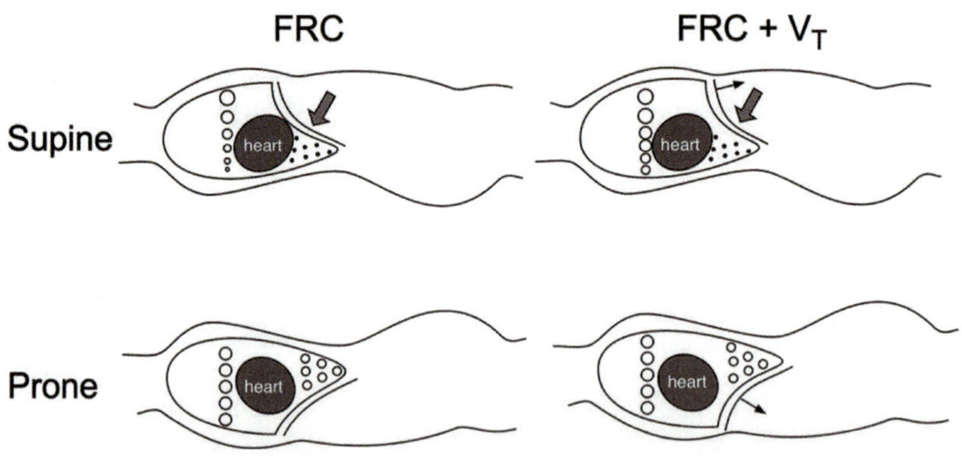

Fig. 25.1 Effect of prone positioning on lung compression and cannula location. (Modified with permission from Johnson NJ et al. [6])

[15, 21]. Future studies like ECMO-PT should provide direction in this area [22]. Estimating the patient's physiologic reserve and anticipating the increased metabolic demand generated by activity is critical to safe mobilization. Even basic patient care activities have been shown to increase oxygen consumption disproportionate to changes in vital signs [23] (Fig. 25.2). As such, adding physiologic stressors may challenge the steady state and put patients at risk for regional organ hypoperfusion and/or global hypoxia. Therefore, prior to mobilization, clinicians should specifically assess the oxygen demands. This can be achieved by assessing surrogate markers of end-organ perfusion, including biochemical markers such as lactate, and physical examination. The stability of this oxygen demand is important to understand the trajectory and stability of the patient. Second, there needs to be consideration of how dependent the patient is on ECMO flow and oxygen delivery from native (including lungs and cardiac output) versus extracorporeal support. There should be an acceptable buffer for both – the patient should not be completely dependent on the ECLS and should have some physiologic reserve to endure the physiologic challenges and transient interruptions of flow and oxygen delivery. Similarly, native cardiac output (of relatively deoxygenated blood) should not easily overwhelm ECLS flows in relation to oxygenation needs. Though there is no limit that can be prescribed, it is important to consider these physiologic states and how the demands induced by mobilization may influence or alter the steady state. Adjustments to flows, sweep, and vasopressors should be made prior to movement with these considerations in mind. During the movement or mobilization, further derangements can be anticipated and mitigated by applying this paradigm. It is important to also recognize that this is a dynamic process depending on metabolic demands and native cardiac function, pulmonary status, and ECLS support.

Simulation Design for Proning, SAT/SBT, and Mobilization on ECLS

Proning, SAT/SBT, and mobilization of adult ECLS patients can be divided into four common phases – pre-movement preparation, movement, post-movement recovery, and inter-movement quiescence. Ideally, each phase should be associated with a checklist of tasks to be performed by members of the interprofessional team. Each phase can also be complicated by a crisis event presenting as a clinical perturbation or "phenotype" in one of four categories: patient related, the ECMO pump or circuit related, other equipment related, or personnel related (Table 25.1). Simulations can be set up to sequentially transition a simu lated patient through all phases, either interrupted by

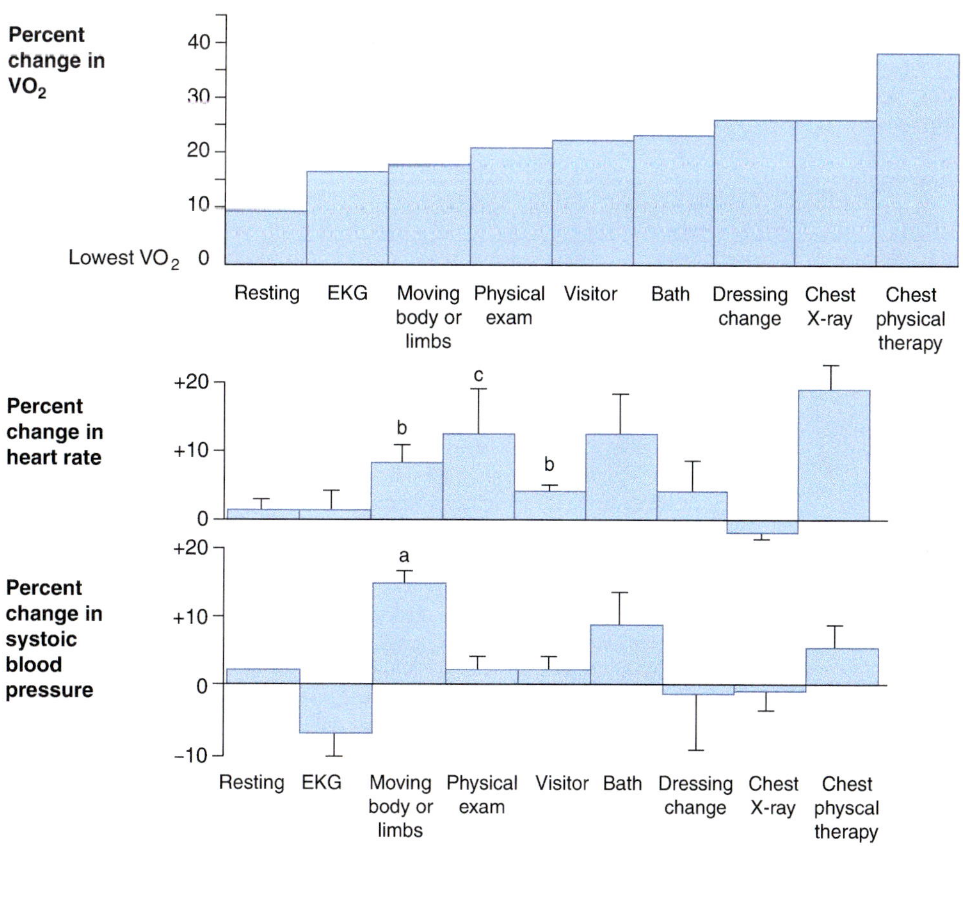

Fig. 25.2 Oxygen consumption and changes in heart rate and systolic blood pressure associated with routine patient care in the intensive care unit. (Modified with permission from Weisman [23])

Table 25.1 Crisis event monitoring and treatment

Crisis event "phenotype" [a]	Crisis event key action item	
Patient	*VV*	*VA*
Cardiac arrest	ACLS protocol should be followed with special attention to protect cannulae.	Maintain full VA support. Consider restoring ejection by increasing inotropic infusions. Consider decreasing afterload to the heart by decreasing flow if cardiac distention is the etiology. Monitor global perfusion and regional oxygen delivery.
Arrhythmia	ACLS algorithm should be followed for stable versus unstable rhythms.	Atrial tachyarrhythmias (atrial fibrillation, SVT) can often be managed with medications for rate control such as amiodarone. If atrial arrhythmia results in loss of effective atrial contractility and loss of native cardiac output, consider DC cardioversion. Ventricular tachycardia may require pharmacologic or electrical cardioversion if there are loss of native cardiac output and LV overdistention.
Hypotension	Hypotension may be managed from perspective of patient and circuit.	Increasing flow may help abate hypotension; however, the source of hypotension needs to be elucidated and fluid or vasoactive medications should be considered. Hypovolemia as a result of bleeding should be considered. With VA, there is systemic support, but in VV, the delivery of flow from the circuit is depending on the native cardiac function and thus there should be a heightened urgency to correct.
New limb ischemia		If limb ischemia is due to local compression or movement, then correction of limb position should be considered. If it is on the side of arterial cannula, a distal perfusion cannula should be considered. If persistent, CT angiogram imaging should be sought.
Fall	If a patient falls, check to assess if ECMO flow is maintained and airway is protected. The patient should be transferred back to bed and assessed for any physical damage from the fall. Imaging is needed to clear head trauma and peripheral damage.	
Decrease in SpO_2	Decrease in SpO_2 is expected but consideration of adequate global oxygen delivery should be considered. If there is hypoxemia, then supplementary oxygen should be considered on increasing FiO_2. If this is not successful, then mobilization should be stopped.	
Acute pain, agitation, delirium	Pain, agitation, and delirium should be managed adequately prior to mobilization. If incurred during mobilization, the activity should be stopped and this should be addressed, likely with the aid of pharmacotherapy. Use of medications will vary between the adult and pediatric population. No reported pediatric/neonatal centers report using propofol as the primary sedative, whereas more than a third of adult centers use this agent primarily (Marhong et al. 2017).	
Vomiting/aspiration	Portable suction to be taken if leaving the bedside.	
Device/ECMO related	*VV*	*VA*
Bleeding from cannula	If minor bleeding, it can often be supported with local compression. If ongoing or increasing bleeding, there is a need to explore the sites and consider holding anticoagulation.	
Cannula displacement/ dislodgement	Maximally ventilate/oxygenate patient with ventilator. Provide analgesia/sedative to prevent further malposition. Assess color and site of ECLS cannula/lines and patient vitals, specifically SpO_2 and SvO_2. Decreasing RPMs may help if cannula malposition is causing chatter or recirculation (VV). Stat X-ray. If displaced, you need to confirm position with radiography. Cease further mobilization should there be suspicion of dislodgement. If confirmed on radiography, then repositioning or alternative cannula strategy needs to be considered.	
Drop in flows	If flows drop, consider local cannula compression and assess integrity of flow. You may consider going up on flows providing that arterial pressures in the ECMO circuit remain in safe range. If low flows persist, then stop mobilization to diagnose the issue that may be challenging the flow.	
Change in venous oxygen saturation(SvO_2)	Increased SvO_2 is suggestive of recirculation. Check for cannulae malposition.	Drop in SvO_2 is expected but if it becomes critically low, consider stopping activity and plan alternative future activity to build up reserve.
Pump failure	Pump failure is a medical emergency and team should immediately stop activity. Reposition patient while simultaneously initiating hand crank protocol as well as attempting to diagnose the etiology of the pump failure. Initiate systemic support cardiopulmonary support.	
Gas failure	Gas failure needs to be immediately recognized and alternative gas source needs to be connected. The mobilization activity should be stopped and patient repositioned in bed.	
Air in circuit	Air in the circuit is a medical emergency. The patient needs to be repositioned in bed. The source of air needs to be immediately identified and emergency deairing protocols need to be instituted. Air in VA is more serious then VV.	

Table 25.1 (continued)

Crisis event "phenotype" [a]	Crisis event key action item	
Circuit line disconnecting or kinking	Disconnection is emergency. Kinking site must be located and unkinked.	
Line displacement, IV, central, chest tubes, feeding tube, and urinary catheter Disconnect of above lines	Discontinue therapy to address medical concern. Lines to be disconnected where possible prior to mobility commencing.	
Unplanned extubation	Emergency airway management	
Personnel	*VV*	*VA*
Limited number of staff	Modify task; if unable to mobilize out of the bed, consider bed mobility/ergometer (Figs. 25.3, 25.4, and 25.5).	
Poor team communication Poor leadership	PT will recommend how ECLS patients are to be mobilized; role and task clarification is to take place prior to mobility with clear goals of therapy session identified.	
Lack of training for staff on how to use equipment	In-service/training on equipment use to all providers.	
Lack of training/ experience mobilizing ECLS patients	Therapists should be ECLS trained with recommended use of a mobilization protocol.	

[a]To occur in context of proning, awakening, or mobilization simulation at instructor discretion

microdebriefs (expert feedback provided during the simulation [24]) or divided into individual phase-specific events. The fidelity of the simulation can be titrated in accordance with the scenario education objectives and learner skill level. For example, the use of high-fidelity simulators embedded in situ within the hospital context utilizing actual equipment and monitoring is ideal for advanced interprofessional teams and can be invaluable at uncovering latent safety threats within a hospital system while improving teamwork and communication [4].

It is important to have clearly articulated scenario objectives directed at tasks and processes of care based on local institutional procedural protocols and checklists. Appendix 25.1 provides an example of a proning protocol which defines the participant roles, tasks, and equipment required (provided courtesy of Vancouver Coastal Health). This can be compared to a proning simulation example template provided as Appendix 25.2. ECLS movement scenarios with multiple team members can be complicated to coordinate; therefore, we recommend starting with a basic clinical narrative and routine progression without a crisis event. This may be followed by a second scenario with a selected crisis event as in Appendix 25.2.

During the movement phase of proning or mobilization on ECLS, pulmonary interventions are frequently necessary. Table 25.2 provides a list of pulmonary interventions, precautions, and management/recommendation which may be included in the simulation.

As a learning team's technical and non-technical skills advance, more complex crisis events can be interjected into routine simulations of prone positioning or mobilization (progressing through SimZones [25] as described in Chap. 4). The crisis event "phenotype" and key action items can be selected from Table 25.1. The instructor can introduce one or more event phenotypes commonly experienced at the institution or rare catastrophic events, depending upon the learner needs. More advanced simulations could also include additional equipment or patient activities depending upon institutional availability such as special beds which verticalize (Fig. 25.3), percuss, vibrate, and partially rotate such as the Hill-Rom TotalCare SpO2RT®, or fully prone such as the ArjoHuntleigh RotoProne, mobilization equipment [26], or exercise and mobilization level and activities (Tables 25.3 and 25.4) [27].

High-performance interprofessional team functioning is especially necessary when mobilizing ECLS patients. The interprofessional team role assignments frequently consist of bedside nurse, a perfusionist/ECMO specialist, a respiratory therapist, and a physical therapist. A physician role should be assigned especially when crisis events are being simulated. The number of staff and choreography of the team will vary depending on the task simulated and whether the simulation involves movements out of the bed [28]. When simulation involves mobilizing away from the bedspace, additional six or more role assignments are necessary depending on cannula location, size of the patient, and room setup as demonstrated in Fig. 25.4.

Percutaneous single-lumen multistage cannulae locations in adult ECLS are typically located in the internal jugular vein (IJV) and femoral veins and artery and bicaval multilumen cannula in the right IJV [29–31]. Many cannulae configurations are possible to simulate including open chest central cannulation, but the selection chosen should be determined by training objectives. Additional patient selection

Table 25.2 Pulmonary and respiratory interventions and management recommendations. Reprinted with permission of Ref. [21]

Intervention	Precautions	Management/Recommendations
Positioning	Position of cannulae, risk of VQ mismatch, patient stability	Positions discussed with ECMO consultant and specialist nurse
Saline	Derecruitment	Instill via dosed suction port
Suction	Airway bleeding and derecruitment	Closed suction, monitoring of platelet level. ACT/APTT ratio
VHI and MHI	Maximum peak pressures should be agreed by ECMO MDT. Consider lung compliance and may not be appropriate if on ultra-protective ventilation (e.g. barotrauma) May not be appropriate with inadequate/unstable ECMO flows. In MHI a manometer should be used to a locally agreed pressure Avoid MHI if PEEP levels are >10 cm H_2O, VHI should be considered	Review lung compliance before commencing treatment Use VHI in patients with high PEEP or use PEEP valve in MHI circuit
Mechanical insufflation: Exsufflation	Consider king volume and compliance Risk of over distention and derecruitment	Review lung compliance before commencing treatment
Manual techniques	Consider cannulae position within vessels May not be appropriate with inadequate/unstable ECMO flows	Commence gentle manual techniques
Nebulisers	Consider appropriateness of breaking circuit and tidal volume for effectiveness of distribution	Discuss with ECMO consultant and specialist nurse Use in circuit nebuliser system
Physiotherapy-assisted flexible bronchoscopy	May not be appropriate with inadequate/unstable ECMO flows	Liaise with ECMO consultant or ICU consultant performing FOB
HFCWO	Arrhythmias, clotting, position of cannulae, wounds	Discuss with ECMO consultant and specialist nurse
Autogenic drainage/ACBT	Consider effect of raising intrathoracic pressure during treatment	Amend treatment plan if adverse changes to cardiovascular system
PEP	Consider lung volumes	Review lung compliance before commencing PEP
IPPB	Consider lung compliance	Review lung compliance before commencing IPPB
Nebulised DNAse	Airway bleeding	Discuss with ECMO consultant and specialist nurse

VQ ventilation-perfusion, *ACT/APTT* activated clotting time/activated partial thromboplastin time, *VHI* ventilator hyperinflation, *MHI* manual hyperinflation, *MDT* multi-disciplinary team, *PEEP* positive end-expiratory pressure, *ICU* intensive care unit, *FOB* fibreoptic bronchoscopy, *HFCWO* high frequency chest wall oscillation, *ACBT* active cycle of breathing techniques, *PEP* positive expiratory pressure, *IPPB* intermittent positive pressure breathing, *DNase* deoxyribonuclease

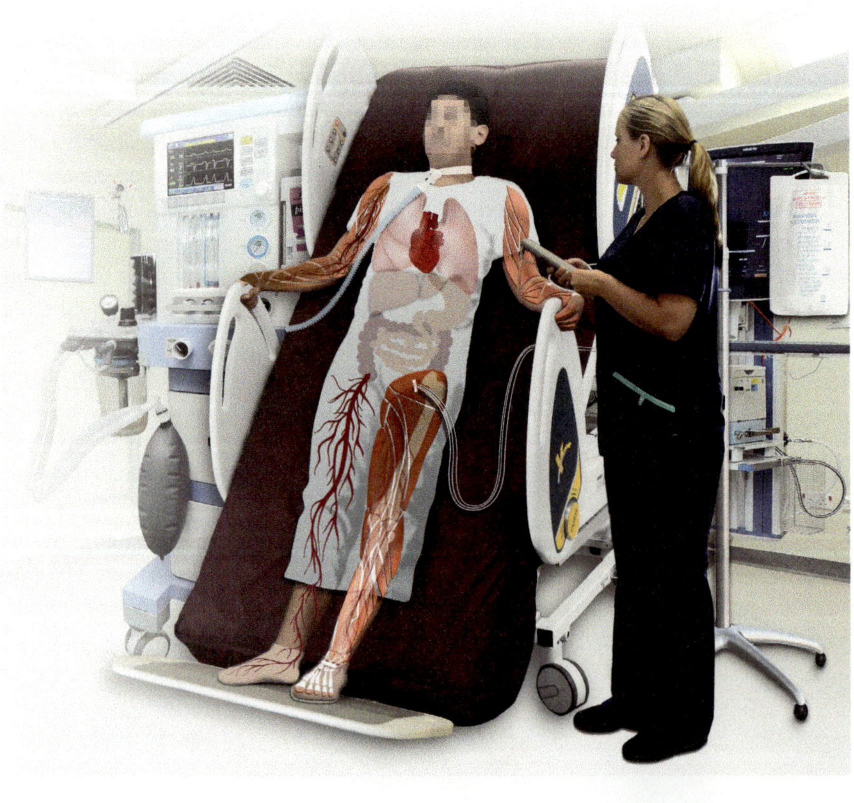

Fig. 25.3 Critical care specialty bed permits transition from supine to standing. Kreg Therapeutics Catalyst Critical Recovery Bed. (With permission from Kreg Therapeutics)

Table 25.3 Level of activity scoring with mobilization [25, 26]

PT level	Level of activity
1	No mobilization or passive range of motion of extremities
2	Turning in bed (including active-assisted range of motion of extremities)
3	Sitting in bed with the head of bed elevated
4	Sitting on the edge of the bed with feet on floor
5	Sitting in a chair
6	Standing
7	Marching in place
8	Ambulation

Table 25.4 Physical therapy interventions

Therapeutic exercises	Range of motion (passive or active), stretching and strengthening exercises, muscle endurance, breathing exercises
Bed mobility	Rolling, supine to sit transfer training, and bridging activities +/− cycling ergometer (Fig. 25.5)
Edge of bed activities	Sitting balance, posture, pre-standing activities, breathing, and coughing
Sit to stand transfer activities	Sit to standing transfers and functional strengthening using sit to stand from the bed or chair
Stand pivot transfers	Patient completing pivot or taking small steps from the bed or chair with purpose to transfer to another surface
Standing activities	Standing balance and tolerance, strengthening, preambulation activities such as weight shifting, marching, and stepping in place +/− tilt table (Fig. 25.4)
Ambulation	Gait training, gait speed, and ambulation tolerance +/− treadmill at the bedside

Adapted from Wells. et al. [3]

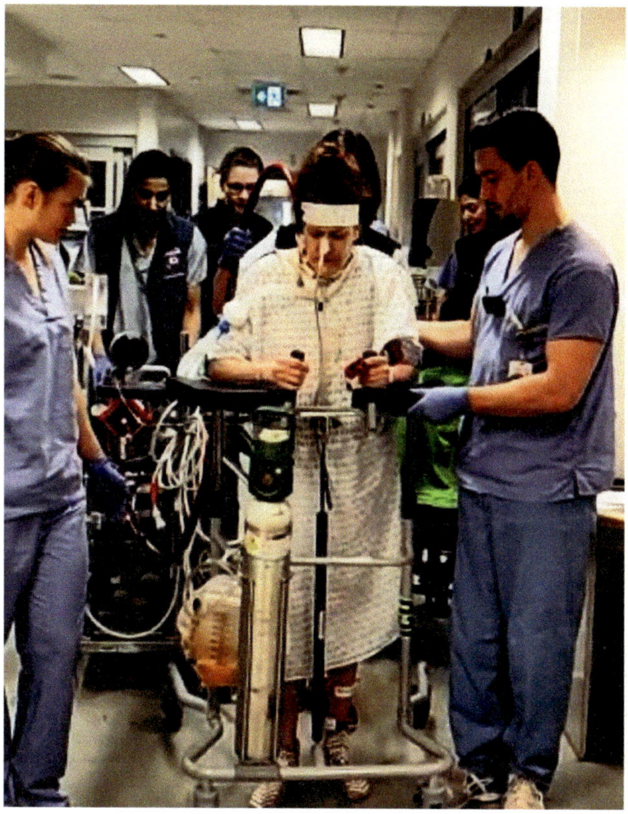

Fig. 25.4 VV ECMO ambulation team:
Roles from front row right to left: Physical therapy, patient, nurse
Role from second row right to left: Perfusionist, nurse behind patient, nurse
Role from back right: Respiratory therapist

criteria should be determined by local institutional criteria. Typical selection criteria and contraindications for proning and mobilization are listed in Table 25.5.

Simulation debriefing templates that include feedback on technical tasks and non-technical skills may be augmented by video debriefing especially when sequencing and details of movement choreography are of interest. Interprofessional collaborative team training principles discussed in other chapters are particularly applicable here with an emphasis on role assignment, communication, coordination, and situational monitoring during patient movement phases. Simulation instructor checklists can be tabular (Table 25.6) or graphical (Fig. 25.5) and can be used to observe for key action items while proning a patient or manikin.

The proning simulation example artifacts include a pre-reading proning protocol (Appendix 25.1), proning simulation (Appendix 25.2), and observers' checklists (Table 25.6 and Fig. 25.5). Key components of an ECLS mobilization simulation are provided in Appendix 25.3 (see also Video 25.1).

Conclusion

Spontaneous awakening/breathing trials, mobilization, and proning of adult ECLS patients, while safe and feasible, are not without risks and require a skilled interprofessional team with knowledge of and attention to various potential therapeutic interactions. Simulation is well suited to meet the training challenges posed by these important and complex tasks.

Table 25.5 SAFER HD (<u>S</u>ecure tubes, <u>A</u>nticoagulation, <u>F</u>iO_2, <u>E</u>KG stable, <u>R</u>ASS, <u>HD</u> hemodynamics) selection criteria

Proning	Mobilization/ambulation
Patient factors	
Contraindications: Intracranial pressure >30 mmHg Massive hemoptysis requiring an immediate procedure Serious facial trauma or facial surgery Cardiac pacemaker inserted in the last 2 days Unstable spine, femur, or pelvic fractures Mean arterial pressure (MAP) < 65 mmHg Pregnant women Single anterior chest tube with air leaks Open abdomen Abdominal compartment syndrome	RASS −1 to +1, awake, cooperative, adequate strength Cardiac stability: HR 50–140 bpm No serious arrhythmias or MI in past 48 hrs Hemodynamic stability SBP 80–180 mmHg MAP > 65 mmHg Low-dose inotropes or vasopressors, stable trend No significant bleeding past 24 hours Plt > 50, INR < 3 Respiratory stability – with stable mechanical ventilator settings Resting FiO_2 < 60% PaO_2 > 60 mmHg PaCO_2 < 80 mmHg pH > 7.30 RR < 30 bpm No other factors Anxiety, vomiting, uncontrolled diarrhea, delirium
ECLS factors	
Contraindications: Active uncontrolled bleeding from cannulation site Inadequate blood flow with cannula site compression	Blood flow 2–5 liters per minute with adequate oxygen delivery per attending physician Gas sweep 0–10 (CO_2 elimination) Activated clotting time levels 160–180 seconds Stable for past 24 hours For femorally cannulated patients: Inability to tolerate transient loss of flow with hip flexion

RASS Richmond Agitation-Sedation Scale, *MAP* mean arterial pressure, *Plt* platelets, *INR* international normalized ratio, *FiO_2* fraction of inspired oxygen, *mmHg* millimeters of mercury, *RR* respiratory rate, *bpm* breaths per minute

Table 25.6 Pre-proning, proning, and supinating Vancouver Coastal Health checklists

Steps	*Complete*
1. Perform hand hygiene & don PPE	
2. RT to:	
(a) Ensure artificial airway position is verified with recent chest X-ray.	
(b) Artificial airway is in situ and firmly secured. Consider using twill ties or low-profile securing device to prevent pressure injury to face/cheeks.	
(c) Ventilator tubing is positioned on side of the mouth furthest from ventilator.	
(d) Emergency airway equipment is at the head of the bed. Consider intubation box at bedside or additional personnel readily available if known difficult airway.	
3. RN to:	
(a) Assess feeding tube – consider post-pyloric.	
(b) Assess lines: Flush and lock any unused lines as per protocol; ensure adequate length. Reposition all lines and tubes that are located above the patient's waist straight upward toward the head of the bed. Reposition all chest tubes as well as lines and tubes that are located below the waist (e.g., bladder catheter, femoral lines, and fecal drainage systems) straight down toward the foot of the bed. Relocate all drainage bags on opposite side of the bed. BE SURE to cross the lines from this drainage bags under the patient and not across their front.	

Table 25.6 (continued)

Steps	*Complete*
4. RN to provide all *anterior body care* if patient is *supine* and all *posterior body care* if *prone*:	
(a) Change any wound dressings, empty ileostomy/colostomy bags, etc.	
(b) Identify areas for potential skin breakdown.	
(c) Wash face and apply barrier cream.	
(d) Perform eye care. Lubricate eyes and close eyes.	
(e) Suction and perform mouth care.	
(f) Ensure tongue is inside patient's mouth; if swollen and/or protruding, monitor it closely.	
(g) Remove patient gown.	
5. Perfusion to:	
(a) Check if cannulae are secure.	
(b) Cannulation sites are clean, with minimal signs of bleeding. Reinforce if needed.	
(c) Tubing length provides enough slack for safe transfer.	
(d) ECLS therapy settings are optimized during procedure.	
(e) Cannula tubings are positioned alongside patient's body toward the head or feet.	
6. MD/RN to:	
(a) Consider additional sedation, analgesics, and paralytics.	
(b) Consider adequacy of baseline systemic oxygen delivery.	
(c) Review contraindications to prone positioning (Appendix 25.1 - Prone Protocol).	
7. Remove headboard and footboard of the bed if able.	
8. Move the bed out from wall to provide access to the head of the bed. Apply brakes.	
9. Administer sedatives and analgesics as needed and consider need for paralytics.	
10. Gather staff members to perform turn as per hospital policy.	
Establishing prone position	
Steps	*Complete*
1. Place linens on top of patient:	
(a) In this order place Dri-Flo pad, one flat sheet, and ceiling lift sling as per unit practice (mesh if on air mattress) over the patient.	
(b) The flat sheet and sling should cover the head to foot of the patient.	
(c) Fold the section of the sheet and sling that is above the shoulders so that the patient's head is not covered up.	
(d) Press MAX-INFLATE if on air mattress.	
2. Ensure patient's head, lines, tubes, etc. are monitored and supported throughout turn.	
3. Tightly roll the sling/sheets on each side of the patient like a burrito to secure patient firmly between the linens.	
4. Slide the patient to the side of the bed away from the ventilator. ECMO cannulae configurations may vary. The access/venous line should be kept upright as to not disrupt the negative flow and to maintain visual of the circuit. Therefore, if access is in the femoral vein, patients may turn away from the ECMO unit depending on room setup providing there is adequate length in the circuit.	
5. To turn patient laterally:	
(a) Hold tightly onto burrito at each side to secure patient.	
(b) Slowly turn patient laterally to face ventilator.	
(c) When patient turned fully laterally, pause.	
(d) Adjust artificial airway and tubing in preparation for final turn.	
(e) Ensure there is no undue tension on lines and tubing. Once confirmed continue with final step of procedure.	
6. To complete the pronation:	
(f) Hold tightly onto burrito at each side to secure patient.	
(g) Gently rotate and prone patient supporting patient's head and neck throughout.	
(h) Remove old linen; straighten out new linens under patient.	
(i) Position patient so their body is in middle of the bed and head is resting on mattress in line with top of the bed.	

(continued)

Table 25.6 (continued)

7. Post-procedure time-out/pause to ensure artificial airway placement, ventilator settings, hemodynamics, ECLS cannula, and therapy settings. As well as assessment of patient response to therapy.	
8. Place V3 lead accurately for prone positioning.	
9. Ensure patient lines and tubes are tension-free and reconnect IV infusions.	
10. Cancel MAX-INFLATE (if on air mattress).	
11. Perfusion to ensure ECLS therapy settings are at baseline, with good SpO_2 and SvO_2. Check cannula positions and circuit flows.	
11. In all positioning of arm, the head of the humerus should not be overstretching and compressing axillary neurovascular bundle.	
12. If patient's status permits, they should be positioned in ¾ prone alternating with fully prone position q2h.	
Establishing supine position	
Steps	*Complete*
1. Always follow directions of the leader.	
2. Ensure patient's head, lines, tubes, etc. are monitored and supported throughout turn.	
3. Place linens on top of patient: (a) In this order place Dri-Flo pad, one flat sheet, and ceiling lift sling as per unit practice (mesh if on air mattress) over the patient. (b) The flat sheet and sling should cover the head to foot of the patient. (c) Fold the section of the sheet and sling that is above the shoulders so that the patient's head is not covered up. (d) Press MAX-INFLATE if on air mattress.	
4. Tightly roll the sling/sheets on each side of the patient like a burrito to secure patient firmly between the linens.	
5. Slide the patient to the side of the bed away from the ventilator.	
6. To turn patient laterally: (a) Hold tightly onto burrito at each side to secure patient. (b) Slowly turn patient laterally to face ventilator. (c) When patient turned fully laterally, pause. (d) Adjust artificial airway and tubing in preparation for final turn. (e) Ensure there is no undue tension on lines and tubing. Once confirmed continue with final step of procedure.	
7. To complete the pronation: (a) Hold tightly onto burrito at each side to secure patient. (b) Gently rotate and prone patient supporting patient's head and neck throughout. (c) Remove old linen; straighten out new linens under patient. (d) Position patient so their body is in middle of the bed and head is resting on mattress in line with top of the bed.	
8. Post-procedure time-out/pause to ensure artificial airway placement, ventilator settings, hemodynamics, ECLS cannula, and therapy settings. As well as assessment of patient response to therapy.	
9. Place V3 lead accurately for supine positioning.	
10. Ensure patient lines and tubes are tension-free and reconnect IV infusions.	
11. Cancel MAX-INFLATE (if on air mattress).	
12. Perfusion to ensure ECLS therapy settings are at baseline, with good SpO_2 and SvO_2. Check cannula positions and circuit flows.	

Reproduced with permission of Vancouver Coastal Health

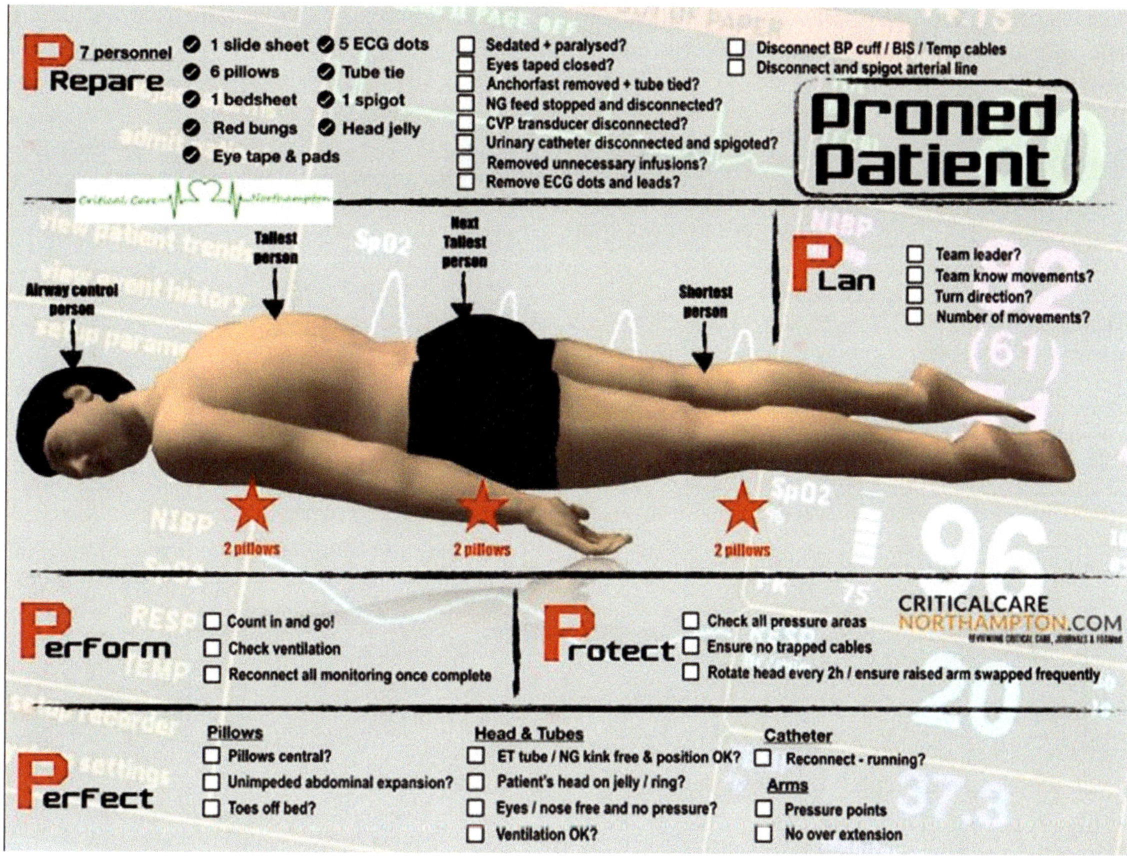

Fig. 25.5 Proning visual checklist. (Source: Criticalcarenorthampton.com, with permission)

Appendix 25.1: Proning Protocol of a Mechanically Ventilated Patient

Site Applicability
VGH – Intensive care unit

Practice Level
RN, RT, and physiotherapists working in VGH ICU

Policy Statement

1. Initiation of proning protocol requires an order from the intensivist. Order should be reviewed daily on rounds.
2. Proning of a patient on ECLS must be done with the perfusionist at the bedside as well as the intensivist. Follow the same directions as outlined below, taking extra care with the ECLS cannulae.

Need to Know

1. *Proning is a planned intervention that requires adequate preparation to ensure patient and staff safety.*
2. Prone position may be indicated in patients in whom conventional ventilator strategies have not been successful in recruiting alveoli and who continue to need maximal ventilator support with marginal oxygenation.
3. The use of prone position is discontinued when the patient no longer shows a positive response to the position change or mechanical ventilation support has been optimized.

4. Exclusion criteria for prone positioning are considered in collaboration with the interdisciplinary team. The criteria include:

Absolute contradindications
Unstable spine, femur, or pelvic fractures
Pregnancy in the third trimester
Endobronchial tubes
Increased intracranial pressure
Serious facial trauma/surgery or eye trauma/injury (e.g., ocular globe rupture) during the previous 15 days
Relative contraindications
Unstable sternum or sternotomy within 2 weeks
Tracheostomy or tracheal surgery within 2 weeks
Major abdominal surgery within 2 weeks
Open abdominal wound and/or ostomy
Open chest
Burns or open wounds on the ventral body surface
Extracorporeal life support
Considerations
CRRT
Temporary pacemaker
Grossly distended abdomen or ischemic bowel
Gross ascites
Difficult intubation

5. Patient should be left in prone position at least 12–16 continuous hours per day unless otherwise ordered.
6. The effect of proning is not immediate and may take several hours to have a measurable positive effect.
7. Proning can have an impact on patient's cardiopulmonary status. Carefully monitor respiratory and hemodynamic status during the entire intervention. If patient's status changes, review intervention with physician or delegate.
8. Turning (prone or supine) should ideally be performed during day hours when staffing/resources are optimal.
9. Prone positioning can be associated with complications including:

Potential complications
Compromising airway security (unplanned extubation, main stem bronchus intubation, artificial airway obstruction, etc.)
Dislodging vascular catheters, tubes, and drains
Hemodynamic instability
Difficulties monitoring patient
Increasing difficulty ventilating patient
Worsening respiratory function
Skin breakdown (pressure sores)
Eye injury due to orbital compression (e.g., conjunctival edema, corneal/sclera abrasion ulceration, retinal ischemia, blindness)
Venous congestion of the head and neck
Nerve compression to brachial plexus and ulnar nerve
Death – secondary to hypoxia and/or hypotension.

Equipment and Supplies *(if Applicable)*

1. Therapulse bed, if available. One should be ordered for patient if not readily available.
2. Wedge cushion.
3. ECG leads.
4. Dri-Flo pads.
5. Flat sheet.
6. Extra pillows.
7. Four to five staff members at a minimum:
   (a) An RT is responsible for the artificial airway and ventilator tubing during the turn.
   (b) An RN should be delegated to monitoring hemodynamics and lines during turns.
   (c) The individual holding the head is the team lead and will coordinate the required steps.
   (d) The remaining individuals will position the limbs and torso.

Practice Guideline

A. *Preparation for supine or prone positioning*

Steps	Rationale
1. Perform hand hygiene as per hospital policy.	
2. Don appropriate PPE.	
3. Ensure physician's order.	
4. Check for contraindications and discuss with intensivist or delegate as appropriate.	
5. Explain procedure and purpose of prone/supine position to patient and family.	
6. *If patient is supine*, transfer to Therapulse bed and weigh patient.	To minimize potential for skin breakdown, e.g., hospital-acquired pressure ulcers
7. *If patient is prone* and not on a Therapulse bed, be sure to transfer when next supine.	Weighing the patient will allow the bed to adjust and optimize mattress pressure for your patient.
8. Apply brakes.	
9. Perform baseline assessment (vital signs, ABG, complete patient head to toe, etc.).	Note: Patient's baseline hemodynamic parameters to assess response to intervention

Steps	Rationale
10. RT to ensure: (a) Artificial airway position is verified with recent chest X-ray. (b) Pre-oxygenate patient on 100% FiO_2. (c) Secretions are managed via suctioning above and below the cuff. (d) Artificial airway is in situ and firmly secured. Consider using twill ties or low-profile securing device to minimize pressure sores to face/cheeks. (e) Ventilator tubing is positioned on side of the mouth furthest from ventilator. (f) Emergency airway equipment is at HOB. Consider intubation box at bedside if known difficult airway.	To minimize potential for extubation and artificial airway displacement during positioning
11. RN to assess *feeding tubes*: (a) Patient should be fed via post-pyloric tube when in prone position. (b) Prior to proning, place post-pyloric feeding tube (inserted by trained RN) if not already in place. If unable to place, attempt placement when patient resumes supine position. (c) Connect large bore gastric tube to suction and empty contents. (d) Leave large bore gastric tube in place.	To minimize potential for aspiration
12. RN to assess *lines:* (a) Check if all IV/arterial lines, drainage tubes, etc. are secure with adequate tubing length (b) Flush and lock any unused lines as per protocol. (c) Reposition all lines and tubes that are located above the patient's waist straight upward toward the head of the bed. (d) Reposition all chest tubes as well as lines and tubes that are located below the waist (e.g., bladder catheter, femoral lines, and fecal drainage systems) straight down toward the foot of the bed. (e) Relocate all drainage bags on opposite side of the bed. BE SURE to cross the lines from this drainage bags under the patient and not across their front.	Placing all lines and tubes in an upward and downward line from the patient facilitates turning. This maneuver prevents the artificial airway and lines from being tangled or caught underneath the patient (where they cause skin breakdown). To ensure the drainage bags end up on the same side as the drain site when patient is positioned. Crossing the lines under the patient prior to turn ensures that the lines are not trapped between the bed and patient after reposition.
13. RN to provide all *anterior body care* if patient is *supine* and all *posterior body care* if *prone*: (a) Change any wound dressings, empty ileostomy/colostomy bags, etc. (b) Identify areas for potential skin breakdown. (c) Wash face and apply barrier cream. (d) Perform eye care. Lubricate eyes and close eyes. (e) Perform mouth care. (f) Suction patient prn. (g) Ensure tongue is inside patient's mouth; if swollen and/or protruding, monitor it closely. (h) Remove patient gown.	To minimize need to return patient to supine position for care To minimize potential for skin breakdown (e.g., hospital acquired pressure injury) by placing pressure relieving dressing (e.g., Mepilex Border) where pressure wound may occur (knees, chest region, forehead, etc.) To minimize the potential for skin maceration to face from increased moisture due to saliva To minimize injury to tongue. Position patient's head to minimize pressure to tongue To minimize pressure injuries from buttons/gown
14. RN to *reposition electrodes*: *If patient is turning supine to prone:* (a) LA lead to left shoulder. (b) RA lead to right shoulder. (c) LL lead to left lower back. (d) RL lead to right lower back. (e) Remove V3 lead from its anterior placement and *place it in posterior position once patient is prone* (see Appendix A: Fig. 25.6). *If patient is turning prone to supine:* (a) Left shoulder lead to LA. (b) Right shoulder lead to RA. (c) Left lower back lead to LL. (d) Right lower back lead to RA. (e) Remove V3 lead from its posterior placement and *place it in anterior position once patient is prone* (see Appendix A: Fig. 25.6).	To minimize pressure points anteriorly when patient is placed prone Pressing Update Lead Set on the GE monitor will reduce beeping until V3 lead can be placed on patient.

Steps	Rationale
15. Administer sedation and analgesics as needed and consider paralytics if appropriate.	To ensure patient comfort
16. Remove headboard and footboard of the bed if able. 17. Move bed out from wall to provide access to the head of the bed. Apply brakes. 18. Gather staff members to perform turn. 19. Staff members to position themselves: (a) The leader at HOB is responsible for the patient's head and directing the turn. (b) The RT at HOB is responsible for artificial airway and ventilator tubing during turn. (c) The remaining 2–3 individuals will position limbs, torso, and equipment throughout turn.	To allow for easier turns
20. Tuck patient's arms along the side of the body with fingers pointing toward toes. Keep arms as close to body as possible. 21. patient's head away from ventilator. 22. *Review procedural steps with entire team prior to initiation of patient turn.* 23. Prior to turning, review the expectations for when to turn (e.g., "we will turn when I say 3 in a 1, 2, 3 count"). 24. Pre-oxygenate with 100% FiO_2. 25. MAX-INFLATE mattress, HOB at 0° as tolerated, and adjust bed to working height.	These positions protect the arms from injury and make turning easier. To ensure patient's face is upward facing throughout turn

B. *Establishing prone position*

Steps	Rationale
1. Ensure you have completed steps outlined in *Preparation prior to turn prone or supine.* 2. Always follow directions of the leader. 3. Ensure patient's head, lines, tubes, etc. are monitored and supported throughout turn	
4. Place linens on top of patient: (a) In this order place Dri-Flo pad, one flat sheet, and ceiling lift sling (mesh if on air mattress) over the patient. (b) The flat sheet and sling should cover the head to foot of the patient. (c) Fold the section of the sheet and sling that is above the shoulders so that the patient's head is not covered up. (d) Press MAX-INFLATE if on Therapulse mattress.	The top linen will become the new bottom linen following proning. This linen will facilitate turning and make the bed in the same step. The head must be uncovered to observe the airway.
5. Tightly roll the sling/sheets on each side of the patient like a burrito to sandwich patient firmly between the linens.	Sandwiching the patient between the sheets helps maintain alignment and protect limbs during turning. The burrito method helps facilitate turning while keeping patient secure.
6. Slide the patient to the side of the bed away from the ventilator.	The patient will be turned to face the ventilator. This provides the most "slack" for the ventilator tubing. Moving the patient away from the ventilator ensures sufficient bed surface for pronation.
7. To turn patient laterally: (a) Hold tightly onto burrito at each side to secure patient. (b) Slowly turn patient laterally to face ventilator. (c) When patient turned fully laterally, *pause.* (d) Adjust artificial airway and tubing in preparation for final turn. (e) Ensure there is no undue tension on lines and tubing. Once confirmed continue with final step of procedure.	By taking a moment to review the steps, all members of the team have the same expectation. This ensures both patient and staff safety and makes the process much more efficient.
8. To complete the pronation: (a) Hold tightly onto burrito at each side to secure patient (b) Gently rotate and prone patient supporting patient's head and neck throughout (c) Remove old linen; straighten out new linens under patient. (d) Position patient so their body is in middle of the bed and head is resting on mattress in line with top of the bed.	Airway positioning must take priority for turning speed. This step poses the greatest risk for the ARTIFICIAL AIRWAY.
9. Perform post-turning care	

C. *Establishing supine position*

Steps	Rationale
1. Ensure you have completed steps outlined in *Preparation to turning prone or supine.*	
2. Always follow directions of the leader.	
3. Ensure patient's head, lines, tubes, etc. are monitored and supported throughout turn.	
4. Place linens on patient: (a) In this order place Dri-Flo pad, one flat sheet, and ceiling lift sling (mesh if air mattress) over the patient. (b) The flat sheet and sling should cover the head to foot of the patient. (c) Fold the section of the sheet and sling that is above the shoulders so that the patient's head is not covered. (d) Press MAX-INFLATE if on Therapulse mattress.	The top linen will become the new bottom linen following proning. This linen will facilitate turning and make the bed in the same step. The head must be uncovered to observe the airway.
5. Tightly roll the sling/sheets together like a burrito to sandwich patient firmly between the sheets.	Sandwiching the patient between the sheets helps maintain alignment and protect limbs during turning. The burrito helps facilitate turning while keeping patient secure.
6. Slide the patient to the side of the bed away from the ventilator.	The patient will be turned to face the ventilator. This provides the most "slack" for the ventilator tubing. Moving the patient away from the ventilator ensures sufficient bed surface for pronation.
7. To turn patient laterally: (a) Turn head *away* from ventilator. To do this gently lift patient's shoulder/upper torso to allow the head to rotate freely. (b) Hold tightly onto burrito at each side to secure patient (c) Slowly turn patient laterally toward the ventilator. (d) When patient turned fully laterally, *pause*. (e) Position artificial airway and tubing in preparation for final turn (f) Ensure there is no undue tension on lines and tubing. Once confirmed continue with final step of procedure.	By taking a moment to review the steps, all members of the team have the same expectation. This ensures both patient and staff safety and makes the process much more efficient. To ensure when patient turned, he/she has space to rotate head toward the ventilator.
8. To complete the supination: (a) Hold tightly onto burrito at each side to secure patient. (b) Gently rotate into supine position supporting head and neck throughout. (c) Remove old linen; straighten out new linens under patient. (d) Position patient so their body is in middle of the bed and head is resting on mattress in line with top of the bed.	Airway positioning must take priority for turning speed.
9. Perform post-proning care	

D. *Post-proning care*

- Place V3 lead accurately for either prone or supine positioning – refer to Appendix A: Fig. 25.6.
- Ensure patient lines and tubes are tension-free. Ensure stopcocks are moved to prevent the patient from lying on them.
- Place BP cuff high on the arm to prevent neuromuscular compression in the antecubital fossa.
- Reconnect IV infusions that were temporarily on hold for the proning.
- Cancel MAX-INFLATE.
- Auscultate patient's chest to ensure proper placement of artificial airway.
- RT to ensure end tidal CO_2 monitoring.
- If patient's status permits, they should be positioned in ¾ prone alternating with fully prone position q2h.
- If intolerant of ¾ prone or severe respiratory compliance issues – position patient fully proned.
- *In all positioning of arm, the head of the humerus should not be overstretching and compressing axillary neurovascular bundle.*
- *DO NOT elevate* upper limbs on pillows or beside tables as this will cause hyper-extension of joints causing torsion of nerves, joints, and vessels.
- Nursing/RT to reposition patient's head and arms q 1–2 hours.
- Follow instructions for prone positioning as outlined below for ¾ and fully proned patients.

Instructions for 3/4 prone positioning	Instructions for fully prone positioning
Turn patient's head to face side that wedge will be placed.	Ensure the head is in line with the spine; face is not turned into mattress and hips parallel to the spine.
Following leader's directions, use ceiling lift and sling (only use sling loops on wedge side of the patient) to lift patient 45° laterally to allow placement of wedge, or manually lift patient laterally to place wedge. Place wedge under patient's torso. Ensure that the head is in line with the spine and the hip parallel to the spine and the patient is not face-down into the mattress. Place patient's arm furthest from wedge at their side (hip level), palm up.	Place patient's arms in a swimmer's position. (a) Arm that patient is facing AWAY from by their side, palm up, and elbow flexed at 30–45 degrees. For example, at hip level with palm up. (b) Arm that patient is facing TOWARD at 75 degrees at shoulder, elbow flexed at 90 degrees, hand toward head of the bed, and fingers extended (if possible). For example, palm down by patient's chin. (c) If tolerated, flex hip and knee on the side patient is facing at <45°. (d) See Appendix A: Fig. 25.7 for positioning.
Gently position arm elevated on wedge at 75 degrees at shoulder while elbow is flexed at 90 degrees, hand toward head of the bed, and fingers extended (if possible). For example, palm down hugging wedge. Flex leg closest to wedge at hip <45° and knee <45° See Appendix A: Fig. 25.7 for positioning.	

Nursing Care and Monitoring of Patient During Prone Position

1. Anticipate potential complications of prone positioning and provide appropriate interventions – please refer to Appendix B.
2. For instructions on how to perform CPR while patient is proned – please refer to Appendix C.

Nursing interventions	Rationale
Reverse Trendelenburg bed to 20°. The head is in a neutral position (not extremely rotated, flexed, or extended). Peri-orbital area and eyes have no pressure on them. For large-breasted women, position breast laterally to reduce pressure on nipples/breast tissues. Male genitalia should hang freely. Foley is positioned between legs. Recalibrate monitoring lines and ensure all parameters and alarms are reviewed.	To minimize incidences of aspiration and decrease venous congestion to head and neck To minimize incidences of pressure injury
Reconnect IV infusions that were temporarily on hold for turning. Assess patient RASS goal is met and maintained along with routine pain assessment using NRS and BPS scales. Assess patient and hemodynamic parameters to ensure tolerance of supine/prone positioning.	Administering analgesia, sedation, and/or paralytics to ensure patient comfort and physiological needs are met
Place gown/blanket/sheet on patient.	Ensure patient is covered as more surface area is exposed for heat loss.
Return side rails to original position and adjust height of the bed into lowest position.	
If patient has a post-pyloric feeding tube, initiate/resume enteral feeds as ordered. Check gastric residuals Q4H. Discard all gastric residuals. (DO NOT ATTACH GASTRIC TUBE TO SUCTION). If GRV > 400 ml/4 h OR contains significant amount of tube feeds, stop feeds and inform physician. Refer to ICU Guideline: Post-pyloric Feeding. If patient does not have a post pyloric feeding tube, hold feeds. Insert post-pyloric feeding tube when next placed in supine position.	To minimize risk of aspiration When administering post-pyloric enteral feeds, gastric tube should not be connected to suction as it may contribute to retrograde flow of post-pyloric feeds.
Assessments as per unit protocol. Follow oxygenation and hemodynamic status closely to monitor for deterioration. Mixed venous gas and ABG as per unit protocol. Perform oral care and suctioning of airway as per protocol and as needed. *WHEN SUPINE*: reposition patient q2h. *WHEN PRONE*: Skin condition should be assessed q2h to face/arms. Head and limb repositioning should be done every 1–2 hours. Please refer to instructions in the following table. *Instructions: Repositioning a patient's head when prone*	To minimize risk of hospital-acquired pressure ulcers

Nursing interventions	Rationale
Follow leader's instructions.	
Pull bed away from wall and remove headboard.	
Ceiling lift technique	To allow enough space to reposition patient toward ventilator.
Leader to hold patient's head at all times and secure artificial airway.	To allow for safe repositioning of patient's head by person at HOB
Attach all sling straps EXCEPT the four straps (two each side) at patient's head/upper body.	
Raise patient 2 inches off bed and slide patient in ceiling lift up the bed so the head is off the bed.	
Leader to rotate patient's head.	
Slide patient in ceiling lift back down the bed so the head is back on the bed. Lower patient onto bed.	
Manual lift technique	To allow enough space to reposition patient toward ventilator
Leader to hold patient's head at all times and secure artificial airway.	To allow for safe repositioning of patient's head by person at HOB
Primary RN and other staff members to boost patient so the head is off the bed.	
Leader to rotate patient's head.	
Primary RN and other staff members to slide patient back down the bed so the head is back on the bed.	
Straighten out linens and position patient so their body is in the middle of the bed.	
Reposition limbs in swimmer's position – refer to Appendix A Fig. 25.7.	

Documentation

1. Documentation must include patient's pre- and post-intervention assessment.
2. Document in the nurses' notes:
   (a) Patient and family education
   (b) Complications during and post-procedure
   (c) Response to proning
   (d) Total length of time in the prone position
   (e) Response once returned to supine position
   (f) Unexpected outcomes
   (g) Nursing interventions
3. Document on critical care flow sheet:
   (a) Amount and type of secretions
   (b) Prone position (fully, left, right)
   (c) Length of time in each position
   (d) Turns to head/arms.
   (e) Eye care and mouth care
   (f) ABG results
   (g) Ventilation and oxygenation.
4. Document on pain, agitation, and delirium record – medications administered during procedure.
5. Document on the Kardex:
   (a) Positioning schedule
   (b) Time proned and expected time to re-supinate

Adapted from similar protocols developed at

- Alberta health Services (Calgary), Critical Care & Cardiac Sciences Unit Manual policy, Prone Positioning of the Ventilated Patient (June 2013)
- London Health Sciences Center, Procedure for turning a ventilated patient prone in CCTC (August 2, 2013). Accessed 30 April 2016 http://www.lhsc.on.ca/Health_Professionals/CCTC/procedures/proning.htm
- Providence Health, St. Paul's Hospital, Prone Positioning of a Ventilated Patient Draft Policy, March 2016.
- Sunnybrook& Women's College Health Science Center, Critical Care Unit, Prone Positioning Protocol (March 2002)

Related Documents

References

- Alsaghir AH, Martin CM. Effects of prone positioning in patients with acute respiratory distress syndrome: a meta-analysis. Crit Care Med, 2008;36(2):603–9.
- American Heart Association Guidelines for Cardiopulmonary Resuscitation and Emergency Cardiovascular Care Science, 2015.
- Balas MC. Prone positioning of patient's with acute respiratory distress syndrome: Applying research to practice. Crit Care Nurse. 2000;20(1):24–36.
- Ball C, Adams J, Boyce S, Robinson P. Clinical guidelines for the use of the prone position in acute respiratory distress syndrome. Intensive Crit Care Nurs. 2001;17: 94–104.
- Dirkes S, Dickson S, Harve R, O'Brien D. Prone positioning: is it safe?. Crit Care Nurs Q 2012;35(1):1–12.
- Goartificial airwayler Goettler CE, Pryor JP, Reilly PM. Brachial plexopathy after prone positioning. Crit Care. 2002;6:540–2.
- Guerin C, Reignier J, Richard JC, Beuret P, Gacoulin A, Boulain T, Mercier E, Badet M, Mercat A, Baudin O, Clavel M, Chatellier A, Jaber S, Rosselli S, Mancebo J, Sirodot M, Hilbert G, Bengler C, Richecoeur J, Gainnier M, Bayle F, Bourdine G, Leray V, Girard R, Baboi L, Ayzac L. Prone positioning in severe acute respiratory distress syndrome. N Engl J Med. 2013;365(23):2159–68.

- Kamel I, Barnette R. Positioning patient's for spine surgery: Avoiding uncommon position-related complications. World J Orthop. 2014;5(4): 425–43.
- Linn DD, Beckett RD, Foellinger K. Administration of enteral nutrition to adult patients in the prone position. Intensive Crit Care Nurs. 2014;31:38–43.
- McCormick J, Blackwood B. Nursing the ARDS patient in the prone position: The experience of qualified ICU nurses. Intensive Crit Care Nurs. 2001;17:331–340.
- Nuri Deniz M, Erakgun A, Sertoz N, Guven Yilmaz S, Ates H, Erhan E. The effect of head rotation on intraocular pressure in prone position: a randomized trial. Rev Bras Anaestesiol. 2012;63(2):209–12.
- Powers J. The five P's Spell positive outcomes for ARDS patients. Am Nurs Today. 2007;2(3):34–38.
- Reignier J, Dimet J, Martin-Lefevre L, Bontemps F, Fiancette M, Clementi E, Lebert C, Renard B. Before-after study of a standardized ICU protocol for early enteral feeding in patient's turned in the prone position. Clin Nutr. 2010;29:210–6.
- Schwarts DR, Malhotra A, Kacmarek RM. Up to date. Prone ventilation. 2014, Nov. Accessed Dec 2014.
- Stewart JA. Resuscitating and idea: prone CPR. Resuscitation. 2002;54:231–6.
- Wei J, Tung D, Sue S, Wu S, Chuang Y, Chan C. Cardiopulmonary resuscitation in prone position: a simplified method for outpatient's. J Chin Med Assoc. 2006;69(5):202–6.
- Wolfe-Citty S. Patient positioning: supine or prone. Mosby's Clinical Review. 2014, Dec. Accessed July 10, 2015 http://mns.elsevierperformancemanager.com/NursingSkills/ContentPlayer/SkillContentPlayerIFrame.aspx?KeyId=668&Id=GN_10_3C&Section=1&bcp=SpecialtyId~0~prone~False&IsConnect=False
- Vollman KM. Prone positioning in the patient who has acute respiratory distress syndrome: the art and science. Crit Care Nurs Clin N Am, 2014;16(3):319–336.

Developed/Revised by

CPD developer lead(s):	**Simmie Kalan, VGH ICU CNE**
	Marta Musa, RN SPH ICU
Other members:	**Jenny O'Mahony, VGH ICU CNE**
	Josephine Cheung, VGH ICU dietician
	Andrea Wnuk, respiratory practice lead
	Jocelyn Ross, physiotherapist
	Rys Chapel, physiotherapist

Appendices: Start separate page with each new appendix – do not list appendices here. Refer to any appendix information within the document so it can be directly linked.

Appendix A: Figures

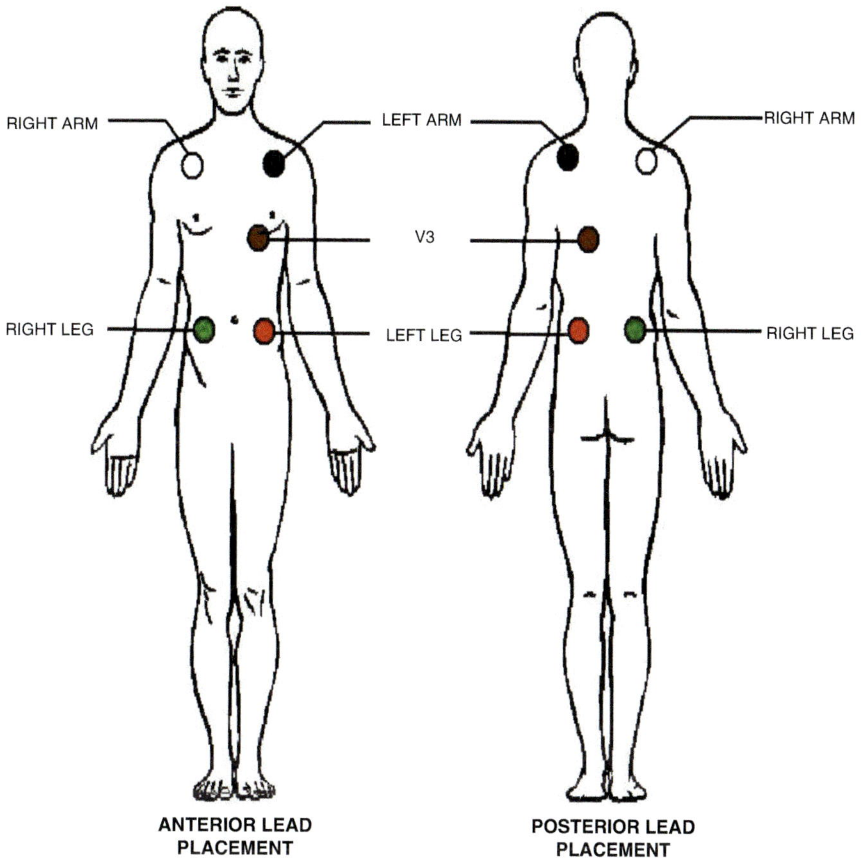

Fig. 25.6 Posterior placement of ECG monitoring leads

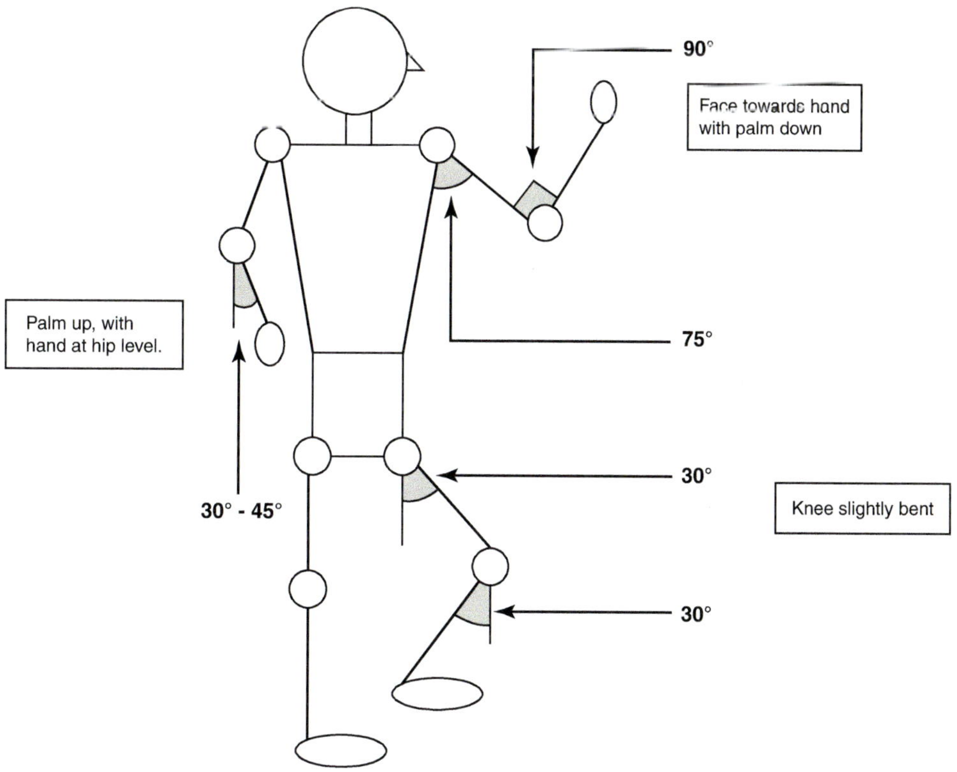

Fig. 25.7 Limb positioning for ¾ and fully proned patients

Appendix B: Potential Complications of Prone Positioning and Interventions

Complication	Prevention and intervention
Skin breakdown: Due to prolonged time between position changes	Inspect skin for any new or additional damage each time patient is repositioned. Reposition patient head q 1–2 hours, turning head side to side and alternating positions of arms accordingly. When repositioning head, ensure: NG/OG is not anchored to patient's cheeks and instead just to nose. Pressure is not placed on Anchor Fast. If patient is tolerant, reposition from full prone to ¾ prone (see procedure outlined above) q 2 hours. If patient intolerant of ¾ prone, make small incremental changes in patient's position q 1–2 hours. Ensure no hard pieces of plastic are under the body and smooth wrinkles from bedding. Ensure wet or soiled linens (e.g., due to oral secretions, wound drainage, etc.) are changed in a timely fashion to minimize skin breakdown. Wash face and apply barrier cream to protect against maceration by saliva.
Eye damage Due to orbital compression when prone resulting in conjunctival edema, corneal scratch, sclera abrasion/ulceration, retinal ischemia, and blindness	Ensure eye is supported free of bed surface. Rotate head laterally when positioned. Eye care q 2 hours. Lubricate and close eyes to prevent corneal drying, abrasion, or infection.
Venous congestion of head and neck: Due to face positioning below level of the heart	Placing bed in a reverse Trendelenburg at 25–30°. Ensure no pillow is under the head. Turning head every 2 hours to ensure adequate arterial perfusion and venous drainage. Avoid over-extension of neck with positioning.
Nerve compression to limbs: Due to improper positioning of limbs	Follow recommended limb positioning techniques. Avoid over-extension of joints with positioning.
Contractures: Due to improper positioning of limbs	Ensure use of therapeutic bed. Follow recommended limb positioning techniques.

Appendix C: CPR on a Prone Patient

1. Follow ACLS protocol.
2. *Do NOT* place patient in a supine position.
3. Emergency deflate bed.
4. Perform prone CPR:
   (a) Place board under patient at the sternum.
   (b) Compressions by rescuer will be performed over thoracic bodies 7–10. To landmark, find inferior border of scapulae and slide your hands medially to T7.

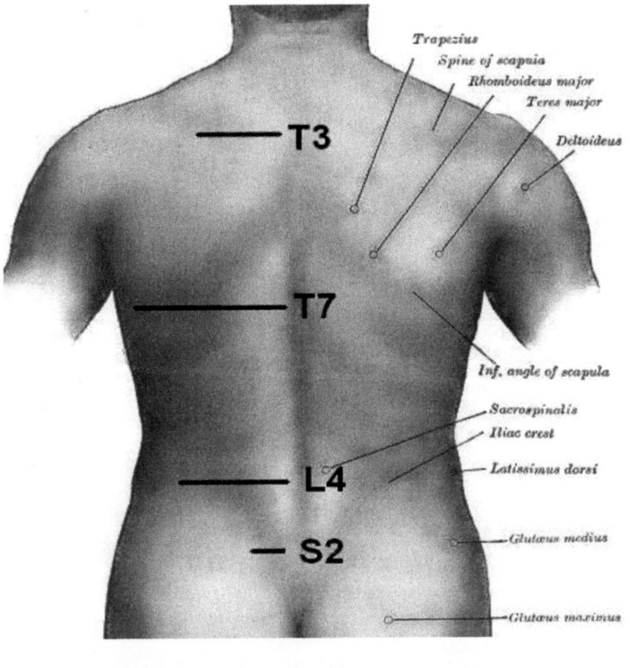

   (c) Place both hands on the patient's spine over T7 and commence compressions using two hands on the spine.
5. Defibrillation/pacing: Place Zoll defibrillator pads anterior/posterior as required.
6. Turn patient supine only if:
   (a) Unable to achieve adequate compressions with CPR.
   (b) There are enough adequately experienced personnel to perform safely.
   Moving a patient from a prone position frantically without proper personnel and preparation may result in unplanned extubation and loss of IV access.
7. https://www.youtube.com/watch?v=AL-ZKsCN_o0.

Appendix 25.2

SIM TEMPLATE:

Vancouver CoastalHealth

COURSE NAME
Scenario Name: PART A: VV ECLS Patient Proning

Learning objectives:
1. Demonstration of crisis resource management skills
2. Use of a standardized protocol or policy on proning/supinating critically ill patients, especially those on ECLS
3. Application of basic ECLS and ventilation/oxygenation theoretical principles to guide decision-making

Pre-reading:
A standardized protocol or policy should be shared with staff prior to simulation and be available for simulation participants to refer to as needed.

Simulation overview:
The goal of simulation scenario is to prone a patient on ECLS and the scenario should begin in patient room with decision to prone already made and all necessary personnel present.
Patient is a stable ECLS VV patient, with minimal infusions to not distract from objectives of the simulation.

Simulation progression:
Part A of scenario/simulation should focus on proning a patient on ECLS without any crisis emergency issues.
Following Part A – debrief to review the proning procedure and team communication skills should be completed.
Following the debrief to Part A – Part B scene should commence with the team now supinating the same patient but with a crisis emergency situation (Table 25.1) arising such as cannula malposition, decrease in SpO_2, airway dislodgement, etc. Limit Part B scenario to one or two major complications.
Following Part B – a debrief regarding the adverse event and management should occur. As well as a review of other adverse events that could occur and primary responsibilities.

Faculty and confederate roles:
SIM tech
  Adjusts vital signs and patient assessments as indicated in simulation scenario and under guidance of clinical expert
Clinical expert (can also be the facilitator)
  Assists SIM tech with changes ad hoc to scenario progression or in response to participants' action
  Helps to direct scenario by providing information to confederate and/or standardized patient
  Has a good understanding of ECLS therapy, proning, and emergency procedures
Facilitator (SIM educator)
  Describes goals of simulation to participants
  Pre-briefing to simulator and environment
  Debriefing with focus on objectives and clarification of clinical take-aways
Confederate
  Provides any details of the case unable to obtain from manikin
  Provides diagnostics as required
  Provides clarification of assessment findings as needed
Standardized patients (when used instead of manikins)
  Provides direct feedback from assessments
  Moves scenario along as per written phases

Audience/participant roles:
ECLS specialists, perfusionist, medical staff, respiratory therapist, and nurse

RN
- Patient monitoring including vitals (specifically SpO_2 and SvO_2), infusions, lines, and overall patient status including pain, agitation, and delirium.
- Ensure lines and drainage tubes are secure with adequate tubing length and position of pumps.
- Flush and lock any unused lines and empty ileostomy/colostomy bags.
- Environmental setup of room and ensuring availability of all required personnel.

PT
- Assess patient's functional and cognitive readiness.
- Functional strengthening program and goal setting, dosage, and frequency.
- Environmental setup of room, equipment to be used, and plan for execution.

RT
- Optimize the ventilator according to patient's current and expected physiologic changes taking into account previous efforts and patient demands.
- Manage secretions via suctioning prior to mobilization and as needed.
- Ensure tube is appropriately positioned and firmly secured.
- Procure emergency airway equipment.
- Identify contingency plan for potential extubation.

Perfusion
- Assure the ECMO lines are secure and confirm the position.
- Monitor and adjust circuit flow and sweep.
- Assure that adequate line length is sufficient to allow mobilization.

MD
- Establish appropriate monitoring parameters.
- Prioritize monitoring and treatment goals.
- Assure communication of plan for any adverse events.

Physical props/equipment:	*References, resources, protocols, algorithms, or evidence-informed practice guidelines:*
SIM manikin and software/laptop and bedside monitor ECLS circuit ECLS cannula ICU/CSICU patient setup, i.e., Art line, CVC, OETT, NG/OG, Foley catheter, and IV pumps with infusions as per scenario Ventilator Safety equipment, i.e., Ambu bag, oral airway, and ECLS emergency supplies Emergency supplies (on ECMO cart) Proning guideline or policy	Proning clinical practice guideline (Appendix 3) Lab work Blood gases Emergency procedural documents if applicable

Monitors:
ECG, ART, SpO_2, NIBP, and CVP

Room setup:	*Medications & fluids:*	*Diagnostics:*	*Documentation forms:*	*Confederates:*
IV pumps with infusions Standard ICU/CSICU room setup BVM at HOB	Access line @ 10 mL/h Heparin 800 u/hr Levophed 10 mcg/min	ABG SvO_2 BW	ECLS flow sheet, Kardex	To confirm assessment findings of manikin and provide diagnostics as needed

Case briefing:

Patient description & diagnosis:

Rena is a 28-year-old, 90-kg female on VV ECMO for H1N1 pneumonia, ARDS. She has a return 31Fr. RIJ. It is day 3 on ECLS; she has had a stable run. It was determined on rounds that patient would need to be proned due to worsening lung function.

Previous assessment:
- RASS +2, follows commands x4 but very agitated and unable to assess orientation. PERL at 3 mm.
- Chest sounds quiet throughout. OETT 7.5 at 24 cm at teeth. Ventilated on ACV 10 × 200, FiO_2 35%, Peep 8. SpO_2 85%.
- VV EMCO: 5.2 Lpm, Sweep flow rate 4.0 Lpm, FiO_2 100%, SvO_2 75%. Pre-oxygenator pressure and post-oxygenator pressures are as displayed on the circuit.
- Warm and well perfused, pulses palpable throughout, CVP 8, Temp 36.8, SR 105, BP 125/85 MAP 95. Heparin infusion at 800 units/hr for PTT of 55. Last INR 1.5, Fib 1.4, AT 0.75, Plts 115, Hgb 86.
- Access line at 10 ml/hr NS.
- GI – NG in place, capped due to the ileus.
- GU – urine output satisfactory with 30 ml/hr.

Time of scene: 1400 in ICU

		Past medical history: Previously healthy *Allergies:* NKA	*Family history:* Not significant *Social history:* Teacher
Vital signs/scenario transitions	*Patient status*	*Effective management*	*Modifiers/triggers*
Phase 1: Team at bedside with all players involved in proning procedure			
HR: Sinus 105 *BP:* 125/85 (95) *CVP*: 8 *Vent*: ACV 10 × 200, FiO_2 35% *SpO_2:* 85% *Temp (C):* 36.8 *SvO_2: 90%* Pre: as on circuit Post: as on circuit Flow: 5.3 Lpm Sweep: 4.0 Lpm FiO_2: 100%	*CNS:* Unchanged *RESP:* Comfortable on vent. *CVS:* Unchanged *ABDO:* Unchanged *GU:* Unchanged *SKIN:* Unchanged *ECMO:* Unchanged	Decision to prone confirmed Team members all accounted for and roles clarified Policy or protocol reviewed	*Modifiers*: Everything stays the same until phase 2. Proceed to phase 2 after 2 minutes.
Vital signs/scenario transitions	*Patient status*	*Effective management*	*Modifiers/triggers*
Phase 2: Patient proned following protocol			
HR: Sinus 105 *BP:* 145/90 (91) *CVP*: 8 *Vent*: ACV 10 × 200, FiO_2 35% *SpO_2:* 93% *Temp (C):* 36.8 *SvO_2:* 97% Pre: As on circuit Post: As on circuit Flow: 5 Lpm Sweep: 4.0 Lpm FiO_2: 100%	Unchanged	Patient safely proned and repositioned Assesses for adequate oxygen delivery (SpO_2 & SvO_2) Team conducts time-out/ pause: Airway placement confirmed Ventilation settings reviewed and weaned/ optimized ECLS settings reviewed ECLS cannula sites assessed Hemodynamics Orders diagnostics (i.e., BW)	VS aren't changed; patient remains stable for objective of goal is the actual prone position. Total time of phase 2: 10 minutes

Debrief points: proning checklist – Appendix 3

Clinical take-home points:

A. Review of proning procedure and adherence to protocol

B. Evaluation of team communication and principles of collaborative care and crisis resource management

Describe

Can someone summarize the case?

Analyze

What do you think you did well?

What would you change and do better next time?

Summarize

1. What were the main issues that you had to deal with?
2. What were your priorities when you first thought about needing to prone the patient?
3. Clarify any actions or roles.

Part B: Supination and Cannula Malposition

- SIM scenario will begin with participants being told to supinate the patient following the same procedure guideline they used earlier.
- Following procedure, patient's SpO_2 decreases drastically whereas the circuit SvO_2 increases – indicating recirculation from cannula malposition. Emergency measures should consist of decreasing RPMs to decrease flow as well as max ventilation/oxygenation using the ventilator.
- Please see template SIM scenario.
- Debrief should include discussion of other adverse events and management strategies.

Adverse event	Management strategies
Cannula malposition	Maximally ventilate/oxygenate patient with ventilator. Provide analgesia/sedative to prevent further malposition. Assess color and site of ECLS cannula/lines and patient vitals, specifically SpO_2 and SvO_2. Decreasing RPMs may help if cannula malposition is causing recirculation. Stat X-ray.
Cardiac arrest	VV – Start CPR and ACLS algorithms. VA – Clamp, hand crank, and ACLS algorithms.
Bleeding from cannula sites	Assess sites. Reinforce securement devices. Bloodwork.
Flow issues on ECLS circuit	Check cannula. Max support from ventilator. Check ECLS lines for kinks, etc.
Artificial airway dislodgement	Full support via ECLS therapy. Prepare to reintubate.
Hemodynamic instability	Titration of vasopressors, inotropes, and fluids as assessed.

SIM TEMPLATE

COURSE NAME

Scenario Name: PART B: VV ECLS Proning

Learning objectives:

1. Demonstration of crisis resource management skills
2. Recognition of patient deterioration and demonstration of emergency management
3. Application of basic ECLS and ventilation/oxygenation theoretical principles to guide decision-making

Audience/Participants:

ECLS specialists, perfusionist, medical staff, respiratory therapist, and nurse

Physical props/equipment:	*References, resources, protocols, algorithms, or evidence-informed practice guidelines:*
SIM manikin and software/laptop and bedside monitor ECLS circuit ECLS cannula ICU/CSICU patient setup, i.e., Art line, CVC, OETT, NG/OG, Foley catheter, and IV pumps with infusions as per scenario Ventilator Safety equipment, i.e., Ambu bag, oral airway, and ECLS emergency supplies Emergency supplies (on ECMO cart) Proning guideline or policy	Lab work Blood gases Emergency procedural documents if applicable

Monitors:

ECG, ART, SpO_2, NIBP, and CVP

Room setup:	*Medications & fluids:*	*Diagnostics:*	*Documentation forms:*	*Confederates:*
IV pumps with infusions Standard ICU/CSICU room setup BVM at HOB	Access line @ 10 mL/h Heparin 800 u/hr Levophed 10 mcg/min	ABG SvO_2 BW	ECLS flow sheet, Kardex	To confirm assessment findings of manikin and provide diagnostics as needed

Case briefing:
Patient description & diagnosis:
SAME PATIENT AS PART A
Time of scene: 0800 in ICU–the next day

Vital signs/scenario transitions	*Patient status*	*Effective management*	*Modifiers/triggers*
Phase 1: Interdisciplinary team at bedside to supinate patient			
HR: Sinus 105 *BP:* 125/85 (95) *CVP:* 8 *Vent:* ACV 10 × 200, FiO_2 35% *SpO_2:* 98% *Temp (C):* 36.8 *SvO_2:* 84% Pre: As on circuit Post: As on circuit Flow: 5.3 Lpm Sweep: 4.0 Lpm FiO_2: 100%	*CNS:* Unchanged *RESP:* Comfortable on vent *CVS:* Unchanged *ABDO:* Unchanged *GU:* Unchanged *SKIN:* Unchanged *ECMO:* Same	Decision to supinate confirmed Team members all accounted for and roles clarified Policy or protocol reviewed Supination completed	*Modifiers*: Everything stays the same until phase 2. Proceed to phase 2 after 4 minutes or at the immediate completion of patient in supine position.

Vital signs/scenario transitions	*Patient status*	*Effective management*	*Modifiers/triggers*
Phase 2: Recirculation due to cannula malposition			
HR: Sinus 120 BP: 145/100 (105) CVP: 8 Vent: ACV 10 × 200, FiO2 35% SpO2: 60% Temp (C): 36.8 SvO2: 97% Pre: As on circuit Post: As on circuit Flow: 5 Lpm Sweep: 4.0 Lpm FiO2: 100%	Sudden decrease in patient SpO_2 and increase in circuit SvO_2	Recognize inadequate oxygen delivery (decreased SaO_2 but high SvO_2 on circuit). Assess for possible reasons why: Cannula position Cardiac function RA size Flow too high Order CxR/ECHO. Assess cannula sites and cannula position. Assess and identify if circuit color in both lines is bright red – recirculation. Decrease flows while troubleshooting cannula malposition. Complete ventilator and oxygenation support taken over by ventilator.	Stop SIM if: Assessment of all possible causes is done & interventions such as complete ventilator support and decreased RPMs done. Identify cause to be cannula malposition. Find CXR with deep IJ placement (into IVC). Total time of phase 2: 8 minutes

Possible debrief points:
Secondary objectives:
Clinical take-home points:
A. Identify urgent risk to patient – decrease oxygenation delivery from ECMO circuit.
B. Evaluation of patient with recirculation on VV ECLS
(a) ECMO access line color is close to/matches return line (bright).
(b) High SvO_2 (e.g., 85% and above) with decrease in SpO_2 (which is dynamic → decreasing flow does the reverse).
C. Review the causes of recirculation.
D. Review of possible complications from cannula malposition (i.e., RA perforation).
E. Need for CXR/ECHO to confirm cannula placement.
F. Effect of flow/access pressure with cannula malposition.
G. Other adverse effects/complications that can occur for ECLS patients being proned/supinated.

Describe

Can someone summarize the case?

Analyze

What do you think you did well?
What would you change and do better next time?

Summarize

1. What were the main issues that you had to deal with?
2. What were your priorities when you first went to the patient?
3. Clarify any actions taken that would be outside of ECLS specialist scope.
4. Refer to relevant CPDs.

I would like to close by having each of you state a take-away that will help you in the future.

Appendix 25.3: Mobilization on ECLS

Title – Simulation Scenario Title and Objectives:
- Mobilization Simulation on VV ECMO (Walking)
- Use of a standardized protocol or policy on mobilizing critically ill patients, especially those on ECLS
- Application of basic ECLS and ventilation/oxygenation theoretical principles to guide decision-making
- Demonstration of interprofessional collaborative practice and crisis resource management skills

Pre-work:
- Reading and ambulation video
- Background literature on ECLS mobilization procedures [3, 26, 27]
- Ambulation video: eAPPENDIX 2

Scenario Overview:
- Goal of simulation scenario is to walk a patient on ECLS.
- Scenario should begin in patient room with decision to mobilize already made and all necessary personal present. Patient is a stable ECLS VV patient, with minimal infusions to not distract from objectives of the simulation. Second phase of simulation can involve a selection of crisis from Table 25.1.

Interprofessional Team Roles:
- When simulating mobilization out of the bed, a perfusionist, physiotherapist, and nurse provide support for a safe transfer, and if ventilated, a respiratory therapist or equivalent is added. When ambulation is remote from the bedspace, additional personnel are needed and can take up to six staff or more depending on cannula location, size of the patient, and room setup (Fig. 25.4).

Registered nurse/ ECLS specialist	Deals with all aspects of patient care Patient monitoring including vitals, infusions, lines, and overall patient state Ensures lines and drainage tubes are secure with adequate tubing length and position of pumps Flushes and locks any unused lines
Physiotherapist	Assesses patient's functional and cognitive readiness Functional strengthening program and goal setting, dosage, and frequency Environmental setup of room, equipment to be used, and plan for execution Conducts the mobility session
Respiratory therapist	Optimizes the ventilator according to patient's current and expected physiologic changes taking into account previous efforts and patient demands Switch to alternate device such as portable ventilator/Ambu bag Manages secretions via suctioning prior to and during mobilization and as needed Ensures airway is appropriately positioned and firmly secured Procures emergency airway equipment if leaving the bedspace Identifies contingency plan for potential extubation
Perfusionist	Ensures the ECMO lines are secure and confirms the position Handles the ECLS cannula and maneuvers the ECLS device as needed Monitors and adjusts circuit flow and sweep Assures that adequate line length is sufficient to allow mobilization
MD	Establishes appropriate monitoring parameters Prioritizes monitoring and treatment goals Assures availability for crisis events

Equipment list:
- Simulation manikin or standardized patient
- Software/laptop to generate vital signs and bedside monitor
- ECLS circuit
- ECLS cannula
- ICU/CSICU patient setup, i.e., Art line, CVC, OETT, NG/OG, Foley catheter, and IV pumps with infusions as per scenario
- Ventilator
- Safety equipment: Ambu bag, suction, oral airway, and ECLS emergency supplies

Mobilization Phases Checklist: Pre-movement Screening, During Movement

Pre-movement phase: Screening checklist for candidacy-criteria to consider (see Table 25.5*)*

Patient:
- RASS −1 to +1, awake, cooperative, adequate
  - strength
- Cardiac stability: HR 50–140 bpm
  - No serious arrhythmias or MI in past 48 hrs
- Hemodynamic stability
  - SBP 80–180 mmHg, MAP > 65 mmHg
  - Low-dose inotropes or vasopressors, stable trend
- No significant bleeding past 24 hrs
  - Plt > 50, INR < 3
- Respiratory stability – with stable mechanical ventilator settings
  - Resting $FiO_2 < 60\%$
  - $PaO_2 > 60$ mmHg, $PaCO_2 < 80$ mmHg, pH >7.30 RR < 30 bpm
- No other factors

  Anxiety, vomiting, uncontrolled diarrhea, delirium

ECMO:
- Blood flow 2–5 liters per min with adequate oxygen delivery per attending physician
- Gas sweep 0–10 (CO_2 elimination)
- Activated clotting time levels 160–180 seconds
- Stable for past 24 hours
- For femorally cannulated patients:

  Inability to tolerate transient loss of flow with hip flexion

Contraindications and precautions checklist:
- Medical instability (max respiratory, inotropic, flows/sweep support at rest or with general nursing care).

- Poor level of consciousness.
- Significant confusion/delirium/anxiety (inability to follow instructions).
- Signs of respiratory or physical intolerance (respiratory distress, exhaustion).
- Coagulopathy – significant bleeding issues.
- Femorally cannulated patients – Care to be taken with hip flexion. Assess the patient lying flat and passively flex the hip to test flows and stability.

Preparation prior to mobility checklist:

- Have a clear goal of the therapy session that has been communicated to the staff as well as the patient. Set the patient up for success and not for failure; this is especially important when considering the patient's psychological well-being. Therapy sessions should include short-term and long-term goal setting ensuring that goals are specific, measureable, achievable, and realistic (SMART) that have been created in collaboration with the patient.
- The therapy session should be led by an advanced trained physical therapist in ECLS who will determine the dose and frequency to improve functional strengthening and mobility.
- Set up the room/hallway and position the ECMO cart/vent where you need them ensuring that you have a complete visual of the circuit. Clear any unnecessary equipment or obstacles.
- Check the fixations of the cannulae; check for clots in the circuit.
- Adequate staffing and clear roles. Task assignment as highlighted prior.
- Observe ventilation parameters and if there is an opportunity to optimize the patient's native lung function. If leaving the bedside, portable suction for pulmonary toileting may be needed.
- Switch to alternate device such as portable ventilator/Ambu bag.
- Intensivist available if needed in the event of unanticipated medical issues or emergencies.
- RN to have rapid analgesia administration medication plan prepared.
- Same as transport, two full oxygen tanks to be taken dedicated to the ECMO circuit.

*Family engagement and education is important when trying to engage the patient and provide motivation.

Movement phase: Ambulation phase checklist

First-name introductions among the team and role recaps.

- Explain to the patient with specific mention to address any fears or anxiety that may impact the treatment session. If unable to talk, identify a clear way for the patient to communicate and if they need to stop treatment and sit down.
- Attach any devices to secure cannulae, e.g., a headstrap.
- Pulmonary toileting prior to ambulating.
- Sit the head of the bed up and progress to then assist the patient to sit on the edge of the bed. If on an air bed, deflate the air mattress to prevent sliding.
- Continuous patient monitoring for ECG, BP, O_2 saturations, ECMO flows, cannula sites, as well as patient subjectively reported symptoms. If the patient is tolerating well, then progress to ambulate with a wheelchair to follow in case the patient needs a physical rest. Once returned to the room and bed, reconnect to previous oxygen support and complete a full circuit check as performed prior to mobility session.

Bibliography

1. Barnes-Daly MA, Pun BT, Harmon LA, Byrum DG, Kumar VK, Devlin JW, et al. Improving health care for critically ill patients using an evidence-based collaborative approach to ABCDEF bundle dissemination and implementation. Worldviews Evid-Based Nurs. 2018;15(3):206–16.
2. Shudo Y, Kasinpila P, Lee AM, Rao VK, Woo YJ. Ambulating femoral venoarterial extracorporeal membrane oxygenation bridge to heart-lung transplant. J Thorac Cardiovasc Surg. 2018;156(3):e135–e7.
3. Wells CL, Forrester J, Vogel J, Rector R, Tabatabai A, Herr D. Safety and feasibility of early physical therapy for patients on extracorporeal membrane oxygenator: University of Maryland Medical Center experience. Crit Care Med. 2018;46(1):53–9.
4. Mayer CM, Cluff L, Lin WT, Willis TS, Stafford RE, Williams C, et al. Evaluating efforts to optimize TeamSTEPPS implementation in surgical and pediatric intensive care units. Jt Comm J Qual Patient Saf. 2011;37(8):365–74.
5. Zakhary BM, Kam LM, Kaufman BS, Felner KJ. The utility of high-fidelity simulation for training critical care fellows in the management of extracorporeal membrane oxygenation emergencies: a randomized controlled trial. Crit Care Med. 2017;45(8):1367–73.
6. Johnson NJ, Luks AM, Glenny RW. Gas exchange in the prone posture. Respir Care. 2017;62(8):1097–110.
7. Kallet RH. A comprehensive review of prone position in ARDS. Respir Care. 2015;60(11):1660–87.
8. Guerin C, Reignier J, Richard JC, Beuret P, Gacouin A, Boulain T, et al. Prone positioning in severe acute respiratory distress syndrome. N Engl J Med. 2013;368(23):2159–68.
9. Bloomfield R, Noble DW, Sudlow A. Prone position for acute respiratory failure in adults. Cochrane Database Syst Rev. 2015;(11):CD008095.
10. Jozwiak M, Teboul JL, Anguel N, Persichini R, Silva S, Chemla D, et al. Beneficial hemodynamic effects of prone positioning in patients with acute respiratory distress syndrome. Am J Respir Crit Care Med. 2013;188(12):1428–33.
11. Guervilly C, Hraiech S, Gariboldi V, Xeridat F, Dizier S, Toesca R, et al. Prone positioning during veno-venous extracorporeal membrane oxygenation for severe acute respiratory distress syndrome in adults. Minerva Anestesiol. 2014;80(3):307–13.
12. Guervilly C, Prud'homme E, Pauly V, Bourenne J, Hraiech S, Daviet F, et al. Prone positioning and extracorporeal membrane oxygenation for severe acute respiratory distress syndrome: time for a randomized trial? Intensive Care Med. 2019;45:1040.
13. Culbreth RE, Goodfellow LT. Complications of prone positioning during extracorporeal membrane oxygenation for respiratory failure: a systematic review. Respir Care. 2016;61(2):249–54.
14. Marra A, Ely EW, Pandharipande PP, Patel MB. The ABCDEF bundle in critical care. Crit Care Clin. 2017;33(2):225–43.

15. Marhong JD, DeBacker J, Viau-Lapointe J, Munshi L, Del Sorbo L, Burry L, et al. Sedation and mobilization during venovenous extracorporeal membrane oxygenation for acute respiratory failure: an international survey. Crit Care Med. 2017;45(11):1893–9.
16. Sen A, Callisen HE, Alwardt CM, Larson JS, Lowell AA, Libricz SL, et al. Adult venovenous extracorporeal membrane oxygenation for severe respiratory failure: current status and future perspectives. Ann Card Anaesth. 2016;19(1):97–111.
17. Epstein SK. How often does patient-ventilator asynchrony occur and what are the consequences? Respir Care. 2011;56(1):25–38.
18. MacIntyre NR, McConnell R, Cheng KC, Sane A. Patient-ventilator flow dyssynchrony: flow-limited versus pressure-limited breaths. Crit Care Med. 1997;25(10):1671–7.
19. EuroELSO. Chattering in ECMO Lines 2018 [cited 2018 November 17]. Available from: http://www.euroelso.net/education-and-simulation/67-chattering-lines-on-ecmo-support.html.
20. Ferreira DDC, Marcolino MAZ, Macagnan FE, Plentz RDM, Kessler A. Safety and potential benefits of physical therapy in adult patients on extracorporeal membrane oxygenation support: a systematic review. Rev Bras Ter Intensiva. 2019;31:227.
21. Eden A, Purkiss C, Cork G, Baddeley A, Morris K, Carey L, et al. In-patient physiotherapy for adults on veno-venous extracorporeal membrane oxygenation – United Kingdom ECMO Physiotherapy Network: a consensus agreement for best practice. J Intensive Care Soc. 2017;18(3):212–20.
22. HodgsonC.A pilot randomised controlled trial in Extracorporeal Membrane Oxygenation Physical Training (ECMO-PT) ClinicalTrials.gov: U.S. National Library of Medicine; 2018. Available from: https://clinicaltrials.gov/ct2/show/NCT03328767.
23. Weissman C, Kemper M, Damask MC, Askanazi J, Hyman AI, Kinney JM. Effect of routine intensive care interactions on metabolic rate. Chest. 1984;86(6):815–8.
24. Taras J, Everett T. Rapid cycle deliberate practice in medical education – a systematic review. Cureus. 2017;9(4):e1180-e.
25. Roussin CJ, Weinstock P. SimZones: an organizational innovation for simulation programs and centers. Acad Med. 2017;92(8):1114–20.
26. Needham DM, Truong AD, Fan E. Technology to enhance physical rehabilitation of critically ill patients. Crit Care Med. 2009;37(10 Suppl):S436–41.
27. Abrams D, Javidfar J, Farrand E, Mongero LB, Agerstrand CL, Ryan P, et al. Early mobilization of patients receiving extracorporeal membrane oxygenation: a retrospective cohort study. Crit Care. 2014;18(1):R38-R.
28. Catchpole KR, de Leval MR, McEwan A, Pigott N, Elliott MJ, McQuillan A, et al. Patient handover from surgery to intensive care: using Formula 1 pit-stop and aviation models to improve safety and quality. Paediatr Anaesth. 2007;17(5):470–8.
29. Colclough E, Ramsey S, Barrett P, Sheffield E, Webster J, Dean D. Mobilization of ECMO patients with various cannulation configurations. J Heart Lung Transpl. 2018;37(4):S59–60.
30. Pasrija C, Mackowick KM, Raithel M, Tran D, Boulos FM, Deatrick KB, et al. Ambulation with femoral arterial cannulation can be safely performed on venoarterial extracorporeal membrane oxygenation. Ann Thorac Surg. 2019;107(5):1389–94.
31. Abrams D, Garan AR, Brodie D. Awake and fully mobile patients on cardiac extracorporeal life support. Ann Cardiothorac Surg. 2018;8(1):44–53.
32. Rowe C. Development of clinical guidelines for prone positioning in critically ill adults. Nurs Crit Care. 2004;9(2):50–7.

The Role of Simulation in Training of ECMO Specialists

26

Paul Shuttleworth, Ozzie Jahadi, and Justin Sleasman

Learning Objectives

After reading this chapter, providers will be able to:

1. Describe the role of simulation in the training of new ECMO specialist candidates.
2. Discuss how ECMO simulation can be utilized as part of an overarching curriculum to train ECMO specialists to understand ECMO, including management and monitoring of the circuit.
3. Demonstrate how ECMO simulation can be utilized to aid ECMO specialists in the recognition of both circuit and patient emergencies, as well as critical decision-making skills around appropriate and timely interventions to address these conditions.

Introduction

Patients with severe respiratory or cardiac failure who are placed on extracorporeal membrane oxygenation require a highly trained ECMO team to manage and troubleshoot ECMO complications. Perfusionists have extensive training and experience in extracorporeal oxygenation and circulation and, as such, are optimal providers to oversee ECMO support. However, given the recent increase in the number of centers providing ECMO, there has been a surge in demand for perfusionists which has resulted in a shortage [1]. This imbalance has driven a change in how ECMO circuits are staffed at some institutions. By developing a comprehensive training program, other qualified hospital staff (including respiratory therapists or registered nurses) can be trained as ECMO "specialists" to assist in filling this gap.

This chapter will illustrate the approach used by one institution as a guide for the selection, initial training, and continuous education for ECMO specialists to ensure that they are able to effectively manage ECMO runs and troubleshoot issues related to patient-ECMO interactions. To make this a successful and safe resource backfill program, extensive training is required to prepare an individual to anticipate and detect possible complications with the ECMO circuit. Current training typically heavily leverages scenario-based simulation drills and bedside debriefings which have been shown to be highly beneficial [2]. Through training in a controlled environment with proper guidance from an experienced team of experts, specialists can be prepared to react quickly and effectively to real-life emergencies.

Utilization of ECMO Simulation Technology to Assist Learning of the ECMO Specialist

Extracorporeal membrane oxygenation (ECMO) remains a complex treatment modality that requires intensive initial training and ongoing education to ensure optimal patient safety and outcomes. The Extracorporeal Life Support Organization (ELSO) provides guidelines for designing training and education programs for ECMO specialists, including didactic courses, water drills, animal laboratory sessions (if possible), and bedside training [3]. Further information on the current training recommendations for ECMO providers can be found in Chap. 12. Given the increasing availability of medical simulation, this modality has been rapidly incorporated into the training of ECMO providers and teams. Multiple authors have described a systematic approach to increasing complexity of training by starting with water drills and progressing toward simulation-based training to incorporate patient-related issues [4–9]. This is

P. Shuttleworth · O. Jahadi
Lucile Packard Children's Hospital, Palo Alto, CA, USA
e-mail: PShuttleworth@stanfordchildrens.org; OJahadi@stanfordchildrens.org

J. Sleasman (✉)
Lucile Packard Children's Hospital, Betty Irene Moore Children's Heart Center, Palo Alto, CA, USA
e-mail: JSleasman@stanfordchildrens.org

L. C. Johnston, L. Su (eds.), *Comprehensive Healthcare Simulation: ECMO Simulation*, Comprehensive Healthcare Simulation,
https://doi.org/10.1007/978-3-030-53844-6_26

particularly relevant to ECMO specialists, as their scope of practice requires them to urgently manage and address circuit-related issues. Water and circuit drills begin the process of preparing the specialist. By following this with simulation-based training, providers can experience activities that require deductive reasoning and problem solving in an environment that can incorporate real-life distractions and interaction with other members of the native interprofessional care team to facilitate development of teamwork and communication skills.

Before being assigned to work in the clinical environment, it is critical for ECMO specialists to develop a comprehensive knowledge of the ECMO platform and circuit, including how the components relate to each other and to the patient [10]. Therefore, following initial learning, there must be opportunities for hands-on practice with situations that will require the specialist to intervene. These interventions might involve component change-outs and de-airing, as well as problem solving, diagnosis, and treatment. Simulation will ensure each learner has the experience to manage both routine and emergency situations that may arise in the clinical setting. As the training process evolves, the learner is given additional opportunities to apply their advancing knowledge and skills to cases of increasing complexity in an environment that may be manipulated to incorporate real-life stressors. Exposure to concepts of crisis resource management and troubleshooting can be increased as the learning progresses, with the ultimate goal of presenting an environment that provides practice of clinical events in an environment that closely mimics a real clinical bedside experience. By structuring training in this manner, educators can assist learners in the process of establishing and maintaining competency as an ECMO specialist.

One way to conceptualize the stages of hands-on/technical training (water drills) and simulation-based training for ECMO specialists is to utilize the concept of SimZones, which is described in detail in Chap. 4. Application of this model to education for an ECMO specialist is presented below.

Zone 0 presents basic skills that a learner needs to master. Ideally, a prerequisite to starting hands-on/technical training should be successful completion of a learning assessment that assures understanding of basic concepts presented in didactic sessions. Although many of these topics are covered in didactic sessions, it is important to provide the learner with dedicated time to visualize and manipulate the circuit. This zone is best conducted individually (through self-study) or in very small groups.

In Zone 1, small groups of specialists are provided with opportunities to practice skills with a functioning circuit that combine cognitive and psychomotor tasks to enhance learning. Ideally, ECMO specialists and interprofessional team members should complete hands-on training sessions related to all critical topics in the curriculum. Functional understanding of resources is introduced by adding further challenges regarding clinical components and resource utilization to the learning exercises.

In Zone 2, scenario-based learning activities are developed to facilitate knowledge growth. Focus areas may include topics such as identification of the need for circuit change, or location and acquisition of necessary supplies and equipment to treat circuit emergencies. In this stage, additional visual cues may be introduced, such as patient monitors and equipment. One monitor may be used to provide the patient history and complete the clinical setting with important data. An additional monitor may be used to mimic the patient dynamics and can incorporate patient data from simulation software. Alternatively, a computer monitor, tablet, or printed image can be utilized to present "screen shots" of patient vital signs. The session will be most useful if the vital signs can be altered in real time with changes in patient status or resulting from learner interventions. Additional monitors or images may be used to mimic the inline blood gas sensor on the ECMO circuit or to provide a screen for laboratory results (Fig. 26.1). Once the scenario is written, the information flow from the monitors is choreographed to provide important facts of the scenario in a realistic manner throughout the progression of the case. More advanced learners may benefit from increasing scenario difficulty. The environment should be realistic, and during scenarios in this zone, participants will continue through the case without interruption, followed by debriefing after the conclusion of the simulation. A list of possible tasks relevant to Zone 2 is included in Box 26.1.

Zone 3 simulations involve members from all disciplines and include technology to create an artificial representation of real-world situations that amplifies experiences in a fully interactive fashion [11]. During these scenarios, the team members are presented with an unanticipated event and must respond as they would in a clinical situation, utilizing institutional protocols and unit processes. The simulation is set up to utilize each member's education and skill set. Sessions should ideally incorporate interprofessional interactions which allow teams to practice non-technical skills, including team behavior, communication, situational awareness, and resource utilization. This allows for the creation of a realistic clinical setting which incorporates many environmental distractions (i.e., alarms, conversations, and noise), but without risk to patients. Many of the scenarios incorporate events that are low frequency and high risk. Zone 3 scenarios are designed to elicit authentic behaviors and promote collaboration among multidisciplinary team members [5]. Once the simulation begins, it should proceed with very little to no external instructor intervention. The interventions, conversations, interactions of players, and the resultant effect of these actions should drive the outcomes. As learners progress from

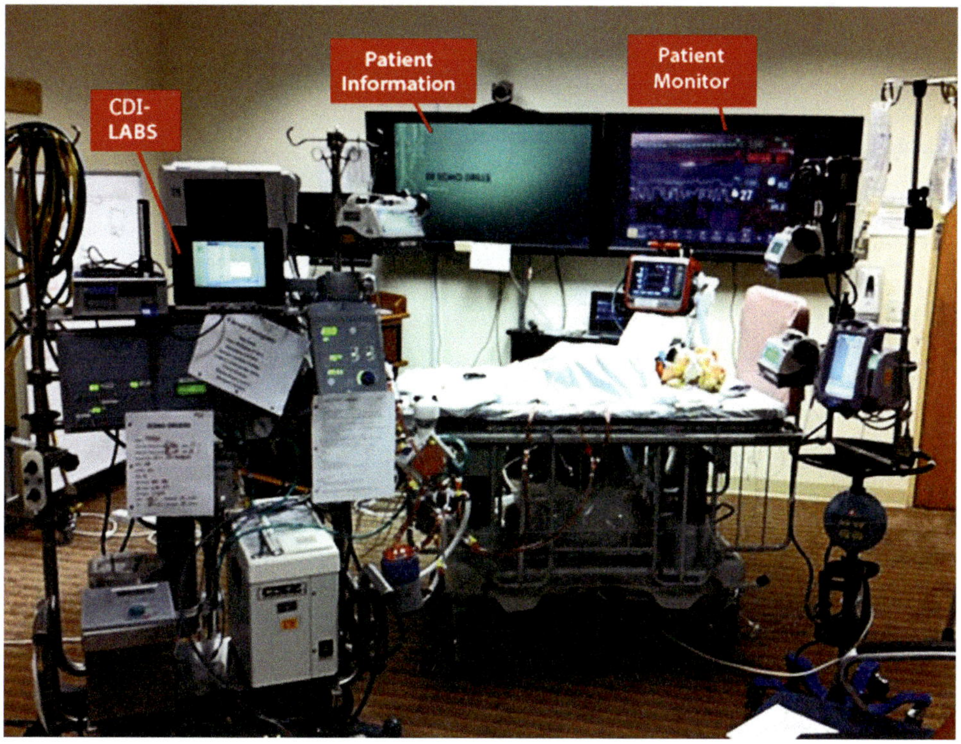

Fig. 26.1 Example ECMO simulation setting with various monitoring displays included and labeled

Box 26.1 Example of Scenarios Relevant for SimZones Zone 2

1. Circuit preload volume deficiencies (low volume status of the patient, poor venous cannula position, kink in the venous tubing, etc.)
2. Circuit afterload resistance
3. Air maneuvers
4. Other examples:
   - Circuit assessment and troubleshooting
   - Drawing circuit gases and flushing pigtails
   - Component change-out
   - Circuit change-out
   - Mechanical problems: Cannula dislodgement and power outage
   - Intrahospital transport (to cath lab/CT/OR)
   - Interhospital transport (via ambulance, helicopter, or fixed-wing)

Zone 0 to Zone 3, the presence of noise or other distractions increases to improve fidelity and further replicate the real-world clinical environment. Team interaction and opportunities for learning occur in post-scenario debriefing sessions. See Table 26.1 for a summary of the SimZones as relevant to the training of ECMO specialists as an integral part of an institutional ECMO team.

SimZones are used to provide a framework to increase the complexity of scenarios in a step-wise fashion, as well as to incorporate all members of the native multidisciplinary treatment team. Norman et al. defined "fidelity" as the extent to which the appearance and behavior of the simulator/simulation match the appearance and behavior of the simulated system [12]. High fidelity does not necessarily imply high technology. Appropriate fidelity can be obtained with low technology depending on the learning objectives. Low-technology simulation allows the learner to develop basic skills that can be built upon to develop complex skills and mental competency [13]. It is mandatory to first master basic skills in order to progress to more difficult scenarios which may be better suited to high-fidelity training. This will combine the patient-ECMO system and full-scale simulation that incorporates stressful unexpected and unplanned events. Management of these simulated cases requires clinical reasoning to identify and enact appropriate interventions, as well as to provide practice that builds confidence in managing ECMO support.

ECMO Specialist Training

From the minute it's decided that a patient should be placed on ECMO, the ECMO specialist and other ECMO team members' responsibility has begun. Selection of right circuit, cannula size, priming medications, and necessary blood products are all within the scope of an ECMO specialist's duty. The requirements to become an ECMO specialist vary across different centers.As an example at one institution, a

Table 26.1 Overview of potential application of the SimZones approach as relevant to the training of ECMO specialists as integral members of an institutional ECMO team

Zone	Objective	Equipment needed	Skills
Zone 0	Understanding of: Circuit configuration Essential equipment Blood path Dexterity skills for circuit repairs Alarms and their purpose Circuit checklists (a) Shift handoff (b) Start of shift checklist (c) Circuit check	ECMO circuit components (a) Tubing set (b) Oxygenator (c) Pump (d) Heater ECMO circuit accessories (a) Connectors (b) Tubing segments (c) Stopcocks (d) Pigtails (e) Transducers ECMO platform (a) Pump (b) Heater (c) Blender	Demonstration of: (a) Connector change-out (b) Tubing applied to connectors (c) Changing of pigtails (d) Safe sampling techniques (e) Stopcock operation (f) Alarm reset (g) Equipment operation
Zone 1	Understanding of: ECMO specialist role Specialist actions when completing checklists Actions required to address circuit events	In addition to Zone 0 Patient monitor Simulation software and equipment	Air evacuation Changing of stopcocks Interpretation of pressure sensors Flow changes and diagnosis of the problem Re-establishing flow after corrections are carried out
Zone 2	Enhance learning Build on techniques and skills in Zone 0 and 1 Utilize protocol-driven activities Addition of unanticipated events Incorporation of team member interaction Role designation	Same as Zone 0 and 1	Incorporation of team events Team treatment of unanticipated events Equipment troubleshooting and failure, with team approach to stabilize condition
Zone 3	Enhance Teamwork Building of skills Communication Critical thinking Confidence Maintain effective treatment with increased distractors	Addition of: Environmental realism Identical room layout and equipment Ventilator Infusion pumps Multidisciplinary teams (eliminate role-playing)	Navigate teamwork elements Manage parent involvement during unexpected event Demonstrate communication during difficult event and distractors

provider seeking to become an ECMO specialist must be a senior registered nurse with at least 3 years of ICU experience and CRRT proficiency. A rigorous training and certification program must exist to ensure ECMO specialists are knowledgeable and experienced in all aspects of the ECMO circuit components and potential complications, as well as relevant changes in patient condition [14]. The ECMO specialist oversees the constant care of the ECMO circuit by performing safety checks on each shift, while keeping a close watch on circuit function and monitoring patient parameters to anticipate and avoid ECMO-related emergencies. Protocols and guidelines which assist in the standardization of care should be instituted and made readily available on the hospital portal to all ECMO team members. A well-developed and enforced competency-based certification program can help to uphold high patient care standards through the use of effective theoretical teachings, water drills, and other scenario-based ECMO activities. ECMO specialists are trained to detect ECMO pitfalls from the most common events, such as venous chatter, to rare situations, such as Harlequin syndrome (differential hypoxia).

Just as the requirements to become an ECMO specialist may vary across institutions, the local training curricula and performance requirements may also differ. For the purposes of this chapter, we will review the training requirements at a single center, where ECMO specialist training consists of five phases:

- Phase I: 12 hours of didactic lectures with a multidisciplinary team of experts to cover fundamental concepts
- Phase II: 4 hours of hands-on small-group wet lab and ECMO emergency drills
- Phase III: 12 hours of proctoring on each circuit with an experienced ECMO specialist

- Phase IV: Testing and certification, including a comprehensive examination (consisting of both written online and oral components) to assess understanding of the circuit, management, and potential emergencies
- Phase V: Continued education and emergency drills twice a year

Phase I: 12 Hours of Didactics

The first phase in ECMO specialist training is to set a solid foundation. The curriculum should be designed to increase the trainee's level of knowledge and awareness about multiple topics, including patient selection for ECMO, analyzing indication and contraindication metrics, as well as ECMO management (considering differences between various modes of support). ECMO specialists are taught to understand interaction between patient conditions and ECMO circuit parameters, including anticipation of and proper reaction to circuit emergencies that may arise. Lectures covering these topics may be given by members of a multidisciplinary team of subject matter experts, including but not limited to physicians, nurses, and perfusionists, who jointly define the course content while following ELSO's ECMO Specialist Training Manual as a source of guidance [3]. A representative sample of the topics covered is provided in Box 26.2. As part of training, actual clinical scenario discussions may be incorporated, allowing learners to think through the encountered problems and complications and come up with proposed resolutions. The goal of this exercise is to link the didactic section to applied knowledge. Time can be allotted between Phase I and Phase II to provide candidates a chance to review, self-study, and reflect upon the material. A reference guide and contact with subject matter experts may be provided.

Box 26.2 Example Didactic Course Lecture Outline from One Institution

1. "What Is ECMO: An Introduction to ECMO" by clinical perfusionist
2. "Management of Pediatric Illnesses & Cardiac Diseases Treated with ECMO" by CVICU cardiologist
3. "VA ECMO Physiology and Patient Management" by PICU intensivist
4. "SVO_2: Supply/Demand" by CVICU cardiologist
5. "VA ECMO Scenarios & VV ECMO Scenarios" jointly by PICU intensivist/clinical perfusionist
6. "End Organ Support" by CVICU cardiologist
7. "Technical Aspects of Cannulation" by cardiovascular surgeon
8. "Anticoagulation for ECMO/Blood Products Required During ECMO" by CVICU cardiologist
9. "Initiation of ECMO (Elective & Emergent)" by clinical perfusionist
10. "CVVH-Prisma/Hemofilter/CDI" by RN ECMO specialist
11. "Circuit Equipment Management" by clinical perfusionist
12. "Transporting on ECMO" by clinical perfusionist
13. "Nursing Care of the ECMO Circuit" by RN ECMO specialist
14. "Weaning" jointly by PICU intensivist/RN ECMO specialist
15. "Trialing Off" Jointly by PICU intensivist/clinical perfusionist
16. "Decannulation Process" Jointly by PICU intensivist/clinical perfusionist
17. "Complications" Jointly by PICU intensivist/clinical perfusionist
18. "Epic/Ordersets" by RN ECMO specialist

Phase II: 4 Hours of Hands on Wet Drills

The second part of training at our example institution includes hands-on scenario-based simulations and water drills. Trainees may be divided into smaller groups of 2–4 individuals, which allows the educators to deliver targeted training and focus on each individual's needs. The main purpose of this section is to familiarize learners with different components of circuits. Instructors should discuss in more detail the functionality and failure modes of each part of the ECMO pumps and circuits that may be involved in a circuit emergency [15]. To confirm understanding, standardized scenario-based drills can be presented to the trainees. Some of the key pitfalls and emergencies in the scenarios are listed below in Box 26.3:

Phase III: 12 Hours of Proctoring

In our example center, following the scenario discussion and hands-on drills, each trainee spends an additional 12 hours on each circuit with an experienced ECMO specialist for bedside education. An ECMO proctoring checklist can be created for each circuit. Educators should focus on every item on the checklist to ensure trainees have a solid understanding of the circuit monitoring and troubleshooting. Pairing of experienced proctors and trainee ECMO specialists allows them to become more acquainted with each other as team members. This close collaboration and partnership is key in future patient safety and quick troubleshooting.

Box 26.3 Potential Topics for Inclusion in Wet Drill

- Pump failure
- Power failure
- Mechanical failure
- Jammed race way
- Malfunctioning motor
- Circuit issues
- Pressures and transducers
- Kinked tubing
- Clots
- Oxygenator failure
- Cannula size and position
- Patient issues
- Preload and afterload
- Tamponade
- Bleeding and clotting

Phase IV: Testing and Certification

An assessment, either written or verbal, should be utilized to measure trainee's understanding of their responsibilities during ECMO management, including a code event. The test should evaluate the learner's knowledge of patient indications, ECMO types, circuit components, and specifications. Trainees are also tested on their ability to understand and differentiate patient and circuit interactions that may cause complications. A minimum passing score should be determined for institutional certification.

Assessment may also include a simulation-based performance assessment to evaluate hands-on troubleshooting skills.

After certification, new trainees may still be paired with and supervised by an experienced ECMO specialist or perfusionist until an adequate level of comfort is achieved. This shadowing opportunity exists not only to answer any remaining questions but also to ensure their initial ECMO experiences are positive and stress-free, allowing them to provide the best care for patients on ECLS support.

Phase V: Continuing Education

To maintain competency, ECMO specialists are required to participate in on-going education. At one example center, this curriculum includes the following activities:

- Manage an ECMO circuit for a period of at least 12 hours/quarter.
- Attend 2 hours of quarterly ECMO meetings where the following topics may be addressed:
  - Review of last-quarter ECMO runs
  - Review of new changes to ECMO guidelines
  - ECMO-related presentations
  - Team building activities
  - Case reviews
- Attend 2 ECMO high-fidelity emergency drills/year.
- Scenarios may include:
  - Air emergency
  - Recirculation on VV
  - Clotted circuit
  - Anticoagulation and bleeding
  - Pump failure
    Mechanical
    Power
  - Patient decompensation or circuit status change

During these sessions, multidisciplinary participants play their role and work as a team to solve problems. Simulation-based training improves patient safety and allows ECMO team members to gain experience without needing to practice on patients [16]. Participants troubleshoot the emergency-related issues and the case is debriefed by the group.

Advancement of Simulation for Training of ECMO Specialists

Organizing an ECMO simulation program is a complex endeavor. No two ECMO programs are alike, but commonalities do exist. A perfusionist, nurse, or respiratory therapist typically has the experience and knowledge base to serve as the ECMO program coordinator. This position has the complex task of being the link between the hospital administrators, surgical and ICU medical leadership, and the numerous specialists required to staff and respond to emergencies. Repetitive institutional dress rehearsals using high-fidelity simulation may offer clarity regarding personnel and role division when applying ECLS in the patient setting. Beyond navigating personnel and the team's development, the ECMO coordinator may also participate in choosing necessary circuitry and following best practice techniques (ELSO database) in applying appropriate ECLS technology [17].

Technology

ELSO data has shown a surge in ECMO programs and overall volume over the last decade (Fig. 26.2). This increased use has served as a catalyst for advances in ECMO simulators, manikins, and the equipment needed to amplify realism and fidelity. Although multiple centers perform less than ten ECMO runs annually, having a robust simulation program will help to maintain the team's ECLS skills between potential pauses of weeks to months between ECMO patients at

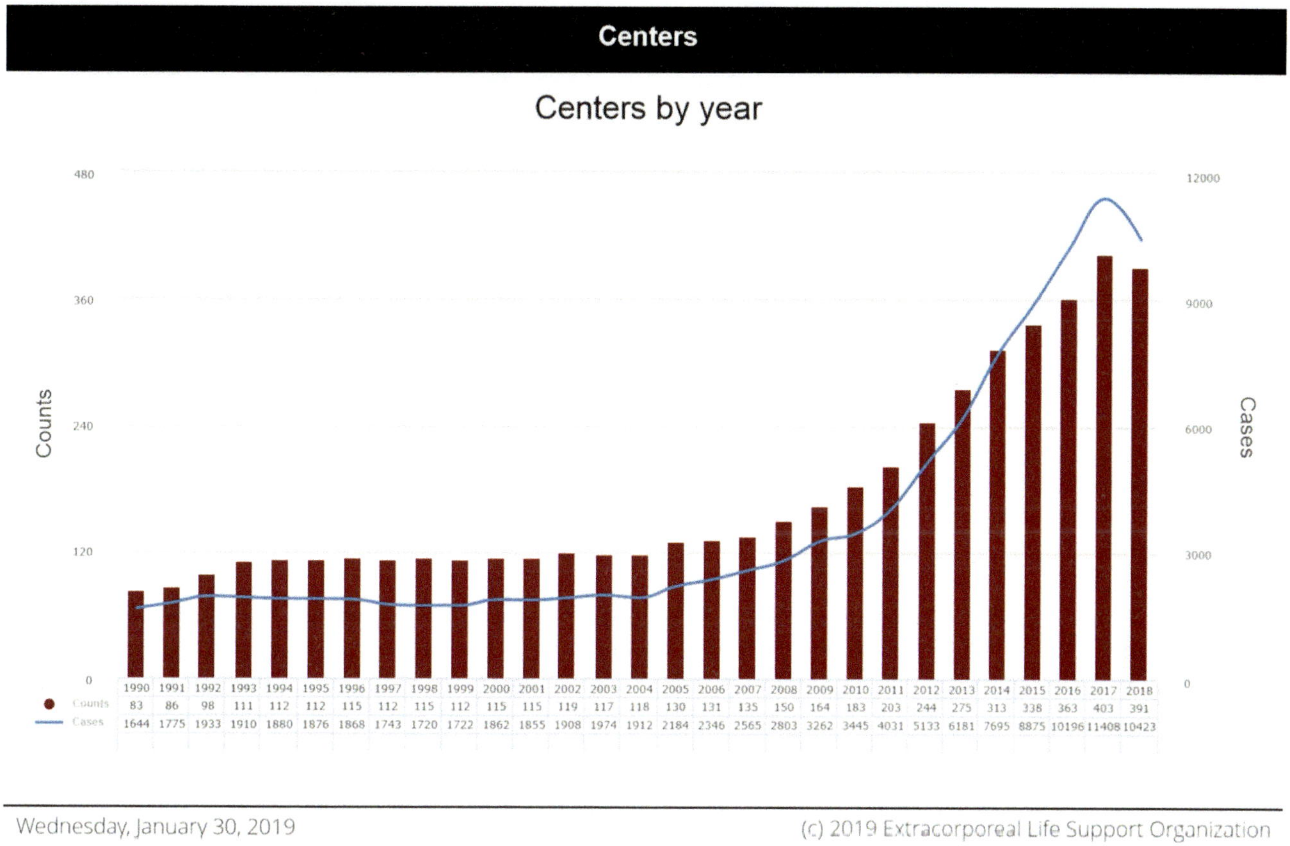

Fig. 26.2 ELSO Registry International Report (January 2019) demonstrating increasing number of ECMO centers and increased case volume. (Reproduced with permission of ELSO)

their institution. Simulators originally invented for training perfusionists in the operating room setting for cardiopulmonary bypass can be modified to allow for high-fidelity ECMO simulation.

The Orpheus Perfusion Simulator (Ulco Technologies, Marrickville, NSW, Australia) has been used by perfusion and ECMO teams alike for high-fidelity training [18]. Landsdowne and colleagues describe the necessary steps needed to adapt the Orpheus System from an open cardiopulmonary simulation system to a closed-loop ECLS option. The Califia 3.0 high-fidelity bypass simulator (Biomed Simulation Inc., San Diego, CA) is another extensively used platform. This system was originally devised for the operating room and is also utilized by multiple certified clinical perfusionist training programs.

Currently, both platforms can be incorporated into ECMO programs to increase realism and enhance clinical decision-making. Along with Orpheus, the Califia 3.0 can be adapted to accommodate all hospital-chosen bypass and ECMO disposable configurations. The Califia 3.0 uses an instructor panel to make changes in system and patient parameters that are viewable on the student panel. Lastly, EigenFlow (Curtis Life Research, Indianapolis, IN) is another simulator option that can be easily adapted to an institution's disposable ECLS circuitry to produce common ECMO complications such as hypovolemia, thrombus, and air emergencies. The EigenFlow uses a wireless iOS platform enabling instructors to alter the circuit from a distance, again, enhancing the realism of the scenario. Each of these companies offers in house demos of their respective product. This provides an opportunity to see if a dedicated ECMO simulator would enhance the ECLS program and, if so, allows the team to determine which option best fits the program's specific needs.

Advancement in manikin technology is another welcome addition to ECMO simulation. Laerdal Medical (Wappingers Falls, NY) and Gaumard Scientific (Miami, FL) are two leaders in advance life support education. Both companies provide tetherless manikins that allow for airway and blood pressure management, adding realism and creating the decision tree of ECLS. Manikin settings can dictate the specific need for ECMO, veno-venous vs. veno-arterial, as well as enhance audience participation. Manikins aid in delineating the roles of the staff supporting the "patient" versus those involved with circuit preparation. As of now, the challenge is the inability to cannulate the manikin, which would allow for real-time alteration in pump parameters translated to manikin physiology.

Cost

Budget considerations are a necessary factor in developing an ECMO simulation program. Centers are devising low-cost techniques to enhance high-fidelity simulation. Disi et al. recently published the application of 3D printing circuit components to cut down on disposable costs [19]. In the same article, the team described the use of ink to differentiate between oxygenated and deoxygenated blood within the ECMO circuit pathway. Expired circuit components such as oxygenators, tubing, and cannulas should be considered for use in simulation if needed to reduce cost.

Environment and Equipment

ECMO, especially ECPR, takes place in various environments within the hospital. In situ ECMO training is just as vital as the technology used to create a worthwhile high-fidelity simulation scenario. The typical locations of ECMO deployment are the operating room, catheterization lab, various intensive care units, and the emergency department. Conducting a high-fidelity simulation in each of these environments benefits the team in fully understanding the capabilities and limitations of their surroundings for process improvement during a true patient ECMO initiation. How quickly a team can get a patient on ECMO has a statistically significant impact on the survival of that patient [20]. Furthermore, there is research showing that the implementation of an ECMO simulation program shortens the length of ECPR resuscitation times [21].

The exact environment will change, but items to incorporate and supplies to bring can be standardized. When practicing in situ high-fidelity ECMO simulation, the first item to check is the power and gas supply of the environment. Each important asset needs to be addressed. Do the outlets in the room have ability to power the ECMO base, heater cooler, and ancillary equipment needed to perform quality ECLS support without an electrical overload? Does the room have the appropriate air and oxygen connectors that are compatible with the ECMO circuit? Does one need to bring air and oxygen splitters to accommodate a shared space with anesthesia or respiratory therapy? Are circuit prime drugs and blood product usage standardized for consistency between specialists? O negative blood should be readily available and the ECMO prime drug kit should be created. Are the correct cannulas and connectors ready for the physician? A cannula legend, kg body weight, should be agreed upon to minimize confusion and increase efficiency (Fig. 26.3).

Lastly, an ECMO mobile case cart should be prepared ahead of time with the necessary surgical tools, Bovie, and headlamps. To minimize the "beehive effect" of unnecessary help, simulation generates an opportunity to create a map of who needs to be in the room and the responsibility of each functional team member (Fig. 26.4). All team members responding to a true ECLS emergency should have a clear understanding of their specific role and physical location within the environment prior to initiation.

Debriefing at the end of each simulation is a vital activity for individual and overall team improvement [22]. Scheduling ample time at the conclusion of simulation facilitates open discussion allowing each participant to discuss hurdles faced and explore solutions.

Circuit-Centered Emergency Scenarios

It has been said cardiopulmonary bypass and extracorporeal membrane oxygenation draw many similarities to the aviation industry. The majority of incidents happen on "take-off" (initiation of ECMO) and "landing" (wean and decannulation) [23]. For this reason, the multidisciplinary team approach again is useful during these two critical events. The common acute emergencies typically fall under air entrainment, clot formation, bleeding, human error, and mechanical failure [24]. ECMO centers should have multiple high-fidelity simulation scenarios created to enhance learning and challenge participants. Scenarios should be continually updated to focus on real patient institutional events in an effort to eradicate human error and improve the efficiency in response to unforeseen clinical emergencies.

Team-Based Approach

Multidisciplinary involvement and buy-in from all team members are the greatest determinants of effective ECMO simulation [25]. Accountability measures, enforced by the ECMO coordinator, need to be in place to ensure ECMO team member attendance. Participants may sign up based on role or specialty, using readily available software such as SignUpGenius (www.signupgenius.com). This is not an exclusive list, but surgeons, cardiologists, intensivists, neonatologists, pharmacists, registered nurses, respiratory therapists, perfusionists, and simulation facilitators are likely candidates to bring fresh perspectives to achieve the ultimate goal of providing quality extracorporeal life support from initiation to decannulation and beyond.

ECPR VA **General Guideline to Cannulation**

Patient Weight	Neck		Groin		Chest		Connector
	Venous	Arterial	Venous Femoral	Arterial Femoral	Venous	Arterial	
≤ 2kg	10 Ven BioMedicus	8 Art Edwards Or Biomedicus	-	-	14 DLP	8 DLP	1/4"
2-2.9 kg	10 Ven BioMedicus	8 Art Edwards Or Biomedicus	-	-	16 DLP	8 DLP	1/4"
3-3.9 kg	12 Ven BioMedicus	8 Art Edwards Or Biomedicus	-	-	16 DLP	10 DLP	1/4"
4-4.9 kg	12 Ven BioMedicus	10 Art Edwards Or Biomedicus	-	-	16 DLP	10 DLP	1/4"
5-5.9 kg	14 Ven BioMedicus	10 Art Edwards Or Biomedicus	-	-	18 DLP	12 DLP	1/4"
6-6.9 kg	14 Ven BioMedicus	10 Art Edwards Or Biomedicus	-	-	18 DLP	12 DLP	1/4"
7-7.9 kg	14 Ven BioMedicus	12 Art Edwards Or Biomedicus	-	-	18 DLP	12 DLP	1/4"
8-8.9 kg	14 Ven BioMedicus	12 Art Edwards Or Biomedicus	-	-	18 DLP	12 DLP	1/4"
9-9.9 kg	14 Ven BioMedicus	12 Art Edwards Or Biomedicus	-	-	18 DLP	12 DLP	1/4"
10-12 kg	14 Ven BioMedicus	12 Art Edwards Or Biomedicus	15 Ven BioMedicus	12 Art Edwards Or Biomedicus	18 DLP	12 DLP	1/4"
13-14 kg	15 Art BioMedicus	14 Art Edwards Or Biomedicus	15 Ven BioMedicus	14 Art Edwards Or Biomedicus	20 DLP	14 DLP	1/4"
15-16 kg	17 Art BioMedicus	14 Art Edwards Or Biomedicus	17 Ven BioMedicus	14 Art Edwards Or Biomedicus	22 DLP	14 DLP	3/8"
17-18 kg	19 Art BioMedicus	15 Art BioMedicus	19 Ven BioMedicus	15 Art BioMedicus	22 DLP	14 DLP	1/4" or 3/8"
19-20 kg	19 Art BioMedicus	15 Art BioMedicus	19 Ven BioMedicus	15 Art BioMedicus	24 DLP	16 DLP	3/8"
21-25 kg	19 Art BioMedicus	15 Art BioMedicus	19 Ven BioMedicus	15 Art BioMedicus	24 DLP	16 DLP	3/8"
26-30 kg	21 Art BioMedicus	15 Art BioMedicus	21 Ven BioMedicus	15 Art BioMedicus	24 DLP	16 DLP	3/8"
31-35 kg	21 Art BioMedicus	15 Art BioMedicus	21 Ven BioMedicus	15 Art BioMedicus	24 DLP	16 DLP	3/8" or 1/2"
36-40 kg	21 Art BioMedicus	17 Art BioMedicus	23 Ven BioMedicus	17Art BioMedicus	28 DLP	16 DLP	3/8" or 1/2"
41-45 kg	23 Art BioMedicus	19 Art BioMedicus	25 Ven BioMedicus	19 Art BioMedicus	28 DLP	16 DLP	3/8" or 1/2"
46-50 kg	23 Art BioMedicus	19 Art BioMedicus	25 Ven BioMedicus	19 Art BioMedicus	28 DLP	18 DLP	3/8" or 1/2"
51-60 kg	23 Art BioMedicus	19 Art BioMedicus	27 Ven BioMedicus	19 Art BioMedicus	30 DLP	18 DLP	3/8" or 1/2"
61-65 kg	23 Art BioMedicus	21 Art BioMedicus	27 Ven BioMedicus	21 Art BioMedicus	30 DLP	20 DLP	3/8" or 1/2"
66-70 kg	23 Art BioMedicus	21 Art BioMedicus	27 Ven BioMedicus	21 Art BioMedicus	30 DLP	20 DLP	3/8" or 1/2"
≥ 70 kg	23 Art BioMedicus	21 Art BioMedicus	27 Ven BioMedicus	23 Art Biomedicus	30 DLP	20 DLP	3/8" or 1/2"

(yellow)	Forest-Squirrel Eqpmt Storage & ECPR Cart
(green)	ONLY 6th & 5th Flr Forest-Squirrel Eqpmt Storage (FA6.112, FA5.112)
(red)	ONLY ECPR Cart

Recommended "Full" Flow	
≤ 7 kg	120-200mL/kg/min
7-10 kg	100-150mL/kg/min
10- 20 kg	80-120 mL/kg/min
20- 25 kg	100 mL/kg/min
≥ 25 kg	80 mL/kg/min

Updated: Aug-18

Fig. 26.3 Example guideline to cannulation. (Reproduced with permission of Seattle Children's Hospital)

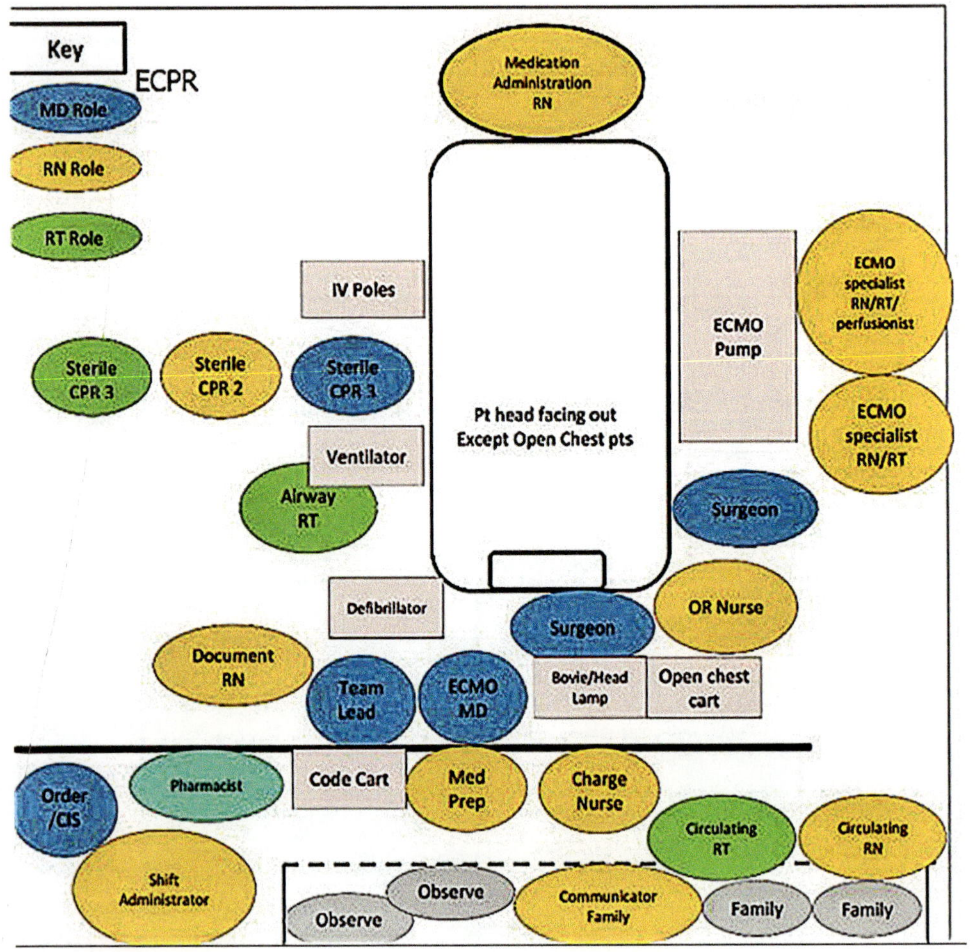

Fig. 26.4 Example of team map for ECPR. (Reproduced with permission of Seattle Children's Hospital)

Conclusion

In conclusion, the ECMO specialist is an integral member of any multidisciplinary ECMO team. When used as part of an institutional training paradigm, simulation can enhance understanding of not only the cognitive and technical aspects of ECMO, but equally important, it can be instrumental in enhancing the teamwork and communication among multidisciplinary providers [26]. In this way, team members can partner together to optimize care of patients requiring ECMO support.

References

1. Ratnani I, Tuazon D, Zainab A, Uddin F. The role and impact of extracorporeal membrane oxygenation in critical care. Methodist Debakey Cardiovasc J. 2018;14(2):110–9. https://doi.org/10.14797/mdcj-14-2-110.
2. Weems MF, Friedlich PS, Nelson LP, Rake AJ, Klee L, Stein JE, et al. The role of extracorporeal membrane oxygenation simulation training at extracorporeal life support organization centers in the United States. Simul Healthcare. 2017;12(4):233–9.
3. ELSO guidelines for training and continuing education of ECMO specialists. 2017. http://www.elso.med.umich.edu/guide.html. Accessed Mar 2017.
4. Chan SY, Figueroa M, Spentzas T, et al. Prospective assessment of novice learners in a simulation-based extracorporeal membrane oxygenation (ECMO) education program. Pediatr Cardiol. 2013;34:543–52.
5. Sakamoto S. Simulation-based training for handling extracorporeal membrane oxygenation emergencies. J Thorac Dis. 2017;9:3649–51.
6. Ogino MT, Froehlich CD, Moore EA. Education and training. In: Brogan TV, Lequier L, Lorusso R, et al., editors. Extracorporeal life support: the ELSO red book. 5th ed. Ann Arbor: ELSO; 2017.
7. Banfi C, Bendjelid K, Giraud R. High-fidelity simulation for extracorporeal membrane oxygenation training, utile or futile? J Thorac Dis. 2017;9:4283–5.
8. Nardo D, et al. Simulation training of ECMO emergencies. J Thorac Dis. 2018;10(6):3409–17.
9. Short BL, Williams L, editors. ECMO specialist training manual. 3rd ed. Michigan: Extracorporeal Life Support Organization; 2010.
10. Brum R, Rajani R, Gelandt E, Morgan L, Raguseelan N, Butt S, et al. Simulation training for extracorporeal membrane oxygenation. Ann Card Anaesth. 2015;18:185–90.
11. Weatherspoon DL, Wyatt TH. Testing computer-based simulation to enjance clinical judgment skills in senior nursing students. Nurs Clin N Am. 2012;46:481–91.
12. Norman G, Muzzin L, Williams R, Swanson D. Simulation in health sciences education. J Instr Dev. 1985;8(1):11–7.

13. Gaba D. The future vision of simulation in health care. Quality Saf Health Care. 2004;13(Suppl 1):2–10.
14. Donaldson L. Safer medical practice: machines, manikins and polo mints, 150 years of the annual report of the chief medical officer: on the state of the public health 2008. London: Department of Health; 2009. p. 49–55.
15. Anderson JM, Boyle KB, Murphy AA, Yaeger KA, LeFlore J, Halamek LP. Simulating extracorporeal membrane oxygenation emergencies to improve human performance. Part I: methodologic and technologic innovations. Simul Healthc. 2006;1:220–7.
16. Gaba D, DeAnda A. A comprehensive anesthesia simulation environment: re-creating the operating room for research and training. Anesthesiology. 1988;69(3):387–94.
17. Yalon L, Sleasman J. ECPR drills and simulation presentation. In: 29th annual ELSO conference. Scottsdale; 2018.
18. Lansdowne W, Machin D, Grant DJ. Development of the orpheus perfusion simulator for use in high-fidelity extracorporeal membrane oxygenation simulation. J Extra Corpor Technol. 2012;44(4):250–5.
19. Al Disi M, Alsalemi A, Alhomsi Y, Bensaali F, Amira A, Alinier G. Revolutionizing ECMO simulation with affordable yet high-Fidelity technology. Am J Emerg Med. 2018;36(7):1310–2.
20. Chen YS, Lin JW, Yu HY, et al. Cardiopulmonary resuscitation with assisted extracorporeal life support versus conventional cardiopulmonary resuscitation in adults with in-hospital cardiac arrest: an observational study and propensity analysis. Lancet. 2008;372:554–61.
21. Su L, Spaeder MC, Jones MB, et al. Implementation of an extracorporeal cardiopulmonary resuscitation simulation program reduces extracorporeal cardiopulmonary resuscitation times in real patients. Pediatr Crit Care Med. 2014;15(9):856–60.
22. Roussin CJ, Weinstock P. SimZones: an organizational innovation for simulation programs and centers. Acad Med. 2017;92(8):1114–20.
23. Statistical summary of commercial jet airplane accidents. 2018. https://www.boeing.com/resources/boeingdotcom/company/about/bca/pdf/statsum.pdf.
24. Puślecki M, Kiel M, Ligowski M, Dąbrowski M, Stefaniak S, Gąsiorowski Ł, Dąbrowska A, Kłosiewicz T, Sip M, Telec W, Karczewski M, Ziemak P, Perek B, Ładzińska M, Misterski M, Urbanowicz T, Stachowiak W, Buczkowski P, Czekajlo M. Prototype of high-fidelity ECMO simulator. Eur J Heart Fail. 2017;19:58–67.
25. Sharma A. From evidence to implementation: introducing neonatal simulation to a tertiary. Open J Pediatr. 2013;3(1):10–6.
26. Anderson JM, Murphy AA, Boyle KB, Yeager KA, Halamek LP. Simulating extracorporeal membrane oxygenation emergencies to improve human performance. Part II: assessment of technical and behavioral skills. Simul Healthc. 2006;1:228–32.

Part VII

Practical Guide

A Practical and Pictorial Guide for Creating ECMO Simulation

27

Loren D. Sacks

Learning Objectives
After reading this chapter, readers will be able to:
1. Define different categories of ECMO simulation and to predict the resources needed as they prepare scenarios.
2. Prepare, set up, and lead standard ECMO simulation scenarios, as defined in the pictorial guide.
3. Design and lead cannulation simulations, including emergency cannulation, in either an in situ or simulation lab environment.
4. Recognize the costs (financial and otherwise) and benefits inherent to the use of specific simulation equipment or settings, allowing for conscientious decision-making when designing a simulation curriculum.

Introduction

Simulation-based training has become the standard method to ensure that members of the multi-disciplinary ECMO team develop and maintain the skills needed to manage patients dependent upon this life-saving technology [1–5]. Moreover, the clinical use of ECMO generates complex and unique interactions between intensive care staff, ECMO specialists, and the technology of the circuit itself [6]. As the demands placed upon team members vary by institution, the development of a simulation program customized to meet the needs and expectations of one's own center is vital. Meeting objectives at each unique program may have varying requirements for the degree of fidelity of the manikins and the clinical setting presented in the simulation environment. Previous chapters have described aspects of simulation training and the learning theories underpinning the education, which are important considerations for those responsible for developing or leading an institutional ECMO simulation program. This chapter will provide a practical guide designed to assist those leaders in the creation of their institution-specific scenarios and to avoid common pitfalls associated with this complex medical simulation.

Basic Simulation: Water Drills

In addition to 24–36 hours of didactic instruction, ELSO guidelines (www.elso.org/Resources/Guidelines.aspx) currently recommend the use of regular, hands-on sessions ("water drills") for both individual and team training. These can serve to introduce new members of the ECMO team to the various components of the ECMO circuit, to refresh existing team members' familiarity with circuit set-up and function, and to provide the opportunity for all team members to practice the skills necessary for circuit emergencies. In addition, mandatory training sessions such as this serve as a convenient touch point for all members of the ECMO team. This can provide programmatic leadership with a venue to effectively disseminate awareness of changes to policies or equipment. If changes to the institution's standard circuit arrangement are planned, for example, those changes can be displayed for members of the team at these sessions. It is recommended by ELSO (see above) that water drills be completed by each team member at least twice per year to ensure ongoing expertise.

The set-up for these sessions should be straightforward. A manikin may be included to visually remind learners of a patient's presence; however, this is not strictly necessary to accomplish the goals of the water drills. Rather, water drills typically focus on the circuit itself and can avoid simulated interactions with patient vital signs, monitors, or other distractors. An ECMO circuit with the institution's standard configuration should be present and, per the

L. D. Sacks (✉)
Department of Pediatrics – Cardiology (CVICU), Stanford University, Palo Alto, CA, USA
e-mail: lsacks@stanford.edu

L. C. Johnston, L. Su (eds.), *Comprehensive Healthcare Simulation: ECMO Simulation*, Comprehensive Healthcare Simulation,
https://doi.org/10.1007/978-3-030-53844-6_27

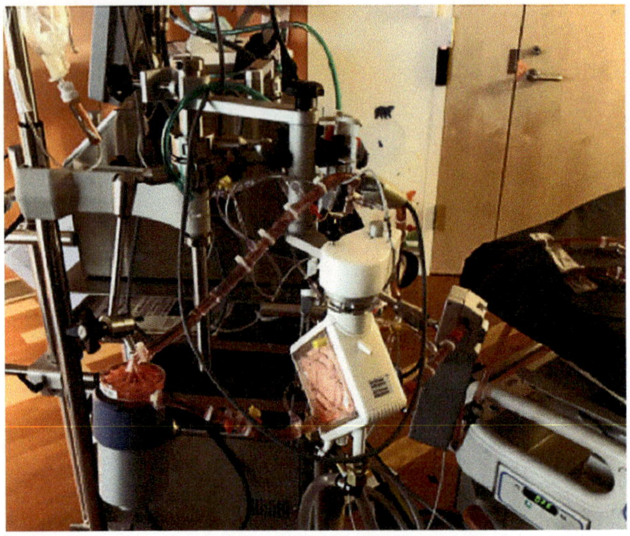

Fig. 27.1 An ECMO circuit primed with red-dyed saline can replicate clinical reality. This circuit, with centrifugal pump shown, can be effectively used for instruction in water drills or more complex simulations

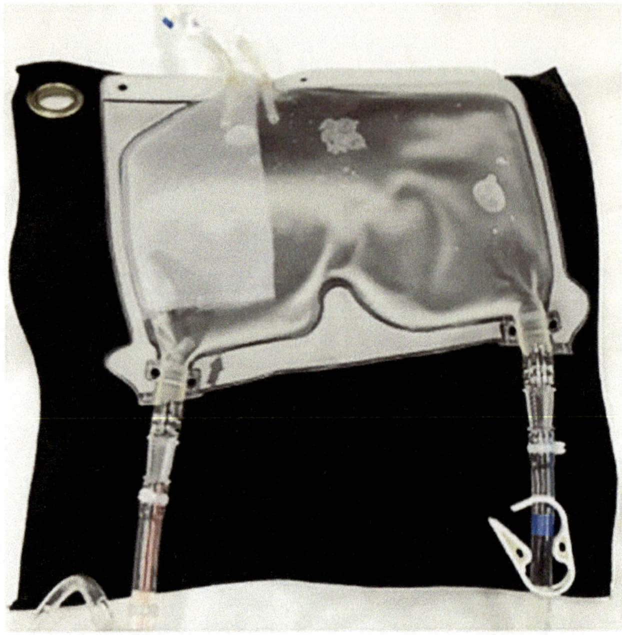

Fig. 27.2 The priming reservoir should remain in-line with the ECMO circuit for simulation purposes. This reservoir will allow for continuous flow through the circuit during training sessions and will serve as a capacitance chamber (replacing the venous capacitance of an actual patient)

ELSO guidelines previously referenced, space should be provided for a maximum of 8–10 learners. It is vital that each learner be provided with "hands-on" time with the circuit; inclusion of greater numbers of trainees will limit the experience for participants and this is to be avoided. The ECMO circuit used for a water drill may be primed with one of several different fluids. Some institutions will utilize expired units of blood, otherwise destined for elimination, for this training purpose. However, the use of this material may increase the cost of the training session and entails risks of blood-borne pathogen exposure to learners. In general, the use of water or saline is entirely sufficient for completing water drill simulations. Red dye or food coloring may be added (Fig. 27.1) to better simulate blood. The use of thickening agents such as corn starch or detergent (frequently used in simulation labs to more closely replicate the viscosity of human blood) should be avoided. These agents will create foam in the ECMO circuit, can impair the circuit's ability to flow, and can therefore impede learners from gaining valuable experience. Finally, a reservoir (Fig. 27.2) should be included in the circuit's pre-formatted set-up to replicate the patient's venous capacitance. With this set-up completed, the ECMO pump will be able to flow normally; flow probes placed in their appropriate positions will effectively monitor fluid flow through the circuit.

Relatively little scenario design is needed to effectively run water drills. Rather, faculty directing these sessions are encouraged to develop a specific list of technical skills that learners are required to demonstrate [7]. Trainees may be provided with a brief clinical history, but the primary objective for these drills should be to practice, achieve, and demonstrate competence in technical skills. Trainees can be tasked to set up and prime the circuit itself, if this is included in the scope of practice for those attending the session. Occlusion settings for roller-head pumps can be checked and all other features of a fully functioning circuit can be reviewed. For emergency skills training, air can be directly introduced into various compartments of the circuit via pigtail connectors (Fig. 27.3; arrow) by the session faculty and trainees can be tasked to remove the air from the circuit under full flow. A Kelly clamp, C-clamp, or other hemostatic devices can be used to occlude a portion of the venous limb of the circuit, simulating obstruction due to thrombus. For example, this intervention may be especially high-yield as learners can be tasked to emergently separate the "patient" from the ECMO circuit using the venous-bridge-arterial sequence of clamping to ensure all flow progresses through the circuit bridge, to hand-pump the circuit so as to disrupt the obstructing thrombus, and to re-establish the ECMO flow to the patient using an arterial-bridge-venous clamping sequence. It should be noted that each of these skills can also be taught in isolation, but the leveraging of a simulated thrombosis event allows them to be combined in a single scenario.

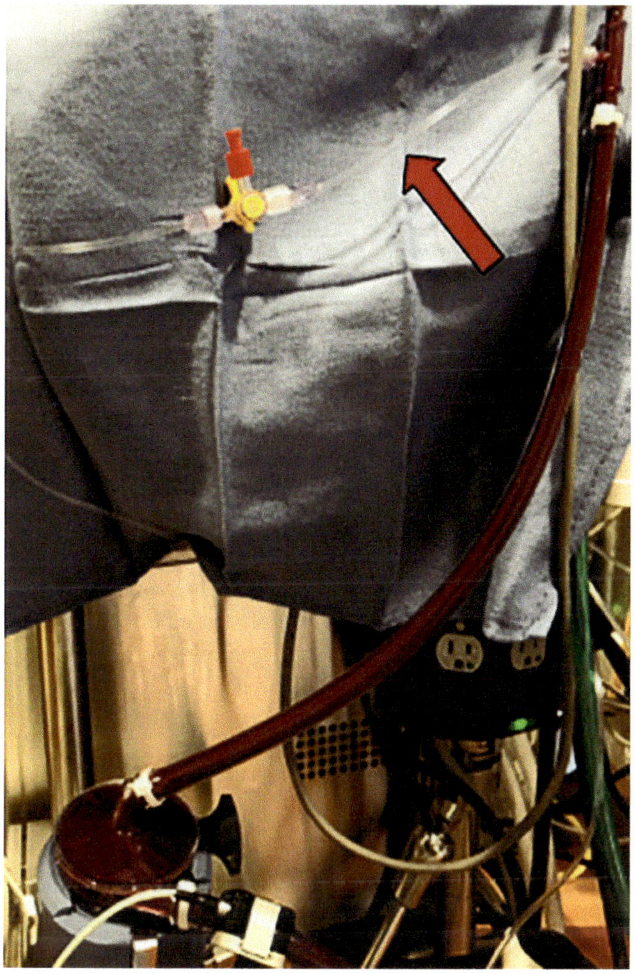

Fig. 27.3 Pigtail connectors (arrow) are commonplace in ECMO circuit design. These ports allow for blood sampling from the circuit and/or pressure transduction. For training purposes, they represent convenient locations to introduce acute change to the circuit, such as the injection of air during simulation sessions

Water drill sessions should be repeated with regularity to allow each member of the ECMO team to participate in a small-group format. Depending on the size of the institution's ECMO team and the number of faculty leaders, this can be a daunting prospect to those designing the simulation training. However, it should be emphasized that these drills do not require specific expertise in medical simulation. Rather, they require a space to host the session, an ECMO specialist to observe learners and correct mistakes in real time, the availability of a training circuit, a standardized list of skills providers are expected to master, and a checklist identifying the proper technique for each of those skills. The use of such a standardized checklist is especially important, as this allows observers to rate learners' performance against an objective standard. Thus, the effort inherent to maintaining this program can be distributed among a larger pool of faculty than those with specific simulation expertise.

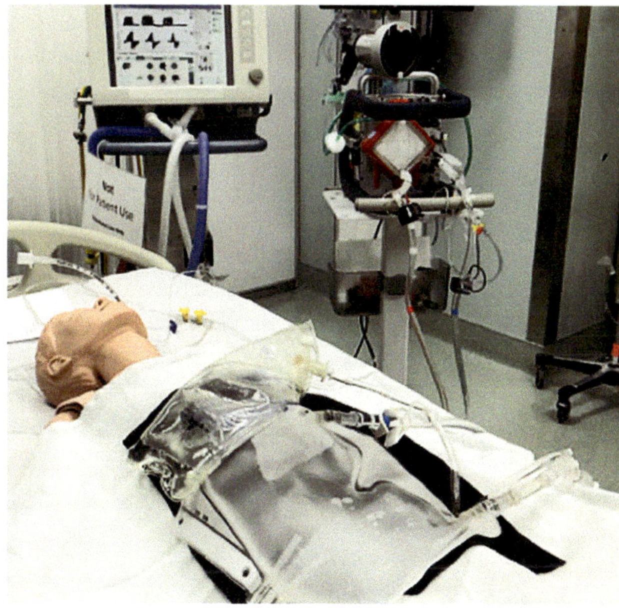

Fig. 27.4 The priming reservoir (shown here atop a high-fidelity manikin) may be hidden beneath the manikin or under blankets. This allows the "connection" of the ECMO circuit to the simulated patient during training sessions

Manikin-Integrated Simulation

In addition to circuit-based technical skill development and maintenance, training on the management of common circuit emergencies is necessary for the ECMO team to develop and maintain competence. Simulation training for these emergency episodes necessitates the integration of a simulation manikin and the ECMO circuit. This can be accomplished using either ¼-inch suction tubing to create a semi-elastic loop between venous and arterial cannulae or by placing a priming reservoir underneath the manikin itself (Fig. 27.4). This will allow the ECMO circuit to flow normally and allow continuous measurement of flow and pre- and post-membrane pressures, as occurs normally in the clinical setting. The circuit can then be manipulated either remotely or by standardized participants staffed within the simulation; outcomes of these manipulations can be reflected in changes to the simulated patient's vital signs and/or the ECMO circuit's function. Included in this section are examples of three types of common emergency scenarios: air entrainment, bleeding/hypovolemia, and circuit thrombosis. Although this list is by no means exhaustive, it serves to illustrate ways in which ECMO specialists and providers can expand simulation training for their institution. These simulations often require extensive preparation and may best be accomplished in a simulation lab setting depending on resources available for in situ simulation. The following guide will include step-by-step instructions for the configuration of these simulations. It should be noted that, for each simulation, a training ECMO circuit will be prepared with the institution's pre-formatted tubing set; this guide will delineate only those additions necessary for each scenario.

Circuit Obstruction/Thrombosis

The need for anticoagulation management is inherent to the use of ECMO technology. However, despite the best efforts of experienced providers, circuit thromboses are common events [8, 9]. These events pose a significant threat not only of thromboembolic insult to patients but also to the integrity of the ECMO circuit itself. A large thrombus may prevent flow through the circuit and require immediate intervention to prevent cessation of flow. It is this aspect, the potential to impact ECMO pump function, that may best be addressed through simulation training. If desired, a program may wish to invest in advanced devices such as the EigenFlow (Curtis Life Research, Indianapolis, IN). This device will allow for on-demand increases in circuit resistance, simulating a building thrombus. The wireless connectivity of this product allows the simulation facilitator to adjust settings without entering into the simulation space. However, this may incur additional costs; similar results can be obtained using a standardized participant as follows:

- Step 1: The ECMO circuit and manikin should first be "connected" by placing the priming reservoir underneath the manikin itself (Fig. 27.4).
- Step 2: A Kelly clamp or other hemostatic devices should be placed across the circuit tubing and covered by blankets or other moulage (Fig. 27.5a).
- Step 3: The clamp itself should be left open as the scenario begins (Fig. 27.5b).
- Step 4: The standardized participant should be cued, during the scenario, to partially obstruct the circuit tubing by closing the Kelly clamp to *only* the first locking point (Fig. 27.5c). This partial occlusion will increase resistance to flow and trigger the ECMO circuit to alarm.
- Step 5: A second cue should be given to the standardized participant to completely close the Kelly clamp (Fig. 27.5d), thereby completely occluding the circuit tubing. This will result in loss of all ECMO flow.

This sequence, when paired with an appropriate scenario (i.e., a circuit maintained without heparin due to patient bleeding), will assist learners in diagnosing a circuit thrombosis event and taking steps to correct this. With partial occlusion, the manikin heart rate should rise noticeably and blood pressure should fall. CVP/RAp (if displayed) should rise slightly. Because the artificial obstruction is actually altering flow in the ECMO circuit, this process will automatically generate changes in circuit pressures (i.e., rising post-pump pressure). With complete occlusion, the ECMO circuit will generate a low-flow alarm and the vital sign trends noted above should acutely worsen. Corrective actions should include separation of the simulated patient from the ECMO circuit, resuscitation of the patient as necessary, and manual cranking of the ECMO pump to dislodge/disrupt the obstructive thrombus. All of these actions can be completed using this configuration; however, care should be taken by the simulation team to un-clamp the hemostatic device used after learners complete the required resuscitation algorithm.

Air Entrainment

A serious potential complication of ECMO support is the entrainment of air bubbles within the circuit. If bubbles are allowed to reach the post-oxygenator portion of the circuit, there is nothing to prevent the active embolism of air into the patient. Therefore, prompt recognition and elimination of air from all regions of the ECMO circuit is a vital skill. For simulation purposes, this can be accomplished by the use of pigtail connections to the ECMO circuit tubing (Fig. 27.3) in the following manner:

- Step 1: Obtain two lengths of small-bore IV tubing and connect them together (Fig. 27.6a). This process can be repeated with additional lengths of tubing as needed to facilitate concealment of this scenario's standardized participant (see below).

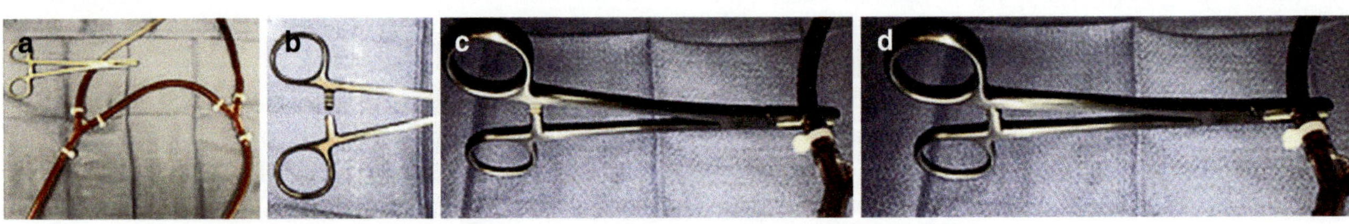

Fig. 27.5 This pictorial guide displays the steps necessary to prepare for and carry out a simulated ECMO circuit thrombosis using standard circuit tubing and a Kelly clamp (**a**). The open clamp (**b**) can be fitted around the circuit tubing. The Kelly can then be closed to the first locking point (**c**) to create partial flow obstruction. If complete circuit flow obstruction is necessary to the simulation, the Kelly clamp may be completely closed (**d**)

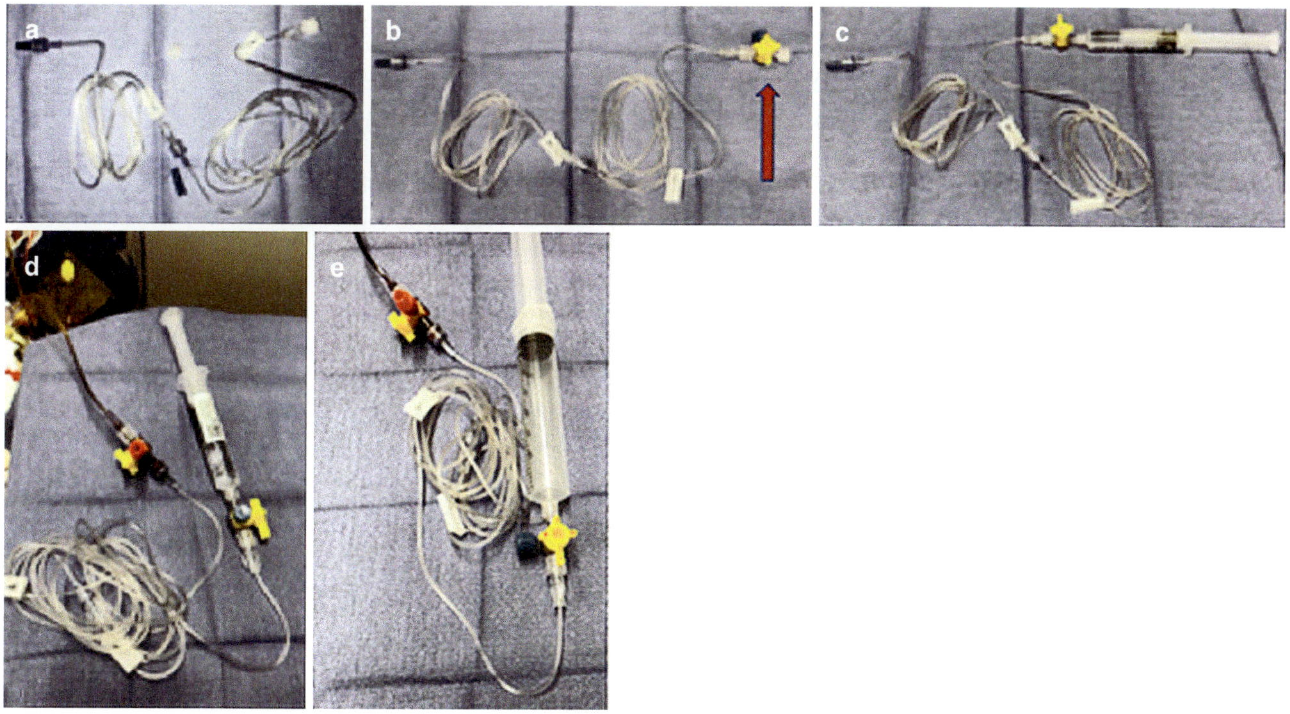

Fig. 27.6 This pictorial guide displays the steps necessary to prepare for and carry out a simulated air embolism while on ECMO. Lengths of small-bore IV tubing can be connected (**a**) as needed to facilitate concealment of a confederate at short distance from the ECMO circuit. A three-way stopcock connector should be added to the distal, "female" end of these tubing sets (**b**; arrow) and the tubing primed using a standard saline flush (**c**). The primed tubing may then be connected to the ECMO circuit via pigtail connectors (**d**), and the saline flush syringe may be exchanged for either a 30-mL or 60-mL syringe filled with air (**e**). When desired, the confederate will be able to directly inject into the ECMO circuit by opening the aforementioned stopcock and fully depressing the plunger of the air-filled syringe

- Step 2: A stopcock adapter should be placed at the distal ("female") end of the IV tubing (Fig. 27.6b, arrow).
- Step 3: Prime the IV tubing using standard saline flush (Fig. 27.6c). Be certain to place the stopcock adapter in the "off" position to the tubing after priming is complete.
- Step 4: Connect the proximal end of the primed IV tubing to a pigtail connector built into the institution's standard ECMO tubing set (Fig. 27.6d). Simulation faculty can choose to connect this IV tubing in the pre-pump, post-pump, or post-oxygenator positions.
- Step 5: Exchange the saline syringe used for priming for a 30-mL or 60-mL syringe filled with air (Fig. 27.6e).
- Step 6: Extend the IV tubing to allow a standardized participant or instructor to remain in a concealed location inside the simulation suite.
- Step 7: During the simulation, when the deemed appropriate by the simulation faculty, the standardized participant should be prompted to inject air. To accomplish this, simply turn the stopcock so that the air-filled syringe can be injected into the IV tubing. After injection, the stopcock should be returned to its original position (i.e., off to the IV tubing) to prevent backflow.

This configuration allows for the addition of air to the region of the ECMO circuit targeted by the simulation facilitator and allows learners to evacuate air as they would during an actual clinical case. Of note, air evacuation will typically require at least brief separation from ECMO support. Therefore, depending on the premise of the simulation scenario, resuscitation of the simulated patient will be required. While the patient is separated from ECMO, it is recommended that the manikin's blood pressure fall rapidly, with an associated rise in CVP/RAp (if this data will be provided for learners). Saturation signal should be lost due to loss of perfusion. If a faculty member was previously designated to act as the voice of the patient, all communication should cease as the manikin loses cerebral perfusion. This aspect has the added benefit of allowing medical teams to practice the coordination of simultaneous patient and circuit resuscitations. All vital signs should revert to normal after air removal and ECMO re-initiation is accomplished.

Bleeding

Due to the necessity of anticoagulation, bleeding risks are inherently elevated for patients receiving ECMO support. Significant blood loss may lead not only to patient instability but also to circuit dysfunction due to profound hypovolemia. Thus, rapid recognition and correction of bleeding is of paramount importance for the ECMO provider. Simulation of this event can take on varying degrees of complexity but should essentially focus on (1) recognition of acute blood loss and (2) administration of blood products to replace volume and halt bleeding. In the simplest form, a simulation can simply include connection of the manikin to an ECMO circuit using the methods previously described and a method to indicate acute, profound bleeding. Thoracostomy tubes or other drains are excellent external locations to demonstrate blood loss and should be included in the set-up for this simulation.

- Step 1: A pigtail or other thoracostomy drains should be affixed to the manikin using adhesive dressings to hold this tubing in place (Fig. 27.7d).
- Step 2: The thoracostomy tubing should be connected to a standard drainage tubing and basin (Fig. 27.7f, g).
- Step 3: Using a blunt-tip needle (Fig. 27.7e), puncture the drainage tubing. This puncture site can then be concealed with opaque tape or other moulage.
- Step 4: Connect a secondary tubing set (Baxter Product #JC7462) to the blunt-tip needle as shown (Fig. 27.7c). Ensure the roller clamp is tightly closed.
- Step 5: Using the spike of the secondary set, access a 500-mL IV bag of red-dyed saline (Fig. 27.7b).
- Note: If a more direct impact on the ECMO circuit is desired, the spike may be used to directly access the priming reservoir of the circuit. If this is done, any volume removed via the secondary set will cause a loss of volume directly to the ECMO circuit.
- Step 6: Place a pressure sleeve around the reservoir of red-dyed saline (Fig. 27.7a) and inflate the sleeve.
- Step 7: Secure the secondary set and red-dyed saline reservoir underneath the manikin's gurney or in another concealed (but easily accessible) location before the simulation begins.
- Step 8: When simulation faculty deem it appropriate to initiate bleeding, a standardized participant should be prompted to open the roller clamp of the secondary set.
- Step 9: The red-dyed solution will flow out of the thoracostomy drain (Fig. 27.7) and visually cue learners to the loss of blood. If the option of connecting the secondary set to the ECMO circuit was taken in Step 5, opening the roller clamp will also trigger low-flow/high-negative pressure alarms, immediately resulting in negative pressure alarms similar to those seen in clinical hypovolemia. However, when making this type of connection, two

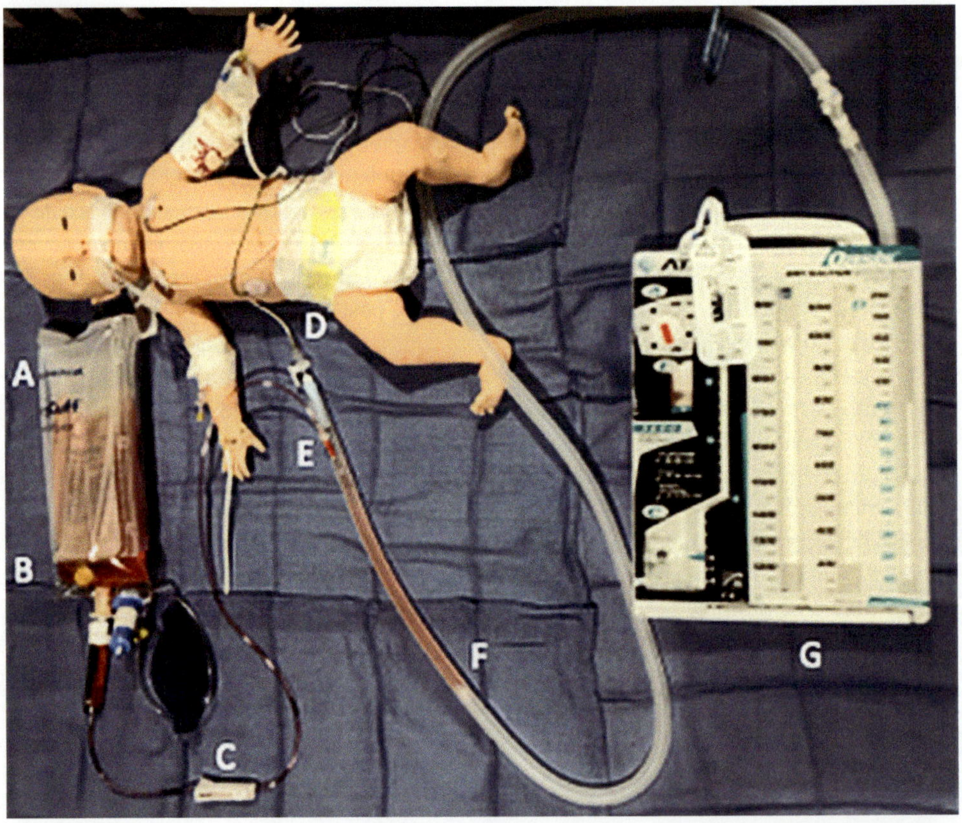

Fig. 27.7 A sample configuration to simulate blood loss via thoracostomy tube. In this configuration, a pressure bag (**a**) is used to drive flow of red-dyed saline from a standard 500-mL bag (**b**). Output can be tightly controlled using the roller clamp (**c**) of a secondary tubing set. This can be mated to a standard thoracostomy drain (**d**) by inserting a blunt-tip needle into the collection tubing (**e**). This will, on release of the roller clamp, allow rapid flow of simulated blood through the tubing (**f**), collecting in a standard drainage basin (**g**)

warnings must be borne in mind. First, it is important that the confederate take great care in opening the roller clamp of the secondary set. The positive pressure of the circuit used in the simulation can lead to rapid, massive transfer of fluid to the drain and risk complete emptying of the ECMO circuit. Second, when using this configuration, all fluid resuscitation performed during the simulation must be achieved by adding fluid directly back to the venous limb of the circuit itself. Only in this way will the circuit be replenished after volume is lost. If fluid or blood product administration to the ECMO circuit is contrary to the institution's guidelines, this configuration is best avoided.

During this scenario, it is recommended that the manikin vital signs be altered such that the heart rate begins to rise *before* the standardized patient is prompted to open the roller clamp. This trend should continue after the clamp is released and blood loss becomes obvious. Similarly, CVP/RAp (if displayed) should begin to fall prior to the initiation of blood loss and should continue to decline as the scenario progresses. If faculty choose not to connect the secondary set directly to the ECMO circuit (see above), learners should be prompted that negative pressure readings on the circuit itself are rising. This may be accomplished either via the standardized participant or by announcement by simulation facilitator. The manikin blood pressure should begin to fall only after blood loss has continued for several minutes. The duration of the resuscitation is left to the discretion of the simulation faculty. When appropriate transfusion/corrective measures are taken, the scenario may be ended by closing the roller clamp to halt visible bleeding and normalizing the circuit flow and manikin vital signs. Alternatively, simulation objectives may include progression to chest exploration; for this option, vital signs should remain abnormal and bleeding should continue until the surgical team is contacted and preparations for bedside surgical exploration are complete.

Preparation for Cannulation/Extracorporeal Cardiopulmonary Resuscitation (eCPR)

Simulation may be used to train team members for both non-emergent and eCPR cannulations. Cannulation scenarios can reinforce the roles necessary for efficient cannulation (under either condition), the appropriate spatial orientation of patient rooms, and the preparation of equipment necessary for the attachment of an ECMO circuit to a live patient. The details of each of these aspects will vary between institutions; however, it is recommended that each institution develop a checklist of roles and actions similar to that used for water drills (above) and train team members based upon the items on that list. In situ simulations within the clinical environment are best suited for this type of training; however, this will rely on the availability of dedicated simulation space. Non-emergent and eCPR scenarios will benefit learner populations differently; therefore, the choice of scenario should be driven by the learning objectives for each individual simulation session.

One of the primary challenges to urgent or emergent initiation of ECMO support is the coordination of resources necessary to prepare both circuit and patient for cannula placement. The addition of the multiple new personnel necessary for ECMO initiation into an environment in which multiple providers are already working to provide emergent care can lead to increased chaos and disorganization. With simulation training, however, the interactions of those personnel can become streamlined and more efficient [5, 10]. Learning objectives for eCPR scenarios should include recognition of the need for ECMO support, establishment of team roles for both resuscitation and cannulation, room organization, and preparation of bedside equipment and the ECMO circuit itself. As with other simulations, center-specific checklists or protocols for cannulation should be used to assess the team and/or guide debriefing. In addition, the time needed to complete cannulation can be easily tracked during the simulated scenario.

It is recommended, for this type of simulation, to create a scenario based on diagnoses that can readily lead to acute, profound decompensation *and* have a reasonably high likelihood of recovery with ECMO support. Examples of this include acute myocarditis [11, 12], sudden and refractory rhythm disturbances [13], heart failure [14, 15], profound ARDS [16], acute pulmonary embolism with right heart stunning [17, 18], and/or sepsis [19]. The scenario should be crafted to avoid uncertainty as to whether ECMO support will be beneficial to the patient in question. This will allow learners to focus on the cannulation process and avoid debates during scenario debriefing as to whether or not ECMO support was indicated. Simulations of this type may be carried out in either a simulation lab or in situ in the clinical setting.

Use of in situ space within the clinical institution often allows for better practice of the actual response systems and room organization needed to effectively perform an emergency cannulation. However, as noted above, this relies on the availability of space which can be unpredictable given the fluctuating occupancy rates of most critical care units. Simulation lab space is more predictable in its availability, but may not adequately replicate the environment encountered by care providers. The pros and cons of each simulation setting must be weighed by simulation faculty, based on resources available at their specific institution. In addition, the availability of learners to participate in the simulation training must be carefully considered. If using in situ space, faculty may consider leveraging staff already present on the unit to participate as learners. However, faculty must be aware that this tactic will pull providers away from actual clinical assignments; this may or may not be acceptable depending on the acuity of the patient care unit on the date of the simulation. Alternatively, faculty may consider scheduling learners to attend the simulation training outside of their normal clinical duties. This will ensure attendance, but may incur additional costs. As with the choice of simulation space, the pros and cons of each option must be weighed carefully by the faculty before committing resources to a specific date and location.

When initiating the eCPR simulation, it may be useful to allow learners to engage in the scenario for 5–7 minutes before progressing to a decompensation that will prompt ECMO cannulation. This lead time simultaneously increases realism and facilitates discussions of appropriate timing for mobilization of the ECMO response team. After this period, the displayed vital signs of the simulated patient should be altered to denote a sudden decompensation. Acute rhythm change, refractory hypoxia, and sudden loss of plethysmograph or arterial BP tracings are useful cues. The simulated patient should not recover from this change despite learners' interventions, and the team leader should mobilize the resources necessary for ECMO support. It is often helpful to include a standardized participant (i.e., a member of the simulation faculty acting as the patient's bedside nurse) with instructions to prompt the team leader if mechanical support is not considered early on in the simulation.

After mobilization of the ECMO team, the specific skills targeted by the simulation team can be assessed. If the simulation is to be performed in situ, the room should be prepared according to the institution's standards for cannulation. At a minimum, the manikin should be positioned to allow surgeons to access the neck or groin while CPR is continued. It may be beneficial to standardize and practice this room preparation if significant adjustment of the patient's position is needed prior to cannulation. Emergent circuit priming can be practiced simultaneously by ECMO specialists utilized at the institution, be they perfusionists or nurses/respiratory therapists with additional training. Staff members required to assist the cannulating surgeon (i.e., scrub RN, circulating RN, surgical assistant) should be brought to the simulation, and bedside staff should prepare equipment such as electrocautery, suction devices, and surgical headlamps.

Depending on the learning objectives, the scenario may be concluded when set-up for cannulation is completed. However, if it is the desire of the simulation team to actually "connect" the manikin to the circuit and initiate flow, several options exist. If a member of the surgical staff will be involved in the simulation, then surgical simulators may be incorporated. This can be accomplished using commercially available products such as those created by 3-Dmed (Franklin, Ohio) or through the use of commercially available products to create a surgical simulator [6, 20]. Alternatively, if surgical skills are not a focus of the training scenario or if the surgeon is not present, a length of ¼-inch suction tubing may be hidden underneath the manikin and used to "connect" to the ECMO circuit. The suction tubing should be primed with saline or other fluids, clamped to prevent leakage, and a standard ¼-inch male-to-male ECMO adapter fitted to each end. When the ECMO circuit is prepared, the ends of the suction tubing may be connected to the venous and arterial limbs and flow will be possible. If using this configuration, it is recommended that a member of the simulation faculty act as a standardized participant and play the role of the surgeon.

Conclusion

The use of ECMO to support critically ill patients requires the commitment of a multidisciplinary team of highly trained providers. Medical simulation, in various forms, presents an ideal modality for establishing and maintaining the expertise necessary for team members. An introduction to circuit "anatomy" and an opportunity to practice technical skills such as air removal or circuit priming may be accomplished during water drill sessions. These small-group sessions require minimal scenario design, but can exponentially improve the team's ability to manipulate the circuit itself. Emergency cannulation scenarios can be used to emphasize the timely application of ECMO support, to streamline the interactions of the multiple teams necessary for cannulation, and to reinforce the logistical steps needed to prepare the workspace for an emergent surgical procedure. These learning objectives best lend themselves to in situ simulation; however, a simulation lab may also suffice and may have advantages in terms of avoiding space/personnel constraints. By integrating a high-fidelity simulation manikin with the ECMO circuit, complex scenarios can be created for high-level training. These scenarios should be crafted with clear emphasis on distinct learning points, and simulation faculty must be prepared to alter the manikin's displayed vital signs and the pressures and flow displayed on the circuit rapidly, in accordance with scenario progression. Corporate entities continue to create devices to allow "interaction" between the manikin and the ECMO circuit, but simple, low-cost solutions can also be employed to achieve realistic results. Leaders of ECMO programs are encouraged to use a mixture of these simulation modalities to provide robust training for all team members; with repeated exposure to varied simulation training, the exceptional skills required of a multidisciplinary ECMO team can be readily developed and maintained.

References

1. Johnston L, Williams SB, Ades A. Education for ECMO providers: using education science to bridge the gap between clinical and educational expertise. Semin Perinatol. 2018;42(2):138–46.
2. Johnston L, Oldenburg G. Simulation for neonatal extracorporeal membrane oxygenation teams. Semin Perinatol. 2016;40(7):421–9.
3. Su L, et al. Implementation of an extracorporeal cardiopulmonary resuscitation simulation program reduces extracorporeal cardiopulmonary resuscitation times in real patients. Pediatr Crit Care Med. 2014;15(9):856–60.
4. Allan CK, et al. Simulation-based training delivered directly to the pediatric cardiac intensive care unit engenders preparedness, comfort, and decreased anxiety among multidisciplinary resuscitation teams. J Thorac Cardiovasc Surg. 2010;140(3):646–52.
5. Di Nardo M, et al. The introduction of a high-fidelity simulation program for training pediatric critical care personnel reduces the times to manage extracorporeal membrane oxygenation emergencies and improves teamwork. J Thorac Dis. 2018;10(6):3409–17.
6. Anderson JM, et al. Simulating extracorporeal membrane oxygenation emergencies to improve human performance. Part II: assessment of technical and behavioral skills. Simul Healthc. 2006;1(4):228–32.
7. Abulebda K, et al. Development of validated checklists to evaluate clinical specialists in pediatric ECMO emergencies using delphi method. ASAIO J. 2019;66(3):314–8.
8. Hastings SM, et al. Sources of circuit thrombosis in pediatric extracorporeal membrane oxygenation. ASAIO J. 2017;63(1):86–92.
9. Fuchs G, et al. Detection of thrombosis in the extracorporeal membrane oxygenation circuit by infrasound: proof of concept. Artif Organs. 2017;41(6):573–9.
10. Whitmore SP, et al. Simulation training enables emergency medicine providers to rapidly and safely initiate extracorporeal cardiopulmonary resuscitation (ECPR) in a simulated cardiac arrest scenario. Resuscitation. 2019;138:68–73.
11. Wolf MJ, et al. Extracorporeal cardiopulmonary resuscitation for pediatric cardiac patients. Ann Thorac Surg. 2012;94(3):874–9; discussion 879–80.
12. Conrad SJ, et al. Extracorporeal cardiopulmonary resuscitation among patients with structurally Normal hearts. ASAIO J. 2017;63(6):781–6.
13. Bell SM, et al. Management of refractory ventricular fibrillation (prehospital and emergency department). Cardiol Clin. 2018;36(3):395–408.
14. Jefferies JL, Morales DL. Mechanical circulatory support in children: bridge to transplant versus recovery. Curr Heart Fail Rep. 2012;9(3):236–43.
15. Goto T, et al. The impact of extracorporeal membrane oxygenation on survival in pediatric patients with respiratory and heart failure: review of our experience. Artif Organs. 2011;35(11):1002–9.
16. Abrams D, et al. ECMO for ARDS: from salvage to standard of care? Lancet Respir Med. 2019;7(2):108–10.
17. Belohlavek J, et al. Veno-arterial ECMO in severe acute right ventricular failure with pulmonary obstructive hemodynamic pattern. J Invasive Cardiol. 2010;22(8):365–9.
18. Sakuma M, et al. Percutaneous cardiopulmonary support for the treatment of acute pulmonary embolism: summarized review of the literature in Japan including our own experience. Ann Vasc Dis. 2009;2(1):7–16.
19. Oberender F, et al. Venoarterial extracorporeal membrane oxygenation versus conventional therapy in severe pediatric septic shock. Pediatr Crit Care Med. 2018;19(10):965–72.
20. Allan CK, et al. An extracorporeal membrane oxygenation cannulation curriculum featuring a novel integrated skills trainer leads to improved performance among pediatric cardiac surgery trainees. Simul Healthc. 2013;8(4):221–8.

Index

L. C. Johnston, L. Su (eds.), *Comprehensive Healthcare Simulation: ECMO Simulation*, Comprehensive Healthcare Simulation,
https://doi.org/10.1007/978-3-030-53844-6